PDxMD

Renal & Genitourinary Disorders

PDxMD Medical Conditions Series is dedicated to health and healing professionals everywhere. We are privileged to be in your service and hope our efforts help you in your quest for better quality-of-life and optimized outcomes for all your patients.

PDxMD

Renal & Genitourinary Disorders

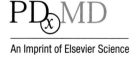

An Imprint of Elsevier Science

Philadelphia ■ St Louis ■ London ■ Sydney ■ New York ■ Toronto

PDxMD
An imprint of Elsevier Science

Publisher: Steven Merahn, MD
Project Managers: Caroline Barnett, Lucy Hamilton, Zak Knowles
Programmer: Narinder Chandi
Production: Aoibhe O'Shea – GMS UK, Alan Palfreyman – PTU
Designer: Jayne Jones
Layout: Alan Palfreyman

NOTICE
Medicine is an ever-changing field. Standard safety precautions must be followed, but as new research and clinical experience broaden our knowledge, changes in treatment and drug therapy may become necessary or appropriate. Readers are advised to check the most current product information provided by the manufacturer of each drug to be administered to verify the recommended dose, the method and duration of administration, and contraindications. It is the responsibility of the licensed prescriber, relying on experience and knowledge of the patient, to determine dosages and the best treatment for each individual patient. Neither the publisher nor the editor assumes any liability for any injury and/or damage to persons or property arising from this publication.

All PDxMD contributors are participating in the activities of PDxMD in an individual capacity, and not as representatives of or on behalf of their individual affiliated hospitals, associations or institutions (where indicated herein), and their participation should not be taken as an endorsement of PDxMD by their individual affiliated hospitals, associations or institutions. Individual affiliated hospitals, associations or institutions are not responsible for the accuracy or availability of information on the product.

Permission to photocopy or reproduce solely for internal or personal use is permitted for libraries or other users registered with the Copyright Clearance Center, provided that the base fee of $4.00 per chapter plus $.10 per page is paid directly to the Copyright Clearance Center, 222 Rosewood Drive, Danvers, MA 01923. This consent does not extend to other kinds of copying, such as copying for general distribution, for advertising or promotional purposes, for creating new collected works, or for resale.

Printed in China by RDC Group

PDxMD
Elsevier Science
The Curtis Center
625 Walnut Street,
Philadelphia, PA 19106

ISBN 1-932141-10-3

The
Publisher's
policy is to use
**paper manufactured
from sustainable forests**

Contents

Introduction

Editorial Faculty and Staff

MediFiles

Contents

Contents

Introduction

What is PDxMD?

PDxMD is a new, evidence-based primary care clinical information system designed to support your judgment with practical clinical information. The content is continuously updated by expert contributors with the latest on evaluation, diagnosis, management, outcomes and prevention – all designed for use at the point and time of care.

First and foremost, PDxMD is an electronic resource. This book gives you access to just a fraction of the content available on-line. At www.pdxmd.com, you will find:

- Over 1400 differential diagnoses for you to search for information according to your patient's chief complaint via a unique signs and symptoms matrix
- Information on more than 450 medical conditions and more than 750 drugs and other therapies, organised in condition-specific 'MediFiles'
- Patient information sheets on 300 topics for you to customize and hand to your patient during consultation

About This Book

The PDxMD Medical Conditions Series is a print version of the comprehensive approach offered on line. Concise information on medical conditions is systematically organized in a consistent MediFile format, our electronic equivalent of chapters.

Each MediFile covers summary information and background on each condition, and comprehensive information on diagnosis, treatment, outcomes, and prevention, and other resources, especially written and designed for use in practice. Each MediFile is organized identically to allow you to find information consistently and reliably for every condition. See the MediFile 'Road Map' inside the back cover for more information.

Ranging from epidemiology to risk assessment and reduction, from diagnostic evaluation and testing to therapeutic options, prognosis and outcomes - you'll find the information that you need is easier to locate with this methodical approach.

How to Use This Book

Find the MediFile for any specific medical condition in the Contents list. Familiarize yourself with the MediFile Road Map (see inside back cover) to rapidly find the precise information you require.

Information on drugs and tests are found within the MediFiles for the specific conditions. For an overview, see the 'Summary of options' sections under DIAGNOSIS and under TREATMENT in the relevant MediFile. Details of tests, drugs and other therapies then follow.

PDxMD believes that physician clinical judgment is central to appropriate diagnostic and therapeutic decision-making. The information is designed to support professional judgment and, accounting for individual patient differences, does not provide direct answers or force specific practices or policies.

Introduction

How is PDxMD created?

PDxMD is created through Collaborative Authoring. This process allows medical information to be reviewed and synthesized from multiple sources – including but not limited to peer-reviewed articles, evidence databases, guidelines and position papers – and by multiple individuals. The information is organized around and integrated into a template that matches the needs of primary care physicians in practice.

Professional medical writers begin the process of reviewing and synthesizing information for PDxMD, working from core evidence databases and other expert resources and with the guidance of Editorial Advisory Board (EAB) members. This first draft is sent to a physician 'clinical reviewer', who works with the writer to make sure the information is accurate and properly organized. A second review by the physician clinical reviewer ensures that appropriate changes are in place.

After these first two levels of clinical review, the files are reviewed and edited by the relevant specialist member of the Editorial Advisory Board. A primary care member of the EAB, who has final sign-off authority, then conducts the final review and edit. Editorial checks are conducted between all review stages and, after primary care sign-off, a pharmacist double checks the drug recommendations prior to a final editorial review.

There are a minimum of three and as many as five physicians involved in each MediFile, and additional clinical reviewers and/or EAB members are added when appropriate (e.g., alternative/complementary medicine experts, or conditions requiring multi-disciplinary approaches). The contributor team for each MediFile is listed in the Resources section.

A complete list of Editorial Faculty and staff of PDxMD is provided below. All Editorial Faculty, and specifically the Editorial Advisory Board members, participate in PDxMD as individuals and not as representatives of, or on behalf of, their affiliated institutions or associations and any indication of their affiliation with a specific institution or association should not be taken as an endorsement of PDxMD or any participation of their institution or association with PDxMD.

Continuous Product Improvement

PDxMD is committed to continuous quality improvement and welcomes any comments, suggestions and feedback from the professional community. Please send any ideas or considerations regarding this volume or any other volume in the PDxMD series via e-mail to feedback.pdxmd@elsevier.com or to PDxMD, Elsevier Science, The Curtis Center, 625 Walnut Street, Philadelphia, PA 19106.

Introduction

Evidence-Based Medicine Policies

PDxMD is committed to providing available and up-to-date evidence for the diagnostic and therapeutic recommendations provided in our knowledge base. All MediFiles begin with a core set of evidence-based references from recognized sources. These are supplemented with extensive searches of the literature and reviews of reference books, peer-reviewed journals, association guidelines and position papers, among others.

Criteria for Evidence-Based Medicine
Evidence Sources

PDxMD has taken the best evidence currently available from the following:

Published Critically Evaluated Evidence

- Cochrane Systematic Reviews – respected throughout the world as one of the most rigorous searches of medical journals with highly structured systematic reviews and use of meta-analysis to produce reliable evidence
- Clinical Evidence – produced jointly by the British Medical Journal Publishing Group and the American College of Physicians–American Society of Internal Medicine. Clinical Evidence provides a concise account of the current state of knowledge on the treatment and prevention of many clinical conditions based on the search and appraisal of the available literature
- The National Guideline Clearinghouse – a comprehensive database of evidence-based clinical practice guidelines and related documents produced by the Agency for Healthcare Research and Quality in partnership with the American Medical Association and the American Association of Health Plans

Evidence Published in Peer-Reviewed Journals

- Association Guidelines and Position Papers

Where evidence exists that has not yet been critically reviewed by one of the sources listed above, for example randomized controlled trials and clinical cohort studies, the evidence is summarized briefly, categorized, and fully referenced.

Clinical Experience

While recognizing the importance of these evidence-based resources, PDxMD also highlights the importance of experience in clinical practice. Therefore, our Editorial Advisory Board also provide advice from their own clinical experience, within Clinical Pearl sections of the MediFiles and elsewhere. Contributing expert physicians are identified in the Resources section of every MediFile.

Introduction

Evaluation of Evidence

PDxMD evaluates all cited evidence according to the AAFP Recommended Basic Model for Evaluating and Categorizing the Clinical Content of CME, based on the model used by the University of Michigan:

Level M   Evidence from either:
                Meta-analysis or
                Multiple randomized controlled trials

Level P   Evidence from either:
                A well-designed prospective clinical trial or
                Several prospective clinical cohort studies with consistent findings (without randomization)

Level S   Evidence from studies other than clinical trials, such as:
                Epidemiological studies
                Physiological studies

References

The information provided by PDxMD is concise and action-oriented. As a result, our editorial policy is to cite only essential reference sources. References and evidence summaries are provided in four areas:

1. In the Diagnostic Decision section under Diagnosis
2. In the Guidelines and Evidence sections under Treatment
3. In the Outcomes section under Evidence
4. In the Key Reference Section under Resources

Where on-line references to the Cochrane Abstracts, BMJ Clinical Evidence and National Guideline Clearinghouse are cited in the text, the internet addresses of the home pages are given. The internet addresses of individual reports are not given.

When references are to association guidelines and position papers, the internet address of the association home page is generally provided. When possible, the internet address of the specific report is provided.

Editorial Faculty and Staff

Executive Committee

Editorial Board

Editorial Faculty and Staff

Editorial Faculty and Staff

Editorial Faculty and Staff

Gary M White, MD
Editorial Board, Dermatology Illustration
Associate Clinical Professor
Dept of Dermatology
University of California, San Diego
San Diego, CA

Basil J Zitelli, MD
Editorial Board, Pediatrics Illustration
Professor of Pediatrics
University of Pittsburgh School of Medicine
Children's Hospital of Pittsburgh
Pittsburgh PA

Clinical Reviewers

Julian N Anthony, MD
Urology
Department of Urology
State University of New York at Buffalo
Buffalo, NY

Thompson H Boyd, III, MD
Primary Care
Clinical Assistant Professor
Physician Liaison - Information Services
Department of Medicine
Hahnemann University Hospital
Philadelphia, PA

Anuj K Chopra, MD
Urology
Private Practitioner
Department of Urology
State University of New York at Buffalo
Buffalo, NY

Ankush Gulati, MD
Nephrology
Nephrology Section
Temple University School of Medicine
Philadelphia, PA

Rakesh Gulati, MD
Nephrology
Assistant Professor of Medicine
Nephrology Section
Temple University School of Medicine
Philadelphia, PA

Robert James, MD
Urology
Santa Rosa, CA

John Pinski, MD
Urology
Amherst, NY

Stewart M Polsky, MD
Urology
Staff Urologist
Department of Urology
Lake Norman Regional Medical Center
Mooresville, NC

Vitaly Raykhman, MD
Urology
Williamsville, NY

Ganesh G Shenoy, MD
Nephrology
Nephrology Section
Temple University Hospital
Philadelphia, PA

Jennifer E Weil, MD
Nephrology
Assistant Professor of Medicine
Nephrology Section
Temple University School of Medicine
Philadelphia, PA

Editorial Faculty and Staff

Writers

Phil D Ambery, MB ChB
Kim S Berman
Liza C Brettingham, MD, JCTGP
Michele Campbell
Rosalyn S Carson-DeWitt, MD
Prasad Devarajan, MD
Robert A Fried, MD
Jacqueline Furnace, BSc MBChB Med
Ewan M Gerard, MB ChB, MSc, MRCGP

Adam Jacobs, MD
Kelly D Karpa, RPh, PhD, BSPharm
Elizabeth Robinson, MB ChB
David T Schwartz, MD, FACS
Mary E Selby, MB ChB, DRCOG, MRCGP
Rosalind N Sulaiman, MD
Chris J Taylor, FRCS
Robyn J S Webber, MB ChB, FRCSEd (Urol)

Staff

Management Team
Fiona Foley, Steven Merahn, MD, Daniel Pollock,
Zak Knowles, Howard Croft, Tanya Thomas,
Lucy Hamilton, Julie Volck, Bill Bruggemeyer,
Andrea Ford

Editorial Team
Anne Dyson, Sadaf Hashmi, Debbie Goring,
Louise Morrison, Ellen Haigh, Robert Whittle,
Claire Champion, Caroline Barnett, Laurie Smith,
Li Wan, Paul Mayhew, Carmen Jones, Fi Ward

Technical Team
Martin Miller, Narinder Chandi, Roy Patterson,
Aaron McGrath, John Wylie, Sarah Craze,
Cameron Sangster

We would also like to acknowledge the
extraordinary contributions of the following
individuals to the conceptualization and
realization of PDxMD over the initial years of its
growth and development:

Tim Hailstone, Jonathan Black,
Alison Whitehouse, Jayne Harris, Angela Baggi,
Sharon Bambaji, Sam Bedser, Layla van den
Bergh, Stuart Boffey, Siobhan Egan, Helen Elder,
Mark Mitchenall, Chris Moodie, Tony Pollard,
Simon Seljeflot, Liz Southey, Tim Stentiford,
Matthew Whyte

AMYLOIDOSIS

SUMMARY INFORMATION

DESCRIPTION

- Rare multisystem disorder
- Diverse family of chronic infiltrative disorders characterized by the presence of extracellular deposits of insoluble fibrillar proteins. Each variety is identified by the immunochemical nature of the amyloid protein fibrils: AL amyloid (primary amyloid) or AA amyloid (secondary amyloid)
- Syndromes at presentation, from most to least common, are nephrotic syndrome or renal failure, carpal tunnel syndrome, congestive heart failure, peripheral neuropathy, orthostatic hypotension
- An important cause of nephrotic syndrome, renal insufficiency, and progressive renal failure. Some manifestations of renal disease are found in more than 75% of patients with amyloid
- Diagnosis is suspected on basis of clinical features and established by biopsy

URGENT ACTION

Patients presenting with signs or symptoms of congestive heart failure or renal failure may need urgent referral to specialist for management of advanced disease.

ICD9 CODE

277.3 Amyloidosis

SYNONYMS

- Primary amyloidosis
- Secondary amyloidosis
- Familial amyloidosis
- Senile amyloidosis
- Dialysis-associated amyloid

CARDINAL FEATURES

- Deposition of amyloid fibrils – insoluble fibrillar proteins – in body tissues; proteins may be AL amyloid (primary amyloid) or AA amyloid (secondary amyloid)
- Amyloid appears homogenous and amorphous under a light microscope, staining pink with hematoxylin and eosin. Usually extracellular; fibrils are insoluble and relatively resistant to proteolytic digestion. Birefringent under polarized light when stained with congo red; electron microscopy shows nonbranching, aggregated fibrils 7.5–10nm wide and of indefinite length
- AL amyloid is due to tissue infiltration of organs by the terminal portion of the variable region of immunoglobulin (Ig) light chains (lambda more commonly than kappa), derived from population of monoclonal plasma cells in the bone marrow (falls in spectrum of plasma cell dyscrasias and distinction from multiple myeloma may be difficult). AA amyloid is the result of a proteolytic cleavage product of serum amyloid A, which is an apolipoprotein acute phase reactant whose synthesis by the liver is increased under the influence of interleukin-1
- Primary amyloidosis accounts for 78% of cases; etiology unknown. The kidney is most frequently affected (50%), followed by heart (40%), carpal tunnel (25%), peripheral polyneuropathy (15–35%) which is commonly associated with autonomic features, liver (16%), and purpuric skin lesions (5–15%)
- Secondary amyloidosis accounts for about 2% of cases; associated with an inflammatory process (e.g. rheumatoid disease, inflammatory bowel disease such as Crohn's disease, or bronchiectasis), infectious disease (e.g. tuberculosis and leprosy), neoplastic diseases (e.g. hypernephroma, macroglobulinemia, multiple myeloma, Hodgkin's disease, or other lymphoma), or other diseases (e.g. familial Mediterranean fever). More than 90% have renal insufficiency or nephrotic syndrome at diagnosis. Gastrointestinal involvement is often manifested as a malabsorption syndrome, and nausea and vomiting from pseudo-obstruction may occur. Heart and peripheral nerves are rarely involved in secondary amyloid (in contrast with primary amyloid)
- Familial amyloidosis accounts for about 6% of cases and can be classified as neuropathic, cardiopathic, or nephropathic. The most common type of FAP, type I, was originally described in Portugal but has been observed in many ethnic groups. It is characterized by sensorimotor peripheral neuropathy beginning in the lower extremities commonly associated with autonomic features. Carpal tunnel syndrome is a major feature of FAP type II where autonomic manifestations are absent. Corneal clouding (lattice corneal dystrophy) with cranial nerve (facial palsy and skin changes) involvement are prominent features of FAP type IV. FAP type III is neurologically similar to type I. Age of onset is variable; some patients do not have symptoms until the sixth or seventh decade
- Characteristic renal presentation is with heavy proteinuria, often with nephrotic syndrome. Progressive renal failure is common especially in patients who have nephritic range proteinuria; up to 20% of such patients develop end stage renal disease. In the earlier stages defects of tubular function, such as renal tubular acidosis, Fanconi syndrome, or defects in urinary concentration, may occur. Rarely, patients (particularly those who have rheumatoid arthritis) develop crescentic glomerulonephritis on top of amyloidosis

- Cardiac involvement causes left ventricular dysfunction and tachydysrhythmias and bradydysrhythmias, and is the cause of death in up to 40% of patients with primary systemic amyloidosis – it is the leading cause of death in these patients. Once heart failure from primary systemic amyloidosis occurs, the median survival is 5 months
- Adrenal failure and autonomic neuropathy may cause orthostatic hypotension
- Infiltration of the gastrointestinal tract and exocrine pancreas may cause malabsorption
- Peripheral neuropathies (PN) occur in 15–35% of the patients and is the presenting manifestation in 10%. Close to 25% of patients develop a superimposed carpal tunnel syndrome. PN without renal involvement may occur

CAUSES
Common causes
Primary- or immunocyte-mediated amyloidosis (AL amyloid):
- Most common type in the US, accounting for 78% of cases
- Etiology unknown

Rare causes
Secondary amyloidosis or systemic reactive amyloidosis accounts for 2% of cases in the US. The major infiltrative protein is AA amyloid. It is associated with a wide variety of conditions, including chronic inflammatory disorders, chronic infectious diseases, neoplastic disorders, most commonly rheumatoid arthritis; however, it is rarely seen in SLE:

(Chronic inflammatory disorders)
- Rheumatoid arthritis
- Ankylosing spondylitis
- Psoriatic arthritis
- Sjögren's syndrome
- Reiter's syndrome
- Behçet's syndrome
- Whipple's disease
- Inflammatory bowel disease (particularly Crohn's disease)
- Systemic lupus erythematosus (rare)
- Polymyositis
- Scleroderma
- Third degree burns
- Takayasu's arteritis

(Chronic infectious diseases)
- Tuberculosis
- Osteomyelitis
- Paraplegia
- Heroin abuse (skin popping associated with chronic suppuration)
- Bronchiectasis
- Leprosy
- Syphilis
- Cystic fibrosis
- HIV
- Xanthogranulomatous pyelonephritis

Chronic granulomatous or bacterial infections (e.g. tuberculosis, osteomyelitis, and bronchiectasis) used to be the most common underlying disorders in secondary amyloidosis. Rheumatoid arthritis, juvenile common rheumatoid, and inflammatory bowel disease (especially Crohn's) are now the most common.

Familial amyloidosis:
- Rarely, familial Mediterranean fever can be associated with amyloid
- Glycogen storage disease type Ib
- Astrocytoma

Dialysis-associated amyloid:
- Beta-2 microglobulin accumulates with long-term dialysis, causing amyloidosis
- Patients on long-term dialysis often have carpal tunnel syndrome and pain involving shoulders, hands, wrists, hips, and knees. Accumulation of amyloid in these patients may also cause cervical myelopathy and cauda equina syndrome

Serious causes
Most serious causes of secondary amyloidosis are neoplastic:
- Hypernephroma
- Macroglobulinemia
- Multiple myeloma
- Hodgkin's or other lymphoma
- Medullary thyroid carcinoma

EPIDEMIOLOGY
Incidence and prevalence
INCIDENCE
- 0.89/100,000 (Minnesota, US)
- Approximately 2450 new cases annually in the US

PREVALENCE
No statistics available.

FREQUENCY
No statistics available.

Demographics
AGE
- Median age at diagnosis is 64 years
- Only 1% of patients are younger than 40 at diagnosis

GENDER
Male:female ratio is approximately 2:1.

GENETICS
Secondary amyloidosis is associated with some familial disorders such as familial Mediterranean fever and familial amyloid polyneuropathy.

GEOGRAPHY
- Renal amyloid is more common in North America than Europe
- Families from Denmark and the Appalachian region of the US may be more commonly affected by cardiopathic amyloid

DIAGNOSIS

DIFFERENTIAL DIAGNOSIS
Multiple myeloma
Multiple myeloma is caused by malignant proliferation of plasma cells.

FEATURES
- Clinical presentation: weakness, anemia, weight loss, severe bone pain, pathologic fractures, symptoms of hypercalcemia
- Laboratory findings: diffuse hypogammaglobulinemia, hypercalcemia, tall homogeneous monoclonal spike (M spike) on protein immunoelectrophoresis

Glomerulonephritis
Glomerulonephritis is caused by alteration in structural or functional integrity of glomerular capillary membrane.

FEATURES
- Clinical presentation: edema, joint pain, dark urine, hypertension
- Urine findings: hematuria, proteinuria, red cell casts

Nephrotic syndrome
Nephrotic syndrome consists of clinical and laboratory abnormalities common to a variety of primary and secondary kidney diseases, each characterized by increased permeability of the glomerular capillary wall to circulating plasma proteins, particularly albumin.

FEATURES
- Most commonly presents in children aged 2–6 years
- Often secondary to membranous glomerulonephritis
- Clinical presentation: edema, ascites, hypertension, pleural effusions, weight gain
- Laboratory findings: proteinuria, urine oval fat bodies, decreased serum albumin, 24h urine protein excretion >3.5g/1.73m^3/24h

Congestive heart failure, restrictive cardiomyopathy
Congestive heart failure and restrictive cardiomyopathies are pulmonary and/or systemic circulatory congestion due to inability of the heart to pump sufficient oxygenated blood to meet the body's metabolic demands.

FEATURES
- The clinical presentation is extremely variable. The most common initial manifestation is congestive heart failure. However, other frequent manifestations are syncope (with AV block or left ventricular outflow tract obstruction), ischemic syndromes due to occlusion of coronary arteries, or sudden cardiac death
- Multiple causes, including: ischemic heart disease; hypertensive cardiovascular disease; primary myocarditis; pericarditis; pericardial effusion; infiltrative myocardial processes, such as neoplasm, amyloid; infectious processes, such as bacterial endocarditis; viral myocarditis
- Clinical presentation (extremely variable): dyspnea on exertion, orthopnea, paroxysmal nocturnal dyspnea, angina, fatigue, lethargy
- Physical findings: pulmonary congestion (rales, wheezing), S3 gallop, jugular venous distention, peripheral edema, cyanosis, hepatomegaly, ascites
- Pathology – microscopic and macroscopic evidence of amyloid infiltration of endocardium, myocardium, and pericardium, as well as valves, coronary arteries, and conduction system. In advanced cases, the ventricular walls are extremely thickened, and the atria are dilated

SIGNS & SYMPTOMS

Signs

- Variable with organ system involvement
- Joint involvement: symmetric polyarthritis, carpal tunnel syndrome
- Neuropathies: sensorimotor peripheral neuropathies (carpal tunnel syndrome in 26% of cases), orthostatic hypotension due to autonomic neuropathy (19% of cases)
- Renal involvement (50% of cases): signs of nephrotic syndrome, edema, proteinuria
- Hypertension occurs in 20–50% of cases
- Lung deposition: as many as 30% of patients may have dyspnea, cough, or both. Plaques and pseudotumors may cause hemoptysis, wheezing, obstruction with atelectasis
- Gastrointestinal involvement: macroglossia (10–20% of patients), malabsorption, hepatomegaly (25% of cases), splenomegaly (5%), weight loss
- Cardiac involvement: common (40%) leads to predominantly right-sided congestive heart failure, jugular venous distention, peripheral edema, and hepatomegaly
- Vascular involvement: easy bleeding, periorbital purpura (raccoon eyes), purpuric skin lesions in 5–15% of cases

Symptoms

- Variable with organ system involvement
- General: weakness, fatigue, and weight loss; lightheadedness, syncope due to autonomic neuropathy; change in the tongue or voice; edema
- Musculoskeletal: jaw or hip claudication, painful or swollen joints
- Neurologic: paresthesias, numbness, or motor weakness, especially in the median nerve distribution or as symmetric paresthesias of the lower extremities
- Pulmonary: dyspnea or cough (30% of patients), hemoptysis
- Gastrointestinal: diarrhea, enlarging tongue (20% of patients), abdominal pain, weight loss, anorexia, nausea, vomiting
- Cardiac (up to 40% of patients): breathlessness and symptoms of right-sided congestive heart failure, such as peripheral edema and abdominal pain
- Vascular: easy bruising or skin lesions, especially around the eyes and on face. Purpuric skin lesions may be present in 5–15% of patients with primary amyloid

ASSOCIATED DISORDERS

Chronic inflammatory disorders:
- Rheumatoid arthritis
- Ankylosing spondylitis
- Psoriatic arthritis
- Sjögren's syndrome
- Reiter's syndrome
- Behçet's syndrome
- Whipple's disease
- Inflammatory bowel disease (particularly Crohn's disease)
- Systemic lupus erythematosus (rare)
- Polymyositis
- Scleroderma
- Third degree burns
- Takayasu's arteritis

Chronic infectious diseases:
- Tuberculosis
- Osteomyelitis
- Paraplegia

- Heroin abuse (skin popping associated with chronic suppuration)
- Bronchiectasis
- Leprosy
- Syphilis
- Cystic fibrosis
- HIV infection
- Xanthogranulomatous pyelonephritis

Neoplastic disorders:
- Multiple myeloma
- Hodgkin's disease
- Renal cell carcinoma
- Medullary carcinoma of thyroid
- Waldenström's macroglobulinemia
- Uterine cervical cancer

Familial disorders:
- Familial Mediterranean fever
- Glycogen storage disease type Ib
- Astrocytoma

Chronic granulomatous or bacterial infections e.g. tuberculosis, osteomyelitis, and bronchiectasis used to be the most common underlying disorders in secondary amyloidosis. Rheumatoid arthritis, juvenile common rheumatoid, and inflammatory bowel disease (especially Crohn's) are now the most common.

CONSIDER CONSULT

- Surgical referral for biopsy of subcutaneous abdominal fat, skin, or gingival, renal, or rectal tissue for diagnosis of amyloidosis
- Referral to neurology for appropriate work-up and management is recommended when nervous system involvement is suspected

INVESTIGATION OF THE PATIENT
Direct questions to patient

Q **How old are you?** More common in older males. Very uncommon under the age of 40.

Q **Do you feel well?** Primary amyloidosis most commonly presents with weakness, fatigue, and weight loss. Fatigue may be misdiagnosed as functional or stress related, particularly in patients with early cardiac amyloid. Other very frequent symptoms include lightheadedness, syncope, change in the tongue or voice, jaw or hip claudication, paresthesias, dyspnea, and edema.

Q **Have you noticed any difficulty eating, talking?** Macroglossia occurs in up to 20% of cases. Pain while eating may suggest jaw claudication and temporal artery involvement.

Q **Have you had any swelling, pain, or tenderness in any of your joints? Any pain when you walk?** Joint involvement may occur in the form of symmetric polyarthritis. Hip claudication may also occur and suggests vascular involvement. Carpal tunnel syndrome may be perceived as wrist pain and be felt as far up the arm as the shoulder.

Q **Have you had any tingling, loss of sensation, or weakness, especially in your hands and feet?** Peripheral sensorimotor neuropathies occur. Carpal tunnel syndrome (compression of the median nerve through the carpal tunnel of the wrist) causes pain (often nocturnal) and paresthesia in the palmar aspect of the radial half of the hand. May also cause median nerve motor weakness (thumb abduction). It occurs in about 26% of cases of primary amyloid. Also common in dialysis-associated amyloid.

Q **Have you had any lightheadedness or fainting spells?** This is a common complaint in amyloid, although nonspecific. Autonomic neuropathy may cause lightheadedness and syncope. May also occur in patients with nephrotic syndrome with significant volume contraction. Patients with cardiac amyloid with a low stroke volume due to inadequate left ventricular filling often have orthostatic hypotension. Presence of exertional syncope is a powerful predictor of imminent sudden death.

Q **Have you noticed any swelling of your feet and legs or of your face?** Could be due to renal involvement or congestive heart failure. Renal involvement is present in more than 90% of patients with secondary amyloidosis at diagnosis and in at least a quarter of those with primary amyloid, and proteinuria may reach nephrotic proportions. Edema in nephrotic syndrome is generalized and commonly affects the face and upper extremities. Edema due to heart failure tends to be in dependent areas, feet, legs, and sacral if patient is bedbound.

Q **Do you have a cough or breathlessness?** May be due to lung or cardiac involvement. As many as 30% of patients may have dyspnea, cough, or both, due to lung deposition. Plaques and pseudotumors may cause hemoptysis, wheezing, and obstruction with atelectasis. Cardiac involvement leads to predominantly right-sided congestive heart failure with breathlessness, peripheral swelling, abdominal pain. Cardiac involvement is common in primary amyloid affecting up to 40% of patients. Secondary amyloid rarely involves the heart.

Q **Have you noticed any weight loss, diarrhea, or abdominal pain?** Gastrointestinal involvement may lead to malabsorption, liver enlargement, diarrhea. Abdominal pain may also occur due to liver distention from right-sided congestive failure.

Q **Have you noticed any easy or spontaneous bruising?** Suggests vascular involvement. Purpuric skin lesions may be present in 5–15% of patients with primary amyloid, especially around the eyes (raccoon eyes) and on face.

Contributory or predisposing factors

Q **Do you have any history of tuberculosis, other chronic lung problems, osteomyelitis, rheumatoid arthritis, Crohn's disease, leukemia, Hodgkin's disease?** Chronic suppurative infection, chronic inflammatory disease, and some neoplastic conditions may be complicated by amyloidosis.

Family history

Q **Is there any family history of amyloid disease?** May be significant in a small proportion of cases e.g. familial Mediterranean fever, Muckle-Wells syndrome.

Examination

A full general physical examination should be performed with attention to the following points (signs may be variable depending on which organ systems are involved, and signs of an underlying disorder may also be prominent):

- **Blood pressure:** hypertension is uncommon given the prevalence of renal insufficiency in this population and occurs in 20–50% of cases. Orthostatic hypotension is common and may be due to autonomic neuropathy or restricted left ventricular filling in cardiac amyloid
- **Enlarged tongue:** about 10% of patients have macroglossia; this is the most specific diagnostic sign but may be difficult to recognize unless there are significant dental indentations on the underside of the tongue
- **Lymph nodes:** submandibular salivary gland involvement is frequently mistaken for lymphadenopathy
- **Examination of the skin:** may show periorbital purpura (raccoon eyes), purpuric skin lesions in 5–15%. If present, can be diagnostic of amyloid. Purpuric lesions occur above the nipple line, particularly in the webbing of the neck, the face, and the eyelids. Frequently subtle and missed unless patient closes eyes
- **General examination:** may also show generalized edema of nephrotic syndrome
- Evidence of weight loss may be apparent

- **Inspection of joints:** may show a symmetric polyarthritis
- **Cardiovascular examination:** may show signs of congestive cardiac failure with jugulovenous distention, peripheral edema, and hepatomegaly
- **Respiratory examination:** may show wheezes or areas of collapse
- **Abdominal examination:** may show hepatomegaly (25% of cases) but rarely beyond 5cm below the costal margin; splenomegaly is uncommon (5% of cases). Renal enlargement may occur but is not particularly useful in diagnosis
- **Neurologic examination:** May show stocking and glove distribution of sensory deficits, autonomic features (postural hypotension, impotence, bladder dysfunction, distal anhidrosis, and abnormal pupils), and muscle weakness, all as manifestations of peripheral neuropathy. Signs of carpal tunnel syndrome (hand pain, Tinel's sign, sensory deficit in the first three fingers, and atrophy with or without weakness of the median innervated muscles) may also be found. Pseudohypertrophy of the muscles due to amyloid deposition might be seen
- **Examination of urine:** will show proteinuria in more than 70% of cases

Summary of investigative tests

- To make the diagnosis of amyloid in a patient with unexplained nephrotic range proteinuria, heart failure, hepatomegaly, or neuropathy, the most appropriate laboratory investigation is immunoelectrophoresis and immunofixation of serum and urine serum. Serum electrophoresis shows monoclonal paraprotein in almost two-thirds of patients and yield increases to 86% when urine is examined also. The finding of a monoclonal immunoglobulin strongly suggests further diagnostic evaluation for amyloidosis
- Investigations likely to be carried out by the primary care physician are those that will aid in the differential diagnosis of nonspecific malaise and characterization of specific amyloid-related syndromes or underlying disease
- Complete blood count/erythrocyte sedimentation rate (ESR): not specifically diagnostic for amyloidosis but may be useful in evaluation of patient presenting with fatigue or weakness. ESR may be raised due to the presence of serum monoclonal protein and result in false diagnosis of polymyalgia rheumatica
- Thyroid function tests: 10–20% of patients with amyloid are hypothyroid. Also useful in evaluation of patient presenting with nonspecific symptoms
- Renal investigations: indicated for all patients suspected of having amyloid, presenting with nonspecific symptoms or nephrotic syndrome. Quantification of proteinuria, tests of renal insufficiency, creatinine, and creatinine clearance should be performed
- Liver function tests: in secondary amyloid, albumin level is reduced in 90%. Alkaline phosphatase is raised in only 14%
- Chest X-ray: indicated for those with cardiac or respiratory symptoms
- Electrocardiogram: indicated for those with cardiac symptoms

Referral to a specialist is likely to be necessary for the following investigations:

- Tissue biopsy for diagnosis: subcutaneous fat pad aspiration is positive in 70–80% of cases and bone marrow biopsy positive in approximately 50%. If these sites are normal then rectal biopsy (positive in 73% of cases), or biopsy of involved organ or sural nerve may be indicated. The sensitivity of renal biopsy in a proteinuric patient approaches 100%. In practice, site-specific biopsies are rarely needed; commonly, when amyloid is suspected, simultaneous fat aspiration biopsy and bone marrow biopsy are performed and one or the other or both is positive in about 90% of amyloid patients. Myocardial biopsy is a reliable means of establishing diagnosis if other means fail
- Echocardiography: 2D Doppler echocardiography is the standard means to diagnose and evaluate cardiac involvement. It is abnormal in two-thirds of patients with primary amyloid. Abnormal features include increased thickness of right and left ventricular walls, abnormal myocardial texture (granular sparkling), atrial enlargement, valvular thickening and regurgitation, pericardial effusion, abnormal diastolic and, ultimately, reduced systolic ventricular function

Pericardial effusions are also frequently observed. Ventricular wall thickness and diastolic function have been demonstrated to be of prognostic usefulness.

- Nuclear imaging with technetium-labeled aprotinin may detect cardiac amyloidosis, but there is lack of sensitivity with this assay
- Detailed biochemical tests on the forms of amyloid proteins are not part of routine clinical practice

DIAGNOSTIC DECISION

- Suspect amyloid when a patient presents with unexplained nephrotic range proteinuria, heart failure, peripheral neuropathy, hepatomegaly
- Pursue diagnosis aggressively by seeking monoclonal protein in serum or urine, performing bone marrow biopsy and fat aspiration biopsy, with site-specific biopsy in the 10% with negative bone marrow or fat aspiration
- Diagnosis of primary amyloidosis depends on demonstration of amyloid deposits in the tissues by congo red staining of biopsies
- Echocardiography will help to determine prognosis

CLINICAL PEARLS

Echocardiography is the primary diagnostic modality for assessment of patients with suspected or proven cardiac amyloid.

THE TESTS
Body fluids
COMPLETE BLOOD COUNT, ERYTHROCYTE SEDIMENTATION RATE (ESR)
Description
Venous blood sample.

Advantages/Disadvantages
Advantage: relatively inexpensive

Disadvantages:
- Associated with mild patient discomfort
- Results not specific to amyloidosis

Normal
- White blood cells: 3.2–9.8x10^9/L
- Red cells: male 4.3–5.9x10^6/mm^3; female 3.3–3x10^6/mm^3
- Hemoglobin: male, 13.6–17–7g/dL (8.4–11.0mmol/L); female, 12–15g/dL (7.4–9.3mmol/L)
- Platelet count 130–400x10^9/L
- ESR: 0–15mm/h (male); 0–20mm/h (female)

Abnormal
Values outside normal range.

Cause of abnormal result
- Anemia is not a prominent feature of primary amyloid but, when present, is usually due to multiple myeloma, renal insufficiency, or gastrointestinal bleeding
- Thrombocytosis occurs among 10% of patients
- ESR may be raised due to the presence of serum monoclonal protein and result in false diagnosis of polymyalgia rheumatica

Drugs, disorders and other factors that may alter results
ESR is raised in collagen vascular disease, infections, myocardial infarction, neoplasms, inflammatory states, thyroid dysfunction, rouleaux formation. It is decreased in sickle cell disease, polycythemia, corticosteroids, spherocytosis, anisocytosis, hypofibrinogenemia, increased serum viscosity.

THYROID FUNCTION TESTS
Description
Serum sample for:
- Thyroid-stimulating hormone (TSH)
- T4, T3

Advantages/Disadvantages
- Advantage: useful in evaluation of patient presenting with nonspecific symptoms
- Disadvantage: results not specific for amyloidosis

Normal
- TSH: 2–11mU/L
- T4: 4–11mcg/dL (51–142nmol/L)
- Free T4: 0.8–2.8ng/dL
- T3: 75–220ng/dL (1.23–3.4nmol/L)

Abnormal
- Hyperthyroidism will cause raised T4, T3, and lower TSH
- Hypothyroidism causes reduced T4, and T3 with increased TSH

Cause of abnormal result
Endocrine dysfunction is rare with primary amyloidosis. Occasionally, hypothyroidism may result from infiltration of the thyroid, pituitary, or other endocrine glands.

Drugs, disorders and other factors that may alter results
TSH may be increased by laboratory error, primary hypothyroidism, lithium or amiodarone, later stages of Hashimoto's thyroiditis, inorganic iodide, recovery phase of severe nonthyroid illness, iodine deficiency, Addison's disease, pituitary TSH-secreting tumor, antibodies interfering with assay, contrast media, amphetamines, high altitudes.

RENAL INVESTIGATIONS
Description
- Urinalysis: proteinuria found in >70% of cases of amyloid
- Quantification of proteinuria: 24h urine collection
- Tests of renal insufficiency: creatinine (serum sample) and creatinine clearance (24h urine sample)

Advantages/Disadvantages
Advantage: relatively inexpensive, noninvasive

Disadvantages:
- Tests not specifically diagnostic for amyloid
- Accurate collection of 24h urine specimen is notoriously difficult
- Creatinine is a good marker for significant renal impairment, but not for early renal disease

Normal
- 24h urinary protein: <150mg/24h
- Creatinine: 0.6–1.2mg/dL
- Creatinine clearance: 75–124mL/min

Abnormal
- Creatinine is higher than 2mg/dL in more than 20% of patients with primary amyloid
- In patients with secondary amyloid more than two-thirds have a raised creatinine level. 87% produce more than 1g of protein in 24h urine collection
- Nephropathic familial amyloid frequently results in nephrotic syndrome and renal insufficiency
- Nephrotic syndrome occurs in the presence of proteinuria >3g/24h

Cause of abnormal result
Renal dysfunction due to amyloid deposits in the kidney.

Drugs, disorders and other factors that may alter results
- Urinary protein elevated in renal disease, congestive heart failure, hypertension, neoplasms of renal pelvis and bladder, multiple myeloma, Waldenström's macroglobulinemia
- Creatinine may be elevated in renal insufficiency, decreased renal perfusion, urinary tract infection, rhabdomyolysis, ketonemia. May be reduced in decreased muscle mass, pregnancy, prolonged debilitation
- Creatinine clearance may be elevated in pregnancy and exercise, and decreased in renal insufficiency, and with drugs such as cimetidine, procainamide, antibiotics, quinidine

LIVER FUNCTION TESTS
Description
Venous blood sample for alanine aminotransferase (ALT; SGPT), aspartate aminotransferase (AST; SGOT), alkaline phosphatase, bilirubin.

Advantages/Disadvantages
Advantages:
- Relatively inexpensive, noninvasive
- May help evaluate severity of disease

Disadvantage: tests not specifically diagnostic for amyloid

Normal
- AST: 0–35U/L
- ALT: 0–35U/L
- Alkaline phosphatase: 30–120U/L
- Bilirubin, direct (conjugated): 0–0.2mg/dL
- Bilirubin, indirect (unconjugated): 0–1.0mg/dL
- Bilirubin, total: 0–1.0mg/dL

Abnormal
Elevations in serum values above the normal range.

Cause of abnormal result
Liver disease secondary to amyloid infiltration or hepatic congestion secondary to congestive heart failure associated with amyloidosis.

Amyloidosis – DIAGNOSIS

13

Drugs, disorders and other factors that may alter results

▪ AST, ALT can be elevated by liver disease, hepatic congestion, infectious process (such as hepatitis, infectious mononucleosis), muscle trauma, malignancy, eclampsia, and drugs (such as antibiotics, narcotics, antihypertensive agents, nonsteroidal anti-inflammatory drugs, phenytoin, amiodarone, and others)

▪ Alkaline phosphatase may be elevated due to biliary obstruction, liver disease, bone disease, hyperparathyroidism, ulcerative colitis, sepsis, neoplastic disease, and drugs such as estrogens, albumin, erythromycin, phenothiazines, and others

▪ Bilirubin values may be elevated due to hepatocellular disease, biliary obstruction, drug-induced cholestasis, some hereditary disorders such as Dubin-Johnson syndrome, Gilbert's syndrome, hemolysis, and drugs such as steroids, phenothiazines, penicillin, erythromycin, captopril, amphotericin B, sulfonamides, azathioprine, allopurinol, indomethacin, oral contraceptives, and others

ELECTROPHORESIS

Description

▪ To make the diagnosis of amyloid in a patient with unexplained nephrotic range proteinuria, heart failure, hepatomegaly, or neuropathy, the most appropriate initial screening investigation is immunoelectrophoresis and immunofixation of serum and urine. The finding of a monoclonal immunoglobulin strongly suggests further diagnostic evaluation for amyloidosis

▪ Immunofixation should be done on both serum and urine because a serum monoclonal protein is absent from the serum in one-third of patients

▪ In patients who do not have detectable monoclonal light chain in the serum or urine, bone marrow in primary amyloid almost always demonstrates a clonal population of plasma cells detectable by immunohistochemistry or immunofluorescence

Advantages/Disadvantages

Disadvantages:

▪ A peak is easy to overlook on the electrophoretic pattern because the monoclonal protein is usually small and the peak may also be obscured by surrounding normal immunoglobulins

▪ In urine, heavy proteinuria may frequently obscure the presence of a small light chain peak

Normal

Serum values:

▪ Albumin: 60–75% or 3.6–5.2g/dL
▪ Alpha-1: 1.7–5% or 0.1–0.4g/dL
▪ Alpha-2: 6.7–12.5% or 0.4–1g/dL
▪ Beta: 8.3–16.3% or 0.5–1.2g/dL
▪ Gamma: 10.7–20% or 0.6–1.2g/dL

Abnormal

Serum electrophoresis shows monoclonal paraprotein in almost two-thirds of patients, and yield increases to 86% when urine is examined also.

Cause of abnormal result

Presence of abnormal paraprotein in serum or urine.

Drugs, disorders and other factors that may alter results

▪ Albumin may be elevated in dehydration and decreased in malnutrition, chronic liver disease, malabsorption, nephrotic syndrome, burns, systemic lupus erythematosus

- Alpha-1 proteins may be elevated in neoplasms and inflammation and decreased in emphysema or nephrosis
- Alpha-2 proteins may be elevated in neoplasms, inflammation, infection, and nephrotic syndrome, and reduced in hemolytic anemias or severe hepatocellular damage
- Beta proteins may be elevated in hypothyroidism, biliary cirrhosis, and diabetes mellitus, and reduced in hypocholesterolemia and nephrosis

Imaging
CHEST X-RAY
Description
Indicated for respiratory or cardiac symptoms.

Advantages/Disadvantages
Advantages:
- Inexpensive
- Noninvasive
- Shows most of gross pathologic changes for infiltrates, fibrosis, bony changes, size of the heart and mediastinum, hilar lymphadenopathy

Disadvantages:
- Nonspecific for cardiovascular abnormalities; additional testing necessary
- Keep in mind the possibility of imaging artifacts

Abnormal
- May show hilar or mediastinal adenopathy
- May show signs consistent with cardiac failure but frequently shows normal cardiac silhouette in amyloid
- Pulmonary infiltrates, pleural effusion

Cause of abnormal result
- Lymph node involvement with amyloidosis
- Congestive heart failure associated with cardiac amyloidosis
- Pulmonary involvement with amyloid

Drugs, disorders and other factors that may alter results
Any nonamyloid cause of lymphadenopathy, congestive heart failure, or pulmonary infiltrates.

ECHOCARDIOGRAM
Description
Primary diagnostic modality for assessment of patients with suspected or proven cardiac amyloid.

Abnormal
- Characteristic features: markedly increased ventricular wall thickness, increased myocardial echogenicity, increased valve thickness, decreased left ventricular cavity size, normal/decreased systolic function, pericardial effusion
- Restrictive pattern of Doppler examination

Cause of abnormal result
Infiltration of endocardium, myocardium, and pericardium.

Other tests
ELECTROCARDIOGRAM
Advantages/Disadvantages
Disadvantages:
- Not specific for amyloidosis
- Subtle changes may frequently be overlooked unless physician is sensitive to the diagnosis

Abnormal
- In primary amyloid may show low voltage or characteristics of anteroseptal infarction, arrhythmia, or heart block
- Pseudoinfarction pattern of QS; QS complexes refer to the ECG findings that mimic Q waves of a myocardial infarction, complexes in precordial leads V1 to V3 frequently lead to interpretation of silent myocardial infarction
- Presence of low QRS voltage can occur in the setting of thickened myocardium by echocardiogram
- Arrhythmias such as atrial fibrillation may be seen
- Sudden death may occur from asystole or ventricular fibrillation

Cause of abnormal result
Amyloid deposits causing wall thickening and a restrictive infiltrative cardiomyopathy.

Drugs, disorders and other factors that may alter results
Any nonamyloid cause of myocardial ischemia, conduction abnormalities, or arrhythmias.

TREATMENT

CONSIDER CONSULT

- Referral to specialist (often hematologist) of primary amyloid patients for consideration of treatments such as alkylating agents and steroids
- Referral of those with progressive renal failure for consideration of dialysis or transplant
- Referral of those with secondary amyloid for assistance with treatment of underlying disorder
- Referral to surgical specialist if renal, cardiac, or liver transplantation is anticipated

PATIENT AND CAREGIVER ISSUES
Forensic and legal issues

Because secondary amyloidosis is sometimes associated with mental status changes, it may be necessary to assess the mental competence of some patients to participate in treatment decisions; in cases of incompetence, appropriate surrogate decision-makers may be needed.

Impact on career, dependants, family, friends

- Ability to carry out professional and personal physical activities may be adversely affected, necessitating significant support and alterations in physically demanding careers
- Frequent visits for medical follow-up, hemodialysis, chemotherapy, and other medical interventions can significantly impact the need for transportation and support

Patient or caregiver request

- Therapy for amyloidosis is aimed at treating the primary disease, together with end-organ effects
- Chemotherapy is often chosen as a treatment for primary amyloidosis; therapy is well tolerated, efficacious, and has minimal side-effects
- In cases of advanced disease, transplantation of the major organ affected (heart, kidney, liver) may be considered, but experience is limited. Diuretic therapy is the mainstay for treatment of heart failure in these patients
- Patients with renal insufficiency or hypotension from amyloidosis may be predisposed to digoxin toxicity or intolerant of vasodilators
- Rarely do patients benefit from cardiac pacing

MANAGEMENT ISSUES
Goals

- Accurate diagnosis
- Appropriate referral for treatment
- Psychologic support of patient and family

Management in special circumstances

Management of amyloidosis may involve administration of chemotherapy in addition to traditional medical therapies aimed at improving end-organ function (e.g. treatment for congestive heart failure, renal failure). Disease management in special patient groups, such as very young or pregnant patients, will require the involvement of a specialist.

COEXISTING DISEASE

Treatment of coexisting disease that actually may be a cause of secondary amyloidosis should be pursued aggressively.

SPECIAL PATIENT GROUPS

- Patients with dialysis-associated amyloid: consider use of newer dialysis membranes that can pass beta-2 microglobulin (called high-flux dialyzers)

- Patients with secondary amyloid: rarely have remissions been reported after antibiotic therapy for underlying infection, chemotherapy for rheumatic disease, or resection of inflammatory bowel disease or neoplasm

PATIENT SATISFACTION/LIFESTYLE PRIORITIES

- Patient lifestyle is most affected by the systemic affects of amyloidosis
- Treatment of amyloidosis itself (e.g. melphalan and prednisone chemotherapy) is well tolerated symptomatically but requires close follow-up and laboratory monitoring, which may limit patient activities
- Treatment of secondary effects of amyloid, such as treatment of congestive heart failure, is aimed at relieving or improving symptoms and may have a positive effect on patient satisfaction and lifestyle
- Treatment of amyloidosis and its secondary effects may have significant economic impact on the patient

SUMMARY OF THERAPEUTIC OPTIONS
Choices

Rational therapy is directed at achieving three goals: reducing precursor protein production, inhibiting synthesis and deposition of amyloid fibrils, and promoting lysis or mobilization of amyloid deposits. Treatment depends on which type of amyloidosis is present.

Primary amyloidosis:
- Chemotherapy with: alkylating agents (such as melphalan), prednisone, or colchicine; iododoxorubicin (may promote amyloid resorption)
- Stem cell transplant and immunosuppressive agents
- Cardiac transplant in certain patients

Secondary amyloidosis (depends on the underlying cause):
- Resorption of amyloid has rarely been reported after treatment for osteomyelitis, tuberculosis or empyema, chemotherapy for rheumatic disease, resection of inflammatory bowel disease, or neoplasms
- Colchicine is useful in preventing attacks of serositis and synovitis in familial Mediterranean fever and in slowing accumulation of amyloid in native kidneys or allografts after transplantation
- Dialysis or renal transplant may be required in up to one-third of patients
- Cardiac transplant may be considered
- Liver transplant may produce a dramatic reduction in variant transthyretin serum level, which should, in theory, stop further deposition of amyloid in familial amyloid polyneuropathy. Only a very small majority of patients would fall in this group and the operation is carried out by a specialist, therefore this will not be dealt with in more detail here
- In reality there may be regression of amyloid deposits in tissues and partial improvement of the neuropathy, but in approximately one-half of the cases the disease progresses, presumably related to the total body amyloid load

Other common supportive treatments include:
- Edema in nephrotic syndrome associated with amyloid may be treated with furosemide and metolazone, although use of these agents is often limited as they produce volume contraction and decreased renal blood flow and frequently precipitate syncopal episodes. Protein and sodium restriction in patients with renal failure is also indicated
- Midodrine can reverse orthostatic hypotension but has sodium-retaining effects and can aggravate edema
- Cardiac amyloid patients with heart failure are frequently treated with diuretic agents and afterload reduction with ACE inhibitors. However, due to low cardiac output and hypotension there is often difficulty in administering therapeutic doses

- Low salt diet in patients with congestive heart failure may be indicated
- Usual measures for conservative management of chronic renal failure

Clinical pearls
- Because of renal insufficiency or hypotension, treatment of congestive heart failure with digoxin or vasodilator therapy is often difficult
- The mainstay of heart failure therapy is diuretics

FOLLOW UP
Follow-up plan will be dependent on which therapies are being used.

Information for patient or caregiver
- Treatment for amyloidosis is aimed at stabilization and/or regression of end-organ effects
- Medical therapy is generally well tolerated
- Not receiving therapy is associated with poor survival, particularly if the patient has cardiac symptoms

DRUGS AND OTHER THERAPIES: DETAILS
Surgical therapy
HEART TRANSPLANT
Heart transplantation for amyloid disease is controversial because of the scarcity of hearts for transplant, the systemic nature of amyloid, and the potential for amyloid deposition in the graft.

Efficacy
Palliative procedure without treatment of the underlying disease.

Risks/Benefits
Risks:
- Postoperative mortality is high (20% in one series)
- Amyloid deposits may recur in graft

Acceptability to patient
May prove acceptable, especially to younger patients – although not curative, it may improve quality of life.

Follow up plan
Regular follow up required, including supervision of immunosuppressants.

Patient and caregiver information
Experience with cardiac transplantation for amyloidosis is very limited.

RENAL TRANSPLANT
- May be considered for end-stage renal failure due to amyloidosis
- Most transplant recipients have secondary (AA) rather than primary (AL) amyloidosis
- Colchicine is used to minimize the risk of recurrence in the allograft in secondary forms of amyloid; its efficacy in primary AL amyloid requires further study
- Contraindicated in presence of malignancy, active infection, patient unfit for general anesthesia, extremes of age
- Recurrent amyloid deposit will occur in 20–23% of the allograft but graft loss is rare

Efficacy
- Dialysis-associated amyloid: renal transplant often leads to dramatic improvement in joint symptoms

- Outcome for renal transplant for amyloidosis has been thought to carry a poorer prognosis than for other causes of renal failure; however, graft survival may be improved with immunosuppression
- Transplant patients with amyloid have shorter survival times than recipients who do not have amyloid

Risks/Benefits
Risks:
- Recurrent amyloid has been reported in allografts and may cause renal failure
- Acute rejection may occur
- Opportunistic infections such as cytomegalovirus and *Pneumocystis* are more prevalent
- There is increased risk of lymphoproliferative disease, skin malignancy, and cervical cancer
- Hypertension and hyperlipidemia are very common after transplant, particularly with cyclosporine therapy
- Transplant patients are at an increased risk of dying because of cardiovascular diseases
- The average length of survival of a cadaveric renal transplant is 6–8 years in the US and 10–12 years for a living related or unrelated transplant

Acceptability to patient
- Releases patient from dialysis
- Requires lifelong immunosuppression with potentially toxic drugs
- Patient with amyloid may feel risks are acceptable as prognosis is otherwise poor

Follow up plan
Regular follow up with assessment of graft function as well as that of disease.

Patient and caregiver information
Transplant experience is limited in amyloidosis.

Chemotherapy

Combined chemotherapy with prednisone and melphalan, with or without colchicine, has been shown to increase median survival in patients with primary amyloidosis.

CHEMOTHERAPY
- Alkylating agent-based chemotherapy, such as melphalan and prednisone and colchicine, may be used with occasionally dramatic responses to treatment seen in primary amyloidosis
- Anecdotal reports suggest that there may be some benefit from colchicine in primary amyloidosis. It is also useful in preventing attacks of serositis and synovitis in familial Mediterranean fever and in slowing accumulation of amyloid in native kidneys or allografts after transplantation
- Iododoxorubicin therapy may promote amyloid resorption in some patients
- Intensive chemotherapy with peripheral stem cell rescue may be useful

Efficacy
- Alkylating agent-based chemotherapy such as melphalan and prednisone may produce a significantly longer survival period than colchicine (18 vs 8.5 months)
- Resolution of nephrotic syndrome and amelioration of progression of chronic renal failure may occur in patients with primary amyloidosis treated with immunosuppressive regimens incorporating melphalan and prednisone

Risks/Benefits
Risks:
- It may take up to a year to achieve an organ response, and in many cases patients do not survive long enough to have an opportunity to respond. Response can be defined as either organ-based or hematologic. One study found mean survival of responders to be 89.4 months compared with 14.7 months in those who failed to respond

- The potential exists for late myelodysplasia or acute leukemia with the use of alkylating agents, and approximately 6.5% of patients exposed to melphalan develop a myelodysplastic syndrome. Because of the age group of many of these patients, myelodysplasia usually results in rapid death with a median survival from onset to death of 8 months
- Melphalan should be administered under the supervision of a qualified physician experienced in the use of cancer chemotherapeutic agents
- As with other nitrogen mustard drugs, excessive dosage will produce marked bone marrow suppression
- Hypersensitivity reactions, including anaphylaxis, have occurred in approximately 2% of patients who received the intravenous formulation and rarely in patients who received oral melphalan
- Secondary malignancies, including acute nonlymphocytic leukemia, myeloproliferative syndrome, and carcinoma have been reported in patients with cancer treated with alkylating agents (including melphalan)
- Dose reduction should be considered in patients with renal insufficiency receiving intravenous melphalan

Acceptability to patient
- Many patients will find treatment acceptable despite the risks, as prognosis for disease left untreated is poor
- Factors impacting patient acceptability include side-effects of medication, discomfort associated with laboratory monitoring of therapy, and the need for frequent physician visits
- Regimens of melphalan and prednisone (with or without colchicine) may be well tolerated, with modifications due to side-effects occasionally required
- Combination therapy has been shown to increase survival
- The most common side-effect is gastrointestinal (usually diarrhea) related to colchicine, which responds well to decreasing colchicine to once-daily dose administration
- 1–3% of patients experience decreased blood counts requiring modification of therapy, and two patients in one study developed infections believed to be secondary to therapy
- Follow-up blood studies are needed approximately every 3 weeks, which may negatively impact lifestyle and patient tolerance

Follow up plan
Follow-up laboratory monitoring of patient red blood cell (RBC), white blood cell (WBC), and platelet counts is required approximately every 3 weeks throughout chemotherapy.

Patient and caregiver information
- Chemotherapy may improve length of survival with amyloid disease
- The term 'chemotherapy' suggests to many patients significant negative side-effects (e.g. nausea, vomiting, hair loss); however, combination prednisone, melphalan, and colchicine therapy is well tolerated, with diarrhea in a minority of patients the only symptomatic side-effect in two studies. Diarrhea was managed with reduction of colchicine dosage
- While median survival in patients with primary amyloid receiving chemotherapy was only 12–18 months, patients presenting without cardiac involvement had significantly longer survival (15% survived >5 years, a few patients >10 years)
- Late development (26–69 months after chemotherapy) of myelodysplasia and leukemia was seen in a small number of patients receiving melphalan therapy for amyloidosis (8/148), half of whom subsequently died. Overall survival rates of amyloidosis were still significantly better than in untreated patients

PREDNISONE
- Dosage should be decided by a specialist and must be individualized
- Studies involving patients receiving combined therapy for primary amyloidosis have used prednisone 0.8–1.5mg/kg/day for 4–7 days

Possible regimens:

- 0.15mg/kg melphalan plus 0.8mg/kg prednisone every day for 7 days; increase melphalan dose by 2mg in each 6-week cycle until midcycle leukopenia or thrombocytopenia develops; repeat cycle every 6 weeks for 2 years or until serious toxicity develops
- 0.15mg/kg melphalan plus 1.5mg/kg prednisone every day for 4 days; repeat cycle every 6 weeks for one year; increase melphalan dose by 2mg in each 6-week cycle until leukopenia or thrombocytopenia develops (not to exceed 0.25mg/kg/dose); limit total melphalan dose over entire treatment regimen to 600mg

Efficacy
Melphalan used in combination with prednisone, with or without colchicine, has been shown to increase survival from 8.5 to 12–18 months in patients with primary amyloidosis.

Risks/Benefits
Risks:

- Use caution in congestive heart failure, diabetes mellitus, glaucoma, and the elderly
- Use caution in renal disease, ulcerative colitis, and peptic ulcer
- Prednisone taken in doses higher than 7.5mg for 3 weeks or longer may lead to clinically relevant suppression of the pituitary-adrenal axis

Side-effects and adverse reactions

- Side-effects are minimized by short duration of therapy
- Cardiovascular system: hypertension, thromboembolism
- Central nervous system: insomnia, euphoria, depression, psychosis, seizures
- Endocrine: adrenal suppression, impaired glucose tolerance, growth suppression in children
- Eyes, ears, nose, and throat: cataract, glaucoma, blurred vision
- Gastrointestinal: dyspepsia, peptic ulceration, esophagitis, oral candidiasis
- Musculoskeletal: proximal myopathy, osteoporosis
- Skin: delayed healing, acne, striae, fragile skin

Interactions (other drugs)

- Aminoglutethimide (increased clearance of prednisone) ▪ Antihypertensives (effects inhibited) ▪ Antidiabetics (hypoglycemic effect inhibited) ▪ Barbiturates (increased clearance of prednisone) ▪ Cardiac glycosides (toxicity increased) ▪ Cholestyramine, colestipol (may reduce absorption of corticosteroids) ▪ Clarithromycin, erythromycin, troleandomycin (may enhance steroid effect) ▪ Cyclosporine (may increase levels of both drugs; may cause seizures) ▪ Diuretics (effects inhibited) ▪ Isoniazid (reduced plasma levels of isoniazid) ▪ Ketoconazole ▪ Nonsteroidal anti-inflammatory drugs (NSAIDs; increased risk of bleeding) ▪ Oral contraceptives (enhanced effects of corticosteroids) ▪ Rifampin (may inhibit hepatic clearance of prednisone) ▪ Salicylates (increased clearance of salicylates) ▪ Warfarin (alters clotting time)

Contraindications

- Systemic infection ▪ Avoid live virus vaccines in those receiving immunosuppressive doses ▪ History of tuberculosis ▪ Cushing's syndrome ▪ Recent myocardial infarction

Acceptability to patient

- Regimens of melphalan and prednisone (with or without colchicine) may be well tolerated, with modifications due to side-effects occasionally required
- Combination therapy has been shown to increase survival
- The most common side-effect is gastrointestinal (usually diarrhea) related to colchicine, which responds well to decreasing colchicine to once-daily dose administration

- 1–3% of patients experience decreased blood counts requiring modification of therapy, and two patients in one study developed infections believed to be secondary to therapy
- Follow-up blood studies are needed approximately every 3 weeks, which may negatively impact lifestyle and patient tolerance

Follow up plan

Follow-up blood studies to detect decreased RBC, WBC, and platelet counts are needed approximately every 3 weeks throughout the duration of therapy.

Patient and caregiver information
- Chemotherapy may improve length of survival with amyloid disease
- The term 'chemotherapy' suggests to many patients significant negative side-effects (e.g. nausea, vomiting, hair loss); however, combination prednisone, melphalan, and colchicine therapy is well tolerated, with diarrhea in a minority of patients the only symptomatic side-effect in two studies. Diarrhea was managed with reduction of colchicine dosage
- While median survival in patients with primary amyloid receiving chemotherapy was only 12–18 months, patients presenting without cardiac involvement had significantly longer survival (15% survived >5 years, a few patients >10 years)
- Late development (26–69 months after chemotherapy) of myelodysplasia and leukemia was seen in a small number of patients receiving melphalan therapy for amyloidosis (8/148), half of whom subsequently died. Overall survival rates of amyloidosis were still significantly better than in untreated patients

MELPHALAN (L-PHENYLALANINE MUSTARD)
- Alkylating agent
- Dosage should be decided by a specialist and must be individualized
- Studies involving patients receiving combined therapy for primary amyloidosis have used melphalan 0.15–0.25mg/kg/day for 4 or 7 days

Possible regimens:
- 0.15mg/kg melphalan plus 0.8mg/kg prednisone every day for 7 days; increase melphalan dose by 2mg in each 6-week cycle until midcycle leukopenia or thrombocytopenia develops; repeat cycle every 6 weeks for 2 years or until serious toxicity develops
- 0.15mg/kg melphalan plus 1.5mg/kg prednisone every day for 4 days; repeat cycle every 6 weeks for one year; increase melphalan dose by 2mg in each 6-week cycle until leukopenia or thrombocytopenia develops (not to exceed 0.25mg/kg/dose); limit total melphalan dose over entire treatment regimen to 600mg

Efficacy

Melphalan used in combination with prednisone, with or without colchicine, has been shown to increase survival from 8.5 to 12–18 months in patients with primary amyloidosis.

Risks/Benefits

Risks:
- Should be administered under the supervision of a qualified physician experienced in the use of cancer chemotherapeutic agents
- As with other nitrogen mustard drugs, excessive dosage will produce marked bone marrow suppression
- Hypersensitivity reactions, including anaphylaxis, have occurred in approximately 2% of patients who received the intravenous formulation and rarely in patients who received oral melphalan

- Secondary malignancies, including acute nonlymphocytic leukemia, myeloproliferative syndrome, and carcinoma have been reported in patients with cancer treated with alkylating agents (including melphalan)
- Dose reduction should be considered in patients with renal insufficiency receiving intravenous melphalan

Benefit: prolongation of life over no therapy at all

Side-effects and adverse reactions – intravenous:
- Cardiovascular system: pulmonary fibrosis
- Gastrointestinal: nausea, vomiting, diarrhea, oral ulceration, hepatotoxicity, including veno-occlusive disease
- Hematologic: bone marrow suppression, hemolytic anemia
- Hypersensitivity: acute hypersensitivity, urticaria, pruritus, edema, tachycardia, bronchospasm, dyspnea, and hypotension
- Skin: hypersensitivity, skin ulceration at injection site, skin necrosis rarely requiring skin grafting, vasculitis, alopecia
- Other: interstitial pneumonitis

Side-effects and adverse reactions – oral:
- Gastrointestinal: nausea, vomiting, diarrhea, oral ulceration
- Hematologic: bone marrow suppression, hemolytic anemia
- Skin: hypersensitivity, vasculitis, alopecia
- Other: pulmonary fibrosis, interstitial pneumonitis

Interactions (other drugs) – intravenous:
- Cyclosporine (severe renal failure has been reported in patients treated with a single dose of intravenous melphalan followed by standard oral doses of cyclosporine) ▪ Cisplatin (may affect melphalan kinetics) ▪ Nalidixic acid (increased incidence of severe hemorrhagic necrotic enterocolitis in pediatric patients)

Interactions (other drugs) – oral:
None listed

Contraindications
- Should not be used in patients whose disease has demonstrated a prior resistance to melphalan. Patients who have demonstrated hypersensitivity to melphalan should not be given the drug ▪ Pregnancy category D ▪ Breast-feeding

Acceptability to patient
Regimens of melphalan and prednisone (with or without colchicine) may be well tolerated, with modifications due to side-effects occasionally required
Combination therapy has been shown to increase survival
The most common side-effect is gastrointestinal (usually diarrhea) related to colchicine, which responds well to decreasing colchicine to once-daily dose administration
1–3% of patients experience decreased blood counts requiring modification of therapy, and two patients in one study developed infections believed to be secondary to therapy
Follow-up blood studies are needed approximately every 3 weeks, which may negatively impact lifestyle and patient tolerance

Follow up plan
Follow-up blood studies to detect decreased RBC, WBC, and platelet counts are needed approximately every 3 weeks throughout the duration of therapy.

Patient and caregiver information
- Chemotherapy may improve length of survival with amyloid disease
- The term 'chemotherapy' suggests to many patients significant negative side-effects (e.g. nausea, vomiting, hair loss); however, combination prednisone, melphalan, and colchicine therapy is well tolerated, with diarrhea in a minority of patients the only symptomatic side-effect in two studies. Diarrhea was managed with reduction of colchicine dosage
- While median survival in patients with primary amyloid receiving chemotherapy was only 12–18 months, patients presenting without cardiac involvement had significantly longer survival (15% survived >5 years, a few patients >10 years)
- Late development (26–69 months after chemotherapy) of myelodysplasia and leukemia was seen in a small number of patients receiving melphalan therapy for amyloidosis (8/148), half of whom subsequently died. Overall survival rates of amyloidosis were still significantly better than in untreated patients

COLCHICINE
- This is an off-label indication
- Studies involving patients receiving combined therapy for primary amyloidosis have used colchicine 0.6mg orally twice daily

Efficacy
Studies found better survival in patients receiving colchicine in combination with prednisone and melphalan than in patients receiving colchicine alone. One study suggests that melphalan and prednisone in combination is as efficacious as melphalan and prednisone combined with colchicine.

Risks/Benefits
Risks:
- Use caution in the elderly and children
- Use caution in alcoholism
- Use caution in gastrointestinal disease, bone marrow suppression, and dental disease

Benefit: may be used in patients who cannot tolerate NSAIDs

Side-effects and adverse reactions
- Central nervous system: peripheral neuropathy, neuritis
- Gastrointestinal: nausea, vomiting, anorexia, abdominal pain, diarrhea, adynamic ileus
- Genitourinary: nephrotoxicity
- Hematologic: blood cell disorders
- Metabolic: hypothyroidism
- Musculoskeletal: myopathy
- Skin: injection site reaction, tissue necrosis, urticaria, angioedema, rashes, alopecia, purpura

Interactions (other drugs)
- Cyclosporine ▪ Ethanol ▪ Macrolide antibiotics ▪ NSAIDs ▪ Tacrolimus ▪ Vitamin B12

Contraindications
- Pregnancy and breast-feeding ▪ Intravenous administration of colchicine ▪ Blood dyscrasias ▪ Severe cardiac, renal, or hepatic impairment ▪ Intramuscular injections

Acceptability to patient
- Regimens of melphalan and prednisone (with or without colchicine) may be well tolerated, with modifications due to side-effects occasionally required
- Combination therapy has been shown to increase survival

- The most common side-effect is gastrointestinal (usually diarrhea) related to colchicine, which responds well to decreasing colchicine to once-daily dose administration
- 1–3% of patients experience decreased blood counts requiring modification of therapy, and two patients in one study developed infections believed to be secondary to therapy
- Follow-up blood studies are needed approximately every 3 weeks, which may negatively impact lifestyle and patient tolerance

Follow up plan

Follow-up blood studies are needed approximately every 3 weeks, which may negatively impact lifestyle and patient tolerance.

Patient and caregiver information

- Chemotherapy may improve length of survival with amyloid disease
- The term 'chemotherapy' suggests to many patients significant negative side-effects (e.g. nausea, vomiting, hair loss); however, combination prednisone, melphalan, and colchicine therapy is well tolerated, with diarrhea in a minority of patients the only symptomatic side-effect in two studies. Diarrhea was managed with reduction of colchicine dosage
- While median survival in patients with primary amyloid receiving chemotherapy was only 12–18 months, patients presenting without cardiac involvement had significantly longer survival (15% survived >5 years, a few patients >10 years)
- Late development (26–69 months after chemotherapy) of myelodysplasia and leukemia was seen in a small number of patients receiving melphalan therapy for amyloidosis (8/148), half of whom subsequently died. Overall survival rates of amyloidosis were still significantly better than in untreated patients

Other therapies
MELPHALAN THERAPY WITH BLOOD STEM CELL TRANSPLANTATION
Efficacy

Remission of blood cell dyscrasia and improvement in nephrotic syndrome has been demonstrated in patients who undergo intensive melphalan therapy combined with autologous stem cell transplantation.

Risks/Benefits

Risks:

- Treatment toxicities include renal failure, mucositis, peripheral edema, bacteremia, pulmonary edema, elevation in liver enzymes, gastrointestinal bleeding, bleeding from other sources
- Mortality is high

Acceptability to patient

Severe side-effects from chemotherapy, together with high mortality rates, may discourage patients from electing for this treatment option.

Follow up plan

Regular follow up to assess end-organ function and bone marrow function will be required.

Patient and caregiver information

- Transplant experience is limited in amyloidosis
- Chemotherapy is associated with significant side-effects and mortality
- Lifelong immunosuppression is not needed after autologous stem cell transplantation

DIALYSIS

- Of patients who are diagnosed with renal amyloid, one-third ultimately require dialysis. Median time from diagnosis to dialysis is approximately 14 months, and median survival from the start of dialysis is 8 months with death usually due to liver or cardiac involvement. There is probably no difference in survival between hemodialysis and continuous ambulatory peritoneal dialysis (CAPD) patients
- CAPD in place of hemodialysis in patients with renal failure may improve hemodialysis amyloidosis by clearing beta-2 microglobulin
- Hemodialysis is most widely used and practically any patient can be treated this way provided access to the circulation is available. This is usually via a radiocephalic arteriovenous fistula. Solute removal occurs by diffusion down a concentration gradient across a semipermeable membrane. Most patients require thrice-weekly treatment with the number of hours dependent on available technology. Synthetic membrane use may produce less amyloid disease than cellulose membranes, but this is not conclusive
- CAPD is increasingly popular worldwide. Requires self-caring patient or reliable assistant. Sterile dialysate is infused into peritoneal cavity via a catheter and left for 1–8h. Solute removal is achieved by diffusion from blood to dialysate and water removal by establishing an osmotic gradient into peritoneal cavity (usually by adding glucose to dialysate)

Efficacy
Hemodialysis and CAPD are equally efficient at solute and water removal.

Risks/Benefits
Risk: peritonitis is a major problem with CAPD.

Acceptability to patient
- Must comply with fluid and salt restrictions
- Hemodialysis requires regular hospital attendance
- CAPD is generally acceptable but requires capable patient or willing assistant at home

Follow up plan
- Principal cause of death in hemodialysis patients is cardiovascular disease; sepsis also occurs and there is an increased relative risk of neoplasia
- CAPD has a limited duration of use and few patients remain on it for more than 10 years, although in the case of amyloidosis this is probably not relevant

Patient and caregiver information
- Hemodialysis requires significant patient/caregiver participation; frequent visits for dialysis (several times per week), significant discomfort from follow-up blood tests, and maintenance of hemodialysis fistula will be required
- CAPD requires meticulous attention to aseptic technique and takes several hours per day
- Both hemodialysis and CAPD will require attention to patient diet with regard to salt and potassium restriction

LIFESTYLE
Dietary restriction of sodium, protein, and possibly potassium may be indicated in patients with cardiac or renal presentation.

RISKS/BENEFITS
Benefit: may benefit patients with edema/congestive heart failure symptomatically and reduce the requirement for diuretics.

ACCEPTABILITY TO PATIENT

Compliance with dietary restriction of sodium, in particular, can be difficult for patients because of effects on palatability of food.

FOLLOW UP PLAN

Follow-up plans will be dictated by patient presentation and severity of symptoms.

PATIENT AND CAREGIVER INFORMATION

Dietary restriction is an important part of therapy for cardiac and renal presentation in amyloid. While the actual progression of disease will be unaffected, the course of development of edema and congestive heart failure can be positively affected. Strict adherence to dietary restrictions may reduce the need for other medications, such as diuretics.

EFFICACY OF THERAPIES

- Patients with primary amyloidosis treated with chemotherapy have a longer survival than those who do not respond to therapy
- Average survival for patients with secondary AA amyloid is approximately 2 years. Resorption of amyloid may occur with successful treatment of the underlying condition, especially infective disorders. Renal transplant improves survival for those with end-stage renal failure
- Colchicine is useful in preventing attacks of serositis and synovitis in familial Mediterranean fever. It may also slow accumulation of amyloid in native kidneys or prevent deposition of amyloid in renal allograft after transplant
- Renal transplant often leads to dramatic improvement in joint symptoms in dialysis-associated amyloidosis
- Cardiac transplant is a palliative procedure

Review period

Periodic review of renal functions, liver function tests, and blood counts of patients receiving chemotherapy for amyloidosis.

PROGNOSIS

- Depends on form of amyloidosis and presence or absence of cardiac involvement
- Cause of death in most patients with primary amyloidosis is cardiac, either through congestive heart failure caused by progressive cardiomyopathy or sudden death from ventricular fibrillation or asystole
- In secondary amyloidosis, eradication of the predisposing disease slows and can occasionally reverse progression. Five- to 10-year survival after diagnosis is not uncommon
- Familial amyloidotic polyneuropathy generally has a prolonged course of 10–15 years
- Amyloidosis associated with immunocytic processes carries the worst prognosis life expectancy (<1 year)
- Progression of dialysis-associated amyloid can be improved by using newer dialysis membranes that can pass beta-2 microglobulin
- Median survival in patients with overt congestive heart failure is approximately 5 months (30 months without congestive heart failure)
- Median survival of patients with primary amyloidosis is 20.4 months with 5-year survival of 19.6%. Presence of congestive cardiac failure, raised serum creatinine level, and interstitial fibrosis on renal biopsy affect overall prognosis unfavorably. Approximately 18% of patients end up dialyzed and median survival for these patients is 8 months after dialysis

Clinical pearls

- In primary systemic amyloidosis, cardiac involvement is the leading cause of death
- Once heart failure from primary systemic amyloidosis occurs, median survival is 5 months

Therapeutic failure

- Patients with primary amyloidosis who do not respond to melphalan-based chemotherapy currently have limited alternatives. Alpha-tocopherol and interferon alpha-2 have been used but not found effective. High-dose dexamethasone with interferon has been reported effective in patients who do not have cardiac involvement
- Heart transplantation may be considered in patients with primary amyloid without extracardiac manifestations of disease and survival times of 69 and 118 months after transplant have been reported
- Intensive chemotherapy with vincristine, carmustine, melphalan, cyclophosphamide, and prednisone has been compared with melphalan and prednisone in patients with primary amyloidosis, but no survival advantage of the five-drug regimen found

- Myeloablative chemotherapy with stem-cell reconstitution has been reported, although no definite conclusions have as yet been drawn. Treatment-related mortality rates of 30–40% and a high rate of gastrointestinal toxicity are reported. This technique may be appropriate in experienced centers in carefully selected patients
- Renal transplant may be considered for end-stage renal failure due to primary amyloidosis without cardiac or liver involvement

Recurrence
May recur in transplanted kidney. Colchicine seems to be beneficial in preventing amyloid deposits in renal allografts after transplantation.

Deterioration
Patients should be referred to a specialist if clinical deterioration occurs on therapy. Alternative therapies, such as intensive chemotherapy, stem-cell transplantation, and major organ transplantation could be considered in patients who deteriorate on conventional therapy.

Terminal illness
Treatment of amyloidosis in the presence of other systemic terminal illness, or in the case of terminally progressive amyloidosis, should be aimed at palliative and symptomatic relief, such as conservative treatment of congestive heart failure, management of renal failure, and symptomatic relief of pain or dyspnea.

COMPLICATIONS
- Dialysis-associated amyloid is the most common cause of pathologic fracture in dialysis patients. Fracture of the femoral neck is the most characteristic. Primary nonunion of the fracture is common as fracture occurs across sites of amyloid deposition
- Amyloidosis is frequently associated with thrombosis of small intrarenal veins, which may subsequently propagate to involve the main renal vein
- Hypokalemic distal renal tubular acidosis reported in amyloid patients. There is an inability to decrease urinary pH below 5.3, even in the presence of severe acidemia. Plasma bicarbonate levels of less than 10mEq/L (10mmol/L) are characteristic. Clinical problems include muscle and skeletal symptoms, weakness, and even paralysis due to associated severe hypokalemia. 50% of patients with this may also suffer recurrent nephrolithiasis with calcium phosphate stones. Alkali therapy is appropriate e.g. with potassium citrate
- Bleeding: factor X deficiency is well recognized, although it occurs in less than 5% of patients
- Those with hepatic amyloidosis may suffer splenic or hepatic rupture, which is usually terminal. Cholestatic jaundice may occur as a preterminal event. Portal hypertension is seen only very occasionally. Ascites is common due to associated nephrotic syndrome rather than portal hypertension
- Steatorrhea occurs in less than 5% of patients. Intestinal pseudo-obstruction may occur, for which surgery is not beneficial. Cisapride has not been reported to be of benefit either

CONSIDER CONSULT
- The management of amyloidosis is complicated, and the majority of cases will benefit from specialist supervision
- Support from a palliative care specialist may be useful to the primary care physician in terminal cases

PREVENTION

There are no particularly useful preventive measures for either primary or secondary amyloid development, except:

- The use of a synthetic membrane in hemodialysis may reduce incidence of dialysis-associated amyloid
- Heroin abusers should avoid 'skin popping', which may lead to chronic suppurative skin infection. Amyloid deposition may reduce the incidence of disease in this population

RISK FACTORS

There is no evidence that lifestyle modification will alter the probability of developing amyloidosis.

PREVENT RECURRENCE

- Chronic, usually unremitting, disease
- Amyloid deposition may occur in a renal allograft after transplant and colchicine may help to prevent this

Reassess coexisting disease

Treatment of coexisting disease, especially if it contributes to secondary amyloidosis, should continue.

ASSOCIATIONS

National Kidney Foundation
30 East 33rd Street, Suite 1100
New York, NY 10016
Tel: (800) 622-9010 or (212) 889-2210
Fax: (212) 689-9261
E-mail: info@kidney.org
www.kidney.org

KEY REFERENCES

- Gertz M, Lacy M, Dispenzieri A. Monoclonal gammopathies and related disorders: amyloidosis. Hematol Oncol Clin North Am 1999;13:1211–33, ix
- Tomson CRV, Plant WD. Key topics in renal medicine. Oxford: BIOS Scientific Publishers, 1997
- Melphalan and prednisone were more effective than colchicine for primary amyloidosis. ACP J Club 1997;127:71
- Dubrey S, Burke M, Khaghani A, et al. Long term results of heart transplantation in patients with amyloid heart disease. Heart 2001;85:202–7 http://heart.bmjjournals.com/cgi/content/abstract/85/2/202
- Tan S, Pepys M, Hawkins P. Treatment of amyloidosis. Am J Kidney Dis 1995;26;267–85
- Keren DF, Alexanian R, Goeken JA, et al. Guidelines for clinical and laboratory evaluation of patients with monoclonal gammopathies. Arch Pathol Lab Med 1999;123:106–7. Available online: http://www.guidelines.gov/FRAMESETS/guideline_fs.asp?guideline=001186&sSearch_string=amyloidosis
- Kyle R, Gertz MA, Greipp PR, et al. A trial of three regimens for primary amyloidosis: colchicine alone, melphalan and prednisone, and melphalan, prednisone, and colchicine. N Engl J Med 1997;336:1202–7
- Skinner M, Anderson J, Simms R, et al. Treatment of 100 patients with primary amyloidosis: a randomized trial of melphalan, prednisone, and colchicine, versus colchicine only. Am J Med 1996;100:290–8
- Isoniemi H, Kyllonen L, Ahonen J, et al. Improved outcome of renal transplantation in amyloidosis. Transpl Int 1994;7(Suppl)1:S298–300
- Kyle RA, Greipp RP. Amyloidosis. Mayo Clin Proc 1983;58;665–83

FAQS

Question 1

What is the duration of therapy necessary with melphalan and prednisone with or without colchicine?

ANSWER 1

Duration of therapy has not been established, but patients underwent 2 years of therapy in one study and were treated with a total of 600mg of melphalan in another (depending on patient weight, this appears to have been 1–1.5 years).

Question 2
What is the leading cause of death in primary systemic amyloidosis?

ANSWER 2
Cardiac involvement.

Question 3
What is the primary diagnostic modality in assessing for suspected cardiac amyloid?

ANSWER 3
Echocardiogram.

Question 4
How do we detect renal involvement in amyloidosis?

ANSWER 4
By checking the urine for protein by a simple dipstick method and or by checking the serum creatinine in every patient.

Question 5
Can these patients undergo renal transplantation and what are the chances of recurrence?

ANSWER 5
These patients can undergo transplant provided there is no evidence of cardiac failure. The chances of recurrence are as high as 20–23% but graft loss is uncommon.

CONTRIBUTORS
Fred F Ferri, MD, FACP
Kara J Quan, MD
Gail A van Norman, MD
Diego A Rielo, MD
Ankush Gulati, MD

BALANITIS AND BALANOPOSTHITIS

DESCRIPTION

- Inflammation of the glans penis (balanitis) and foreskin (balanoposthitis)
- Balanoposthitis occurs in uncircumcised men only
- Tends to be relapsing and recurring
- Affects all ages

URGENT ACTION

If paraphimosis complicates balanoposthitis, urgent surgical treatment by dorsal slit or circumcision may be required.

KEY! DON'T MISS!

Assess patency of urinary meatus and vascular supply to the glans. If either is significantly compromised urgent surgical referral is needed.

ICD9 CODE
112.2 Balanitis

CARDINAL FEATURES
- Inflammation of the foreskin and glans penis
- Balanoposthitis occurs in uncircumcised men only
- Tends to be relapsing and recurring
- Affects all ages
- Characterized by redness of glans, local edema, discharge, pain
- May cause difficulty with urination

CAUSES
Common causes
The cause is often not ascertained, but common causes include:
- Candida infection
- Bacterial infection
- Intertrigo
- Irritant dermatitis
- Maceration injury
- Postcoital hypersensitivity
- Trauma
- Allergy
- Reiter's syndrome
- Associated with sexually transmitted diseases (gonorrhea, trichomoniasis, chlamydia, mycoplasma, and nonspecific urethritis)
- Irritation by smegma, urine, and alkalis
- Poor hygiene

Rare causes
- Secondary syphilis (NB primary chancre not a recognized cause of balanitis)
- Balanitis xerotica obliterans (localized form of lichen sclerosis)
- Anaerobic infection such as with Vincent's organisms (causing tissue destruction)

Serious causes
- Syphilis (may cause local tissue destruction and systemic illness)
- Balanitis xerotica obliterans (if untreated leads to obliteration of subprepucial space and scarring of the meatus)
- Anaerobic infection such as with Vincent's organisms (causing tissue destruction)

Contributory or predisposing factors
- Presence of a foreskin (especially if large and redundant)
- Tight foreskin (prepuce)
- Poor genital hygiene
- Sexual contact (with or without infection)
- Recent antibiotic treatment
- Coexisting debilitating or chronic disease (anemia and diabetes mellitus, HIV/AIDS, etc.)
- Coexisting malignancy (other than carcinoma of the penis) causing generalized debility

EPIDEMIOLOGY
Incidence and prevalence
This is a common, often subclinical condition, the exact incidence and prevalence of which are not known.

Demographics
AGE
- Variable – occurs in all ages
- Balanitis xerotica obliterans is more common in older men

GENDER
Males only.

RACE
All races affected.

GENETICS
No genetic factors.

GEOGRAPHY
Worldwide.

SOCIOECONOMIC STATUS
- Poor hygiene due to ignorance and social deprivation may exacerbate the condition
- Crowded living may contribute to spread of infective causes

DIFFERENTIAL DIAGNOSIS
Psoriasis
Chronic skin disorder characterized by excessive proliferation of keratinocytes resulting in the formation of thick scaly plaques and localized inflammation.

FEATURES
- Very common (1%–3% of world population)
- Positive family history (association with HLA types B13, B17, and B27)
- Sharply demarcated silver-scaled patches
- Tends to develop on extensor surfaces, but flexural variant favors skin creases including the coronal sulcus
- Often exacerbated by stress
- Pruritus is variable but uncommon
- Multiple drop-like lesions in guttate psoriasis (preceded by streptococcal pharyngitis)

Lichen planus
Chronic idiopathic skin disorder characterized by violaceous papular rash that can coalesce into scaling plaques.

FEATURES
- Fairly common
- No family history
- Shiny surface interrupted by white streaks (Wickham's striae)
- Pruritus is common

Balanitis xerotica obliterans
Slowly progressive localized genital form of lichen sclerosus et atrophicus, producing non-ulcerative atrophy of skin and mucous membranes of unknown etiology.

FEATURES
- Affects all ages but commoner in older men
- May affect glans, prepuce, and terminal urethra
- Skin atrophy and depigmentation (white patches)
- Later forms scars and contractures
- May cause obliteration of prepucial space and phimosis
- May lead to meatal obstruction and affect urinary flow
- Clinical diagnosis requires biopsy to confirm

Bowen's disease
Premalignant skin condition that occurs on the penis in a rare variant called erythroplasia of Queyrat.

FEATURES
- Rare
- Non-invasive on the penis
- Characteristic velvety plaques
- Very rarely can progress to squamous cell carcinoma
- Diagnosis confirmed by biopsy

Reiter's syndrome
Seronegative spondyloarthropathy associated with urethritis (and/or cervicitis, dysentery, inflammatory eye disease, and mucocutaneous lesions).

FEATURES
- Circinate balanitis
- Arthritis is present by definition
- May occur after dysentery
- Genetic susceptibility (HLA B27)
- Clinical syndrome with no diagnostic test

Fixed drug reactions
Rare idiopathic consequence of use of various therapeutic and diagnostic drugs, including allopurinol, barbiturates, chlordiazepoxide, NSAIDs (naproxen, phenacetin, phenylbutazone, salicylates, sulindac, tolmetin), phenolphthalein, sulfonamides, and tetracycline.

FEATURES
- Rare
- Well-defined erythematous plaques, may be multiple
- Crusting, scaling, and pigmentation may occur as lesions heal
- Exacerbations at same site occur with repeat use of causative drug

Secondary syphilis
Localized or diffuse mucocutaneous lesions with generalized lymphadenopathy occuring in cases where primary syphilis is untreated.

FEATURES
- Occurs usually 4–6 weeks after primary chancre
- Rashes are usually multifocal
- Spontaneous resolution occurs in 1 week to 12 months

Squamous cell carcinoma
Squamous cell carcinoma is a malignant tumor of the skin arising in the epithelium.

FEATURES
- Occurs on the penis (about 1% of all male malignancies in USA)
- Circumcision confers almost total protection against squamous cell carcinoma
- Preceding phimosis, balanoposthitis, and sexually transmitted diseases all may predispose to squamous cell carcinoma
- Primary lesion may have scaly erythematous macule or plaque

Leukoplakia
Rare premalignant condition resembling leukoplakia of the oral mucosa.

FEATURES
- Usually preceded by chronic or recurring balanoposthitis
- Lesions are discrete white or bluish-white flat papules
- Erosions and ulcers with adhesions may occur
- Intense pruritus is common
- Diagnosis is confirmed by biopsy

SIGNS & SYMPTOMS
Signs
Local genital signs:
- Redness
- Local edema
- Exudate
- Urethral discharge
- Rarely, ulceration
- Swelling of prepuce
- Scarring between glans and prepuce causing phimosis

Regional signs:
- Regional lymph node enlargement
- Rarely, palpable bladder

Symptoms
Acute symptoms:
- Pain and tenderness
- Itching
- Pain on urination
- Inability to urinate

Chronic symptoms:
- Changed appearance
- Scarring with or without palpable nodule

ASSOCIATED DISORDERS
- Urethritis (feature of sexually transmitted diseases)
- Diabetes (may predispose to infection including causative organisms of balanoposthitis)

KEY! DON'T MISS!
Assess patency of urinary meatus and vascular supply to the glans. If either is significantly compromised urgent surgical referral is needed.

CONSIDER CONSULT
- Signs of dysplasia or carcinoma
- Suspected sexually transmitted disease
- Associated diabetes or debilitating disease
- Complications at presentation such as retention and meatal stricture
- When paraphimosis is present and cannot be reduced by primary care physician

INVESTIGATION OF THE PATIENT
Direct questions to patient
Q Are you circumcised? Excludes balanoposthitis as diagnosis and makes carcinoma very unlikely.

Q Do you regularly clean your penis and foreskin? Lessens likelihood of infective cause, and increases possibility of irritant cause.

Q Are you sexually active? Tell me about your contacts. Postcoital sensitivity and infection are possible causes of balanitis.

Q Have you ever had a sexually transmitted disease?

Q Do you have any history or family history of skin disease? May alert to psoriasis.

Q Do you have any history of joint problems? May suggest diagnosis of Reiter's syndrome.

Q Has there been recent diarrhea? Suggestive of Reiter's syndrome.

Q Do you use condoms, bath additives, etc.? Alerts to allergy and hypersensitivity reactions.

Q Can you think of any other irritants that could be involved? Detergents used on underwear, unguents used in sexual play, etc.

Q What medications have you used, both prescribed and over-the-counter? Many constituents of common creams may cause skin reactions and other drugs cause possible fixed drug reactions.

Contributory or predisposing factors

Q Do you have a tight or nonretractable foreskin? This tends to trap urine and smegma, leading to infection.

Q Are you sexually active? Trauma, infection, and postcoital sensitivity can lead to balanitis.

Q Do you have any underlying disease such as diabetes, HIV, or malignancy? Debilitation makes infection more likely to occur.

Q Any past or current history of sexually transmitted disease?

Q Any recent diarrhea or arthritis? May suggest Reiter's syndrome.

Q Are you sensitive to soaps, etc.? Allergic individuals may produce local skin reactions.

Q Do you have allergic reactions to condoms or any medications? Allergic individuals may produce local skin reactions, and fixed drug reactions often affect genital areas.

Q Do you have a urinary catheter? Infections are associated.

Q Have you had any trauma to the genitals? Suggests mechanical cause of local symptoms.

Family history

Q Do you have anyone in your family with:

- Psoriasis? Association with HLA types B13, B17, and B27
- Diabetes? Positive family history alerts to possibility of new diagnosis presenting as balanitis

Examination

General examination:

- Are there signs of systemic disease including anemia, skin disease, or signs of debilitating disease? Keratoderma blenorrhagica in Reiter's syndrome
- Is eye inflammation, mouth lesions, or joint signs present? May be present in Reiter's syndrome
- Is there any local or general lymphadenopathy? Indicates infection locally or debilitating disease

Specific examination of the genital area:

- Is there redness of the glans and foreskin (prepuce)?
- Is there local edema of the prepuce (and the glans in some cases)? Occurs in acute phimosis and paraphimosis
- Is any exudate present? Suggests sexually transmitted disease
- Is there any obvious urethral discharge? Suggests sexually transmitted disease
- Is there any ulceration? Rare sign of more serious disease
- Is there scarring between glans and prepuce causing phimosis? Indicates condition is chronic or recurring

Summary of investigative tests

Tests to identify infective causes where present:

- Microscopy of discharge (wet mount preparation), can give quick evidence of infection with *Treponema pallidum, Trichomonas vaginalis,* or Vincent's organisms
- Microscopy of Gram stain smear, used to identify *Neisseria gonorrhea* or *Candida albicans* infection
- Microbial culture (fungal, bacterial, and viral), used to identify infective organism(s) and likely best choice of antibiotic treatment

Tests to identify any underlying disease:

- Random serum glucose, to exclude diabetes
- Treponeme-specific serology for syphilis
- Chlamydia serology
- Biopsy (normally performed by a specialist)

DIAGNOSTIC DECISION

Likely cause depends on age and sexual activity:

- Nonsexually active boys tend to have minor self-limiting infections only
- Sexually active men are at risk of sexually transmitted diseases, other infections (e.g. candida), trauma, and allergy
- Older men are at risk of dysplastic and neoplastic disease, especially if uncircumcised
- Diagnostic decision is based on results of tests for infection and (if relevant) tests for underlying disease

CLINICAL PEARLS

- Balanitis is an acute or chronic inflammation of the glans penis
- Posthitis refers to an inflammation of the mucous surface of the prepuce
- Balanoposthitis refers to an inflammation of the penile skin

Fusospiral organisms are normally abundant in the foreskin of the prepuce and are described as normally saprophytic. However, under conditions of lowered local or general resistance, these organisms can become pathogenic.

There are different types of balanoposthitis [1]

- Circinate erosive balanitis: a short-lived mucosal form of Reiter's disease. It manifests as a circinate edge that extends on to the edge of the glans and prepuce
- Acute infectious balanitis: manifests as erythema of the glans, coronal sulcus, and preputial surface. The erythema and edema can cause phimosis
- Candidal balanitis: caused by *Candida albicans*
- Trichomonal balanitis: seen in young men who may have associated urethritis. The redundant foreskin predisposes to this condition. It manifests as a superficial or erosive balanitis. Responds to metronidazole
- Amebic balanitis: caused by *Entamoeba histolytica*. Circumcision is curative
- Mycoplasmal balanitis: may be accompanied by lesions on the penis. Swabs from the lesions should be carbon typed to avoid inhibition. Tetracycline is the treatment of choice
- Micaceous and pseudoepitheliomatous balanitis: starts as a coronal balanitis, which changes appearance, with micaceous crusts and horny masses appearing on the glans. The glans appears atrophic and there is loss of elasticity of the preputial skin. Histologically, we see striking hyperkeratosis and pseudoepitheliomatous hyperplasia as well as acanthosis. It is thought that this condition arises as a response to infection. Circumcision is not effective. Topical cytotoxic agents have been used to treat this
- Syphilitic balanitis: caused by *Treponema pallidum*
- Chlamydial balanitis: caused by *Chlamydia trachomatis*, specifically the D through K serotypes. Tetracycline is the treatment of choice
- Plasma cell balanitis: also known as Zoon's balanitis and pseudoerythroplasic balanitis. Presents in middle aged and elderly men with a well-circumscribed plaque on the glans penis that is shiny and smooth on the surface. The surface is slightly moist and stippled with minute red specks – the 'cayenne pepper' spots. Diagnosis is confirmed with biopsy
- Erythroplasia of Queyrat or Bowen's disease of the glans penis
- Balanitis xerotica obliterans

THE TESTS
Body fluids
MICROSCOPY OF DISCHARGE
Description
- Specimen obtained from discharge or exudate of terminal urethra or glans (may require irrigation under foreskin) suspended in saline
- Placed on clean glass microscope slide
- Mixed with a drop of 10% potassium hydroxide
- Covered with coverslip
- Gently heated to fix
- Examined under light microscope in bright field

Advantages/Disadvantages
Advantages:
- Quick
- Inexpensive
- Non-invasive
- Can be performed in physician's office
- Result available immediately

Disadvantages:
- Messy and fiddly
- Variable patient acceptability (intimate samples)
- Depends upon microscopy skills of doctor
- May be inconclusive
- Risk of nosocomial infection (gloves should be worn)
- Consider need for chaperone

Normal
No abnormal microorganisms seen.

Abnormal
- Presence of microorganisms (e.g. elongated spiral spirochetes)
- May be difficult to identify which organism on this test
- Keep in mind the possibility of a falsely abnormal result

Cause of abnormal result
Presence of specific bacteria:
- *Treponema pallidum*
- Vincent's organisms
- *Trichomonas vaginalis*

Drugs, disorders and other factors that may alter results
- Specific or coincidental treatment with antibiotics may alter numbers of microorganisms seen
- Poorly taken and prepared specimen may yield falsely low numbers of microorganisms
- Lack of microscopy skills in examining physician

MICROSCOPY OF GRAM STAIN SMEAR
Description
- Specimen obtained from urethral swab
- Smeared on glass slide
- Fixed by gentle heating
- Stained by Gram's method
- Examined under light microscope

Advantages/Disadvantages
Advantages:
- Quick
- Inexpensive
- Non-invasive
- Can be performed in physician's office
- Result available rapidly

Disadvantages:
- Messy and fiddly
- Variable patient acceptability (intimate samples)
- Depends upon microscopy skills of physician
- Difficult to perform Gram stain outside laboratory
- May be inconclusive
- Risk of nosocomial infection (gloves should be worn)
- Consider need for chaperone

Normal
No abnormal microorganisms seen.

Abnormal
- Presence of microorganisms
- Gram-negative diplococci (*Neisseria gonorrhea*)
- Keep in mind the possiblity of a falsely abnormal result

Cause of abnormal result
Gonococcal infection.

Drugs, disorders and other factors that may alter results
- Specific or coincidental treatment with antibiotics may alter numbers of microorganisms seen
- Poorly taken and prepared specimen may yield falsely low numbers of microorganisms
- Lack of microscopy skills in examining physician

MICROBIAL CULTURE
Description
- Most physicians will take samples for culture and arrange their processing at a suitable laboratory
- Specimens for culture are taken using moist cotton swabs, gently rubbed on the sample area and placed immediately in a suitable transport medium (e.g. Stuart's medium)

Advantages/Disadvantages
Advantages:
- Quick to take sample
- Inexpensive
- Relatively non-invasive
- Can be performed in physician's office
- Aids definitive therapeutic choice

Disadvantages:
- Messy and fiddly
- Technique consistency important
- Delay between sampling and result from laboratory
- Transport time (delays may impair result)
- Variable patient acceptability (intimate samples)

- May be inconclusive
- Risk of nosocomial infection (gloves should be worn)
- Consider need for chaperone

Normal
No microorganisms grown.

Abnormal
- Pathological microorganisms identified, plus antibiotic sensitivities
- Keep in mind the possibility of a falsely abnormal result

Cause of abnormal result
Infection by pathogenic microorganisms (e.g. *Neisseria gonorrhea*, *Candida albicans*).

Drugs, disorders and other factors that may alter results
- Specific or coincidental treatment with antibiotics may alter numbers of microorganisms seen
- Poorly taken and prepared specimen may yield falsely low numbers of microorganisms
- Technical problems in the laboratory

RANDOM SERUM GLUCOSE
Description
Standard venous blood sample taken at random time and processed in laboratory.

Advantages/Disadvantages
Advantages:
- Quick and simple
- Easy to interpret
- Not dependent on fasting state

Disadvantages:
- Requires venipuncture (invasive)
- Laboratory turnaround variable

Normal
Less than 140mg/dl (7.8mmol/l).

Abnormal
- Greater than 140mg/dl (7.8mmol/l)
- Keep in mind the possibility of a falsely abnormal result

Cause of abnormal result
Impaired glucose tolerance.

Drugs, disorders and other factors that may alter results
- Diabetes mellitus
- Stress
- Infections
- Cushing's syndrome
- Acromegaly
- Glucagonoma
- Hemochromatosis
- Drugs (glucocorticoids and diuretics)

SYPHILIS SEROLOGY

Description
- Standard venous blood sample processed in laboratory
- The most useful test is a treponeme specific antibody test such as TPHA (*T. pallidum* hemagglutination) or FTA/ABS (fluorescent treponemal antibody), but none have high diagnostic specificity

Advantages/Disadvantages
Advantages:
- Quick and simple
- Easy to interpret
- Not dependent on fasting state

Disadvantages:
- Requires venesection (invasive)
- Laboratory turnaround variable

Normal
Negative antibody test, but false negatives do occur.

Abnormal
- Positive antibody test
- Keep in mind the possibility of a falsely abnormal result

Cause of abnormal result
Current or recent/treated syphilis.

Drugs, disorders and other factors that may alter results
False positive results occur in:
- Lyme disease
- Autoimmune disease, including systemic lupus erythematosus
- Collagen vascular diseases

NONCULTURE TESTS FOR CHLAMYDIA TRACHOMATIS

Description
- Direct culture tests for *Chlamydia trachomatis* are expensive and technically highly demanding (specialized training and laboratory techniques required) and are, therefore, not recommended for PCPs
- Nonculture tests are a more practical alternative for PCPs, although they are limited by lower specificity, often giving false positives. It is necessary to refer patients with positive results for confirmatory *Chlamydia* culture tests, ideally to a genitourinary clinic with specialized laboratory facilities
- Several commercial tests exist (for example MicroTrak Registered DFA [Syva] and Chlamydiazyme Registered EIA [Abbott] test), and their instructions for specimen collection should be followed. In addition, there are simple qualitative rapid test kits available for use in physicians' offices, etc. In each case the sample required in male patients is a urethral swab

Advantages/Disadvantages
Advantages:
- Rapid results (in the office in the case of Rapid Chlamydia Test kits)
- Ease of use
- Usually acceptable to patient

Disadvantages:
- False-positive result necessitates further testing
- Nosocomial infection is possible; precautions must be observed when taking specimens

TREATMENT

CONSIDER CONSULT
- Recurrent episodes for consideration of circumcision
- When anaerobic infection has been demonstrated
- When disease is refractory to treatment

IMMEDIATE ACTION
- Refer if an anaerobic infection is suspected
- If severe phimosis with an inability to void, may require prompt slit drainage
- Refer for biopsy if lesions are not healing (to rule out malignancy)

PATIENT AND CAREGIVER ISSUES
Patient or caregiver request
- Do I have a sexually transmitted disease?
- Am I infectious?
- Is there any thing that I could have done to prevent it occurring?
- Will it recur?
- Will it impair sexual function?
- Will I need circumcision?

Health-seeking behavior
- Have you tried to self medicate, or tried alternative therapies? Allergic individuals may produce local skin reactions
- Have you tried to self clean the area? Trauma from scrubs, etc.

MANAGEMENT ISSUES
Goals
- Relieve symptoms
- Treat underlying disorder
- Educate on genital hygiene
- Prevent recurrence

Management in special circumstances
- Diabetics may need evaluation of their disease control or referral if a new diagnosis
- Young boys need reassurance and hygiene measures usually suffice
- Scarring as a consequence of recurrent attacks may impair sexual function or ability to void, and may require referral for circumcision

COEXISTING DISEASE
- Underlying disease such as diabetes or malignancy will need appropriate treatment, but balanitis management should be started concurrently
- Good control of diabetes can reduce the frequency of candidal or bacterial infection in a diabetic patient
- Balanitis may be the presenting symptom of diabetes especially in the elderly patient

COEXISTING MEDICATION
Very unlikely to have any impact on management choices.

SPECIAL PATIENT GROUPS
- Young boys will often need nothing more than reassurance and good advice on retraction of the foreskin and hygiene, and encouragement to maintain good fluid intake
- Patients with catheters have a special need for scrupulous catheter and penile hygiene, preferably as close to aseptic technique as possible

PATIENT SATISFACTION/LIFESTYLE PRIORITIES
Patients with disability or extreme age may require nursing assistance to ensure that adequate topical treatment and hygiene for balanitis is carried out.

SUMMARY OF THERAPEUTIC OPTIONS
Choices
In addition to the following therapies, all patients should be encouraged to adopt certain lifestyle measures.

Drug treatment is chosen according to etiology:
- **Candidal infection:** first choice is a broad spectrum topical antifungal such as 1% clotrimazole cream
- **Bacterial infection:** first choice is a topical antibacterial such as Bacitracin or Neosporin ointment
- **Bacterial infection:** second choice (in more severes cases) is a systemic antibiotic such as oral cephalexin that may be needed in addition to topical therapy
- **Dermatitis:** first choice is topical weak steroid 1% hydrocortisone
- **Dermatitis:** second choice is topical steroid in conjunction with other antifungal or antibacterial treatments if dermatitis severe

Nondrug treatments:
- Dorsal slit drainage may be used to relieve severe phimosis or irreducible paraphimosis, which may complicate balanoposthitis (usually performed by a specialist)
- Circumcision may relieve recurrent episodes of balanitis
- Castellani's paint can be used as a drying agent although its effectiveness may only be marginal

Clinical pearls
- When faced with an individual with balanitis, treat first with local therapies (improved hygiene, etc.) and topical remedies if applicable
- More serious presentations in which there may be secondary bacterial/fungal infection are treated with a combination of topical, local, and oral antibiotics/oral antifungal agents
- In these two presentations, the patient and the practitioner should work together to develop a short-term treatment plan to address the acute flare up, and a long-term plan to keep the problem from recurring
- If the patient can avoid a circumcision and live comfortably, they will opt for and follow the more conservative plan. When there is compromise to urination, increasing pain, and loss of function, surgical intervention is required

Never
Never initiate topical steroids alone unless infection has been ruled out.

FOLLOW UP
- Review within 5 days and plan further review as appropriate
- Sexually transmitted diseases will require prolonged follow-up usually under a specialist

Plan for review
- Check response to treatment; patient to call if no better in 1 day or if worsening
- Check compliance with hygiene advice
- Look for complications such as scarring

Information for patient or caregiver
- Self-help measures – most important is meticulous genital hygiene
- Recurrence is always possible and should be promptly reported

DRUGS AND OTHER THERAPIES: DETAILS
Drugs
TOPICAL ANTIFUNGALS
For example, clotrimazole cream 1% over-the-counter.

Dose
Apply 1cm squeezed length, twice daily to affected area.

Efficacy
Treats *Candida albicans*, but requires up to a 2-week course to eliminate risk of immediate recurrence.

Risks/Benefits
Risks:
- Occasional allergic reaction to cream
- Recurrence if full course not completed
- Risk of affecting the reliability of latex contraceptives

Benefits:
- Good results
- Straightforward treatment

Side-effects and adverse reactions
- Gastrointestinal: nausea, abdominal pain (oral administration)
- Skin: burning, rash, urticaria, stinging
- Genitourinary: dyspareunia, urinary frequency

Interactions (other drugs)
No known interactions with topical clotrimazole

Contraindications
Previous allergic reaction to the cream

Acceptability to patient
Usually very acceptable unless the patient has difficulty in using a cream.

Follow up plan
Review after the end of the course to check that there is no recurrence.

Patient and caregiver information
- Completion of the course is vital for success
- Sexual partner may need treatment too in order to prevent reinfection
- Treatment can interact with latex condoms

TOPICAL ANTIBACTERIALS
For example, Bacitracin or Neosporin ointment, which are available as combinations with other antibiotics. (Some preparations are available over-the-counter.)

Dose
Apply 1cm squeezed length, four times daily to the affected part.

Efficacy
Usually good antibacterial cover for likely causative organisms.

Risks/Benefits

Risks:

- Occasional allergic reaction to cream
- Recurrence if full course not completed
- Use caution in cutaneous tuberculosis
- Systemic absorption can occur if applied to denuded skin

Benefits:

- Good results
- Straightforward treatment
- Easy to apply

Side-effects and adverse reactions

Systemic side-effects:

- Gastrointestinal: nausea, vomiting, diarrhea
- Eyes, ears, nose and throat: poor corneal wound healing, visual disturbances
- Skin: rashes
- Genitourinary: tubular and glomerular necrosis leading to renal failure

Interactions (other drugs)

Systemic:

- Aminoglycosides ▪ Amphotericin B ▪ Cisplatin ▪ Cyclosporine ▪ Foscarnet ▪ Loop diuretics ▪ Pentamidine ▪ Tacrolimus ▪ Vancomycin

Contraindications

- Fungal or viral infections ▪ Aminoglycoside hypersensitivity ▪ Neomycin hypersensitivity ▪ Severe renal disease ▪ Ocular application

Acceptability to patient

Usually very acceptable unless the patient has difficulty in using a cream.

Follow up plan

Review after the end of course to check that there is no recurrence.

Patient and caregiver information

- Completion of the course is vital for success
- Sexual partner may need treatment too in order to prevent reinfection

SYSTEMIC ANTIBIOTICS

Cephalexin orally.

Dose

250–500mg orally every 6 hours.

Efficacy

Good broad spectrum antibiotic for likely pathogens.

Risks/Benefits

Risks:

- Hypersensitivity: approximately 10% of penicillin-sensitive patients will be allergic to cephalosporins
- Use caution in renal impairment
- Use caution in history of gastrointestinal disease

Benefit: rapid simple course of treatment

Side-effects and adverse reactions
- Gastrointestinal: anorexia, nausea, diarrhea, abdominal pain, vomiting
- Central nervous system: headache, sleep disturbance, confusion, dizziness
- Hematologic: blood cell disorders
- Skin: rashes, erythema multiforme, pruritus
- Genitourinary: nephrotoxicity
- Anaphylaxis

Interactions (other drugs)
- Vancomycin ■ Aminoglycosides ■ Loop diuretics ■ Probenecid ■ Polymixin B ■ Warfarin
- Penicillins

Contraindications
- Cephalosporin hypersensitivity ■ Porphyria ■ Infants less than 1 month old

Acceptability to patient
Generally acceptable, although some patients may be reluctant to take antibiotics for various reasons.

Follow up plan
Review after the end of course to check that there is no recurrence.

Patient and caregiver information
- Complete the prescribed course
- Report any possible reactions immediately
- Warn of common side-effects such as diarrhea
- Take cephalexin on an empty stomach

TOPICAL CORTICOSTEROIDS
For example, hydrocortisone 1% cream or ointment over-the-counter.

Dose
- Apply 1cm squeezed length, twice daily (may be increased to four times)
- Not recommended for use in excess of 2 weeks (as cutaneous side-effects can occur)
- Recommended amount for an adult per week is 15–30g for treatment of groin and genital area

Efficacy
Good, with symptomatic relief and as an anti-inflammatory agent.

Risks/Benefits
Risks:
- Flare up of infection may be precipitated
- Skin atrophy with prolonged use
- Hypersensitivity to other cream components leading to contact dermatitis
- Systemic absorption may reach significant levels in prolonged or extensive use, leading to adrenal suppression
- Exacerbation of local infection, especially viral
- Rebound flare up of dermatitis following withdrawal after prolonged use
- Use caution in elderly due to risk of diabetes and osteoporosis
- Use caution in patients with psychosis, seizure disorders, or myasthenia gravis
- Use caution in congestive heart failure, hypertension
- Use caution in ulcerative colitis, peptic ulcer, or esophagitis

Benefit: relieves allergic dermatitis quickly

Side-effects and adverse reactions
In mild steroid preparation use it is rare to see systemic effects.

Systemic side-effects:
- Gastrointestinal: dyspepsia, peptic ulceration, esophagitis, oral candidiasis, nausea, vomiting
- Cardiovascular system: hypertension, thromboembolism
- Central nervous system: insomnia, euphoria, depression, psychosis, seizures
- Endocrine: adrenal suppression, impaired glucose tolerance, growth suppression in children
- Musculoskeletal: proximal myopathy, osteoporosis
- Skin: delayed healing, acne, striae
- Eyes, ears, nose and throat: cataract, glaucoma, blurred vision

Interactions (other drugs)
No known interactions for topical hydrocortisone

Contraindications
- Untreated fungal or bacterial infection ▪ Continuous prophylactic use ▪ Use in childhood needs rigorous control ▪ Previous sensitivity to drug

Acceptability to patient
- Usually very acceptable as good response
- Some patients reluctant to use any steroid (bad publicity)

Follow up plan
Review after 2–3 weeks to exclude rebound post-treatment flare up.

Patient and caregiver information
- Do not continue medication after prescribed course
- Do not allow anyone else to use your medication
- Make sure hands are clean before applying cream, and washed afterwards
- Creams can stain clothing

Surgical therapy
- Dorsal slit may be needed in an emergency for paraphimosis
- Circumcision may be advisable in recurrent or sclerotic disease
- It is to be performed only by qualified, well trained individuals. It is a reason for specialist referral

DORSAL SLIT DRAINAGE
- This is an emergency surgical procedure to relieve severe phimosis or irreducible paraphimosis, which may complicate balanoposthitis
- It may be performed under local or general anesthesia

Efficacy
Confers immediate relief of pain and constriction of urinary flow and blood flow to the glans.

Risks/Benefits
Risks:
- Uncontrolled bleeding
- Postoperative infection
- Noncosmetic result with scarring
- Adverse reaction to anesthesia

Benefits:
- Immediate pain relief
- Rapid reduction of threat to vascular supply to glans

Acceptability to patient

While dorsal slit drainage produces relief of acute pain due to paraphimosis, it leaves an unsightly end result that most patients will want corrected by an elective circumcision at a later date.

Follow up plan

- Normal surgical follow-up to confirm healing should be after 2–3 weeks
- Consideration should be given to elective circumcision

Patient and caregiver information

Patient must be advised that dorsal slit is an emergency procedure and does not leave a good cosmetic result.

CIRCUMCISION

- This surgical procedure may be performed electively to relieve established phimosis or recurrent episodes of balanitis
- It may also be performed as an emergency in skilled hands to relieve paraphimosis
- It may be performed under local or general anesthesia

Efficacy

- Circumcision cures phimosis and markedly reduces the chance of future balanitis
- Further episodes of balanoposthitis are eliminated
- The risk of penile carcinoma is reduced to near zero

Risks/Benefits

Risks:

- Uncontrolled bleeding
- Postoperative infection
- Unsightly result and scarring
- Adverse reaction to anesthesia

Benefits:

- Cures phimosis and recurrent balanoposthitis
- Reduces the chance of future balanitis
- Risk of penile carcinoma is reduced to near zero

Acceptability to patient

Patients may need to be reassured that sexual potency and fertility remain unaffected by circumcision.

Follow up plan

Normal surgical follow-up to confirm healing should be after 2–3 weeks.

Patient and caregiver information

- Careful postoperative wound care is necessary to avoid infection and unsightly scarring
- Patients should be warned the glans will be very sensitive for several days but will gradually settle to an acceptable level

Other therapies
CASTELLANI'S PAINT
This is a drying agent, which may be applied under the foreskin.

Efficacy
Probably only of marginal benefit.

Risks/Benefits
Risks:
- Possible hypersensitivity
- Failure to improve balanoposthitis

Benefit: Aids speed of resolution of balanoposthitis

Acceptability to patient
The manual dexterity required may preclude some patients using this method.

Follow up plan
Review in the physician's office after 1–2 weeks is desirable.

Patient and caregiver information
The use of the Castellani's paint does not obviate the need for good hygiene.

LIFESTYLE
- Regular retraction of the foreskin to help glans and keep prepuce dry
- Meticulous hygiene in Sitz baths encourages resolution of balanoposthitis and minimizes recurrence
- Strict glycemic control in diabetics reduces the chances of further infection and encourages healing

RISKS/BENEFITS
Risks:
- Overzealous washing, etc. can traumatize the glans and in itself predispose to infection
- Hypersensitivity may occur with washing agents

Benefits:
- Better hygiene improves personal confidence
- Improved diet and glycemic control enhances diabetic lifestyle and prevents other complications

ACCEPTABILITY TO PATIENT
Compliance good if wash facilities allow.

FOLLOW UP PLAN
- Reassurance especially important in boys, therefore, review is beneficial
- Follow up is optional and may be on an 'open door' basis

EFFICACY OF THERAPIES

In young boys it usually resolves in 3–5 days with hygiene advice only and no other treatment.

In men response varies according to cause:
- Simple bacterial and candidal infection resolve quickly with appropriate treatment
- Treatment of underlying sexually transmitted disease and Reiter's syndrome is more prolonged and, therefore, response is more dictated by compliance

Review period
- For simple balanitis and balanoposthitis, follow up in 1–2 weeks (if necessary)
- Balanitis other than that caused by local infection will need more prolonged follow-up
- Balanitis caused by sexually transmitted disease will need careful follow-up and possible contact tracing
- If a sexually transmitted disease is found it may need to be reported to the local health department

PROGNOSIS
- Simple balanoposthitis resolves completely with no after-effects
- The condition is often recurrent and relapsing
- Some types require circumcision to enable resolution and prevent recurrence

Therapeutic failure
- Re-evaluate possibility of underlying disease
- Referral to a specialist urologist recommended

Recurrence
Referral recommended for consideration of circumcision.

Deterioration
Referral recommended.

COMPLICATIONS
Complications arise as a result of scarring:
- Secondary phimosis
- Retention of urine
- Strangury
- Ascending urinary tract infection
- Severe tissue damage if anaerobic infection missed and not treated promptly

CONSIDER CONSULT
Signs of post-infective scarring that impair function warrant referral.

RISK FACTORS

- **Poor hygiene:** predisposes to infection spread
- **Uncircumcised:** predisposes to infection due to build up of smegma
- **Sexual behavior, multiple partners:** predisposes to sexually transmitted diseases
- **Anatomical phimosis:** predisposes to infection due to build up of smegma
- **Underlying disease:** may predispose to infection in general or local conditions similar to balanitis
- **Use of over-the-counter creams:** may produce local reactions

MODIFY RISK FACTORS
Lifestyle and wellness
Those who are circumcised for reasons of custom, religion, or choice are at much lower risk of developing balanitis and balanoposthitis than the uncircumcised.

SEXUAL BEHAVIOR
- Encouragement of safe sex reduces the risk of sexually transmitted diseases and HIV
- Careful choice of condoms and other sexual aids minimizes irritant causes

ENVIRONMENT
General standards of hygiene should be promoted and specific genital hygiene included.

PREVENT RECURRENCE

- Consider elective circumcision
- Retract tight foreskin (prepuce)
- Encourage good genital hygiene
- Education regarding safe sexual contact
- Optimize management of debilitating or chronic disease including diabetes

Reassess coexisting disease
Monitor glycemic control in diabetic patients to minimize chance of infection.

ASSOCIATIONS

American Urological Association
1120 North Charles Street
Baltimore
MD 21201
Tel 410 727 1100
Fax 410 223 4370
http://www.auanet.org

Evidence references and guidelines

1   Vohra S, Badlani G: Balanitis and balanoposthitis. Urol Clin North Am 1992; 19:142–147.

FAQS
Question 1
Why does fungal balanitis recur?

ANSWER 1
It has been noted that, despite successful local therapy, at least 10% of the patients experience recurrent episodes. It has been suggested that intestinal or urethral reservoirs of *Candida* are responsible.

Question 2
In which types of balanitis should I investigate the partner and treat?

ANSWER 2
In those cases of chlamydial, fungal, mycoplasma, syphilitic, and trichomonal balanitis.

Question 3
When do we biopsy or refer out for biopsy?

ANSWER 3
When there are lesions that do not respond to local and systemic therapies. When the lesion(s) increase(s) in size, or demonstrates an invasive appearance.

Question 4
Will circumcision cure my patient of his balanitis?

ANSWER 4
In the overwhelming number of cases, circumcision will cure the balanitis. It will not cure the underlying cause of the balanitis (i.e. sexually transmitted disease).

Question 5
Isn't circumcision in the adult a morbidly painful experience?

ANSWER 5
Circumcision is a safe procedure that when performed in the proper setting by a skilled clinician can afford the patient relief from the pain and embarrassment of balanitis and the secondary foreskin response to acute and chronic inflammation and infection. While the first week postoperatively can be trying, the combination of the surgical cure, antibiotics, local therapy, and analgesics makes the short-term patient discomfort worth the long-term healthcare gain realized by the patient.

CONTRIBUTORS

Gordon H Baustian, MD
Philip J Aliotta, MD, MHA, FACS
John Pinski, MD

BENIGN PROSTATIC HYPERPLASIA

SUMMARY INFORMATION

DESCRIPTION

- An almost universal finding in older men
- Typically presents with urinary outflow obstruction or bladder irritability (or both)
- The symptoms of prostate cancer can be identical to those of benign prostatic hyperplasia (BPH)
- Treatment choices include watchful waiting, pharmacotherapy, and surgery

URGENT ACTION

- Urgent referral for any patient who has retention of urine or evidence of compromised renal function
- Catheterize patients who are in acute retention or who have obstructive renal failure (if the facilities are available) while arranging referral

KEY! DON'T MISS!

Slowly developing urinary retention may be difficult to recognize clinically.

ICD9 CODE
600 Hyperplasia.

SYNONYMS
- Benign prostatic hypertrophy
- BPH

CARDINAL FEATURES
- An almost universal finding in older men
- Etiology unknown
- No relationship between the degree of prostatic enlargement and the severity of a patient's symptoms
- May be asymptomatic
- Typically present with a mixture of outflow obstruction and bladder irritability
- Obstructive symptoms include decreased force and caliber of urinary stream, hesitancy and postmicturition dribble
- Irritative symptoms include urinary frequency, urgency and nocturia
- 'Postrenal' or obstructive renal failure may develop in severe cases
- Symptoms of prostate cancer may be identical, and this diagnosis always needs to be excluded
- Treatment choices include watchful waiting, pharmacotherapy, and surgery

CAUSES
Common causes
- Exact etiology unknown
- Popular theories involve the influence of hormones and/or growth factors

Contributory or predisposing factors
- Increasing age
- Intact testes: at least one functioning testis must be present for a patient to develop benign prostatic hyperplasia

EPIDEMIOLOGY
Incidence and prevalence
FREQUENCY
- Seen almost universally in older men
- More than 20% of men have required either medical or surgical therapy for benign prostatic hyperplasia by age 75
- 80% of men have evidence of the disease by age 80

Demographics
AGE
- Rare in men under 40 years of age
- Seen in approximately 50% of men over 50
- Seen in approximately 80% of men over 80

GENDER
Men only.

RACE
No strong evidence for a racial predisposition to BPH. (This is different from prostate cancer, which does have a racial predisposition.)

GENETICS
May play a role, but currently no conclusive proof.

DIAGNOSIS

DIFFERENTIAL DIAGNOSIS

- The most important differential diagnosis is prostate cancer, which requires prompt referral, so that the patient's disease may be staged and appropriate treatment begun
- Other common differential diagnoses include prostatitis, urethral stricture, bladder neck contracture, carcinoma of the bladder, neurogenic bladder, and interstitial cystitis

Prostate cancer

Symptoms of prostate cancer may be identical to those of benign prostatic hyperplasia.

FEATURES

- Patients may have a palpable abnormality of the prostate on digital rectal examination
- Patients may have an elevated prostate-specific antigen (PSA)
- Incidence increases with age; 80% of patients are aged 65 years or more at the time of diagnosis
- Bone pain, pathological fractures, neurological deficits may be seen in advanced disease and may be presenting symptoms

Prostatitis

Prostatitis may be an acute or chronic condition.

FEATURES

- Acute prostatitis is often seen in younger patients (30–50 years of age) than those with benign prostatic hyperplasia
- Chronic prostatitis is usually seen in men over 50 years of age
- Perineal, scrotal, penile pain
- Urinary frequency and urgency
- Dysuria
- Acute urinary retention occasionally occurs
- Caliber of urinary stream may be reduced
- Hematospermia
- Presentation may include fever and chills
- Digital rectal examination may reveal a tender boggy prostate

Urethral stricture

FEATURES

- May have history of infection, trauma or urethral instrumentation, including catheterization
- Reduction in caliber and/or force of stream
- Acute retention occasionally seen

Bladder neck contracture

FEATURES

- May be congenital or acquired
- If acquired, may follow surgery, especially retropubic prostatectomy, or radiation
- Reduction in caliber and/or force of stream

Bladder cancer

The features of bladder cancer are as follows:

FEATURES

- Hematuria; either gross painless hematuria or microhematuria
- Frequency, urgency, dysuria
- Abdominal or bone pain in advanced disease
- Cigarette smoking, chemical occupational exposure thought to be involved in the etiology

SIGNS & SYMPTOMS
Signs
- May be minimal, even with a markedly enlarged prostate
- Enlarged prostate
- Abdominal distension, which may be marked in chronic retention
- Palpable bladder after voiding
- Post-void urinary residual (>100mL)
- Signs of obstructive uropathy (edema, pallor, ecchymoses)

Symptoms
Benign prostatic hyperplasia may be asymptomatic.

Obstructive symptoms:
- Decrease in force and/or caliber of urinary stream
- Urinary hesitancy
- Postmicturition dribble
- Sensation of incomplete voiding
- Overflow incontinence
- Acute or chronic retention of urine – acute retention of urine is of sudden onset and is usually painful; chronic retention develops gradually and tends to be painless

Irritative symptoms:
- Frequency
- Urgency
- Urge incontinence
- Nocturia

Other symptoms:
- Hematuria
- Symptoms of obstructive uropathy with decrease in renal function (tiredness, anorexia, nausea, malaise)

ASSOCIATED DISORDERS
- Prostate cancer
- Prostatitis

KEY! DON'T MISS!
Slowly developing urinary retention may be difficult to recognize clinically.

CONSIDER CONSULT
- Refer if there is doubt over the diagnosis
- Refer patients with evidence of compromised renal function or suspected sepsis
- Refer patients with evidence of acute or chronic retention of urine, particularly when associated with decreased renal function or sepsis
- Refer patients who are severely symptomatic

INVESTIGATION OF THE PATIENT
Direct questions to patient
Q Do you have trouble starting or stopping the stream of urine? Patients may complain of hesitancy, difficulty in initiating micturition, and/or terminal dribbling at the end of micturition.
Q Do you think the force or caliber of the stream has changed? Do you have to sit to urinate? The force of the stream may become weaker, and the caliber more narrow.
Q Do you have to get up at night to pass urine? And if so, how many times? Nocturia, often many times per night, is common.

Q Do you pass urine more often during the day than you used to? Frequency is common.

Q Do you ever wet yourself? Incontinence of urine may be seen either as an aspect of severe terminal dribbling, or in cases of chronic retention, where overflow incontinence may occur.

Q Have you ever had any surgery for urinary problems in the past? Previous instrumentation of the urinary tract may predispose to a urethral stricture or bladder neck contracture.

Q Have you ever had any trauma to the urinary tract or genitalia, or have suffered a pelvic fracture? Trauma may predispose to the development of a urethral stricture.

Q Do you take any medications? Certain medications may mimic symptoms or make them worse; e.g. anticholinergic agents, which may impair bladder contractility; or sympathomimetic agents, which may impair bladder outflow resistance.

Contributory or predisposing factors

Q How old are you? Incidence increases with age.

Q Have you ever had any operations on your testicles? At least one functioning testis must be present for a patient to be able to develop the disease. If both testicles are absent and were not removed surgically, a referral is needed.

Family history

Q Have your father or brothers had the same symptoms? Is there a family history of prostate cancer? It is thought that genetic factors may play a role.

Examination

- Abdominal examination: for signs of a palpable bladder
- Genital examination: if the patient has a severe phimosis or a meatal stenosis, this may be the cause of, or contributing to, any obstructive symptoms. At least one testis must be present for a patient to be able to develop benign prostatic hyperplasia
- Neurological examination: both general (for obvious abnormalities, e.g. paraplegia, hemiplegia) and focused (perianal sensation, anal sphincter tone and control). An underlying neurological abnormality may be contributing to a patient's symptoms
- Digital rectal examination: assess the size and consistency of the prostate
- Check the patient's clothing: for evidence of urinary incontinence. Patients may deny this if they are confused or embarrassed
- Assess patient's overall condition: if pale, confused, generally unwell, may have obstructive renal failure

Summary of investigative tests

- Renal function should be checked since it may be abnormal (e.g. if patient has obstructive uropathy)
- Urine dipstick should be performed in all patients; it provides a rapid confirmation of a variety of abnormalities, including microscopic hematuria
- Urine culture should be carried out if the urine dipstick examination is abnormal
- Urine cytology should be performed if the patient has symptoms of bladder irritability, frank hematuria, a history of smoking, or possible occupational exposures
- International Prostate Symptom Score (IPSS) should be performed in all patients, since it helps in decisions about treatment
- Prostate-specific antigen (PSA) is an optional test, but it is recommended (to help exclude prostate cancer) in Caucasian men over 50 years of age, in African-Americans over 40 years of age, and in patients with a positive family history of prostate cancer
- Uroflowmetry is an optional test that provides an indication of the degree of obstruction; it may help in decisions about management
- Postmicturition urinary residual volume should be measured in patients in whom urinary obstruction is suspected. It may be performed either alone or as part of a renal or abdominal ultrasound scan. Persistently high residual volumes may indicate more advanced disease
- Renal tract ultrasound can be performed to confirm or exclude hydronephrosis if there is a suspicion of renal impairment

- Cystometrography measures urine flow versus voiding pressure. It is an optional test that may be performed in patients in whom pharmacologic management has failed and who may require surgical intervention. It is performed by a specialist only
- Intravenous urography is an optional test that tends to be performed by a specialist; it may be performed for specific indications (e.g. in patients with hematuria to exclude malignancy or calculous disease)
- Cystoscopy is performed if the diagnosis is in doubt, or as part of the work-up for prostatic surgery or part of the procedure. It is performed by a specialist only
- Transrectal ultrasound scan gives a general estimate of prostatic volume and may demonstrate any abnormal areas within the prostate that may be malignant. It is often combined with a needle biopsy. It is performed by a specialist only
- Prostatic biopsy is performed if there is any suspicion of prostatic malignancy (e.g. elevated prostate-specific antigen [PSA] or palpable abnormality on digital rectal examination). It is performed by a specialist, often with transrectal ultrasound guidance

DIAGNOSTIC DECISION

Although the precise diagnosis is based on pathology, a clinical diagnosis is reached on the basis of a patient's signs and symptoms and the results of relevant investigations, particularly the International Prostate Symptom Score (IPSS) and uroflowmetry.

CLINICAL PEARLS

- The strongest predictors of retention are an enlarged prostate by digital rectal examination, moderate symptoms, a flow rate below 15mL/s, and an elevated prostate-specific antigen (PSA)
- Recent studies have shown a strong age-dependent relationship between prostate volume and serum PSA among men with BPH, in whom serum PSA is a sufficiently accurate indicator of prostate enlargement for use in decision-making
- Age-specific criteria to detect men with prostate volumes of greater than 40mL have been proposed, with a specificity of 70% and a sensitivity of 65–70%. The relevant PSA values are >1.6ng/mL for men in their 50s, >2.0ng/mL for men in their 60s, and >2.3ng/mL for men in their 70s

THE TESTS
Body fluids
RENAL FUNCTION TESTS
Description
Cuffed venous blood sample to measure blood urea nitrogen and creatinine; this can be combined with a measurement of serum potassium.

Advantages/Disadvantages
Advantages:
- Indicates whether renal function is impaired
- Simple, inexpensive test

Normal
- Blood urea nitrogen: 8–25mg/dL (3.3–6.7mmol/L)
- Creatinine: 0.6–1.2mg/dL (60–120mcmol/L)
- Potassium: 3.8–5.0mEq/L (3.8–5.0mmol/L)
- Note that reference ranges can vary; check with local laboratory

Abnormal
- Blood urea nitrogen: >25mg/dL (>6.7mmol/L)
- Creatinine: >1.2mg/dL (>120mcmol/L)
- Potassium: >5.0mEq/L (>5.0mmol/L)

Cause of abnormal result
Impaired renal function, usually secondary to outflow obstruction in benign prostatic hyperplasia.

Drugs, disorders and other factors that may alter results
Renal function may be impaired by many drugs.

SERUM PROSTATE-SPECIFIC ANTIGEN (PSA)
Advantages/Disadvantages
Advantage: useful screening test for prostate cancer

Disadvantages:
- May not be diagnostic of prostatic cancer, especially in men with benign prostatic hyperplasia, as a variety of other conditions may also cause an elevation in serum PSA
- May result in increased use of more expensive and invasive diagnostic testing

Normal
- <4.0ng/mL (must consider age and race of patient – there is some evidence for age- and race-specific PSA levels)
- Note that reference ranges vary; check with local laboratory

Abnormal
- >4.0ng/mL
- PSA may increase slightly with age, this may make the significance of a mildly elevated PSA difficult to interpret in an elderly patient

Drugs, disorders and other factors that may alter results
- Prostate cancer – elevated prostate-specific antigen (PSA) may be seen
- Prostatitis – elevated PSA may be seen
- Acute retention of urine – elevated PSA may be seen
- Urinary tract instrumentation – elevated PSA may be seen
- Prostatic infarction – elevated PSA may be seen
- Digital rectal examination – elevated PSA may be seen (controversial)
- Finasteride – PSA levels may be reduced by up to 50%; patients taking finasteride should have their PSA levels measured at least every 6 months; if PSA levels rise, referral is needed

URINE DIPSTICK
Description
Midstream urine specimen.

Advantages/Disadvantages
Advantages:
- Quick and simple to perform at office level
- Provides information about a variety of urinary constituents very quickly

Disadvantage: very nonspecific – whether normal or abnormal, does not confirm or refute the diagnosis

Normal
No red blood cells, white blood cells, or protein identified.

Abnormal
- Red and/or white blood cells, and/or protein present
- Dipstick tests can be highly sensitive, and a false-positive result is possible

URINE CULTURE
Description
Midstream urine specimen.

Advantages/Disadvantages
Advantages:
- Confirms or excludes diagnosis of urinary tract infection
- Identifies the bacteria responsible

Normal
No bacteria cultured.

Abnormal
Bacteria cultured, suggestive of a urinary tract infection.

Cause of abnormal result
Presence of infection.

Drugs, disorders and other factors that may alter results
Urine sample may be contaminated, e.g. by skin or bowel commensal organisms.

URINE CYTOLOGY
Description
Midstream urine sample.

Advantages/Disadvantages
- Advantage: simple screening test for bladder carcinoma
- Disadvantage: false-negative results may occur, especially if bladder carcinoma is of low grade

Normal
No atypical or malignant cells present.

Abnormal
Atypical or malignant cells present.

Cause of abnormal result
Bladder carcinoma.

Drugs, disorders and other factors that may alter results
- Urinary tract infection
- Chronic irritation of the bladder (e.g. presence of urinary catheter or bladder stone)

Tests of function
UROFLOWMETRY
Description
Measurement of urine volume voided per unit time.

Advantages/Disadvantages
Advantages:
- Simple to perform
- Result available immediately

Disadvantages:
- May be time-consuming (if there is need to wait until the patient's bladder is full)
- Patient needs to fully understand what he needs to do, and elderly or confused patients may not be able to perform the test adequately

- A patient with severe symptoms may not be able to tolerate a sufficient volume of urine within their bladder for the test result to be valid
- False-positive and false-negative results may occur
- Special equipment required

Normal
- Peak flow rate >15mL/s
- Peak flow rate 10–15mL/s may be considered equivocal, depending on the clinical setting

Abnormal
- Peak flow rate <10mL/s
- Keep in mind the possibility of a false-positive or false-negative result

Cause of abnormal result
Bladder outflow obstruction.

Drugs, disorders and other factors that may alter results
- If the patient has a urethral stricture, the flow trace may be abnormal, exhibiting a typical 'box shape'
- Result may be normal if a patient with bladder outlet obstruction is able to generate a high bladder pressure when voiding
- Abdominal straining during voiding creates an artificially high peak flow and spurious elevations in the average flow rate, resulting in a false-negative result
- A false-positive result may be seen if a patient has no obstruction but has a hypotonic bladder
- Patients taking anticholinergic agents may have a false-positive result owing to impairment of bladder contractility
- Patients taking sympathomimetic agents may have a false-positive result owing to increased bladder outflow resistance
- If voided volume is <150mL, result may not be valid (particularly if flow rate is low), since a false-positive result may be obtained
- If voided volume is >500mL, result may not be accurate if flow rate is slow, because the bladder may be overdistended and contractility may be impaired; a false-positive result may be obtained

POSTMICTURITION URINARY RESIDUAL VOLUME
Description
- Measurement of the volume of urine present in the bladder after micturition
- Usually measured by ultrasound, may also be measured following insertion of a urethral catheter

Advantages/Disadvantages
Advantages:
- Simple and quick to perform
- May be performed at office level

Disadvantages:
- Special equipment (e.g. ultrasonic bladder scanner) required for more definitive measurement
- False-positive results may occur
- Catheterization can result in trauma and/or introduction of infection

Normal
<100ml of urine in bladder 5–10min after micturition.

Abnormal
>100ml residual urine in bladder after micturition.

Cause of abnormal result
- Bladder outlet obstruction
- Hypotonic bladder

Drugs, disorders and other factors that may alter results
If bladder is overfull before micturition, it may not empty completely.

Imaging
ULTRASOUND OF RENAL TRACT
Advantages/Disadvantages
Advantages:
- Noninvasive
- No ionizing radiation exposure
- Postmicturition urinary residual volume may be measured concurrently

Disadvantage: in a patient suspected of having obstructive uropathy, the delay required to organize this investigation may not be acceptable

Normal
No hydronephrosis or hydroureter.

Abnormal
- Hydronephrosis
- Hydroureter

Cause of abnormal result
Significant bladder outflow obstruction.

Drugs, disorders and other factors that may alter results
Hydronephrosis or hydroureter may be due to other diagnoses, e.g. ureteropelvic junction obstruction, ureteric calculus, pelvic malignancy.

Special tests
INTERNATIONAL PROSTATE SYMPTOM SCORE (IPSS)
Description
A questionnaire that provides an indication of the severity of a patient's symptoms.

Advantages/Disadvantages
Advantages:
- Has been extensively tested and validated
- Information gained helps in making decisions about treatment
- Provided that the patient is capable of answering the questions, the questionnaire form may be completed by caregiver if necessary (e.g. if the patient is blind)

Disadvantages:
- Is subjective; requires truthful, accurate answers from the patient
- Results may not be of use in patients with confusion or significant impairment of memory

Normal
Symptom score of 0.

Abnormal
Symptom score of:
- 1–7 indicates mild symptoms
- 8–19 indicates moderate symptoms
- 20–35 indicates severe symptoms

Cause of abnormal result
Bladder outlet obstruction.

Drugs, disorders and other factors that may alter results
- If patient is untruthful or incapable of filling in the questionnaire
- If patient has urethral stricture
- Anticholinergic agents, which may impair bladder contractility
- Sympathomimetic agents, which may increase bladder outflow resistance

CONSIDER CONSULT
- Refer patients who have failed conservative treatment, including pharmacotherapy
- Refer if prostate cancer cannot be confidently excluded (elevated prostate-specific antigen [PSA] and/or an abnormal prostate exam)
- Refer if another urological disorder (e.g. bladder cancer, urethral stricture) cannot be excluded

IMMEDIATE ACTION
Patients with acute retention or with obstructive renal failure should be catheterized as soon as possible and before reaching hospital if there is likely to be any delay in treatment.

PATIENT AND CAREGIVER ISSUES
Patient or caregiver request
- **Is it possible that my symptoms may be due to cancer?** Patients may be concerned that they have prostate cancer
- **Will the treatment make me impotent?** Patients may have heard or read that treatment frequently results in impotence

Health-seeking behavior
- **Has patient waited too long before presenting?** Patients may ignore or not recognize the severity of their symptoms until they have developed acute or chronic retention
- **Has the patient self-medicated?** Self-medication with complementary therapies (e.g. saw palmetto) may have been successful, so the patient may delay consulting his doctor

MANAGEMENT ISSUES
Goals
- Improve patient's symptoms and quality of life
- Identify and reduce the risk that renal function become compromised
- Identify those patients who have prostate cancer rather than benign prostatic hyperplasia

Management in special circumstances
COEXISTING DISEASE
- Prostate cancer: treatment of prostate cancer should take precedence and may make treating coexisting benign prostatic hyperplasia unnecessary
- Prostatitis: treat concurrently

COEXISTING MEDICATION
If a patient is already taking an antihypertensive agent, extreme care must be taken if he is started on an alpha-blocking medication because there is a slightly increased risk of hypotension.

SPECIAL PATIENT GROUPS
Elderly men:
- Many patients with benign prostatic hyperplasia are elderly
- Treatment choices may be influenced by the presence of coexisting disease and by medications that a patient is already taking

PATIENT SATISFACTION/LIFESTYLE PRIORITIES
- Patient's priority is likely to be symptomatic relief, and thus improvement in quality of life
- Symptoms such as frequency and incontinence particularly may affect a patient's ability to continue with employment and/or social activities, and thus relief of these symptoms is especially important

SUMMARY OF THERAPEUTIC OPTIONS
Choices

- In patients with mild symptoms, watchful waiting is an option, although the patient must be followed-up because for many patients the disease will progress and intervention may be required
- An alpha-adrenergic blocking agent is usually the drug of first choice. A highly selective agent such as tamsulosin is preferable, but other choices include terazosin and doxazosin
- Hormonal manipulation, most commonly with the 5-alpha reductase inhibitor finasteride may be considered, especially for patients with larger prostates
- Complementary therapy may be an option in some men. The most common agent is saw palmetto
- Surgery may be required if pharmacotherapy is unsuccessful, or if the patient is severely symptomatic. Transurethral resection of the prostate (TUR) is currently still the 'gold standard' of treatment, but other options include transurethral incision of the prostate, laser prostatectomy, open prostatectomy, transurethral microwave thermotherapy, or transurethral needle ablation
- For patients who are unfit for any form of surgery, and for whom pharmacotherapy is either contraindicated or has been unsuccessful in the past, a prostatic stent or balloon dilatation of the prostate may be considered, although balloon dilatation is no longer generally offered as a therapy for outlet obstruction

Clinical pearls

- Balloon dilatation of the prostate enjoyed a very brief period of enthusiasm but has not proven effective over the long term. It is generally no longer offered as a legitimate therapy for outlet obstruction
- If cancer and compromise of renal function can be ruled out, treatment should be directed by the patient's symptoms and willingness to deal with them. Some patients may have a very high tolerance of symptoms such as nocturia

FOLLOW UP
Plan for review

- Review every 3–6 months with an International Prostate Symptom Score (IPSS) and uroflowmetry
- Annual digital rectal examination
- Annual prostate-specific antigen (PSA) estimation

DRUGS AND OTHER THERAPIES: DETAILS
Drugs
TAMSULOSIN
Dose
0.4–0.8mg/day orally, 30min after a meal.

Efficacy
In one trial, 74–81% of patients showed improvement on the International Prostate Symptom Score (IPSS) (56% of patients on placebo showed improvement).

Risks/Benefits
Risks:
- Use caution in patients with renal impairment and in the elderly
- Use caution in patients receiving calcium channel blockers, beta-blockers, and diuretics

Benefit: since tamsulosin is a selective alpha-1 adrenergic antagonist, risk of 'first dose' phenomenon may be less than with nonselective medications

Side-effects and adverse reactions
- Gastrointestinal: nausea, vomiting, dry mouth, abdominal pain
- Genitourinary: erectile and ejaculation dysfunction, urinary frequency, incontinence
- Central nervous system: asthenia, headache, depression, dizziness, drowsiness, vertigo
- Ears, eyes, nose, and throat: rhinitis, pharyngitis, sinusitis
- Cardiovascular system: tachycardia, orthostatic hypotension, palpitations
- Skin: rashes, angioedema

Interactions (other drugs)
- Alpha-blockers ■ Beta-blockers ■ Cimetidine ■ Warfarin

Contraindications
- Orthostatic hypotension and syncope ■ Severe liver impairment ■ Prostate carcinoma
- Women

Evidence
Alpha-blockers are effective in the management of benign prostatic hyperplasia (BPH).
- A systematic review compared the efficacy of alpha-blockers in the management of BPH. Most randomized controlled trials found alpha-blockers to be more effective than placebo in improving lower urinary tract symptoms. There is comparable efficacy between the different antagonists (alfuzosin, terazosin, doxazosin and tamsulosin). Tamsulosin is one of the better tolerated alpha-blockers [1] *Level M*
- A systematic review assessed the efficacy of the 5-alpha adrenergic blockers and finasteride (an antiandrogen) in the management of BPH. Both classes of medication were found to be effective for symptom reduction, and there was similar efficacy with all alpha-adrenergic blockers [2] *Level M*

Acceptability to patient
- Once-daily dosage is easy to remember
- If hypotension is significant it may cause patients distress, and/or put them at risk of a fall leading to injury
- The biggest problem is the ejaculatory disturbances caused by this drug

Follow up plan
- After starting treatment, patients should be reviewed soon afterwards (within 4 weeks) in case side-effects are a major problem
- Once a patient is being treated satisfactorily he should be reviewed every 3–6 months, with a repeat International Prostate Symptom Score (IPSS) and uroflowmetry

Patient and caregiver information
Take care, especially in the first 12h after starting the medication, in case you feel dizzy or faint.

TERAZOSIN
Dose
- Initially, 1mg at bedtime for 3–7 days, increased to 2mg for one week, then increased to 5mg and to 10mg as tolerated
- Many patients may be unable to tolerate doses as high as 10mg per day and may be at risk of syncope and falls; dose is titrated against efficacy and side-effects in each patient
- Initial dose is given at bedtime to reduce the 'first dose' effect; once a patient is stabilized on terazosin it can be taken in the morning or at bedtime

Efficacy
- More effective than placebo. In studies reporting patient satisfaction, 71% of patients showed some improvement
- Terazosin has been shown to decrease symptoms more than finasteride

Risks/Benefits
Risks:
- Likely to induce postural hypotension or syncope, therefore avoid dangerous tasks
- Use caution in patients with renal impairment, the elderly, and in patients with angina
- Use caution coadministering with antihypertensive drugs

Side-effects and adverse reactions
- Gastrointestinal: nausea, vomiting, constipation, diarrhea
- Genitourinary: urinary frequency, priapism, incontinence
- Respiratory: dyspnea, nasal congestion, sinusitis
- Central nervous system: dizziness, lethargy, fatigue, headache, drowsiness, nervousness
- Cardiovascular system: postural hypotension, palpitations, peripheral edema, tachycardia
- Skin: sweating, rashes

Interactions (other drugs)
- ACE inhibitors ▪ Adrenergic neurone blockers (both alpha and beta) ▪ General anesthetics
- Alcohol ▪ Aldesleukin ▪ Alprostadil ▪ Amifostine ▪ Angiotensin-II receptor antagonists
- Antihypertensives (clonidine, diazoxide, methyldopa, minoxidil, nitrates, nitroprusside)
- Antipsychotics ▪ Anxiolytics and hypnotics ▪ Calcium channel blockers ▪ Corticosteroids
- Diuretics ▪ Levodopa ▪ Non-steroidal anti-inflammatory agents (NSAIDs)
- Skeletal muscle relaxants (baclofen, tizanidine)

Contraindications
No known contraindications

Evidence
Terazosin is effective in the management of benign prostatic hyperplasia (BPH).
- A double-blind randomized controlled trial (RCT) compared terazosin with placebo in the management of men with moderate to severe symptoms of BPH. A significant improvement in symptoms was noted in the treatment group, which was maintained for 12 months [3] *Level P*
- A systematic review compared the efficacy of alpha-blockers in the management of BPH. Most RCTs found alpha-blockers to be more effective than placebo in improving symptoms of the lower urinary tract. There was comparable efficacy between the different antagonists (alfuzosin, terazosin, doxazosin and tamsulosin) [1] *Level M*
- A systematic review assessed the efficacy of the 5-alpha adrenergic blockers and finasteride (an antiandrogen) in the management of BPH. Both classes of medication were found to be effective for symptom reduction, and there was similar efficacy with all alpha-adrenergic blockers [2] *Level M*
- A prospective trial compared terazosin and finasteride (alone and in combination), in the management of BPH. Terazosin therapy was associated with a greater reduction in symptoms than finasteride. Combination therapy was not found to be superior to terazosin alone [4] *Level P*

Acceptability to patient
- Complex initial dosage regime may be confusing
- If hypotension is significant it may cause the patient distress or put him at risk of a fall, leading to injury

Follow up plan
- After commencing treatment, patient should soon be reviewed (within 4 weeks), in case side-effects are a major problem
- Once a patient is being treated satisfactorily, he should be reviewed every 6 months and given a repeat International Prostate Symptom Score (IPSS) at each visit; a uroflowmetry should only be performed to document persistent voiding difficulty and failure to respond to drug therapy

Patient and caregiver information
Take care, especially when commencing the medication or changing the dose, in case you feel dizzy or faint. The very first dose must be taken at night, before you go to bed.

DOXAZOSIN
Dose
- 1mg at bedtime, initially
- May increase gradually (by doubling the dose at weekly intervals) to a maintenance dose of 5–10mg per day
- Many patients may be unable to tolerate doses as high as 10mg per day and may be at risk of syncope and falls

Efficacy
- Alpha-blockers are more effective than placebo in improving lower urinary tract symptoms in men with BPH
- These drugs work to reduce the effect of alpha-adrenergic stimulation on the bladder neck
- Alpha-blockers reduce the risk of acute urinary retention in men with larger glands

Risks/Benefits
Risks:
- Orthostatic hypotension, particularly in patients taking other antihypertensive, diuretic, or vasodilator medications
- Use caution in patients with hepatic disease, in nursing mothers, and in children

Benefit:
- Improved bladder control

Side-effects and adverse reactions
- Gastrointestinal: abdominal cramps, dry mouth, vomiting, constipation, diarrhea
- Genitourinary: urination difficulties
- Respiratory: dyspnea
- Skin: rash
- Central nervous system: dizziness, headache, fever, paresthesia, vertigo, fatigue, somnolence
- Cardiovascular system: edema, chest pain, palpitations, hypotension (particularly orthostatic), dysrhythmia
- Eyes, ears, nose, and throat: visual disturbances, tinnitus, rhinitis

Interactions (other drugs)
- ACE inhibitors ▪ Adrenergic neurone blockers (both alpha and beta) ▪ Corticosteroids
- Alcohol ▪ Aldesleukin ▪ Alprostadil ▪ Amifostine ▪ Angiotensin-II receptor antagonists
- Antihypertensives (clonidine, diazoxide, methyldopa, minoxidil, nitrates, nitroprusside)
- Antipsychotics ▪ Anxiolytics and hypnotics ▪ Calcium channel blockers ▪ Diuretics
- General anesthetics ▪ Levodopa ▪ Non-steroidal anti-inflammatory drugs (NSAIDs)
- Skeletal muscle relaxants (baclofen, tizanidine)

Contraindications
None in this setting

Evidence
Alpha-blockers are effective in the management of benign prostatic hyperplasia (BPH).
- A systematic review compared the efficacy of alpha-blockers in the management of BPH. Most randomized controlled trials (RCTs) found alpha-blockers to be more effective than placebo in improving lower urinary tract symptoms. There is comparable efficacy between the different antagonists (alfuzosin, terazosin, doxazosin and tamsulosin) [1] *Level M*

- A systematic review assessed the efficacy of the 5-alpha adrenergic blockers and finasteride (an antiandrogen) in the management of BPH. Both classes of medication were found to be effective for symptom reduction, and there was similar efficacy with all alpha-adrenergic blockers [2] *Level M*

Acceptability to patient
- Complex initial dosage regimen may be confusing
- If hypotension is significant, may cause patient distress or put him at risk of a fall, leading to injury

Follow up plan
- When commencing treatment, patient should be reviewed soon afterwards (within 4 weeks), in case side-effects are a major problem
- Once a patient is being treated satisfactorily, he should be reviewed every 6 months, given a repeat International Prostate Symptom Score (IPSS) at each visit, and uroflowmetry only to document persistent voiding difficulty and failure to respond to drug therapy

Patient and caregiver information
Take care, especially when commencing the medication or changing the dose, in case you feel dizzy or faint. The very first dose must be taken at night, before you go to bed.

FINASTERIDE
Dose
5mg/day.

Efficacy
- More effective than placebo in improving lower urinary tract symptoms and reducing complications in men with benign prostatic hyperplasia (BPH), particularly men with larger prostates (in excess of 40g)
- Benefit in smaller prostates is doubtful

Risks/Benefits
Risks:
- Use caution in patients with hepatic disease and obstructive uropathy
- Condoms should be used if partner is pregnant or likely to become pregnant (finasteride is excreted in the semen)
- Women of childbearing age should avoid handling crushed or broken tablets

Side-effects and adverse reactions
- Genitourinary: decreased libido, impotence, ejaculation disorders, breast tenderness and enlargement
- Hypersensitivity reactions

Interactions (other drugs)
No known interactions

Contraindications
- Children - Women

Evidence
Finasteride may be effective in the management of BPH, and is especially useful for men with large prostates.
- A meta-analysis compared finasteride with placebo. A significantly greater reduction in symptom scores was noted in the treatment group, especially in men with large prostates [5] *Level M*

- A systematic review found a significantly greater reduction in symptom scores with finasteride than placebo in men with BPH [2] *Level M*
- A large randomized controlled trial compared finasteride with placebo in men with symptomatic BPH. Finasteride significantly reduced symptoms and reduced the risk of acute urinary retention or the need for prostatectomy [6] *Level P*
- A prospective trial compared terazosin and finasteride (alone and in combination), in the management of BPH. Terazosin therapy was associated with a greater reduction in symptoms than finasteride. Combination therapy was not found to be superior to terazosin alone [4] *Level P*

Acceptability to patient
- Simple, once-daily dose that does not require adjustment
- May not be acceptable to very symptomatic patients, since it can be some time before an effect is seen
- Not suitable for men with partners of childbearing age if the partner wishes to become pregnant, as such women should not be exposed to the semen

Follow up plan
- After commencing treatment, patient should soon be reviewed (within 4 weeks), in case side-effects are a major problem
- Once a patient is being treated satisfactorily, he should be reviewed every 6 months, using a repeat International Prostate Symptom Score (IPSS). A uroflow should be performed at 6 months to assess adequacy of the drug. Further uroflow testing should be based on patient IPSS score and the patient's complaints. Re-evaluate for any change in patient status
- Need continued prostate-specific antigen (PSA) evaluations every 6 months; a referral is needed if PSA is rising while on finasteride

Patient and caregiver information
- The medication may need to be taken for at least 3 months before you will experience any effect
- If your partner is of childbearing age, you must use a condom during intercourse, even if you are already using another form of contraception
- If you and your partner are planning a pregnancy, you must tell your doctor beforehand, as you will need to discontinue this medication and possibly take an alternative drug

Surgical therapy
TRANSURETHRAL RESECTION OF PROSTATE (TURP)
Efficacy
Generally provides good symptom relief.

Risks/Benefits
Risks:
- Incontinence: complete incontinence afterwards is rare, but significant incontinence can occur in 5% of patients
- Hemorrhage – although the need for blood transfusion is extremely rare
- Urethral stricture
- Sexual dysfunction – in up to 20% of patients, varying from soft erections to complete impotence
- Retrograde ejaculation

Benefits:
- Symptomatic relief
- Mortality rate <1%
- Prostatic tissue available for histological examination

Evidence

There is limited evidence for the treatment of benign prostatic hyperplasia (BPH) with TURP.

- A randomized controlled trial (RCT) compared TURP with watchful waiting in men with moderate symptoms of BPH. Symptomatic improvement was achieved in 90% of men who were treated with TURP and 39% of the watchful waiting patients. At 5 years, the treatment failure rate was 21% for TURP and 10% for watchful waiting; and 36% of men from the watchful waiting group had changed to the surgery group [7] *Level P*
- Another RCT found that TURP significantly improved International Prostate Symptoms Score (IPSS) when compared with conservative management [8] *Level P*

Acceptability to patient

- Invasive procedure
- Risks of incontinence, retrograde ejaculation, infertility and sexual dysfunction may be unacceptable to some patients

Follow up plan

Review 3 months postoperatively with an International Prostate Symptoms Score (IPSS) and uroflowmetry. This may be done by a specialist.

TRANSURETHRAL INCISION OF PROSTATE (TUIP)

Efficacy

- More effective than watchful waiting in patients with moderate symptoms, but may not be as effective as transurethral resection
- May be procedure of choice in patients who are critically ill and who cannot tolerate full resection of the prostate

Risks/Benefits

Risks:

- Retrograde ejaculation and infertility (less common than with transurethral resection)
- Bladder neck contracture
- The majority of prostatic tissue is left behind, and so a further procedure may be required in the future, and patients continue to be at risk of prostate cancer
- No tissue available for histological examination

Benefits:

- Can be performed under local anesthetic as an outpatient procedure
- Symptomatic relief
- Lower incidence of complications than with transurethral resection

Evidence

Several randomized controlled trials have found similar efficacy for TUIP and transurethral resection of the prostate (TURP) in the symptomatic management of men with smaller prostates [9] *Level P*

Acceptability to patient

- Minimally invasive procedure compared to transurethral resection
- May be preferred by some patients because of the lower incidence of retrograde ejaculation

Follow up plan

Review 3 months postoperatively with an International Prostate Symptom Score (IPSS) and uroflowmetry. This may be done by a specialist.

TRANSURETHRAL MICROWAVE THERMOTHERAPY (TUMT)
Efficacy
Effective, but it is unclear whether transurethral microwave thermotherapy (TUMT) is as effective as transurethral resection.

Risks/Benefits
Risks:
- No tissue available for histology
- Hematuria (usually slight)
- Acute urinary retention

Benefits:
- Outpatient procedure performed under topical anesthesia
- Low incidence of urethral stricture
- Little effect on ejaculation
- Little or no incontinence
- Has been effectively used in catheter-bound patients who are medically unstable and who would not normally tolerate an anesthetic or the fluid shifts that occur with surgery
- Can be safely done in an office-based surgicenter as well as in ambulatory and hospital settings

Evidence
TUMT is more effective than sham treatment for the treatment of BPH.
- A blinded randomized controlled trial (RCT) compared TUMT with sham treatment. International Prostate Symptom Score (IPSS) was significantly reduced in patients treated with TUMT at 6 months following treatment [10] *Level P*
- Two RCTs found no significant difference in symptomatic improvement between TUMT and TURP at 2.5 year follow-up [9] *Level P*
- Another RCT found improved symptoms in patients treated with TURP compared with TUMT. Significantly more patients treated with TURP suffered from sexual dysfunction postoperatively [11] *Level P*
- One RCT compared TUMT with terazosin. TUMT lead to significantly improved IPPS at 6 months [12] *Level P*

Acceptability to patient
Outpatient procedure, no general anesthetic and few complications may make this very acceptable to some patients.

Follow up plan
Patient should be monitored especially in the first few postoperative days, as he may develop acute retention of urine.

Patient and caregiver information
- Improvement in symptoms, and International Prostate Symptom Score (IPSS), will be slow initially, but will continue to improve over weeks to a few months
- Contact your doctor if you have any difficulty passing urine, especially in the first few days after treatment

TRANSURETHRAL NEEDLE ABLATION (TUNA)
Efficacy
- Limited follow-up data suggest that transurethral needle ablation (TUNA) is effective in improving symptoms, but not as effective as transurethral resection of the prostate (TURP) in improving peak urinary flow
- May require further intervention later (e.g. TURP, pharmacotherapy)

Risks/Benefits
Risks:

- No tissue available for histological examination
- Some patients will require further intervention in the future

Benefits:

- Low incidence of side-effects (anejaculation, erectile dysfunction, incontinence)
- Some patients do not require postoperative catheterization
- Can be used for patients who would ordinarily not tolerate an anesthetic and surgery
- Can be performed in an office-based surgicenter, an ambulatory center, or a hospital

Evidence
A randomized controlled trial compared TUNA with TURP in the management of benign prostatic hyperplasia (BPH). There was a significantly greater benefit noted for patients treated with TURP at one year. TUNA was associated with less bleeding and retrograde ejaculation than TURP [13]
Level P

Acceptability to patient
Outpatient procedure requiring no anesthetic may make this acceptable to patients wishing to avoid more invasive surgery.

Follow up plan
Review 3 months postoperatively and obtain an International Prostate Symptom Score (IPSS) and uroflowmetry. This may be done by a specialist.

TRANSURETHRAL LASER PROSTATECTOMY
Efficacy

- Increasing efficacy as laser technology improves, although still said to be less effective than transurethral resection. Different types of laser (e.g. Indigo, Nd:YAG, holmium:YAG) have been used. Holmium may be the most efficacious; although some surgeons will operate on larger prostates (>80g)
- Interstitial laser therapy (insertion of a laser fiber into the prostate, with subsequent tissue necrosis) has also been tried, but is now rarely used. It can, however, be performed as an office procedure by a urologist
- Effective for smaller prostates

Risks/Benefits
Risks:

- Urethral stricture
- Some prostatic tissue remains, and therefore there is a risk of regrowth of benign prostatic hyperplasia or of the later development of prostate cancer

Benefits:

- Very good hemostasis, and suitable for patients on anticoagulants
- Hospital stay usually shorter than after transurethral resection
- Shorter catheterization postoperatively than after transurethral resection

Acceptability to patient
Shorter hospital stay may make this highly acceptable to some patients.

Follow up plan
Review 3 months postoperatively and obtain an International Prostate Symptom Score (IPSS) and uroflowmetry. This may be done by a specialist.

OPEN PROSTATECTOMY
Also known as retropubic prostatectomy and suprapubic prostatectomy.

Efficacy
Highly effective, especially for prostates that are too large for transurethral resection (e.g. >80g).

Risks/Benefits
Risks:
- Open surgical procedure
- Midline incision required
- Longer recovery time than after transurethral resection
- Hemorrhage may occur postoperatively

Benefits:
- Complete removal of prostate under direct vision
- Useful for large prostate glands (50–75g) in which the ureteral orifices are difficult to see
- Useful when there is a large median lobe or a large intravesical extension of the prostate
- Useful when there is concomitant bladder disease (e.g. diverticuli, stones) that cannot be managed transurethrally
- Useful in patients who cannot be placed in the dorsal lithotomy position necessary for a transurethral resection (e.g. those with inguinal hernia or ankylosis of the hips)
- Does not carry the risk of dilutional hyponatremia, which may be seen after transurethral resection

Acceptability to patient
Open procedure with longer recovery period, so this technique may be less acceptable than some others.

Complementary therapy
SAW PALMETTO
Extract of the American saw palmetto (*Serenoa repens*) or dwarf palm plant.

Efficacy
Unknown – there is no regulation over the manufacture of this product.

Risks/Benefits
Risks:
- Not thought to be as effective as other medication
- Unknown mechanism of action
- Poorly regulated dosage in available preparations

Evidence
Symptoms of benign prostatic hyperplasia (BPH) may be effectively treated with saw palmetto.
- A systematic review found that *Serenoa repens* improves urologic symptoms and flow measures compared with placebo, and compared with finasteride [14] *Level M*
- A nonsystematic review found that saw palmetto improved nocturia compared with placebo [15] *Level P*
- A randomized controlled trial compared saw palmetto herbal blend with placebo in patients with symptomatic BPH. A nonsignificant symptomatic improvement was noted with saw palmetto [16] *Level P*

Acceptability to patient
For men who wish to try complementary therapy, it may be highly acceptable.

Follow up plan

- Review every 3–6 months with International Prostate Symptom Score (IPSS) and uroflowmetry based on patient's scores
- Annual digital rectal examination
- Annual prostate-specific antigen estimation

Patient and caregiver information

As this treatment is not thought to be as effective as some others, your treatment may need to be changed if your symptoms worsen.

Endoscopic therapy
PROSTATIC STENT
Efficacy

- Good, particularly because stent technology has improved
- Improvement in approximately 90% of patients
- Useful for patients who are not fit enough for a surgical procedure, either on a temporary or permanent basis
- Evidence is unclear whether it should be used in acute or chronic retention

Risks/Benefits

Risks:

- 'Older' style stents (which epithelialize) may be difficult to remove
- May cause discomfort
- May dislodge
- Incontinence
- No tissue available for histological examination
- Expensive
- Stent may fail and need to be replaced
- Can only be placed where the prostatic urethra is 2.0cm or longer
- May be associated with infection, intractable frequency

Benefits:

- Minimally invasive procedure, performed under local anesthetic with flexible cystoscope
- No bleeding
- Newer, nonepithelializing stents can be readily changed if necessary

Acceptability to patient

- Degree of safety may make the procedure more acceptable to old and frail patients
- May be unacceptable if the stent causes significant discomfort

Follow up plan

Review every 3–6 months to assure patient is not having any problems related to the stent.

Patient and caregiver information

See your doctor if you experience increasing discomfort, incontinence, or difficulty in passing urine, as the stent may need to be changed or removed.

BALLOON DILATATION OF PROSTATE
Efficacy
- Effective in selected patients, but relapse is common after 2–3 years
- Not often used at present

Risks/Benefits
Risks:
- No prostatic tissue available for histological examination
- Likely to need a further procedure in 2–3 years

Benefits:
- Minimally invasive procedure
- Minimal or no bleeding
- Suitable for elderly, frail patients

Acceptability to patient
- High degree of safety may make this acceptable to elderly, frail patients
- Younger, fitter patients may find the need for repeat procedures unacceptable

Follow up plan
- Review every 6 months with International Prostate Symptom Score and uroflowmetry. Be aware that a repeat procedure is likely to be required if symptoms deteriorate
- Annual digital rectal examination
- Annual prostate-specific antigen

Patient and caregiver information
Although this procedure may relieve your symptoms, it is likely that it will need to be performed again in 2–3 years.

Other therapies
WATCHFUL WAITING
Risks/Benefits
Risks:
- Symptoms may worsen
- No tissue for histological examination

Benefits:
- No medical or surgical therapy
- No side-effects

Acceptability to patient
Lack of surgery or side-effects from medication may make this highly acceptable.

Follow up plan
Review every 3–6 months as symptoms may worsen, and treatment may then be required.

Patient and caregiver information
Your symptoms may become worse in the future. If that happens, treatment such as tablets or surgery may be required.

LIFESTYLE

Avoiding caffeinated and alcoholic beverages and highly spiced foods may lead to some improvement in symptoms.

RISKS/BENEFITS

Risk:

■ Improvement in symptoms may not be maintained, especially if patient is not on any treatment

Benefits:

■ Useful adjunct to watchful waiting or pharmacotherapy
■ Symptomatic improvement

ACCEPTABILITY TO PATIENT

Patients may find avoiding caffeinated and alcoholic beverages in particular very restrictive.

PATIENT AND CAREGIVER INFORMATION

Although avoiding certain foods and drinks may make you feel better for a while, your symptoms may well worsen in the future.

EFFICACY OF THERAPIES
Evidence

- Alpha-blockers are more effective than placebo in improving lower urinary tract symptoms in men with benign prostatic hyperplasia (BPH). There is comparable efficacy among the different antagonists (alfuzosin, terazosin, doxazosin and tamsulosin) [1] *Level M*
- 5-alpha adrenergic blockers and finasteride have been found to be effective for symptom reduction in BPH, with similar efficacy noted for all alpha-adrenergic blockers [2] *Level M*
- A meta-analysis compared finasteride with placebo. A significantly greater reduction in symptom scores was noted in the treatment group, especially for men with large prostates [5] *Level M*
- Terazosin therapy has been associated with a greater reduction in symptoms than finasteride [4] *Level P*
- Transurethral resection of the prostate (TURP) has been found to significantly improve International Prostate Symptom (IPSS) score when compared with conservative management [8] *Level P*
- Several randomized controlled trials have found similar efficacy for transurethral incision of the prostate (TUIP) and TURP in the symptomatic management of men with smaller prostates [9] *Level P*
- International Prostate Symptom Score (IPSS) and peak flow rate were significantly reduced in patients treated with transurethral microwave thermotherapy (TUMT) at 6 months compared with placebo [10] *Level P*
- There is conflicting evidence comparing the short-term efficacy of TUMT with TURP [9]
- A significantly greater benefit was noted for patients treated with TURP compared with transurethral needle ablation (TUNA) in a randomized controlled trial, although TUNA was associated with less bleeding and retrograde ejaculation than TURP [13] *Level P*
- *Serenoa repens* improves urologic symptoms and flow measures compared with placebo, and compared with finasteride [14] *Level M*

PROGNOSIS
Varies, but some patients' symptoms will not deteriorate, even without treatment.

Clinical pearls

- In the absence of risk of cancer or obstruction, treatment should be guided by the patient's decision. Patients may be willing to tolerate quite severe symptoms and opt for no intervention
- Men with prostate glands in excess of 40g, elevated International Prostate Symptom Score (IPSS), and elevated age-related prostate-specific antigen (PSA) are at increased risk of acute urinary retention
- In patients with prostate glands that weigh 40g or more, the combination of an alpha-blocker and a 5-alpha reductase inhibitor can be used effectively and with few side-effects
- In young men with a moderately raised IPSS and voiding complaints, the use of saw palmetto is an effective first step. Start with this, and an alpha-blocker may be added if the patient does not realize a measurable benefit within 3 months. Test the efficacy with the use of the IPSS and uroflowmetry
- Balloon dilatation of the prostate is ineffective

Therapeutic failure

- If watchful waiting fails, consider commencing pharmacotherapy, or refer for surgery
- If pharmacotherapy fails, consider referring for surgery

Recurrence
Patient should be referred to a urologist if symptoms recur after pharmacotherapy or surgery.

Deterioration

If a patient's symptoms deteriorate despite active treatment, he should be referred if this has not been done already.

COMPLICATIONS

■ Obstructive renal failure may develop if bladder emptying is poor. This complication should improve or resolve when the obstruction is relieved

■ Hypotonic or atonic bladder may develop if the patient has high post micturition residuals for a considerable time. This may not improve after obstruction is relieved, and patient may continue to have high post micturition residuals

■ Urinary tract infection or bladder calculi may occur if bladder emptying is poor

CONSIDER CONSULT

■ Refer patients with high urinary residuals

■ Refer patients with renal failure

■ Refer if prostate-specific antigen (PSA) is high, even if the patient clinically does not appear to have prostate cancer

PREVENTION

The development of benign prostatic hyperplasia is thought to be a part of the aging process. Currently prevention is not possible and screening for detection of early disease is not appropriate.

ASSOCIATIONS
National Kidney and Urologic Diseases Information Clearinghouse
Box NKUDIC
Bethesda
MD 20893
Tel: (301) 468-6345
http://www.niddk.nih.gov/

KEY REFERENCES
- Walsh PC. Campbell's Urology, 7th edn. Philadelphia: Harcourt, 1998
- Marks LS. Effects of a saw palmetto herbal blend in men with symptomatic benign prostatic hyperplasia. J Urol 2000;163(5):1451–6
- Lepor H. The efficacy of terazosin, finasteride, or both in benign prostatic hyperplasia. Veterans Affairs Cooperative Studies Benign Prostatic Hyperplasia Study Group. N Engl J Med 1996;335:8 533–9
- Blaivas JG. Obstructive uropathy in the male. Urol Clin North Am 1996;23:373–384
- Ramsey EW. Office treatment of benign prostatic hyperplasia. Urol Clin North Am 1998;25:571–580
- Guthrie R. Benign prostatic hyperplasia in elderly men. What are the special issues in treatment? Postgrad Med 1997;101:141–3,148:151–4
- Ball AJ, Feneley RCL, Abrams PH. The natural history of untreated 'prostatism'. Br J Urol 1981;53:613–616
- McConnell JD, Barry MJ, Buskewitz RC, et al. Benign prostatic hyperplasia: diagnosis and treatment. Clinical Practice Guidelines, no. 8. AHCPR publication number 94–0582. Rockville, Maryland. The Agency for Health Care Policy and Research, Public Health Service, US Department of Health and Human Services, 1994
- Moody JA, Lingeman JE. Holmium laser enucleation of the prostate with tissue morcellation: initial United States experience. J Endourol 2000;14:219–223
- Roehrborn CG, Boyle P, Gould AL, et al. Serum prostate specific antigen as a predictor of prostate volume in men with benign prostatic hyperplasia. Urology 1999;53:581–9
- Djavan B, Marberger M. A meta-analysis on the efficacy and tolerability of alpha-1 adrenoceptor antagonists in patients with lower urinary tract symptoms suggestive of benign prostatic obstruction. Eur Urol 1999;36:1–13
- Boyle P, Gould AL, Roehrborn CG. Prostate volume predicts outcome of treatment of benign prostatic hyperplasia with finasteride. Urology 1996;48:398–405
- Roehrborn CG, Oesterling JF, Auerbach S, et al. The Hytrin community assessment trial study. Urology 1996;47:159–168
- Wasson, J, Reda D, Bruskewitz RC, et al. A comparison of transurethral surgery with watchful waiting for moderate symptoms of benign prostatic hyperplasia. N Engl J Med 1995;332:75–79
- Orandi A. Transurethral resection of the prostate. J Urol 1973;110:229–231
- Miller J, Edyvane KA, Sinclair GR, et al. A comparison of bladder neck incision and transurethral prostatic resection. Aust N Z J Surg 1992;62:116–122
- Ahmed M, Bell T, Lawrence WT, et al. Transurethral microwave thermotreatment compared to transurethral resection of the prostate for BPH; a randomized controlled parallel study. Br J Urol 1997;79:181–185
- Francisca EA, D'Ancone FC, Meuleman EJ, et al. Sexual function following high energy microwave thermotreatment. J Urol 1999;161:486–490
- Roehrborn C, Preminger G, Newhall P, et al. Microwave thermotherapy for BPH; results of a randomized, controlled, double blind multicenter sham-controlled trial. Urology 1998;51:19–28
- Thomas PJ, Britton JP, Harrison NW. The ProstaKath stent; four years experience. Br J Urol 1993;71:430–432
- Isogawa Y, Ohmori K. Application of urethral stents under metal bougie guidance. Hinyokika Kiyo 1993;39:231–235

Evidence references

1 Djavan B, Marberger M. A meta-analysis on the efficacy and tolerability of alpha-1 adrenoceptor antagonists in patients with lower urinary tract symptoms suggestive of benign prostatic obstruction. Eur Urol 1999;36:1–13. Reviewed in Clinical Evidence 2001;5:588–598.

2 Clifford GM, Farmer RD. Medical therapy for benign prostatic hyperplasia: a review of the literature. Eur Urol 2000;38:2–19. In: Clinical Evidence 2001;5:588–598.

3 Roehrborn CG, Oesterling JE, Auerbach S, et al. The Hytrin Community Assessment Trial study: a one-year study of terazosin versus placebo in the treatment of men with symptomatic benign prostatic hyperplasia. HYCAT Investigator Group. Urology 1996;47:159–68. Reviewed in: Clinical Evidence 2001;5:588–598.

4 Lepor H, Williford WO, Barry MJ. The efficacy of terazocin, finasteride, or both in benign prostatic hyperplasia. Veterans Affairs Cooperative Studies Benign Prostatic Hyperplasia Study Group. N Engl J Med 1996;335:533–9. Medline

5 Boyle P, Gould AL, Roehrborn CG. Prostate volume predicts outcome of treatment of benign prostatic hyperplasia with finasteride: meta-analysis of randomised clinical trials. Urology 1996;48:398–405. Reviewed in: Clinical Evidence 2001;5:588–598.

6 McConnell J, Bruskewitz R, Walsh P, et al. The effect of finasteride on the risk of acute urinary retention and the need for surgical treatment among men with benign prostatic hyperplasia. N Engl J Med 1998;338:557–563. Reviewed in: Clinical Evidence 2001;5:588–598.

7 Wasson JH, Reda DJ, Bruskewitz RC, et al. A comparison of transurethral surgery with watchful waiting for moderate symptoms of benign prostatic hyperplasia. The Veterans Affairs Cooperative Study Group on Transurethral Resection of the Prostate. N Engl J Med 1995;332:75–79. Reviewed in: Clinical Evidence 2001;5:588–598.

8 Donovan JL, Peters T, Neal DE, et al. A randomized trial comparing transurethral resection of the prostate, laser therapy and conservative treatment of men with symptoms associated with benign prostatic enlargement: the ClasP study. J Urol 2000;164:65–70. Reviewed in: Clinical evidence 2001;5:588–598.

9 Barry M, Roehrborn C. Benign Prostatic hyperplasia. Men's health. In: Clinical Evidence 2001;5:588–598. London: BMJ Publishing Group.

10 Roehrborn CG, Preminger G, Newhall P, et al. Microwave thermotherapy for benign prostatic hyperplasia with the Dornier Urowave: results of a randomized, double blind, multicenter, sham-controlled trial. Urology 1998;51:19–28. Reviewed in: Clinical Evidence 2001;5:588–598.

11 Francisca EA, d'Ancona FC, Meuleman EJ, et al. Sexual function following high energy microwave thermotherapy: results of a randomized controlled study comparing transurethral microwave thermotherapy to transurethral prostatatic resection. J Urol 1999;161:486–490. Reviewed in: Clinical Evidence 2001;5:588–598.

12 Djavan B, Roehrborn CG, Shariat S, et al. Prospective randomized comparison of high energy transurethral microwave thermotherapy versus alpha blocker treatment of patients with benign prostatic hyperplasia. J Urol 1999;161:139–143. Reviewed in: Clinical Evidence 2001;5:588–598.

13 Bruskewitz R, Issa M, Roehrborn C, et al. A prospective, randomized 1-year clinical trial comparing transurethral needle ablation to transurethral resection of the prostate for the treatment of symptomatic benign prostatic hyperplasia. J Urol 1998;159:1588–1594. Reviewed in: Clinical Evidence 2001;5:588–598.

14 Wilt T, Ishani A, Stark G, et al. Serenoa repens for benign prostatic hyperplasia (Cochrane Review). In: The Cochrane Library, 4, 2001. Oxford: Update Software.

15 Boyle P, Robertson C, Lowe F, Roehrborn C. Meta–analysis of clinical trials of Permixon in the treatment of benign prostatic hyperplasia. Urology 2000;55:533–539. Reviewed in: Clinical Evidence 2001;5:588–598.

16 Marks LS, Partin AW, Epstein JI, et al. Effects of a saw palmetto herbal blend in men with symptomatic benign prostatic hyperplasia. J Urol 2000;163:1451–6. Medline

FAQS
Question 1
What is the role of the prostate?

ANSWER 1
- Unclear
- Known to provide the major portion of the ejaculate
- Nutritional aspects for spermatozoa function and survival
- Proteases that liquefy the ejaculate

Question 2
What is zonal anatomy of the prostate?

ANSWER 2
Described by McNeal, the prostate consists of a combination of glandular tissues (which make up 66% of the prostate) and fibromuscular structures (which make up 33% of the prostate).

There are the following zones of glandular tissue:
- The peripheral zone, which is the site of most cancers of the prostate
- The transition zone, which is the source of benign prostatic hypertrophy and 20% of the cancers
- The periurethral glands, which are involved in the growth of the middle lobe
- The central zone, which surrounds the ejaculatory duct, is relatively resistant to cancers (10% occurrence)
- The fibromuscular structures, which include the anterior fibromuscular stroma, the pre- and postprostatic sphincters, and longitudinal smooth muscle

Question 3
What is the basic diagnostic testing required to assess bladder outlet obstruction?

ANSWER 3
- The International Prostate Symptom Score
- Uroflow with bladder scan for postvoiding residual volume

Question 4
What are the long-term effects of untreated BPH?

ANSWER 4
- Recurrent urinary tract infection
- Bladder decompensation, leading to urinary retention
- Bladder stones
- Vesicoureteral reflux
- Hydroureteronephrosis
- Chronic renal failure
- Acute renal failure

Question 5
Where do alpha-blockers work in patients with BPH?

ANSWER 5
- In the alpha receptors of the trigone of the bladder
- In the fibromuscular stroma of the prostate

CONTRIBUTORS
Randolph L Pearson, MD
Phillip J Aliotta, MD, MHA, FACS
John Pinski, MD

BLADDER INJURY

DESCRIPTION

Bladder injury can occur as a result of either blunt trauma or penetrating trauma. It is usually classified as:

- Contusion – a diagnosis of exclusion. The diagnosis is made in the patient with a history of trauma but negative radiographic studies of the upper tracts, negative cystogram with normal bladder contours, and in patients presenting with gross hematuria after a long-distance run
- Intraperitoneal rupture
- Extraperitoneal rupture
- Both intraperitoneal and extraperitoneal

Also:

- Hematuria is an almost universal finding
- May not be recognized at time of injury
- Minor injuries may be managed by a urinary catheter alone
- Major injuries require open repair, and may be fatal

URGENT ACTION

All patients with suspected bladder injury should be referred urgently to the hospital for further investigation and appropriate management.

KEY! DON'T MISS!

If blood is present at the urethral meatus, suspect urethral injury. Do not attempt to pass urethral catheter, and arrange for urgent transfer to the hospital.

ICD9 CODE
596.9 Unspecified disorder of bladder

SYNONYMS
- Bladder trauma
- Bladder contusion and bladder rupture indicate degrees of severity of injury

CARDINAL FEATURES
- May be caused by blunt or penetrating trauma
- May follow transurethral bladder procedures
- Bladder rupture can be intraperitoneal or extraperitoneal
- May not be recognized at time of injury
- Hematuria is an almost universal finding
- Minor injuries may be managed by urinary catheterization
- Major injuries require open repair, and may be fatal in some cases

CAUSES
Common causes
Easy acronym to identify cause: IS IT?
- I = Iatrogenic-Instrumental: a recent history of cystoscopy, laparoscopy, intra-abdominal or vaginal surgery, catheterization, or self-instrumentation
- S = Spontaneous: usually occurs in association with intermittent catheterization, bladder augmentation, or known bladder dysfunction
- I = Intoxicated: any patient with acute or chronic alcohol abuse history who presents with any one of the following three findings; inability to void, hematuria, or a history of trauma (regardless of the severity)
- T = Traumatic: blunt lower abdominal trauma, pelvic fracture, proximal femoral fracture, and penetrating wound(s) to the abdomen or back

Blunt trauma (86%):
- Blow to abdomen
- Motor vehicle accident, especially if wearing a seatbelt
- Pelvic fracture: shearing force of injury may tear bladder, or a spicule of bone may lacerate it

Penetrating trauma (14%):
- Stab wound
- Gunshot wound
- Operative injury following abdominal or pelvic surgery, especially transurethral procedures

Rare causes
- Migration and erosion of foreign materials, especially surgical drains, intrauterine contraceptive devices, hip prostheses, urinary catheters
- Spontaneous rupture: usually the patient has pre-existing bladder pathology (e.g. chronic retention); most likely associated with minor blunt trauma

Serious causes
Major trauma.

Contributory or predisposing factors
State of bladder filling:
- Empty bladder is more susceptible to extraperitoneal rupture
- Full bladder is more susceptible to intraperitoneal rupture

EPIDEMIOLOGY
Incidence and prevalence
FREQUENCY

Frequency of bladder rupture by mechanism of injury is:

- External trauma 82%
- Iatrogenic 14%
- Intoxicated 2.9%
- Spontaneous <0.1%

Of all bladder injuries, 60–85% are caused by blunt trauma and 15–40% are caused by penetrating injury.

Demographics
AGE

- May occur at any age
- Incidence of intraperitoneal rupture is higher in children because of predominantly intra-abdominal location of bladder before puberty
- The adult bladder is mostly an extraperitoneal organ located deep within the pelvis and is protected by the bony pelvis laterally, the symphysis pubis anteriorly, the pelvic floor inferiorly, and the rectum posteriorly
- The pediatric bladder is primarily an intraperitoneal organ that lies just beneath the anterior abdominal wall and is therefore more vulnerable to external trauma. With age the bladder descends into the true pelvis. The bladder is in the adult position by the end of the sixth year

DIFFERENTIAL DIAGNOSIS
Bladder injury must be distinguished from injuries to other intrapelvic and abdominal organs. Such injuries may coexist in multiple trauma cases.

SIGNS & SYMPTOMS
Signs
Classic triad for bladder injury:
- Suprapubic or perineal pain and tenderness – bruising over suprapubic or pelvic region; abdominal tenderness
- Difficulty or inability to void – low urine output
- Hematuria: hematuria is an almost universal finding; gross hematuria is seen in >95% cases

Other signs:
- Hypotension may be present, but rarely caused by bladder injury alone; suspect coexisting injuries
- Abdominal distension – if recognition of injury is delayed, urinoma may develop
- Absent bowel sounds, especially in intraperitoneal rupture
- Rectal examination may reveal distorted landmarks due to pelvic hematoma

Symptoms
- May initially be asymptomatic
- Difficulty in passing urine: patient may complain of difficulty or inability to void
- Lower abdominal pain
- Shoulder tip pain due to diaphragmatic irritation if intraperitoneal urine collects under diaphragm

ASSOCIATED DISORDERS
- Associated intra-abdominal or pelvic trauma is common
- Patients with bladder injury caused by gunshot wounds have associated bowel injuries in up to 83% cases
- Vascular injuries are reportedly as high as 82% in patients with penetrating bladder injury
- Concurrent urethral injury in 10% of male patients
- Concurrent renal injury in 2% of patients
- Concurrent pelvic fracture in 90% of patients

KEY! DON'T MISS!
If blood is present at the urethral meatus, suspect urethral injury. Do not attempt to pass urethral catheter, and arrange for urgent transfer to the hospital.

CONSIDER CONSULT
- All patients with suspected bladder injury should be referred on an urgent basis to a urologist or trauma specialist
- Speed of transfer to the hospital will be influenced by patient's overall condition

INVESTIGATION OF THE PATIENT
Direct questions to patient
Q Do you remember anything about your accident? Mechanism of injury may give a clue to diagnosis.
Q Have you had any recent surgery on your bladder or prostate? A recent resection of prostate or bladder tumor may have caused bladder perforation.
Q Have you passed urine since the accident? If patient has been able to pass urine, then the presence of severe bladder or urethral injury is less likely.

Contributory or predisposing factors

Q **Have you any history of bladder problems?** Patients with pre-existing bladder pathology may be at risk for spontaneous rupture.

Examination

- **Check temperature:** pyrexia may be present; in the context of bladder injury, this may suggest peritonitis, which is more likely if injury is diagnosed late
- **Check pulse and blood pressure:** tachycardia and hypotension may be present; if marked, suspect additional injuries
- **Examine the abdomen:** for evidence of distension and/or tenderness, which may be diffuse or localized suprapubically
- **Auscultate the abdomen:** bowel sounds may be absent due to ileus
- **Examine the external genitalia:** blood at the urethral orifice (especially in males) suggests urethral injury
- **Examine the urine:** gross hematuria is usually present. If not, perform urinalysis. If no hematuria of either type present, then bladder injury is the less likely diagnosis
- **Check the prostate:** a free-floating prostate is an indication of prostatomembranous urethral disruption. No attempt at catheter passage and immediate referral to urologist or trauma specialist

Summary of investigative tests

- Urinalysis: dipstick test should be performed regardless if gross hematuria is not seen
- Complete blood count (CBC): low hemoglobin may indicate acute blood loss. Leukocytosis with a left shift may also indicate rupture
- Creatinine and blood urea nitrogen (BUN) estimation: acute renal failure may be present; serum BUN and creatinine may rise if patient with intraperitoneal rupture has significant volume of urine lying in the peritoneal cavity
- Cystogram: will diagnose majority of bladder injuries. Normally performed by a specialist
- If concurrent urethral injury is suspected, then retrograde urethrogram must be performed before attempting to insert a urinary catheter. A specialist normally performs this test
- Abdominal and pelvic ultrasound: will provide rapid assessment of most intra-abdominal and pelvic organs and will identify whether any 'free fluid' (e.g. urine) is present within the abdomen. A specialist normally performs this test
- Abdominal and pelvic CT scan: provides detailed assessment of intra-abdominal and pelvic organs. May identify the presence of free fluid within the abdomen, but may not identify bladder rupture if bladder is not distended with contrast material. Normally performed by a specialist
- Cystoscopy: occasionally performed to identify and evaluate size and extent of injury. Performed by a specialist

DIAGNOSTIC DECISION

Bladder injury should be suspected in a patient with gross hematuria and a history of recent trauma. Diagnosis is usually confirmed on the basis of cystogram findings.

CLINICAL PEARLS

- The superior surface or dome of the bladder is the weakest and least supported part of the bladder and is the only surface completely covered by the peritoneum
- Extraperitoneal rupture is more common than intraperitoneal rupture
- It has been estimated that pressures $>300 cmH_2O$ are required to rupture a normal bladder
- In patients with an acute bladder laceration, laboratory evaluations other than urinalysis are rarely of any benefit. In contrast, if the time from bladder rupture to clinical presentation is prolonged, serum electrolyte determination, renal function testing, and a complete blood cell count may help in establishing the diagnosis of bladder injury

- Intraperitoneal extravasation can lead to absorption if urine producing hyperchloremic metabolic acidosis, hypernatremia, azotemia, and leukocytosis with a left shift. Although the majority of these laboratory abnormalities take several hours to develop, azotemia secondary to an intraperitoneal rupture may occur within 30min of the injury

THE TESTS
Body fluids
URINALYSIS (DIPSTICK)
Description
Urine specimen. Usually midstream, but in context of trauma may be catheter specimen.

Advantages/Disadvantages
Advantages:
- Quick and simple to perform at office level
- If no hematuria present, then bladder injury is very unlikely to be present

Disadvantages:
- Nonspecific; not diagnostic of bladder trauma
- Presence of a urinary catheter may lead to spurious results

Normal
No red or white blood cells, or protein present.

Abnormal
- Red and/or white blood cells, and/or protein present
- Keep in mind the possibility of a false-positive result

Cause of abnormal result
Blood from traumatized bladder released into urine.

Drugs, disorders and other factors that may alter results
- Urinary catheter can produce a false-positive result, caused by either trauma of passing catheter, or irritant nature of catheter within bladder
- Menstruation may lead to a false-positive result
- Certain foods and medications may lead to false-positive results

COMPLETE BLOOD COUNT (CBC)
Description
Venous blood sample.

Advantages/Disadvantages
Advantages:
- Confirms or excludes anemia
- Mandatory for evaluating severity of acute blood loss (although this may not be appropriate in the primary care situation)

Disadvantages:
- Does not indicate underlying cause of anemia
- Children especially may find venipuncture distressing

Normal
Hemoglobin:
- Men – 15+/-2g/dL (150+/-20g/L)
- Women – 13.5+/-1.5g/dL (135+/-15g/L)

Abnormal
Hemoglobin:
- Men – <15+/-2g/dL (<150+/-20g/L)
- Women – <13.5+/-1.5g/dL (<135+/-15g/L)

Cause of abnormal result
Acute blood loss.

Drugs, disorders and other factors that may alter results
Anemia is seen as part of many disorders, and may be unrelated to bladder trauma.

SERUM BLOOD UREA NITROGEN (BUN) AND CREATININE
Description
Venous blood sample.

Advantages/Disadvantages
Advantage: mandatory for assessing whether renal function is impaired

Disadvantages:
- Abnormal findings are not diagnostic of any particular type of trauma
- Children especially may find venipuncture distressing

Normal
- Urea (BUN): 10–20mg/dL (3.6–7.1mmol/L)
- Creatinine: <1.5mg/dL (<133mcmol/L)

Abnormal
- Urea (BUN): >20mg/dL (>7.1mmol/L)
- Creatinine: >1.5mg/dL (>133mcmol/L)

Cause of abnormal result
- Acute renal failure in patients with severe injuries
- In patients with urinoma formation, resorption of nitrogenous waste products may occur in the peritoneal cavity. Typically, BUN is increased proportionally greater than creatinine
- Keep in mind the possibility of a falsely abnormal result

Drugs, disorders and other factors that may alter results
Laboratory technique can affect results.

Imaging
RETROGRADE URETHROGRAM
Description
Diluted contrast medium is injected into distal urethra and radiographic images obtained of urethra and bladder.

Advantages/Disadvantages
Advantage: detects urethral injury

Disadvantages:
- Involves exposure to ionizing radiation
- Experience required to perform examination correctly

Normal
Intact urethra and bladder.

Abnormal
- Extravasation of contrast if urethra injured
- Distorted bladder outline if contusion present

Cause of abnormal result
Urethral or bladder injury.

Drugs, disorders and other factors that may alter results
- Operator experience may affect results
- Not recommended for primary care provider or any other healthcare provider without appropriate training

CT SCAN OF ABDOMEN AND PELVIS
Description
Computed tomographic (CT) scan of abdomen and pelvis, often first test performed on patients with blunt abdominal trauma.

Advantages/Disadvantages
Advantages:
- Provides detailed information about most abdominal and pelvic organs
- May identify multiple injuries, if present
- Will identify free fluid if present in abdomen or pelvis
- CT cystogram may be done concurrently with 300mL of contrast in bladder

Disadvantages:
- Involves exposure to ionizing radiation
- Requires expertise to perform and interpret
- May not adequately delineate the bladder unless it is forcibly distended

Normal
Normal appearance of abdominal and pelvic organs.

Abnormal
Trauma to individual organs may be identified.

Drugs, disorders and other factors that may alter results
If bladder is empty (which may be the case if it has ruptured) it may be difficult to assess accurately.

Other tests
CYSTOSCOPY
Description
Endoscopic examination of bladder.

Advantages/Disadvantages
Advantages:
- Provides visual assessment of bladder injury
- Can be performed under local anesthetic if necessary

Disadvantages:

- Must be performed by specialist
- Bladder irrigant fluid may leak out of bladder, adding to that already extravasated

Normal
Intact bladder.

Abnormal
Bladder contusion(s) or rupture.

PATIENT AND CAREGIVER ISSUES
Forensic and legal issues
Particularly in the presence of multiple and/or life-threatening injuries, emergency treatment may need to begin without the patient's consent.

Impact on career, dependants, family, friends
Impact varies depending on severity of bladder injuries, any associated injuries, and any underlying pathology (e.g. bladder tumor). May be of no or minimal impact, but if injuries are severe and/or significant other pathology is present, then they may have significant and long-lasting impact on patient's ability to attend school, work, or undertake social activities.

Health-seeking behavior
Has patient delayed seeking medical attention? Patients with blunt trauma may delay seeking medical attention because they do not recognize the potential severity of their injuries, or they may not remember the accident taking place.

MANAGEMENT ISSUES
Goals
- Early identification of bladder injury so that patient can be referred and treated appropriately with a minimum of delay
- Identification of any coexisting injuries so that they may be treated appropriately

Management in special circumstances
SPECIAL PATIENT GROUPS

Multiple trauma: if patient has intra-abdominal injuries requiring laparotomy, then it may be appropriate to perform an open repair of any bladder injury, even if it would be managed with a urethral catheter if it was the only injury present.

PATIENT SATISFACTION/LIFESTYLE PRIORITIES

Patients want treatment that, on recovery, will allow a normally functioning bladder.

SUMMARY OF THERAPEUTIC OPTIONS
Choices
Choices to be made by the urologist or trauma specialist:
- The choice of treatment is based on mechanism of injury (blunt or penetrating) and type of injury (intraperitoneal or extraperitoneal)
- Oftentimes, individuals with a bladder contusion may have associated injuries that make monitoring outputs necessary with a catheter
- All penetrating injuries require urgent surgical exploration
- All intraperitoneal ruptures caused by penetrating trauma, and the majority of those caused by blunt trauma require surgical exploration and repair
- Extraperitoneal rupture due to blunt trauma in many cases may be managed conservatively with catheter drainage for 7–10 days. If there is evidence of a large tear on cystography, other imaging, or cystoscopy, open repair should be performed. Other indications for open exploration after a conservative trial with Foley catheter drainage are persistent extravasation, severe bleeding, and sepsis
- In follow-up, a voiding cystogram should be performed to rule out injury to the bladder neck and urethra

Clinical pearls

- If the fluid from a urinary source in the abdomen shows a fluid-to-creatinine ratio greater than a factor of 1, it is strongly suggestive of urinary extravasation
- Instillation of methylene blue into the catheter located in the bladder, in the absence of vesicoureteral reflux, with resultant leakage of blue from the incision, confirms injury to the bladder and not the ureter
- There is controversy regarding the adequacy of CT vs cystogram to make the diagnosis of bladder laceration/rupture. The biggest problem in making the diagnosis is the adequacy of bladder filling. Underfilling of the bladder leads to a misdiagnosis. To prevent misdiagnosis: fill the bladder with contrast material via gravity from a height of 75cm above the level of the pelvis; instill a minimum of 400mL of contrast in the adult; in children instill 60mL plus an additional 30mL per year of age up to a maximum of 400mL; and instill contrast until a bladder contraction occurs
- Obtain the following films at the time of evaluation: precontrast kidney-ureter-bladder (KUB); an anteroposterior (AP) view with the bladder distended; an oblique view with the bladder distended; and another AP view with the bladder drained. Note: from a clinical perspective, more often than not in the case of a pelvis fracture, the oblique view is not practical because of the degree of pain
- In the case of spontaneous rupture, a CT scan is advocated in place of because of the small perforation that typically occurs and spontaneously seals prior to instillation of contrast. The CT scan while failing to show the leak will document free air or fluid in the peritoneum

Never

- Never catheterize a patient if urethral injury is suspected. In an emergency situation, a suprapubic tube placed percutaneously can be performed only by trained personnel
- Ideally, discuss all patients with admitting surgeon before catheterization

FOLLOW UP
Plan for review

- Following discharge from the hospital, most patients will be kept under review by their surgeon
- Duration of review period depends on patient's individual circumstances

Information for patient or caregiver

- Patients with bladder injury usually require hospital admission for assessment and observation
- Patients with serious injuries usually require surgery to repair the bladder

DRUGS AND OTHER THERAPIES: DETAILS
Surgical therapy
LAPAROTOMY AND OPEN REPAIR OF BLADDER INJURY
Any large tear in the bladder, and most intraperitoneal ruptures, will require open repair.

Efficacy
High.

Risks/Benefits
Risks:
- General anesthetic required
- Fistula formation

Benefits:
- Definitive closure of bladder tear
- Any other injuries can be dealt with concurrently

Acceptability to patient
Most seriously ill or injured patients will accept the need for surgery.

Follow up plan
Patient will remain in the hospital until recovering. After discharge, may be reviewed by surgeon; patients with underlying pathology (e.g. bladder tumor) will have life-long follow-up.

Patient and caregiver information
Patient will have a urinary catheter in place while bladder is healing. It should only be removed on advice of surgeon.

Other therapies
URINARY CATHETER
Efficacy
Highly effective for treatment of minor bladder injuries.

Risks/Benefits
Risks:
- Not suitable for large tears in the bladder. Clinical judgment necessary to decide whether surgery is more appropriate
- May provide focus for infection

Benefits:
- Nonoperative treatment
- Patient may be allowed to go home from the hospital with catheter in place, if well enough

Acceptability to patient
Patient may find catheter uncomfortable.

Follow up plan
When catheter is removed (usually following a cystogram), the patient requires a period of close observation (usually in the hospital) to ensure that he/she is passing urine adequately and without pain. Further follow-up after discharge will depend on the individual patient's circumstances. For trauma cases, this may be until patient is fully recovered. If patient has underlying pathology (e.g. bladder tumor), follow-up will be life-long.

Patient and caregiver information
Catheter needs to remain in place while bladder is healing. It should only be removed on advice of physician.

OUTCOMES

EFFICACY OF THERAPIES
- Urinary catheterization is highly effective treatment for minor injuries, but is of no or minimal benefit in serious bladder trauma. The duration of time the catheter needs to remain in situ varies with surgeon preference; minimum length of time would be several days, but often it needs to remain in for over 7 days
- Open repair is highly effective, but length of time to recovery depends on many factors, including any associated injuries, and overall health of patient

Review period
- Varies with patient's circumstances
- Patients with bladder injury alone will be discharged from review when fully recovered
- Patients with more severe injuries or underlying pathology may require life-long follow-up

PROGNOSIS
In general, complete recovery from an isolated minor bladder injury is to be expected. If patient has multiple injuries, or some underlying pathology, recovery period will depend on each individual patient's circumstances. In cases of multiple traumas, mortality rate may be up to 44%.

Clinical pearls
- Voiding cystourethrography (VCUG) is performed in the follow-up phase to assure that there is no disruption occurring at the bladder neck and urethra
- The individual with a pelvic fracture should be considered to have a bladder laceration until it is proved otherwise

Therapeutic failure
- If a bladder injury fails to heal with urinary catheterization, open repair is required
- If an open repair fails to heal, and urinary extravasation occurs, further laparotomy and repair are required
- In exceptional circumstances, the bladder may be too badly damaged to be repaired, and cystectomy may be required

COMPLICATIONS
- Urinary tract infection may occur, particularly if an indwelling catheter is present
- Peritonitis and sepsis: especially if intraperitoneal rupture is diagnosed late. May initially be a chemical peritonitis caused by urine, but infection may supervene
- Injuries involving the bladder neck and urethra may result in incontinence
- Hemorrhage with hypovolemic shock

CONSIDER CONSULT

- All patients should have been referred at the time of presentation and will be managed by specialists

PREVENTION

- In general, prevention of bladder injury in the community is not possible
- For patients undergoing surgical procedures in which bladder injuries may occur, such injuries are best prevented by careful surgical technique

MODIFY RISK FACTORS
SCREENING
Screening is not appropriate for bladder injury.

PREVENT RECURRENCE
Reassess coexisting disease
Patients who undergo regular cystoscopy for bladder tumor survcillance are at risk for repeated bladder injury. Prevention of recurrent injury is by careful surgical technique. Prevention is not possible in other groups.

RESOURCES

KEY REFERENCES

- Corriere JN Jr. Trauma to the lower urinary tract. In: Gillenwater JY, Grayback JT, Howards SS, Duckett JW, eds. Adult and pediatric urology. St Louis: Mosby, 1998, p563–9
- Peters PC, Sagalowsky AI. Genitourinary trauma. In: Walsh PC, ed. Campbell's urology, 7th edn. Philadelphia: WB Saunders, 1998, p316–328
- Cass AS. The multiple injured patient with bladder trauma. J Trauma 1984; 24:731
- Corriere JN Jr, Sandler CS. Mechanisms of injury, patterns of extravasation and management of extraperitoneal rupture due to blunt trauma. J Urol 1988;139:43
- Spirnak JP. Pelvic fracture and injury to the lower urinary tract. Surg Clin North Am 1988;68:1061

FAQS

Question 1

What types of bladder perforation may occur?

ANSWER 1

Bladder perforation can be intraperitoneal, extraperitoneal, or both.

Question 2

Do patients with a pelvic fracture and microscopic hematuria require formal bladder evaluation?

ANSWER 2

All patients with a history of pelvic fracture are assumed to have a bladder injury until proven otherwise.

Question 3

How are gunshot and/or stab wounds to the abdomen and pelvis treated?

ANSWER 3

All penetrating injuries to the abdomen and pelvis require surgical exploration by a qualified team of trauma specialists.

Question 4

What is the mechanism for intraperitoneal bladder perforation in patients with blunt abdominal trauma?

ANSWER 4

It is assumed that the bladder is full or near full and the individual suffers an abrupt increase in the intravesical pressure (in excess of 300cm H_2O), causing the bladder to perforate at its weakest point, which in most cases is the dome.

Question 5

How does extraperitoneal rupture occur?

ANSWER 5

Rupture can occur with pelvic fracture and perforation of the bladder from the bony fragments occurring near the bladder neck. It can also occur as a result of significant increase in the intravesical pressure from the traumatic event.

CONTRIBUTORS

Fred F Ferri, MD, FACP
Philip J Aliotta, MD, MHA, FACS
Anuj K Chopra, MD

BLADDER TUMORS

SUMMARY INFORMATION

DESCRIPTION

- Three main histologic types: transitional cell carcinoma, squamous carcinoma, and adenocarcinoma; transitional cell carcinoma is the most common in the US (>90%)
- May be asymptomatic until disease is advanced
- Majority of patients develop hematuria (microscopic or gross)
- Prognosis varies depending on how aggressive the disease is

URGENT ACTION

Patients with profuse hematuria, especially if accompanied by a palpable bladder and difficulty in micturition, should be transferred urgently to specialist care.

KEY! DON'T MISS!

Always investigate even a single episode of hematuria in an appropriate manner, as a single episode may be presenting sign of an underlying malignancy.

ICD9 CODE
- 188.9 Primary
- 198.1 Secondary
- 233.7 CIS
- 223.3 Benign
- 239.4 Uncertain behavior

SYNONYMS
- Bladder tumor
- Bladder neoplasm

CARDINAL FEATURES
- Three main histologic types: transitional cell carcinoma, squamous carcinoma, and adenocarcinoma
- Cigarette smoking is associated with the development of transitional cell carcinoma
- May be asymptomatic until disease is advanced
- Majority of patients develop hematuria (microscopic or gross)
- Pain is a late feature, indicating advanced disease
- Choice of treatment is influenced by histologic type and degree of invasiveness
- Prognosis varies depending on how aggressive the disease is

CAUSES
Common causes
Transitional cell carcinoma of the bladder:
- Cigarette smoking
- Industrial exposures

Squamous cell carcinoma of the bladder:
- Schistosomiasis: infection with *Schistosoma haematobium* (and also, less commonly, transitional cell carcinoma)
- Urinary calculi, if present for many years
- Indwelling catheters, if used for many years
- Bladder diverticula

Adenocarcinoma of the bladder:
- Neurogenic bladder
- Metastases from other primary malignancies
- Urachal remnant

Rare causes
Transitional cell carcinoma of the bladder:
- Occupational exposure: workers in dye, textile, tire, rubber, and petroleum industries
- Chemical exposure: O-toluidine, 2-naphthylamine, benzidine, 4-aminobiphenyl, nitrosamines

Adenocarcinoma of the bladder:
- Bladder extrophy
- Endometriosis
- Urachal abnormalities
- Secondary site for tumors from other organs, e.g. colon

Miscellaneous causes of bladder cancer:

- Phenacetin abuse: heavy consumption of analgesics containing phenacetin has been linked with the development of urothelial cancer
- Pelvic irradiation following, for example, radiotherapy for cervical cancer
- Tuberculosis

Serious causes
All causes may be classified as serious.

Contributory or predisposing factors
Spinal cord-injured patients with bladder neuropathy requiring long-term bladder drainage with a Foley catheter – long-term indwelling catheters are a risk for developing bladder cancer, usually squamous cell carcinoma.

EPIDEMIOLOGY
Incidence and prevalence
INCIDENCE

- Age 65–69: men 1.3/1000; women 0.35/1000
- Age 85 and over: men 2.85/1000; women 0.67/1000

FREQUENCY
Because many patients with bladder cancer experience recurrences, but do not die from the disease, it is the second most important malignancy in middle-aged and elderly men.

Demographics
AGE
Incidence increases with age: high >60 years; low <40 years.

GENDER

- Men: fourth most common cancer, accounting for 10% of all tumors
- Women: eighth most common cancer, accounting for 4% of all tumors
- Male:female ratio is 3:1

RACE

- Incidence in African-American males is about 50% of that for Caucasian males
- Bladder cancer is rare in Asians, Hispanic-Americans, and Native Americans

GENETICS

- Etiology is thought to be multifactorial, involving both genetic and environmental factors
- No epidemiologic evidence for a hereditary cause in most cases
- Familial clusters have been reported

GEOGRAPHY

- Incidence reported to be higher in the American north compared with the south
- Common in the US, Great Britain, and industrialized countries
- Rare in Japan and Finland

SOCIOECONOMIC STATUS

- An occupational link is well recognized and is thought to be due to exposure to a variety of chemicals, mainly aromatic amines
- Depending on frequency of exposure, there is a latent period of up to 50 years
- Occupations associated with development of bladder cancer include: autoworkers, painters, truck drivers, drill press operators, leather workers, metal workers, machinists, dry cleaners, paper manufacturers, rope and twine makers, dental technicians, barbers, beauticians, physicians, workers in apparel manufacturing, plumbers, and those in the tire industry

DIFFERENTIAL DIAGNOSIS
- A variety of conditions may mimic bladder cancer and may also be present concurrently
- Most important differential diagnosis is prostate cancer, which requires urgent referral so that patient's disease may be staged and appropriate treatment commenced

Urinary tract infection
The term urinary tract infection encompasses a broad range of clinical entities that have a positive urine culture in common.

FEATURES
- More common in women
- Patient may be generally ill with pyrexia, suprapubic discomfort, and loin pain
- Hematuria (gross or microscopic) may be present
- Often frequency and dysuria
- Can also be seen as a presenting complaint in patients with bladder cancer

Frequency-urgency syndrome
The need to pass urine with little warning and very frequently.

FEATURES
- More common in women
- Gross hematuria uncommon

Interstitial cystitis
Interstitial cystitis is characterized by frequent bouts of symptoms of urinary infection (burning, frequency and urgency of urination) without a bacterial infection actually being present.

FEATURES
- More common in women (10:1)
- Severe frequency and urgency
- Pain with full bladder, which resolves on bladder emptying

Bladder calculus
Calculi in the bladder are also called vesical calculi.

FEATURES
- Frequency, terminal dysuria, and hematuria
- May occur in men with bladder outflow obstruction
- If present for a long period, patient may develop squamous metaplasia, and subsequently squamous carcinoma of the bladder

Endometriosis
Endometriosis is the presence of functioning endometrial glands and stroma outside the uterine cavity.

FEATURES
- Most common in women <30 years
- Commonly symptoms of dysmenorrhea, dyspareunia, infertility
- Pelvic pain, if present, may be severe

Neurogenic bladder
A dysfunction that results from interference with the normal nerve pathways associated with urination.

FEATURES

- Seen in patients with a neurologic disorder, e.g. multiple sclerosis, spinal cord injury
- May be asymptomatic
- Some patients may be able to pass urine spontaneously, but be unable to fully empty their bladder
- Frequency, urgency, urge incontinence

Prostate cancer

Neoplasms involving the prostate are known as prostate cancer; >99% are adenocarcinomas.

FEATURES

- Symptoms may be identical to benign prostatic hyperplasia
- Palpable abnormality of the prostate on digital rectal examination (90%)
- Elevated prostate-specific antigen (PSA) (80%)
- Incidence increases with age: 80% of patients are aged 65 or more at the time of diagnosis
- Bone pain, pathologic fractures, and neurologic deficits seen in advanced disease

Benign prostatic hyperplasia

Benign prostatic hyperplasia is an almost universal finding in older men.

FEATURES

- May be asymptomatic
- Typically presents with a mixture of outflow obstruction and bladder irritability

SIGNS & SYMPTOMS
Signs

- Hematuria – either gross or microscopic – occurs in 80%
- Abdominal mass: bladder may be palpable if filled with blood clot or if a large tumor mass is present
- Anemia due to acute or chronic blood loss
- Cachexia in advanced disease

Symptoms

- May initially be asymptomatic
- Urinary frequency and urgency
- Dysuria
- Anorexia, weight loss in advanced disease
- Abdominal and bone pain in advanced disease
- Flank pain from ureteral obstruction or retroperitoneal metastasis

ASSOCIATED DISORDERS

- Urinary tract infection – may be a presenting feature
- Benign prostatic hyperplasia – may be a comorbid finding
- Prostatic cancer – may coexist and produce symptomatic complaints

KEY! DON'T MISS!

Always investigate even a single episode of hematuria in an appropriate manner, as a single episode may be presenting sign of an underlying malignancy.

CONSIDER CONSULT

- All patients with suspected bladder cancer should be referred urgently to an urologist
- Patients with profuse hematuria may require urgent admission to hospital

INVESTIGATION OF THE PATIENT
Direct questions to patient

Q **Do you smoke cigarettes? How long have you been smoking? How much do you smoke in a day?** Cigarette smoking is associated with bladder cancer.

Q **Have you seen any blood in your urine?** Gross hematuria is highly suggestive of a serious urinary tract disorder, especially if it is painless.

Q **Is it painful to pass urine and are you passing urine more often?** Frequency and dysuria are symptoms of many bladder disorders.

Q **Have you lost any weight recently?** Weight loss may be seen in advanced malignancy.

Q **Do you have any pain?** Pelvic pain suggests locally advanced disease; bone pain suggests metastatic spread.

Contributory or predisposing factors

Q **What type of tobacco do you use?** Cigarette smokers are at greater risk when compared with pipe, cigar, and chewing tobacco.

Q **What kind of work have you done in your lifetime? Any chemical exposures?** Workers in a number of industries (dye, textile, tire, rubber, and petroleum) or with a history of exposure to certain chemicals (O-toluidine, 2-naphthylamine, benzidine, 4-aminobiphenyl, nitrosamines) are at risk of developing bladder cancer.

Q **What foreign countries have you visited?** Risk of exposure to schistosomiasis.

Q **Have you ever had any exotic ('tropical') diseases?** Specifically schistosomiasis.

Q **Have you ever had chemotherapy?** Patients who have had cyclophosphamide are at increased risk of developing transitional cell carcinoma.

Q **Have you ever had tuberculosis?** Patients with a history of tuberculosis of the urinary tract are at increased risk of malignancy.

Q **Have you ever had radiotherapy to your pelvis?** Patients who have had radiotherapy for other conditions are at increased risk of malignancy.

Q **Have you ever had a kidney or bladder stone?** Patients who have had a stone for many years may develop squamous metaplasia due to irritation by the stone; malignant change may subsequently take place.

Q **Have you ever taken excessive amounts of painkillers?** Excessive consumption of phenacetin is associated with the development of transitional cell carcinoma.

Q **Were you born with a bladder abnormality?** Bladder extrophy or a patent urachus are associated with squamous carcinoma.

Q **Do you have an indwelling urinary catheter?** Patients with long-term catheters (e.g. paraplegics) are at increased risk of, particularly, squamous carcinoma.

Examination

- **Examine for signs of anemia:** pallor, pale conjunctiva
- **Examine pulse and blood pressure,** especially in patients with profuse hematuria as they may be at risk of hypovolemia
- **Examine abdomen for signs of a mass:** rare unless patient has advanced disease
- **Perform bimanual examination for signs of a bladder mass** and to assess if it is mobile or fixed (latter suggests more advanced disease)

Summary of investigative tests

- Urinalysis (dipstick): should be performed in patients who do not have gross hematuria. May confirm presence of microscopic hematuria and/or proteinuria
- Urinary cytology: optional for PCPs, but performed by urologic specialists in patients who have symptoms of bladder irritability, present with hematuria (microscopic or gross), have industrial exposures, or are heavy tobacco users
- Urine culture: should be performed, as urinary tract infection may be associated with bladder cancer

- Full blood count: should be performed in all patients, as anemia may be present
- Serum blood urea nitrogen (BUN) and creatinine: should be performed in all patients, as renal failure may be present
- Serum potassium: should be checked, especially if renal function is abnormal
- Liver function tests: should be performed if metastatic spread is suspected
- Intravenous urogram: should be performed, either prior to referral or by a specialist, for assessment of kidneys and ureters. May be contraindicated if renal function is abnormal or if patient is taking metformin hydrochloride.
- Renal tract ultrasound: alternative imaging method for assessing the renal tract. Particularly useful for determining presence or absence of hydronephrosis
- Computed tomography (CT) of abdomen and pelvis: if invasive or metastatic disease is suspected (normally performed by a specialist)
- CT scan of chest if invasive bladder cancer is suspected
- Cystoscopy and biopsy: cystoscopy is mandatory if bladder cancer is suspected (performed by a specialist)
- Retrograde pyelogram: if filling defects are seen in kidneys or ureters (performed by a specialist)
- Bone scan: if metastatic disease suspected (performed by a specialist)

Staging of bladder cancer is usually accomplished by the urologic specialist after the tumor is resected and the pathologic type and level of bladder penetration is identified. Classification requires pathologic classification, an assessment of the nodal status, and an assessment of distant metastatic potential.

DIAGNOSTIC DECISION
Bladder cancer is usually diagnosed by histologic examination of bladder biopsy.

TNM staging
Pathologic stage:
- T0: no tumor in specimen
- Tis: carcinoma *in situ*
- Ta: papillary TCCa noninvasive
- T1: papillary TCCa into lamina propria
- T2: TCCa invasive of superficial ms
- T3a: invasive of deep ms
- T3b: invasive of perivesical fat
- T4a: invasive of adjacent pelvic organ
- T4b: invasive of pelvic wall with fixation

Nodal status:
- N0: no nodal involvement
- N1–3: pelvic nodes
- N4: nodes above bifurcation
- Nx: unknown

Metastatic status:
- M0: no distant metastases
- M1: distant metastases
- Mx: unknown

CLINICAL PEARLS
- Area around an identified tumor should be biopsied to determine if there is any form of urothelial dysplasia, i.e. intraurothelial neoplasia types I–III, or carcinoma *in situ*. The presence of these dysplasias serves as a strong predictor of tumor recurrence

- When patients who present with lower urinary tract irritability, i.e. frequency, pelvic pressure, and urgency, fail to respond to standard treatment protocols, an aggressive evaluation should be initiated to rule out dysplasia and/or carcinoma *in situ*
- Aggressive evaluation with a specialist is recommended for patients who suffer from symptoms that resemble urinary tract infection and have negative culture results

THE TESTS
Body fluids
URINALYSIS (DIPSTICK)
Description
Midstream urine specimen.

Advantages/Disadvantages
Advantages:
- Quick and simple to perform in office setting
- Provides information about a variety of urinary constituents very quickly

Disadvantages:
- Not diagnostic, as microscopic hematuria may be intermittent
- Very nonspecific: any abnormalities found are not diagnostic of a particular disorder

Normal
No red or white blood cells or protein identified.

Abnormal
- Red or white blood cells or protein identified
- Keep in mind the possibility of a false-positive result

Cause of abnormal result
Bladder tumors are often friable, leading to bleeding into the urine.

Drugs, disorders and other factors that may alter results
If the patient is a woman of childbearing age, check she is not menstruating, as this may lead to a false-positive result.

URINARY CYTOLOGY
Advantages/Disadvantages
- Advantage: simple screening test for bladder carcinoma
- Disadvantage: false-negative results may occur, especially if bladder carcinoma is of low grade

Normal
No atypical or malignant cells present.

Abnormal
Atypical or malignant cells present.

Cause of abnormal result
Bladder carcinoma.

Drugs, disorders and other factors that may alter results
- Urinary tract infection
- Chronic irritation of the bladder, e.g. presence of a urinary catheter or bladder stone

URINE CULTURE
Advantages/Disadvantages
- Advantage: confirms or refutes diagnosis of urinary tract infection and identifies bacteria responsible
- Disadvantage: identifying the presence of a urinary tract infection does not confirm or refute diagnosis of bladder carcinoma

Abnormal
Bacteria cultured.

Cause of abnormal result
Presence of infection.

Drugs, disorders and other factors that may alter results
Urine sample may be contaminated, e.g. by bowel or skin commensal organisms.

FULL BLOOD COUNT
Advantages/Disadvantages
Advantages:
- Confirms or excludes anemia
- Mandatory for evaluating severity of acute blood loss (this may not be appropriate in the primary care situation)

Disadvantage: does not indicate underlying cause of the anemia

Normal
Hemoglobin:
- Men: 13–17g/dL (130–170g/L)
- Women: 12–15g/dL (120–150g/L)

Abnormal
- Men: <13g/dL (<130g/L)
- Women: <12g/dL (<120g/L)

Cause of abnormal result
- Acute or chronic blood loss
- Chronic disease (of many types)

Drugs, disorders and other factors that may alter results
Anemia is seen as part of many disorders.

SERUM BLOOD UREA NITROGEN AND CREATININE
Advantages/Disadvantages
Advantage: indicates whether renal function is abnormal.

Normal
- Urea (BUN): 10–20mg/dL (3.6–7.1mmol/L)
- Creatinine: <1.5mg/dL (<133mcmol/L)

Abnormal
- Urea (BUN): >20mg/dL (>7.1mmol/L)
- Creatinine: >1.5mg/dL (>133mcmol/L)

Cause of abnormal result
Impaired clearance of nitrogenous waste products from the blood.

Drugs, disorders and other factors that may alter results
Laboratory technique can affect results.

SERUM POTASSIUM
Description
Cuffed venous blood sample (can be combined with measuring BUN and serum creatinine).

Advantages/Disadvantages
Advantage: identifies hyperkalemia, which has an important bearing on patient's cardiovascular status.

Normal
3.5–5.5mEq/L (3.5–5.5mmol/L).

Abnormal
- <3.3mEq/L or >5.5mEq/L (<3.3mmol/L or >5.5mmol/L)
- Keep in mind the possibility of a false-positive result

Cause of abnormal result
Impaired clearance of excess potassium from the blood.

Drugs, disorders and other factors that may alter results
- Hemolyzed blood sample
- Significant delay between taking and analyzing sample

LIVER FUNCTION TESTS
Description
Cuffed venous blood sample.

Advantages/Disadvantages
- Advantage: provides information on liver function
- Disadvantage: results are mainly nonspecific and not diagnostic of a particular disorder

Normal
- Alkaline phosphatase: 30–120U/L (0.5–2.0mckat/L)
- Alanine aminotransferase: 0–35U/L (0–0.58mckat/L)
- Albumin: 3.5–5.5g/dL (35–55g/L)
- Bilirubin: direct 0.1–0.3mg/dL (1.7–5.1mcmol/L); indirect 0.2–0.7mg/dL (3.4–12mcmol/L); total 0.3–1.0mg/dL (5.1–17mcmol/L)

Abnormal
- Alkaline phosphatase: >120U/L (>2.0mckat/L)
- Alanine aminotransferase: >35U/L (>0.58mckat/L)
- Albumin: <3.5g/dL (<35g/L)
- Bilirubin: direct >0.3mg/dL (>5.1mcmol/L); indirect >0.7mg/dL (>12mcmol/L); total >1.0mg/dL (>17mcmol/L)
- Keep in mind the possibility of a falsely abnormal result

Cause of abnormal result
Abnormal liver function.

Drugs, disorders and other factors that may alter results
- Excessive alcohol consumption
- Many disease processes

Imaging
INTRAVENOUS UROGRAM
Description
Radiograph series using radio-opaque contrast to outline urinary tract.

Advantages/Disadvantages
Advantages:
- Identifies filling defects at all levels of the urinary tract
- May identify other possible pathologies, e.g. renal or ureteric tumor

Disadvantages:
- Significant dose of radiation
- Requires experience to interpret
- On its own, not normally diagnostic and further investigations are usually required to confirm diagnosis
- Risk of allergy to radio-opaque contrast
- May be contraindicated in patients with poor renal function
- If normal, does not completely exclude presence of a small tumor

Abnormal
- Filling defect in bladder
- Hydronephrosis – may be unilateral or bilateral (occurs if ureteric orifice(s) are obstructed by tumor)

Cause of abnormal result
Presence of tumor.

Drugs, disorders and other factors that may alter results
- If prostate projects into the bladder in men with prostatic enlargement, this may mimic a bladder tumor
- If patient has gross hematuria, blood clot anywhere in the urinary tract will appear as a filling defect and mimic a tumor

RENAL TRACT ULTRASOUND
Description
Ultrasound scan of kidneys, ureters, and bladder.

Advantages/Disadvantages
Advantages:
- Noninvasive
- No exposure to radiation
- May be repeated as often as required with no risk to patient
- Provides a rapid assessment of entire urinary tract

Disadvantages:
- Specialist knowledge required for interpretation
- Small bladder tumors may not be seen

Abnormal
- Mass in bladder
- Hydronephrosis – may be unilateral or bilateral (occurs if ureteric orifice(s) are obstructed by tumor)

Cause of abnormal result
Presence of bladder tumor.

Drugs, disorders and other factors that may alter results
- If prostate projects into the bladder in men with prostatic enlargement, this may mimic a bladder tumor
- If patient has gross hematuria, blood clot anywhere in the urinary tract will appear as a filling defect and mimic a tumor

TREATMENT

IMMEDIATE ACTION
- Stop active bleeding by immediate referral to an urologic surgeon
- Correct renal failure if secondary to obstructive uropathy with immediate urologic referral

PATIENT AND CAREGIVER ISSUES
Impact on career, dependants, family, friends
- Bladder cancer is a serious disease which requires repeated investigations ('check' cystoscopy) and in some cases major surgery (cystectomy)
- Many patients with superficial disease maintain an essentially normal lifestyle, but those with more extensive disease are incapacitated for significant periods of time and are unable to work or take part in family or social activities
- Patients requiring cystectomy have a significant alteration in their body image (even if they have an orthotopic substitution) and this may impact especially on their relationship with their partner
- In some cases, patients and their families and friends have to come to terms with their having a terminal disease. This group particularly requires a great deal of support

Patient or caregiver request
Stop smoking and limit second-hand smoke exposure.

Health-seeking behavior
Have you had your symptoms for a long time? Has patient delayed seeing a doctor either through fear or not understanding the potential significance of their symptoms?

MANAGEMENT ISSUES
Goals
- To refer patient with appropriate degree of urgency
- To recognize signs and symptoms of recurrent disease so that appropriate action may be taken
- To provide appropriate advice and support for those patients with advanced, possibly terminal, disease

Management in special circumstances
COEXISTING DISEASE
Patients with significant comorbidity (particularly cardiac and respiratory problems) may not be fit enough for major surgery (e.g. cystectomy). This is frequently an issue as a significant number of these patients are heavy smokers.

SPECIAL PATIENT GROUPS
Some elderly patients with advanced (muscle-invasive) disease will not be physically fit enough to undergo radical surgery. Treatment options may be limited to radiotherapy or transurethral resection for smaller tumors.

PATIENT SATISFACTION/LIFESTYLE PRIORITIES
As far as is practicable, patients require treatment likely to maximize their chances of preserving their bladder and prolonging life.

SUMMARY OF THERAPEUTIC OPTIONS
Choices
Choice of treatment modality depends on histologic type and extent of tumor (i.e. superficial, invasive, or metastatic).

Transitional cell carcinoma:
- Superficial lesions are resected endoscopically, either by biopsy and cystodiathermy or transurethral resection of bladder tumor (TURBT). If they are multiple or recur frequently, intravesical mitomycin, thiotepa, doxorubicin hydrochloride, epirubicin, or bacille Calmette-Guérin (BCG) may be used. BCG is the treatment of choice for recurrent superficial transitional cell carcinoma
- Carcinoma *in situ* may be treated endoscopically, and requires treatment with intravesical BCG. A few patients ultimately require cystectomy
- Muscle invasive disease is treated by radical cystectomy; in selected patients an orthotopic substitution may be performed. Patients who are not fit enough or do not wish to undergo cystectomy may be treated with aggressive TURBT plus radiotherapy plus combination chemotherapy, most commonly M-VAC (methotrexate, vinblastine, doxorubicin, cisplatin), CMV (cisplatin, methotrexate, vinblastine), or CISCA (cisplatin, cyclophosphamide, doxorubicin)
- Metastatic disease may be treated with combination chemotherapy: CMV, M-VAC, or CISCA
- Prognosis has improved dramatically with institution of cyclophosphamide treatment

Squamous cell carcinoma:
- Preferred treatment is radical cystectomy; some centers recommend preoperative radiotherapy

Adenocarcinoma:
- Radical cystectomy is usually recommended as these tumors tend to be resistant to radiotherapy and chemotherapy

Clinical pearls
Adenocarcinoma of the bladder that manifests itself as a solitary lesion confined to the dome of the bladder can in some cases be treated with partial cystectomy.

Indications for urethrectomy:
- *En bloc* urethrectomy for obvious involvement of the anterior or posterior urethra in males
- *En bloc* or delayed (within 2 months) urethrectomy for patients with pTis of the prostatic urethra or tumor involvement of the prostate (pT4)
- Positive urethral cytologies in patients with proven pTis
- Immediate urethrectomy for patients developing bloody urethral discharge or if a perineal or urethral mass is detected on physical examination
- *En bloc* urethrectomy is always indicated in a woman undergoing cystectomy and cutaneous diversion. Alternatively, the distal two-thirds of the urethra can be preserved in orthotopic diversions

FOLLOW UP
Plan for review
- All patients with an intact bladder require regular repeat ('check') cystoscopies to ensure disease has not recurred. Interval between cystoscopies may be lengthened if patient repeatedly has no evidence of recurrence
- Because transitional cell carcinoma may also develop in the ureters or renal pelvis, some recommend that patients have an intravenous urogram every few years, but this is controversial

DRUGS AND OTHER THERAPIES: DETAILS
Surgical therapy
RADICAL CYSTECTOMY
Efficacy
Excellent local control of disease provided there is no extravesical spread.

Risks/Benefits

Risks:

- Major operative procedure requiring a long general anesthetic
- Some patients have difficulty coping with their altered body image, which can lead to psychologic problems
- Technically more demanding procedure if performed after radiotherapy, with a greater risk of intra- and postoperative complications

Benefit: curative in some patients

Acceptability to patient

Removal of the bladder leads to a major change in body image, regardless of whether or not the patient has an orthotopic replacement. Some find this difficult or impossible to accept.

Follow up plan

Patients require lifelong follow up, particularly those with transitional cell carcinoma who are at risk of developing transitional cell carcinoma of the ureter or renal pelvis.

Patient and caregiver information

- This is a major procedure with a long recovery period. It may necessitate several months off work
- If patient has a urostomy they will need to learn to care for the stoma and may wish a family member or caregiver to be involved with this
- Family members and caregivers need to be aware that a major period of adjustment may be required by the patient after such surgery, and that their support may be vital to the recovery process

Radiation therapy
RADIOTHERAPY

Efficacy

- Effective treatment for muscle-invasive transitional cell carcinoma and as an adjunct to cystectomy in squamous cancer
- Adenocarcinoma is radioresistant and radiotherapy therefore should not be used

Risks/Benefits

Risks:

- Short- and long-term side-effects occur, including frequency and dysuria, hematuria, diarrhea
- If tumor recurs, patient may require 'salvage cystectomy', which is a more technically demanding procedure

Benefits:

- Bladder is preserved
- May be used as a palliative treatment for inoperable tumors

Acceptability to patient

Generally, patients find radiotherapy acceptable, although it may cause erectile dysfunction in men.

Follow up plan

- Patients usually require repeat ('check') cystoscopies on a regular basis
- Interval between cystoscopies can be lengthened if patient repeatedly has no evidence of recurrence

Patient and caregiver information
- Cystoscopies need to be carried out regularly – often for the rest of the patient's life
- It is important for the patient to attend for cystoscopies regularly so that any recurrence can be treated promptly

Chemotherapy

Use of combination chemotherapy in the treatment of bladder cancer is complex and a variety of regimens have been utilized. The two most common are probably M-VAC and CMV.

M-VAC
- Treatment regimen combining methotrexate, vinblastine, doxorubicin, and cisplatin
- Used to treat locally advanced disease (i.e. extension into perivesical fat or pelvic lymph node metastases) and metastatic disease in an attempt to improve survival
- Two to three cycles are usually given

Efficacy
Variable – response of primary tumor correlates with overall treatment outcome.

Risks/Benefits
Risks
General:
- Significant toxicity may occur, which can delay or preclude cystectomy
- Cystoscopic restaging after treatment may not be accurate
- In patients who respond completely, it is not certain whether cystectomy is always required, but not performing cystectomy carries a significant risk of recurrence
- Must be administered under specialist supervision

Methotrexate:
- Use caution in infection and bone marrow depression
- Use caution in peptic ulceration and ulcerative colitis
- Use caution in renal and hepatic impairment
- Use caution in the elderly

Vinblastine:
- For intravenous use only
- Use caution in hepatic impairment
- Acute shortness of breath and severe bronchospasm have been reported
- Use of small amounts of vinblastine sulfate daily for long periods is not advised

Doxorubin:
- Typically causes nausea, vomiting, tiredness, fall in white cell count, hair loss, and neuropathy
- Special attention must be given to cardiotoxicity induced by doxorubicin
- Cardiomyopathy and/or congestive heart failure may be encountered several months or years after discontinuation of doxorubicin therapy

Cisplatin:
- Should not be used in patients with hearing impairment
- Should not be used in myelosuppressed patients
- Use caution with renal impairment
- Peripheral blood counts should be monitored weekly

Benefit: may downstage tumor in some patients prior to cystectomy, which can improve survival rates

Side-effects and adverse reactions

- Central nervous system: headache, seizures, dizziness, drowsiness, peripheral neurotoxicity
- Eyes, ears, nose, and throat: visual disturbances, tinnitus, conjunctivitis, and lacrimation
- Gastrointestinal: abdominal pain, diarrhea, hepatotoxicity, nausea, vomiting, stomatitis, mucositis
- Genitourinary: renal failure, urinary retention, depression of and defective spermatogenesis, hematuria
- Hematologic: blood cell disorders, secondary acute myeloid leukemia
- Hypersensitivity reactions: fever, chills, urticaria
- Musculoskeletal: osteoporosis, muscle pain and wasting
- Respiratory: pulmonary fibrosis, shortness of breath
- Skin: rashes, acne, dermatitis, alopecia, hyperpigmentation, vasculitis, severe cellulitis, vesication and tissue necrosis

Interactions (other drugs)

- Aminoglycosides ▪ Antimalarials ▪ Binding resins ▪ Co-trimoxazole ▪ Cyclosporine
- Ethanol ▪ Etretrinate ▪ Live vaccines ▪ Nonsteroidal anti-inflammatory drugs (NSAIDs)
- Omeprazole ▪ Penicillins ▪ Probenicid ▪ Salicylates ▪ Sulfinpyrazone ▪ Phenytoin
- Drugs that inhibit cytochrome P-450 isoenzymes in the CYP 3A subfamily

Contraindications

- Nursing mothers, pregnancy, and conception should be avoided for 6 months after stopping
- Safety and effectiveness in pediatric patients have not been established, other than in cancer chemotherapy ▪ Severe renal and hepatic impairment ▪ Hearing impairment
- Profound bone marrow depression

Acceptability to patient

Systemic chemotherapy is often feared by patients because of well known side-effects such as nausea, vomiting, and hair loss. If reassured that nausea and vomiting can be minimized with modern antiemetics, patients will generally accept this treatment.

Follow up plan

- Postchemotherapy follow up depends on intended future treatment
- Most patients undergo a restaging cystoscopy, followed by either a partial or total cystectomy, or regular repeat ('check') cystoscopies

Patient and caregiver information

- Because this is a very complex treatment regimen, it is important for the patient to follow all instructions given by their specialist
- Patient will be monitored very closely during their treatment
- Many of the side-effects of chemotherapy can be treated successfully

CMV

- Treatment regimen combining cisplatin, methotrexate, and vinblastine
- Used to treat metastatic disease in an attempt to improve survival

Efficacy

Cisplatin-based combination chemotherapy may improve survival in patients with metastatic bladder cancer, although this is still under investigation.

Risks/Benefits

Risks

General:

- Must be administered under specialist supervision
- Should not be used in myelosuppressed patients

- Use caution in renal impairment
- Peripheral blood counts should be monitored weekly

Cisplatin:
- Should not be used in patients with hearing impairment

Methotrexate:
- Use caution in peptic ulceration and ulcerative colitis
- Use caution in the elderly

Vinblastine:
- For intravenous use only
- Acute shortness of breath and severe bronchospasm have been reported
- Use of small amounts of vinblastine sulfate daily for long periods is not advised

Benefit: may improve survival

Side-effects and adverse reactions
- Cardiovascular system: hypertension
- Central nervous system: numbness of digits (paresthesias), loss of deep tendon reflexes, peripheral neuritis, mental depression, headache, convulsions
- Gastrointestinal: constipation, anorexia, nausea, vomiting, abdominal pain, ileus, vesiculation of the mouth, pharyngitis, diarrhea, hemorrhagic enterocolitis, bleeding from an old peptic ulcer, rectal bleeding
- Hematologic: leukopenia, anemia, thrombocytopenia
- Skin: alopecia, photosensitivity

Interactions (other drugs)
- Phenytoin ▪ Drugs that inhibit cytochrome P-450 isoenzymes in the CYP 3A subfamily
▪ Aminoglycosides ▪ Antimalarials ▪ Binding resins ▪ Co-trimoxazole ▪ Cyclosporine
▪ Ethanol ▪ Etretrinate ▪ Live vaccines ▪ NSAIDs ▪ Omeprazole ▪ Sulfinpyrazone
▪ Penicillins ▪ Probenicid ▪ Salicylates ▪ Pyridoxine plus hexmethylmelamine (may affect response duration)

Contraindications
- Hypersensitivity to any component of treatment ▪ Profound bone marrow depression
▪ Pregnancy and breast-feeding ▪ Cachexia or ulcerated areas of the skin surface
▪ Bacterial infections ▪ Hearing impairment

Acceptability to patient
Systemic chemotherapy is often feared by patients because of well known side-effects such as nausea, vomiting, and hair loss. If reassured that with modern antiemetics nausea and vomiting can be minimized, patients will generally accept this treatment.

Follow up plan
- Postchemotherapy follow up depends on intended future treatment
- Most patients undergo a restaging cystoscopy, followed by either a partial or total cystectomy, or regular repeat ('check') cystoscopies

Patient and caregiver information
- Because this is a very complex treatment regimen, it is important for the patient to follow all instructions given by their specialist
- Patient will be monitored very closely during their treatment
- Many of the side-effects of chemotherapy can be treated successfully

DOXORUBICIN HYDROCHLORIDE

- Anthracycline antibiotic
- Interferes with cell function by binding to base pairs of DNA
- Usually instilled at doses of 30–100mg dissolved in 50mL saline
- Administered either weekly or every 3 weeks, although number of treatments has varied between different studies
- Should be retained in the bladder for 1–2h

Efficacy
Mixed results have been reported, especially with respect to prophylaxis against recurrence of papillary transitional cell carcinoma.

Risks/Benefits
Risks:

- Must be administered under specialist supervision
- Typically causes nausea, vomiting, tiredness, fall in white cell count, hair loss, and neuropathy
- Special attention must be given to the cardiotoxicity induced by doxorubicin
- Cardiomyopathy and/or congestive heart failure may be encountered several months or years after discontinuation of doxorubicin therapy

Side-effects and adverse reactions

- Cardiovascular system: cardiotoxicity, phlebosclerosis
- Central nervous system: acute nausea and vomiting, mucositis, peripheral neurotoxicity
- Eyes, ears, nose, and throat: conjunctivitis, lacrimation
- Hematologic: secondary acute myeloid leukemia
- Hypersensitivity reactions: fever, chills, urticaria
- Genitourinary: red coloration to the urine for 1–2 days after administration
- Skin: severe cellulitis, vesication, and tissue necrosis

Interactions (other drugs)
- **Paclitaxel** ■ **Progesterone** ■ **Verapamil** ■ **Cyclosporine**

Contraindications
■ Previous treatment with complete cumulative doses of doxorubicin, daunorubicin, idarubicin, and/or other anthracyclines and anthracenes ■ Marked myelosuppression induced by previous treatment with other antitumor agents or by radiotherapy ■ Pregnancy category D and breast-feeding

Acceptability to patient
Mostly acceptable, although some may find the insertion of a urethral catheter uncomfortable.

Follow up plan

- At completion of the course of treatment, patient commences repeat ('check') cystoscopies at regular intervals
- Interval between cystoscopies can be lengthened if patient repeatedly has no evidence of recurrence

Patient and caregiver information

- Cystoscopies need to be carried out regularly – often for the rest of the patient's life
- It is important for the patient to attend regularly for treatment and follow-up cystoscopies so that any recurrence can be treated promptly

CYCLOPHOSPHAMIDE
Prognosis has improved dramatically with institution of cyclophosphamide treatment.

Risks/Benefits
Risks:
- Must be administered under specialist supervision
- Risks of hemorrhagic cystitis, confusion, and coma
- Use caution with renal impairment

Benefit: prognosis has improved dramatically with institution of this therapy

Side-effects and adverse reactions
- Cardiovascular system: cardiotoxicity, hypotension, hypertension
- Central nervous system: toxicity, somnolence, confusion, hallucinations, coma, fever
- Gastrointestinal: nausea, vomiting, anorexia, constipation
- Genitourinary: urotoxic side-effects, hemorrhagic cystitis
- Hematologic: severe myelosuppression, hematuria
- Metabolic: renal impairment, liver impairment
- Skin: alopecia, dermatitis, delayed wound healing

Interactions (other drugs)
None listed

Contraindications
- **Known hypersensitivity to ifosfamide**
- **Severely depressed bone marrow function**
- **Pregnancy and breast-feeding**
- **Safety and efficacy in children have not been established**

THIOTEPA
- Alkylating agent inducing cross–linking between DNA, RNA, nucleic acids and proteins, inhibiting nucleic acid synthesis
- Usually instilled at doses of 30–60mg dissolved in 30–60mL distilled water
- Administered weekly for 6–8 weeks, then monthly for up to one year
- Should be retained in bladder for 2h
- Because myelosuppression may occur, a white blood cell and platelet count should be performed before each instillation

Efficacy
- Highly effective for treating superficial transitional cell carcinoma
- Especially useful when extensive or multiple superficial tumors are present

Risks/Benefits
Risks:
- Death after intravesical administration, caused by bone marrow depression from systematically absorbed drug
- Death from septicemia and hemorrhage as a direct result of hematopoietic depression by thiotepa
- Thiotepa has a low molecular weight (189Da) and is easily absorbed into the systemic circulation: myelosuppression occurs in up to 20% of patients
- Serious complication of excessive thiotepa therapy, or sensitivity to the effects of thiotepa, is bone marrow depression

Side-effects and adverse effects
- Central nervous system: dizziness, headache, blurred vision
- Eyes, ears, nose, and throat: conjunctivitis
- Genitourinary: amenorrhea, interference with spermatogenesis, dysuria, urinary retention. Rare reports of chemical or hemorrhagic cystitis following intravesical, but not parenteral, administration of thiotepa

- Respiratory: prolonged apnea
- Skin: dermatitis, alopecia (skin depigmentation has been reported following topical use), contact dermatitis, pain at the injection site
- Hypersensitivity reactions: allergic reactions, rash, urticaria, laryngeal edema, asthma, anaphylactic shock, wheezing

Interactions (other drugs)
Other alkylating agents

Contraindications
- Pregnancy category D and breast-feeding ▪ Safety and efficacy in pediatric patients have not been established ▪ Concurrent radiotherapy

Acceptability to patient
Mostly acceptable, although some may find the insertion of a urethral catheter uncomfortable.

Follow up plan
- At completion of the course of treatment, patient commences repeat ('check') cystoscopies at regular intervals
- Interval between cystoscopies can be lengthened if patient repeatedly has no evidence of recurrence

Patient and caregiver information
- Before each treatment, a blood test will be performed to ensure that it is safe for the patient to have their treatment
- Cystoscopies need to be carried out regularly – often for the rest of the patient's life
- It is important for the patient to attend regularly for treatment and follow-up cystoscopies so that any recurrence can be treated promptly

INTRAVESICAL MITOMYCIN C
- An intracellular antibiotic isolated from *Streptomyces caespitosus*
- Usually instilled at doses of 40mg dissolved in 30–50mL of sterile water
- Administered weekly for 6–8 weeks; some use a monthly maintenance instillation for 6–12 months
- Should be retained in the bladder for 2h

Efficacy
- Highly effective in treating superficial transitional cell carcinoma
- Especially useful when extensive or multiple superficial tumors are present
- May be effective in some patients who have not responded to intravesical thiotepa

Risks/Benefits
Risks:
- Must be administered under specialist supervision
- Use caution in renal and hepatic impairment
- Risk of bone marrow suppression, notably thrombocytopenia and leukopenia
- Risk of acute shortness of breath and severe bronchospasm

Benefit: can be instilled on an outpatient basis

Side-effects and adverse reactions
- Cardiovascular system: pulmonary toxicity, cardiac toxicity
- Central nervous system: fever, anorexia

- Gastrointestinal: nausea, vomiting
- Hematologic: thrombocytopenia and/or leukopenia, hemolytic uremic syndrome
- Metabolic: renal toxicity
- Skin: cellulitis, extravasation, delayed erythema

Interactions (other drugs)
None listed

Contraindications
- History of hypersensitivity or idiosyncratic reaction to mitomycin C ■ Safety of use in pregnancy has not been established ■ Thrombocytopenia, coagulation disorder, or an increase in bleeding tendency due to other causes

Acceptability to patient
Largely acceptable, although some find the insertion of a urethral catheter uncomfortable.

Follow up plan
- At completion of the course of treatment, patient commences repeat ('check') cystoscopies at regular intervals
- Interval between cystoscopies can be lengthened if patient repeatedly has no evidence of recurrence

Patient and caregiver information
- Cystoscopies need to be carried out regularly – often for the rest of the patient's life
- It is important for the patient to attend regularly for treatment and follow-up cystoscopies so that any recurrence can be treated promptly

EPIRUBICIN
- Derivative of doxorubicin
- Interferes with DNA replication and transcription, thus inhibiting protein synthesis
- Usually instilled at doses of 50mg dissolved in 50mL saline
- Administered weekly for 8 weeks
- Should be retained in bladder for one hour

Efficacy
Effective for treating superficial transitional cell carcinoma.

Risks/Benefits
Risks:
- Should be administered only under the supervision of qualified physicians experienced in the use of cytotoxic therapy
- Risk of cardiotoxicity
- Some patients develop chemical cystitis
- Occasionally hypersensitivity reactions may occur
- Decrease in bladder capacity may be seen; this is usually reversible

Benefit: can be instilled on an outpatient basis

Side-effects and adverse reactions
- Central nervous system: lethargy, fever
- Eyes, ears, nose, and throat: conjunctivitis
- Gastrointestinal: nausea, vomiting, mucositis, anorexia
- Hematologic: leukopenia, neutropenia, anemia, thrombocytopenia
- Other: infection

Interactions (other drugs)
- Cimetidine (delayed epirubicin clearance)

Contraindications
- History of hypersensitivity to epirubicin
- Baseline neutrophil count <1500 cells/mm^3 (<1.5x10^9/L)
- Pharmacokinetics of epirubicin in pediatric patients have not been evaluated
- Severe myocardial insufficiency or recent myocardial infarction
- Previous treatment with anthracyclines up to the maximum cumulative dose
- Severe hepatic dysfunction
- Concurrent treatment with other anthracyclines, or anthracenediones

Acceptability to patient
Generally acceptable, although some may find insertion of a urethral catheter uncomfortable.

Follow up plan
- At completion of the course of treatment, patient commences repeat ('check') cystoscopies at regular intervals
- Interval between cystoscopies can be lengthened if patient repeatedly has no evidence of recurrence

Patient and caregiver information
- Cystoscopies need to be carried out regularly – often for the rest of the patient's life
- It is important for the patient to attend regularly for treatment and follow-up cystoscopies so that any recurrence can be treated promptly

INTRAVESICAL BACILLE CALMETTE-GUÈRIN (BCG)
- Attenuated form of *Mycobacterium bovis*; originally developed as a vaccine against tuberculosis
- Anticancer properties
- Usually given following a bladder biopsy or transurethral tumor resection
- This is an off-label indication

Efficacy
Effective treatment for superficial bladder cancer, especially carcinoma *in situ*.

Risks/Benefits
- Risk: severe systemic reactions may occur
- Benefit: can be instilled on an outpatient basis

Side-effects and adverse reactions
- Central nervous system: flu-like symptoms, fever
- Genitourinary: dysuria, urinary frequency, hematuria, cystitis, urgency, nausea, vomiting
- Musculoskeletal: arthralgia
- Skin: alopecia

Interactions (other drugs)
Immunosuppressants and/or bone marrow depressants

Contraindications
- Concurrent radiotherapy
- Concurrent febrile illness, urinary tract infection, or gross hematuria
- Immunosuppressed patients or persons with congenital or acquired immune deficiencies
- Asymptomatic carriers with a positive HIV serology and patients receiving steroids at immunosuppressive therapies
- Positive Mantoux test (only contraindicated if there is evidence of an active tuberculosis infection)
- Safety and efficacy in pregnancy, breast-feeding, and children have not been established

Acceptability to patient
Mostly acceptable, although some may find the insertion of a urethral catheter uncomfortable.

Follow up plan
- At completion of the course of treatment, patient commences repeat ('check') cystoscopies at regular intervals
- Interval between cystoscopies can be lengthened if patient repeatedly has no evidence of recurrence

Patient and caregiver information
- Cystoscopies need to be carried out regularly – often for the rest of the patient's life
- It is important for the patient to attend regularly for treatment and follow-up cystoscopies so that any recurrence can be treated promptly

Endoscopic therapy
BIOPSY AND CYSTODIATHERMY
Efficacy
- Highly effective for small papillary tumors and small areas of carcinoma *in situ*
- First-choice treatment

Risks/Benefits
Risks:
- Tumor may not be completely excised
- Biopsy may cause bladder perforation

Benefits:
- Biopsy allows histologic examination of the tumor
- Additional biopsies from macroscopically normal urothelium can be taken if desired
- Minimally invasive

Acceptability to patient
Patients usually find this treatment acceptable, although the repeated visits to hospital (and for some, the need for repeated general anesthetics) may be inconvenient.

Follow up plan
- Patients usually require repeat ('check') cystoscopies on a regular basis
- Interval between cystoscopies may be lengthened if patient repeatedly has no evidence of recurrence

Patient and caregiver information
- Cystoscopies need to be carried out regularly – often for the rest of the patient's life
- It is important for the patient to attend for cystoscopies regularly so that any recurrence can be treated promptly

TRANSURETHRAL RESECTION OF BLADDER TUMOUR (TURBT)
Efficacy
Effective treatment for superficial papillary tumors.

Risks/Benefits
Risks:
- Bladder perforation may occur
- Requires general or spinal anesthetic
- Profuse hematuria may occur

Benefits:

- Often possible to resect tumor completely
- For extensive tumors likely to require more radical treatment; allows the taking of multiple large biopsies

Follow up plan

- Patients usually require repeat ('check') cystoscopies on a regular basis
- Interval between cystoscopies may be lengthened if patient repeatedly has no evidence of recurrence

Patient and caregiver information

- Cystoscopies need to be carried out regularly – often for the rest of the patient's life
- It is important for the patient to attend for cystoscopies regularly so that any recurrence can be treated promptly

EFFICACY OF THERAPIES

In patients with superficial bladder cancer, 70% will respond to intravesical therapy while 30% will fail and develop a recurrence or progress to invasive disease.

PROGNOSIS

Prognostic indicators include tumor grade, depth of tumor penetration, multifocal tumors, frequency of recurrence, tumor size, presence of carcinoma *in situ*, lymphatic invasion, and papillary or solid tumor configuration.

Based on cystoscopic and pathologic findings, patients are classified into two groups: low risk and high risk for recurrence and progression.

Low risk:
- Patients present with either a bladder tumor for the first time or after a long interval of time without recurrence
- On cystoscopy they may have up to three lesions
- Lesions can be as big as 3.0cm
- Papillary configuration
- Lesions do not invade the lamina propria (stage Ta)
- Lesions are well or moderately differentiated (grade I or II)

High risk:
- Patients present with a bladder tumor for the first time, or they may have had multiple recurrences in a short period of time
- More than three lesions
- Lesions >3.0cm
- Lesions are less papillary and more sessile
- Presence of urothelial dysplasia (IUN-1, 2, 3)
- Presence of carcinoma *in situ*
- Tumors are high grade (II–III)
- Pathologically, tumors are invasive of lamina propria (T1)

Recurrence

Transitional cell carcinoma:
- Superficial: if patient develops multiple superficial recurrences after transurethral tumor resection, treatment with intravesical bacille Calmette-Guérin (BCG) is the standard of care. Other agents include mitomycin. Rarely requires cystectomy
- Carcinoma *in situ*: if patients fail to respond to treatment with intravesical BCG, the course may be repeated, and if this is still not successful, Intron A (interferon alfa-2b), or valrubicin can be tried. Cystectomy may be required in the face of tumor persistence
- Muscle invasive disease: if this recurs after radiotherapy, radiotherapy plus chemotherapy, then patient may require salvage cystectomy

Squamous carcinoma:
- If carcinoma recurs after radiotherapy, patient may require 'salvage' cystectomy. This is often a technically difficult procedure due to radiation fibrosis

Terminal illness

Bladder cancer is a terminal illness for a proportion of patients, usually those with muscle invasive disease. In addition to symptoms normally associated with advanced malignancy (anorexia, weight loss), problems specifically relating to bladder carcinoma may be encountered:

- Hematuria: may be profuse and recurrent, possibly leading to clot retention. If severe, may require admission to hospital for possible blood transfusion, and in some cases cystoscopy, bladder washout, and cystodiathermy or tumor resection
- Obstructive renal failure: management is controversial and may depend on patient's overall condition. If patient is reasonably well otherwise, treatment may be by insertion of unilateral or bilateral nephrostomies and/or insertion of ureteric stent(s). If patient's overall condition is poor, it may be appropriate to treat this conservatively, in which case it may be a terminal event
- Pain: pelvic or bone pain may require strong (often opiate) analgesia

COMPLICATIONS

- Obstructive renal failure: may occur if ureteric orifices or ureters are occluded by tumor
- Anemia: due to acute or chronic blood loss

CONSIDER CONSULT

- Patients with suspected tumor recurrence should be referred for further investigation, including cystoscopy
- Patients with gross, recurrent hematuria who are at risk of anemia and clot retention should be referred. Blood transfusion and/or cystoscopy with bladder washout and/or cystodiathermy may be needed
- Patient's whose renal function deteriorates often need to be referred, as unilateral or bilateral nephrostomies and/or insertion of ureteric stents may be required. A renal ultrasound scan should be performed; presence of hydronephrosis suggests obstructive renal failure
- Patients with advanced bladder cancer and severe pelvic or bone pain that cannot be controlled easily should be referred (or at least advice sought)

PREVENTION

RISK FACTORS

- **Cigarette smoking**: up to 60% of bladder cancers in industrialized countries may be due to smoking
- **Occupational exposure**: especially to aromatic amines; long latent period
- **Phenacetin**: excessive consumption is associated with the development of transitional cell carcinoma
- **Cyclophosphamide**: link to bladder cancer in humans is strongly suspected, but not proven
- **Indwelling catheter**: if used on a prolonged (many years) basis

MODIFY RISK FACTORS

Indwelling catheter: for patients (especially paraplegics) who require an indwelling catheter, it may not be possible to modify this risk.

Lifestyle and wellness

TOBACCO

Stopping smoking is thought to reduce risk by 30–60%, although risk never returns to the level of nonsmokers.

ENVIRONMENT

Occupational exposure: those in at-risk occupations should minimize their exposure to chemical carcinogens.

DRUG HISTORY

- Phenacetin: consumption should be minimized
- Cyclophosphamide: for patients who have been treated with cyclophosphamide, it may not be possible to reduce their risk of developing bladder cancer. Maintain a high index of suspicion and arrange early referral for any patient with symptoms suggestive of bladder cancer

SCREENING

- Routine screening for bladder cancer is not recommended
- People who work in high-risk occupations may be eligible for screening, but its benefit has not been determined

PREVENT RECURRENCE

Prompt appropriate treatment may reduce the chance and/or frequency of recurrences, especially of superficial disease. As with the majority of malignancies, it is not possible entirely to prevent recurrence.

ASSOCIATIONS
American Cancer Society
1599 Clifton Road, NE
Atlanta, GA 30322
Tel: (800) ACS-2345
www.cancer.org

American Foundation for Urologic Disease
1128 North Charles Street
Baltimore, MD 21201
Tel: (800) 242-2383
E-mail: admin@afud.org
www.afud.org

National Cancer Institute (NCI)
National Institutes of Health (NIH)
NCI Public Inquiries Office
Building 31, Room 10A31
31 Center Drive, MSC 2580
Bethesda, MD 20892–2580
Tel: (800) 4-CANCER (800-422-6237)
www.nci.nih.gov

KEY REFERENCES
- Hudson MA, Catalona WJ. Urothelial tumors of the bladder, upper tracts and prostate. In: Gillanwater JY, Grayhack JT, Howards SS, Duckett JW, eds. Adult and pediatric urology. 3rd edn. New York: Mosby, 1995
- Petrivich Z, Jozsef G, Brady LW. Radiotherapy for carcinoma of the bladder: a review. Am J Clin Oncol 2001;24:1
- Hayter CR, Paszat LF Groome PA, et al. A population based study of the use and outcome of radical radiotherapy for invasive bladder cancer. Int J Rad Oncol Biol Phys 1999;45:1239–45
- Splinter TAW, et al. The prognostic value of the pathological response to combination chemotherapy before cystectomy in patients with invasive bladder cancer. J Urol 1992;147:606
- Splinter TAW, et al. Neoadjuvant chemotherapy of invasive bladder cancer: the prognostic value of local tumor response. In: Murphy GP, Khoury S, eds. Therapeutic progress in urological cancers. New York: Alan R Liss, 1989:541–7
- Denis L, Hendricks G, Keuppens F. Preoperative chemotherapy for T3/T4-NX-M0 bladder cancer (abstract). J Urol 1986;135:222A
- Shipley WU, et al. Cisplatin and full-dose irradiation for patients with invasive bladder carcinoma: a preliminary report of tolerance and local response. J Urol 1984;132:899
- Herr HW, et al. Neoadjuvant chemotherapy in invasive bladder cancer: the evolving role of surgery. J Urol 1990;144:1083
- Maffezzini M, et al. Systemic preoperative chemotherapy with cisplatin, methotrexate and vinblastine for locally advanced bladder cancer: local tumor response and early followup results. J Urol 1991;145:741
- Advanced Bladder Cancer Overview Collaboration. Neoadjuvant cisplatin for advanced bladder cancer. (Cochrane Review). In: The Cochrane Library, 4, 2001. Oxford: Update Software
- Shelley MD, Barber J, Mason MD. Surgery versus radiotherapy for muscle invasive cancer (Cochrane Review) In: The Cochrane Library, 4, 2001. Oxford: Update Software

FAQS
Question 1
What is the most common histology of bladder cancer in the US?

ANSWER 1
Transitional cell carcinoma accounts for >90% of bladder cancers in the US. Other rarer types include squamous cell carcinoma (5%) and adenocarcinoma (<2%).

Question 2
What are the most common symptoms with bladder cancer?

ANSWER 2
From most to least common:
- Painless hematuria (microscopic or gross)
- Irritative symptoms (frequency, urgency, dysuria)
- Flank pain from ureteral obstruction or retroperitoneal metastasis, bone pain from metastasis
- Pelvic mass

Question 3
What is the natural history of noninvasive and invasive transitional cell carcinoma?

ANSWER 3
- 70–75% of transitional cell carcinoma are superficial, noninvasive tumors at presentation, and most low-grade tumors are destined to remain so. However, most patients, depending upon tumor size, grade, focality, ploidy, and other factors, are prone to multiple recurrences over time and in other bladder sites
- 10–15% of noninvasive tumors, usually those of higher grade and with documented invasion of the lamina propria, progress to muscle invasion
- Most invasive tumors are invasive at the time of diagnosis, and 50% have occult metastatic disease. Untreated invasive disease predictably results in patient death within about 2 years

Question 4
What are the clinical features of carcinoma *in situ*?

ANSWER 4
- Carcinoma *in situ* may be asymptomatic or produce irritative urinary symptoms (urgency, frequency, bladder pain) which are often confused with prostatism, infection, interstitial cystitis, or neurogenic bladder
- Occurs more commonly in men and may occur alone or in association with noninvasive papillary or invasive transitional cell carcinoma
- Symptomatic carcinoma *in situ* is typically due to diffuse urothelial involvement. When associated with other tumors, it is usually more focal and may surround the base of a high-grade papillary tumor. The occurrence of carcinoma *in situ* in conjunction with papillary tumors indicates a higher likelihood of recurrence and progression to invasive disease
- Urinary cytology is almost universally positive in the presence of carcinoma *in situ* because of tumor cell slough from the basement membrane of the lamina propria

Question 5
What is the ideal imaging study in evaluating patients with transitional cell carcinoma?

ANSWER 5
- The ideal study should evaluate renal function, test for the presence of renal parenchymal abnormalities, and visualize the upper tract urothelium
- This is best achieved with an intravenous urogram, although renal ultrasound and retrograde pyelograms yield similar information but without functional details
- Computed tomography (CT) scan of the abdomen and pelvis is not indicated in patients with noninvasive tumors because of the low likelihood of extravesical disease
- Magnetic resonance imaging cannot distinguish depth of tumor invasion
- In patients with invasive tumors, a CT scan of the abdomen and pelvis is helpful in determining tumor extent and the presence of macroscopically enlarged lymph nodes, but a 'negative' scan does not rule out the presence of microscopic lymphatic metastasis

CONTRIBUTOR
Philip J Aliotta, MD, MHA, FACS

EPIDIDYMITIS

SUMMARY INFORMATION

DESCRIPTION

- Inflammation of the epididymitis
- Can present at any age
- Common causative agent varies with age of patient
- Infection may spread to involve the testis
- Most cases can be treated adequately with oral antibiotics
- Complications include infertility, abscess formation, and chronic epididymitis

URGENT ACTION

Commence empirical therapy with a suitable antibiotic.

KEY! DON'T MISS!

Prepubertal boys presenting with epididymitis need to be investigated for congenital abnormalities of the urinary tract (e.g. vesicoureteral reflux). All should be referred.

BACKGROUND

ICD9 CODE
- 604.0 Epididymitis with abscess
- 604.90 Epididymitis (nonvenereal)
- 604.99 Acute epididymitis
- 098.2 Chronic epididymitis

SYNONYMS
- Nonspecific bacterial epididymitis
- Sexually transmitted epididymitis
- If testis is also involved, may be referred to as epididymo-orchitis

CARDINAL FEATURES
- May be unilateral or bilateral
- Can present at any age
- Common causative agent varies with age of patient
- Prepubertal boys with epididymitis must be assessed for underlying congenital abnormalities of the urinary tract
- May spread to involve testis
- Most cases can be treated adequately with oral antibiotics
- Severe cases will require hospital admission for parenteral antibiotics
- Complications include infertility, abscess formation, and chronic epididymitis

CAUSES
Common causes
Usually because of a bacterial infection, common causative organisms vary with age group.

Prepubertal boys:
- *Escherichia coli*

Men <35 years:
- *Chlamydia trachomatis*
- *Neiserria gonorrheae*

Men >35 years:
- *Escherichia coli*
- *Pseudomonas* species

Rare causes
- *Staphylococcus epidermidis*
- *Staphylococcus aureus*
- In association with intravesical chemotherapy for bladder cancer
- Cytomegalovirus (CMV): in patients with HIV
- *Salmonella* species: in patients with HIV

Serious causes
Mycobacterium tuberculosis: often associated with orchitis.

Contributory or predisposing factors
- Orchitis
- Urinary tract infection (in both children and adults)
- Prostatitis

- Indwelling urethral catheter
- Recent urethral instrumentation or surgery
- Urethral stricture
- Congenital abnormalities of the urinary tract, e.g. vesicoureteral reflux, ectopic urethra, especially in prepubertal boys
- Immunocompromised, e.g. HIV

EPIDEMIOLOGY
Incidence and prevalence
FREQUENCY

- Common, although precise data unavailable
- Cause of >600,000 visits to physicians per year in the US

Demographics
AGE

- May occur at any age
- Less common in prepubertal boys
- Common in men of all ages, although causative organisms differ

GENDER
Males only.

DIFFERENTIAL DIAGNOSIS

- The most important differential diagnoses are testicular torsion, testicular tumor, and Fournier's gangrene, all of which require urgent referral
- Other differential diagnoses include torsion of the testicular appendages, orchitis, epididymal cyst, and hydrocele

Testicular torsion

The main features of testicular torsion are as follows

FEATURES

- Commonest at ages 12–18 years, but can occur at any age
- Usually present with testicular pain and swelling of sudden onset
- 10% have painless testicular swelling
- May have had previous episodes of testicular pain that settled spontaneously
- Refer immediately to urologist for scrotal exploration and detorsion
- If detorsion within 12h of onset, 80% chance of salvaging testis

Testicular tumor

The main features of testicular malignancies are as follows

FEATURES

- Commonest in young adults, but can occur at any age
- Higher incidence in patients with undescended testicle (even if surgically corrected), previous contralateral testis tumor or intersex disorders
- Painless swelling of the testis
- Usually no other symptoms, unless has metastasized

Fournier's gangrene

FEATURES

- Necrotizing fasciitis of the scrotum
- Variety of organisms may be responsible
- Risk factors include recent scrotal trauma or surgery, or a history of diabetes mellitus
- Scrotal pain
- Foul smell
- Fever, tachycardia
- Dark discoloration of scrotal skin
- Crepitation may be felt if responsible organism is gas-producing
- Urgent surgical intervention required
- High mortality rate

Torsion of the testicular appendages

FEATURES

- Commonest in prepubertal boys
- Severe testicular pain
- Scrotal swelling
- May be clinically indistinguishable from testicular torsion
- Torted appendage may be visible through skin ('blue dot sign')
- If sure of diagnosis, treat conservatively
- If any doubt, will require scrotal exploration

Orchitis

The main features of orchitis are as follows

FEATURES

- May be bacterial or viral
- If no associated involvement of epididymis, cause most likely viral
- Can occur at any age
- May be clinically indistinguishable from epididymitis
- No specific treatment for viral orchitis
- Bacterial orchitis treated with antibiotics
- Occasionally surgical exploration of scrotum required

Epididymal cyst

FEATURES

- Commonest in men over 40 years
- Palpable lump separate from testis
- No treatment required unless large or painful
- Treatment, if necessary, is by excision

Hydrocele

The main features of hydrocele are as follows

FEATURES

- Occurs at any age
- Congenital or acquired
- Congenital hydrocele usually presents in childhood and requires surgical repair
- Acquired hydrocele does not require treatment if asymptomatic and underlying testis is normal

SIGNS & SYMPTOMS

Signs

- Pyrexia
- Tachycardia
- Swelling of the epididymis and possibly testis also
- Urethral discharge
- Signs of urinary tract infection: cloudy urine, hematuria
- Reactive hydrocele
- Discrete areas of thickening of vas deferens ('string of beads') in tuberculous epididymitis
- Scrotal erythema and induration

Symptoms

- Scrotal pain: may extend into groin
- Symptoms of urinary tract infection: frequency, dysuria
- Obstructive urinary symptoms

KEY! DON'T MISS!

Prepubertal boys presenting with epididymitis need to be investigated for congenital abnormalities of the urinary tract (e.g. vesicoureteral reflux). All should be referred.

CONSIDER CONSULT

- All young boys
- Patients in whom the diagnosis is in doubt
- Patients with systemic sepsis
- Patients suspected of having infection with an unusual organism
- Patients suspected of having tuberculous epididymitis
- Immunocompromised patients (e.g. those with HIV)

INVESTIGATION OF THE PATIENT
Direct questions to patient
Q How old are you? In young men and boys, testicular torsion and tumor must be excluded early.

Q Have you had any discharge from your penis? Presence of a discharge indicates that an infection with *Chlamydia trachomatis* or *Neiserria gonorrheae* is most likely.

Q If yes, what did the discharge look like? Serious discharge suggests chlamydial infection, purulent discharge suggests gonococcal infection.

Q Have you had urethritis or a urethral discharge in the past? Both *Chlamydia trachomatis* and *Neiserria gonorrheae* may be carried for long periods before the patient develops epididymitis.

Q Have you been passing urine more frequently than normal and has it been painful? A recent urinary tract infection or episode of urethritis may contribute to the development of epididymitis.

Q Have you had any aching of the scrotum or pain on ejaculation? An episode of prostatitis may lead to the development of epididymitis.

Q Have you recently had any surgery on your urinary tract? Instrumentation of the urinary tract may predispose to urinary tract infection.

Q Have you ever had any trauma to your urinary tract or genitalia? Trauma may predispose to the development of a urethral stricture.

Q Do you think the strength of your flow when you urinate has changed at all? A slow flow may indicate the presence of a stricture or benign prostatic hyperplasia.

Contributory or predisposing factors
Q Any history of predisposing factors? For example recent episode of orchitis, prostatitis, urinary tract infection (children, adults), chlamydia, gonorrhea.

Q Any history of serious illness? Especially tuberculosis, HIV.

Family history
Q Has anyone in the family had tuberculosis? If so, tuberculosis may need to be considered as a diagnosis, even if the patient is not known to have had it in the past.

Examination
- **Check temperature:** may be elevated
- **Take pulse:** may be tachycardic
- **Measure blood pressure:** if patient is hypotensive, with signs of systemic sepsis, suspect septic shock
- **Examine the penis:** crusting around the meatus suggests the patient may have a urethral discharge
- **Examine the scrotum:** the epididymis may be tender and indurated. If the testis is involved, it will be hard, swollen, and possibly surrounded by a reactive hydrocele. In some cases, the entire hemiscrotum may be swollen and erythematous

Summary of investigative tests
- Urinalysis (dipstick): should be performed in all patients, the presence of protein and/or leukocytes especially is suggestive of infection
- Gram stain: of urethral discharge, if this is present
- Urine culture: should be performed, as urinary tract infection may coexist
- Full blood count: if patient is systemically unwell. Raised white cell count suggestive of significant infection
- Ultrasound scan of scrotal contents: to check for abscess, or any other pathology, particularly tumor
- Doppler ultrasound to assess arterial and venous blood flow
- Radionuclide scan of scrotal contents: to exclude torsion. Would usually be performed by specialist

DIAGNOSTIC DECISION

Diagnosis based on clinical examination, supported by laboratory tests and ultrasound.

Guidelines

National guideline for the management of epididymoorchitis [1] Available online at the National Guideline Clearinghouse

CLINICAL PEARLS

- If there is ever a question of torsion, referral to a specialist is mandatory. If the specialist feels that it is a case of torsion, exploration without radionuclide scanning is the standard of care
- Acute epididymitis can occur after vigorous work, strenuous exercising, and forceful coughing. The etiology of this is vague. There is some suggestion that reflux of an acid urine into an alkaline vas creates distal obstruction of the vas and obstruction with secondary epididymitis. Others have suggested that there is subclinical bacterial infection from the prostate. These patients do improve on antibiotic and anti-inflammatory/analgesic medications

THE TESTS

Body fluids

URINALYSIS (DIPSTICK)

Description

Mid-stream urine specimen.

Advantages/Disadvantages

Advantages:

- Quick and simple to perform at office level
- Provides information about a variety of urinary constituents very quickly

Disadvantages:

- Whether normal or abnormal, does not confirm or refute the diagnosis
- Is very nonspecific

Normal

No red or white blood cells, or protein identified.

Abnormal

- Red and/or white blood cells, and/or protein present
- Dipstick tests can be highly sensitive, a false-positive result is possible

GRAM STAIN OF URETHRAL DISCHARGE

Description

Swab of urethral discharge.

Advantages/Disadvantages

Advantages:

- Confirms if infection is present
- If Gram-negative diplococci seen, highly likely to be *Neiserria gonorrheae*

Normal

No organisms seen.

Abnormal

- Organisms seen
- Keep in mind the possibility of a falsely abnormal result

Cause of abnormal result
Presence of infection.

Drugs, disorders and other factors that may alter results
Specimen may be contaminated by skin or bowel commensals.

URINE CULTURE
Description
Mid-stream urine specimen.

Advantages/Disadvantages
Advantages:
- Confirms or refutes diagnosis of urinary tract infection
- Identifies bacteria responsible

Disadvantage: takes 36–48h

Normal
No bacteria cultured.

Abnormal
- Bacteria cultured
- Keep in mind the possibility of a falsely abnormal result

Cause of abnormal result
Presence of infection.

Drugs, disorders and other factors that may alter results
Urine sample may be contaminated, e.g. by skin or bowel commensal organisms.

FULL BLOOD COUNT
Description
Cuffed venous blood sample.

Advantages/Disadvantages
Disadvantage: nonspecific

Normal
White blood cell count 4.0–11.0x10^9/L.

Abnormal
- White blood cell count >4.0–11.0x10^9/L
- Keep in mind the possibility of a falsely abnormal result

Drugs, disorders and other factors that may alter results
- Many infections
- Some hematologic disorders
- Depending on the severity of the abnormality, may need investigation in its own right

Imaging
ULTRASOUND SCAN OF SCROTAL CONTENTS

Advantages/Disadvantages
Advantages:
- No exposure to ionizing radiation
- Identifies a variety of pathologies, e.g. abscess, tumor, torsion
- Doppler ultrasound can evaluate blood supply to testis
- Can be repeated as often as desired

Disadvantages:
- Often does not provide conclusive proof of a diagnosis
- If testicular torsion suspected, delay involved in organizing ultrasound will be unacceptable

Normal
Normal testes.

Abnormal
- Hypoechoic or hyperechoic area may be seen
- Considerable experience required to interpret scan

Drugs, disorders and other factors that may alter results
Scarring or atrophy of testis owing to previous trauma or infection.

DOPPLER ULTRASOUND
Advantages/Disadvantages
Advantages:
- No exposure to ionizing radiation
- Easy to perform
- Noninvasive, no patient discomfort
- Relatively inexpensive

Disadvantages:
- Nonspecific
- Operator dependent

Normal
Flow within normal guidelines.

Abnormal
- Increased flow: inflammation, e.g. epididymitis
- Decreased flow: torsion

TREATMENT

CONSIDER CONSULT
- Patients who fail to respond to oral antibiotics
- If a scrotal abscess is suspected
- Solitary testicle

IMMEDIATE ACTION
Commence empirical therapy with an appropriate antibiotic, selected to cover the most likely causative organism.

PATIENT AND CAREGIVER ISSUES
Patient or caregiver request
- The patient may be concerned that he has a sexually transmitted disease
- The patient may be concerned that he has testicular cancer
- The patient may be concerned that he will be left infertile

Health-seeking behavior
Has the patient waited too long before presenting? Possibly out of fear or embarrassment.

MANAGEMENT ISSUES
Goals
- Treat infection
- Early recognition of the presence of a sexually transmitted disease
- Reduce pain and swelling
- Reduce chances of permanent sequalae
- Early recognition of need for specialist referral

Management in special circumstances
COEXISTING DISEASE
- Orchitis: treat concurrently
- Chlamydia: treat concurrently
- Gonorrhea: treat concurrently
- HIV: these patients often require complex care and specialist advice should be sought

PATIENT SATISFACTION/LIFESTYLE PRIORITIES
- If infection is due to chlamydia or gonorrhea, it will have implications for both the patient and his sexual partner(s)
- A small proportion of patients may be rendered infertile, this will have major implications if they wish to have children in the future
- In patients who subsequently develop orchitis, a few will require orchidectomy, which may lead to psychological distress

SUMMARY OF THERAPEUTIC OPTIONS
Choices
- Epididymitis requires antibiotic therapy in most cases. If severe systemic sepsis present, patient should be admitted to hospital for parenteral antibiotics. Often treatment needs to be commenced before the causative agent is identified
- Choice of antibiotic depends on suspected causative organism
- If chlamydial or gonorrheal infection is suspected, suitable antibiotics are doxycycline, tetracycline, or ofloxacin
- If *Escherichia coli* is suspected, suitable antibiotics are trimethoprim-sulfamethoxazole, ciprofloxacin, levofloxacin, norfloxacin, or ofloxacin

- Analgesia is often required. Useful agents include NSAIDs (e.g. naproxen, ibuprofen) and acetominophen
- Occasionally patients require surgical exploration of the scrotum, or rarely, epididymo-orchiectomy
- Wearing a scrotal support may increase patient comfort

Guidelines:

- National guideline for the management of epididymoorchitis [1] Available online at the National Guideline Clearinghouse

Clinical pearls

- Warm-to-hot tub soaks can be highly effective at reducing the pain and inflammation that occurs with epididymitis
- One other rule of thumb to advocate for men with epididymitis is to empty the bladder at regular intervals and always before doing anything that requires exertion and/or force
- Occasionally, a person's stress level and lifestyle may contribute toward occurrence and recurrence

Never

Never commence a patient on antituberculous therapy without specialist referral.

FOLLOW UP
Plan for review

Review every 2–3 days until patient shows obvious improvement.

Information for patient or caregiver

Notify physician immediately if condition worsens or infection spreads.

DRUGS AND OTHER THERAPIES: DETAILS
Drugs
DOXYCYCLINE
Tetracycline antibiotic.

Dose
Adults: 100mg twice daily orally for 10 days

Efficacy
- Effective against a wide range of Gram-positive and Gram-negative organisms
- Recommended for treatment of chlamydial infections

Risks/Benefits
Risks:
- Compliance can be a problem
- Use caution in patients with hepatic impairment
- Use caution with repeated or prolonged doses

Benefits: inexpensive compared with azithromycin

Side-effectss and adverse reactions
- Cardiovascular system: pericarditis, angioedema
- Central nervous system: fever, headache
- Gastrointestinal: abdominal pain, diarrhoea, heartburn, nausea, hepatotoxicity, vomiting, pseudomembraneous colitis

- Hematologic: blood cell disorders
- Skin: pruritus, rash, photosensitivity, exfoliative dermatitis

Interactions (other drugs)
- Antacids (magnesium, calcium) ▪ Anticonvulsants (barbiturates, carbemazepine, phenytoin) ▪ Bismuth ▪ Cholestyramine ▪ Ethanol ▪ Mineral supplements (iron, zinc) ▪ Oral contraceptives ▪ Penicillins ▪ Warfarin

Contraindications
- Pregnancy ▪ Nursing mothers ▪ Children less than 8 years

Evidence
Doxycycline is one of the recommended treatments for epididymo-orchitis, which is most probably due to infection with gonococci, chlamydia, or nongonococcal, nonenteric organisms [1] *Level C*

Acceptability to patient
High.

Follow up plan
Review every 2–3 days until clear evidence of improvement.

Patient and caregiver information
- Take tablets regularly
- Finish the course, even if you are feeling better
- Take tablets with food
- Do not take antacids or iron products at the same time as your antibiotic

TETRACYCLINE
Tetracycline antibiotic.

Dose
- Adults: 500mg, four times daily, orally, for 10 days
- Children: not indicated

Efficacy
- Effective against a wide range of Gram-positive and Gram-negative organisms
- Recommended for treatment of chlamydial infections

Risks/Benefits
Risks:
- Compliance can be a problem
- Use caution in patients with hepatic impairment
- Use caution with repeated or prolonged doses

Side-effectss and adverse reactions
- Cardiovascular system: pericarditis
- Central nervous system: headache, paresthesia, fever
- Gastrointestinal: abdominal pain, diarrhoea, heartburn, hepatotoxicity, vomiting, nausea, dental staining, anorexia
- Genitourinary: polyuria, polydipsia, azotemia
- Hematologic: blood cell dyscrasias
- Skin: pruritus, rash, photosensitivity, changes in pigmentation, angioedema, stinging

Interactions (other drugs)
- Antacids ▪ Atovaquone ▪ Barbiturates ▪ Bismuth subsalicyclate ▪ Cholesytramine, colestipol ▪ Cephalosporins ▪ Calcium, iron, magnesium, zinc ▪ Carbamazepine ▪ Digoxin ▪ Ethanol ▪ Methoxyflurane ▪ Oral contraceptives ▪ Penicillins ▪ Phenytoin ▪ Quinapril ▪ Sodium bicarbonate ▪ Vitamin A ▪ Warfarin

Contraindications
- Pregnancy ▪ Nursing mothers ▪ Children less than 8 years ▪ Severe renal disease

Acceptability to patient
High.

Follow up plan
Review every 2–3 days until clear evidence of improvement.

Patient and caregiver information
- Take tablets regularly
- Finish the course, even if you are feeling better
- Take tablets with food
- Take tablets with a whole glass of water
- Do not take antacids or milk products for 2h before or after taking tetracycline tablets

TRIMETHOPRIM-SULFAMETHOXAZOLE
Co-trimoxazole.

Dose
- Adults: 160mg/800mg, twice daily, orally, for 10–14 days
- Children: 8mg trimethoprim/kg/day orally in divided doses, every 12h for 10–14 days

Efficacy
- Effective against a wide range of Gram-positive and Gram-negative organisms
- Ineffective against *Pseudomonas* species

Risks/Benefits
Risks:
- Use caution in renal and hepatic function impairment
- Use caution in elderly patients receiving diuretics
- Use caution in patients with G 6 PD deficiency
- Risk of streptococcal pharyngitis

Benefit: can be used in children

Side-effectss and adverse reactions
- Central nervous system: seizures, anxiety, aseptic meningitis, ataxia, chills, depression, fatigue, headache, insomnia, vertigo
- Hematologic: agranulocytosis, aplastic anemia, thrombocytopenia, leukopenia, neutropenia, hemolytic anemia, megaloblastic anemia, hypoprothrombinemia, methemoglobinemia, eosinophilia
- Gastrointestinal: hepatitis (including cholestatic jaundice and hepatic necrosis), elevation of serum transaminase and bilirubin, pseudomembranous enterocolitis, pancreatitis, stomatitis, glossitis, nausea, emesis, abdominal pain, diarrhea, anorexia.
- Genitourinary: renal failure, interstitial nephritis, BUN and serum creatinine elevation, toxic nephrosis with oliguria and anuria, and crystalluria.

- Musculoskeletal: arthralgia, myalgia
- Respiratory: pulmonary infiltrates
- Skin: Stevens-Johnson syndrome, erythema multiforme, exfoliative dermatitis, generalized skin eruptions, photosensitivity, pruritus, urticaria, rash. Periarteritis

Interactions (other drugs)
- Dapsone (may cause increased serum concentrations of both dapsone and trimethoprim-sulfamethoxazole) - Disulfiram, metronidazole - Methotrexate (increases methotrexate level) - Oral anticoagulants (increases hypoprothrombinemic response) - Oral hypoglycemics (may cause hypoglycemia) - Phenytoin (may increase phenytoin concentration to toxic levels) - Procainamide (increases procainamide level)

Contraindications
- Megaloblastic anemia secondary to folate deficiency - Neonates under 2 months of age - Renal disease manifested by serum creatinine <15 ml/min - Should not be used in breastfeeding woman or in pregnant women near term

Acceptability to patient
High.

Follow up plan
Review every 2–3 days until clear evidence of improvement.

Patient and caregiver information
- Drink plenty of fluids
- Take tablets regularly
- Finish the course, even if you are feeling better

CIPROFLOXACIN
Fluoroquinolone antibiotic.

Dose
- Adults: 250–500mg, twice daily, orally, for 10–14 days
- Children: not recommended

Efficacy
- Effective against a wide range of Gram-positive and Gram-negative organisms
- Effective against most *Pseudomonas* species

Risks/Benefits
Risks:
- History of allergy
- Not suitable for children or growing adolescents
- Use caution in pregnancy, epilepsy, G6PD deficiency
- Use caution in renal disease

Side-effectss and adverse reactions
- Central nervous system: anxiety, depression, dizziness, headache, seizures
- Eyes, ears, nose, and throat: visual disturbances
- Gastrointestinal: abdominal pain, altered liver function, anorexia, diarrhoea, heartburn, vomiting
- Skin: photosensitivity, pruritus, rash

Interactions (other drugs)

■ Antacids ■ Beta-blockers ■ Cyclosporine ■ Caffeine ■ Didanosine ■ Diazepam ■ NSAIDs ■ Mineral supplements (zinc, magnesium, calcium, aluminium, iron) ■ Opiates ■ Oral anticoagulants ■ Phenytoin ■ Theophylline ■ Warfarin

Contraindications

■ Use is not recommended in children because arthropathy has developed in weight-bearing joints in young animals ■ Pregnancy category B. Compatible with breast feeding

Evidence

Ciprofloxacin is one of the recommended treatments for epididymo-orchitis most probably due to gonoccal infection [1] *Level C*

Acceptability to patient

High.

Follow up plan

Review every 2–3 days until clear evidence of improvement.

Patient and caregiver information

■ Take tablets regularly
■ Finish the course, even if you are feeling better
■ Do not take antacids or preparations containing iron or zinc for several hours before and after taking your tablet
■ Avoid sunbathing or using a sunbed while you are taking the treatment

LEVOFLOXACIN

Fluoroquinolone antibiotic.

Dose

■ Adults: 250mg, daily, orally, for 10–14 days
■ Children: not recommended

Efficacy

■ Effective against a wide range of Gram-positive and Gram-negative organisms
■ Effective against most *Pseudomonas* species

Risks/Benefits

Risks:

■ Use caution in children and adolescents
■ Use caution in patients with a history of epilepsy and other seizure conditions, myasthenia gravis
■ Use caution in renal disease
■ Use caution in diabetes mellitus

Side-effectss and adverse reactions

■ Central nervous system: anxiety, depression, dizziness, headache, seizures
■ Eyes, ears, nose, and throat: visual disturbances
■ Gastrointestinal: abdominal pain, altered liver function, anorexia, diarrhoea, heartburn, pseudomembraneous colitis, vomiting
■ Genitourinary: monoliasis, vaginitis
■ Skin: photosensitivity, pruritus, rash

Interactions (other drugs)
- Antacids ■ Anti-ulcer agents (cimetidine, famotidine, lansoprazole, nizatidine, omeprazole, ranitidine, sucralfate) ■ Cyclosporine ■ Didanosine ■ Estrogens ■ Iron, aluminium, magnesium, calcium, zinc ■ NSAIDs ■ Theophylline ■ Typhoid vaccine ■ Warfarin ■ Zolmitriptan

Contraindications
- Pregnancy ■ Nursing mothers

Acceptability to patient
High, once-daily dose.

Follow up plan
Review every 2–3 days until clear evidence of improvement.

Patient and caregiver information
- Drink plenty of fluids
- Take tablets regularly
- Finish the course, even if you are feeling better
- Do not take antacids or preparations containing iron or zinc for several hours before and after the time of taking your tablet
- Avoid sunbathing or using a sunbed while you are taking this treatment

NORFLOXACIN
Fluoroquinolone antibiotic.

Dose
- Adults: 400mg, twice daily, orally, for 10–21 days
- Children: not recommended

Efficacy
- Effective against a wide range of Gram-positive and Gram-negative organisms
- Effective against most *Pseudomonas* species

Risks/Benefits
Risks:
- Use caution in the elderly
- Use caution in renal disease and dehydration
- Use caution in seizure disorders

Side-effectss and adverse reactions
- Central nervous system: headache, dizziness, seizures, fatigue, anxiety
- Eyes, ears, nose, and throat: visual disturbances
- Gastrointestinal: nausea, vomiting, diarrhea, constipation, altered liver function tests, abdominal pain
- Genitourinary: crystalluria
- Hematologic: blood cell disorders
- Skin: rashes

Interactions (other drugs)
- Aluminium, calcium, magnesium, iron, zinc ■ Antacids ■ Antipyrine ■ Caffeine ■ Diazepam ■ Foscarnet ■ Metoprolol, propanolol ■ Pentoxyfilline ■ Phenytoin ■ Ropinirole ■ Sodium bicarbonate ■ Theobromine ■ Theophylline ■ Warfarin

Contraindications
- Pregnancy ▪ Nursing mothers ▪ Children

Acceptability to patient
High.

Follow up plan
Review every 2–3 days until clear evidence of improvement.

Patient and caregiver information
- Drink plenty of fluids
- Take tablets regularly
- Finish the course, even if you are feeling better

OFLOXACIN
Fluoroquinolone antibiotic.

Dose
- Adults: 300mg, twice daily, orally, for 14 days
- Children: not recommended

Efficacy
Effective against most common causative organisms including *Chlamydia trachomatis, Neiserria gonorrheae,* and *Escherichia coli.*

Risks/Benefits
Risks:
- Use caution with the elderly and children
- Use caution in renal disease and seizure disorders
- Not approved for use in pregnancy or children less than 8 years

Side-effectss and adverse reactions
- Central nervous system: dizziness, headache, anxiety, depression, seizures
- Eyes, ears, nose, and throat: visual disturbances
- Gastrointestinal: vomiting, altered liver function, anorexia, diarrhea, heartburn, abdominal pain, pseudomembraneous colitis
- Skin: rash, photosensitivity, pruritus

Interactions (other drugs)
- Aluminium, magnesium, iron, zinc, calcium ▪ Antacids ▪ Didanosine ▪ Procainamide
- Sodium bicarbonate ▪ Sulcrafate ▪ Warfarin

Contraindications
- Pregnancy ▪ Nursing mothers

Evidence
- Ofloxacin is a recommended treatment for epididymo-orchitis most probably due to enteric organisms [1] *Level C*
- Ofloxacin is the recommended treatment for epididymo-orchitis of all causes when the patient is allergic to cephalosporins and tetracyclines [1] *Level C*

Acceptability to patient
High.

Follow up plan
Review every 2–3 days until clear evidence of improvement.

Patient and caregiver information
- Take tablets on an empty stomach (an hour before or 2h after meals)
- Drink plenty of fluids
- Take tablets regularly
- Finish the course, even if you are feeling better
- Do not take antacids or preparations containing iron or zinc for several hours before and after taking your tablet
- Avoid sunbathing or using a sunbed while you are taking the treatment

NAPROXEN
NSAID.
Dose
Adults:
- Mild pain: 220mg, orally, every 12h
- Mild to moderate pain: 250mg, orally, every 6–8h

Efficacy
Effective analgesic.

Risks/Benefits
Risks:
- Use caution in hepatic, renal and cardiac disorders
- Use caution in elderly
- Use caution in bleeding disorders
- Use caution in porphyria

Benefits:
- Effective pain relief
- Propionic acids are effective and better tolerated than most other NSAIDs

Side-effectss and adverse reactions
- Cardiovascular system: congestive heart failure, dysrhythmias, edema, palpitations, dyspnea
- Central nervous system: headache, dizziness, drowsiness, vertigo
- Gastrointestinal: constipation, heartburn, diarrhea, vomiting, nausea, dyspepsia, peptic ulceration, stomatitis
- Genitourinary: acute renal failure
- Hematolgic: thrombocytopenia
- Hypersensitivity: rashes, bronchospasm, angioedema
- Skin: pruritis, ecchymoses, sweating, purpura

Interactions (other drugs)
- Aminoglycosides ▪ Anticoagulants ▪ Antihypertensives ▪ Corticosteroids ▪ Cyclosporine ▪ Digoxin ▪ Diuretics ▪ Lithium ▪ Methotrexate ▪ Phenylpropanolamine ▪ Probenecid ▪ Triamterene

Contraindications
- Not recommended for children in this instance ▪ Peptic ulceration ▪ Coagulation defects
- Hypersensitivity to NSAIDs ▪ Do not use naproxen and naproxen sodium concomitantly

Evidence
Nonsteroidal anti-inflammatory treatment may be helpful in the management of epididymo-orchitis [1] *Level C*

Acceptability to patient
Good, but significant incidence of gastrointestinal side-effectss will make this unacceptable to some.

Patient and caregiver information
- Avoid aspirin and aspirin-containing medications
- Avoid alcohol
- Take with food, milk, or antacid to reduce the chance of indigestion or stomach upset
- If your stools turn black, see your doctor promptly

IBUPROFEN
NSAID.

Dose
Adults:
- 200–800mg, orally, four times daily (not to exceed 3200mg/day)
Children:
- 20–40mg/kg/day, orally, divided 3–4 times daily

Efficacy
Effective analgesic.

Risks/Benefits
Risks:
- Use caution in elderly
- Use caution in hepatic, renal and cardiac failure
- Use caution in bleeding disorders
- May cause sever allergic reactions including hives, facial swelling, asthma, shock

Benefits:
- May be used in children
- Inexpensive

Side-effectss and adverse reactions
- Cardiovascular system: hypertension, peripheral edema
- Central nervous system: headache, dizziness, tinnitus
- Gastrointestinal: anorexia, nausea, dyspepsia, peptic ulceration, bleeding
- Genitourinary: nephrotoxicity
- Hematologic: blood cell disorders
- Hypersensitivity: rashes, bronchospasm, angioedema

Interactions (other drugs)
- Aminoglycosides ■ Anticoagulants ■ Antihypertensives ■ Baclofen ■ Corticosteroids ■ Cyclosporine, tacrolimus ■ Digoxin ■ Diuretics ■ Lithium ■ Methotrexate ■ Warfarin ■ Phenylpropanolamine

Contraindications
- Peptic ulceration
- Hypersensitivity to any pain reliever or antipyretic (including NSAIDs)
- Coagulation defects
- Severe renal or hepatic disease

Evidence
Nonsteroidal anti-inflammatory treatment may be helpful in the management of epididymo-orchitis [1] *Level C*

Acceptability to patient
Good, although incidence of gastrointestinal side-effectss may make this unacceptable to some.

Patient and caregiver information
Take tablets either with food or an antacid.

ACETAMINOPHEN
Para-aminophonol analgesic.

Dose
- Adults and children >14 years:
325–1000mg, orally, every 4h, as required (not more than 4g/day)
- Children <14 years:
10–15mg/kg, orally, every 4h, as required (not more than 5 doses per 24h)

Efficacy
Effective analgesic.

Risks/Benefits
Risks:
- Use caution in hepatic and renal impairment
- Overdosage results in hepatic and renal damage unless treated promptly
- Overdose may lead to multiorgan failure and may be fatal
- Accidental overdosage can occur if over-the-counter (OTC) preparations containing acetaminophen are taken with prescribed drugs that contain acetaminophen

Benefits:
- May be used in children
- Reduces fever and malaise

Side-effectss and adverse reactions
- Acetaminophen rarely causes side-effectss when used intermittently
- Gastrointestinal: nausea, vomiting
- Hematologic: blood disorders
- Metabolic: acute hepatic and renal failure
- Skin: rashes
- Other: acute pancreatitis

Interactions (other drugs)
- Alcohol
- Anticoagulants
- Anticonvulsants
- Isoniazid
- Cholestyramine
- Colestipol
- Domperidone
- Metoclopromide

Contraindications
Known liver dysfunction

Acceptability to patient
High.

Patient and caregiver information
- Avoid alcohol
- Read labels of other over-the-counter drugs, many contain acetaminophen and may cause toxicity if taken concurrently

Surgical therapy
SCROTAL EXPLORATION
Efficacy
Highly effective.

Risks/Benefits
Benefits:
- Can drain infected material, or abscess if present
- If torsion or tumor present, will be identified and treated appropriately

Acceptability to patient
Moderate, will require admission to hospital and a general anesthetic.

Follow up plan
Daily review until clear evidence that infection settling, then review weekly to fortnightly until wound healed.

Patient and caregiver information
- Wear scrotal support after your operation until pain and swelling settle
- If your stitches are dissolvable, do not spend a long time in the bath until the wound has healed, take a short bath or shower instead

EPIDIDYMO-ORCHIDECTOMY
Efficacy
Highly effective.

Risks/Benefits
- Risks: Patient left with a single testis, and if he develops epididymo-orchitis in remaining testis, could be left anorchic

- Benefits: Infected organ removed, symptoms should now resolve

Acceptability to patient
Low, as most men would not wish removal of a testicle, even though in the presence of severe infection this may be inevitable.

Follow up plan
Daily review until clear evidence that infection is settling, then review weekly to fortnightly until wound has healed.

Patient and caregiver information

- The infected testis and epididymis has been severely damaged, and probably has little or no function
- Normal sexual function and fertility are possible with a single testis
- A prosthetic testis can be inserted (later, when the infection has resolved), to produce a more normal appearance
- Do not take any long baths until your wound is properly healed. A shower is better

Other therapies
SCROTAL SUPPORT
Efficacy
Highly effective for improving patient comfort, but does not influence course of infective process.

Risks/Benefits
Benefit: increased patient comfort

Evidence
Scrotal support is recommended in the management of epididymo-orchitis [1] *Level C*

Acceptability to patient
Generally acceptable.

Patient and caregiver information
Wear the support all the time, except when washing, until scrotal swelling and pain has resolved. An ice pack to the groin may decrease discomfort.

EFFICACY OF THERAPIES

- Pain and swelling generally resolve within 2–4 weeks with appropriate antibiotics and analgesia
- Resolution of epididymal induration may require several weeks

Evidence

PDxMD are unable to cite evidence that meets our criteria for evidence.

PROGNOSIS

Most patients make a full recovery, but some will be rendered infertile (especially with epididymitis owing to *Chlamydia trachomatis* or *Neiserria gonorrheae*) or develop chronic epididymitis.

Therapeutic failure

All patients failing antibiotic therapy should be referred urgently to a urologist.

Recurrence

Any patient suffering from recurrent epididymitis should be referred to a urologist.

Deterioration

If the patient's condition deteriorates, they should be referred urgently for admission to hospital for parenteral antibiotics and possible surgical exploration of the scrotum.

COMPLICATIONS

Orchitis, abscess formation (especially in gonococcal epididymitis), chronic epididymitis, and infertility may occur.

RISK FACTORS

- Presence of congenital abnormality of the urinary tract: especially in prepubertal boys. Often will be corrected surgically, reducing the subsequent risk of urinary tract infection or epididymitis
- Infection with *Chlamydia trachomatis* or *Neiserria gonorrheae*: incidence of infection can be reduced (by using barrier methods of contraception), thereby reducing risk of subsequently developing epididymitis
- Presence of indwelling catheter or need for urinary tract surgery places patient at risk of developing epididymitis

MODIFY RISK FACTORS
Lifestyle and wellness
SEXUAL BEHAVIOR

The use of condoms helps to reduce the spread of sexually transmitted diseases, including chlamydia and gonorrhea, and may thus reduce the risk of subsequent development of epididymitis.

CHEMOPROPHYLAXIS

Patients undergoing catheterization or surgery on the urinary tract should have prophylactic antibiotics. In most cases a single preprocedure dose of an intravenous antibiotic will be sufficient to prevent a bacteremia or bacteriuria leading to epididymitis.

PREVENT RECURRENCE

In general, the prevention of recurrence is not possible in this disorder.

RESOURCES

ASSOCIATIONS

American Urological Association
1120 N Charles St.
Baltimore, MD 21201
Phone: 410-727-1100
Fax: 410-223-4373
http://www.amuro.org

KEY REFERENCES

- Ball TP, Seidmon JE, Hanno PM. Current urologic therapy. Philadelphia: W.B. Saunders, 1994
- Berger RE. Campbell's urology. Philadelphia: W.B. Saunders, pp.672–673, 1997
- Holmes HK et al. Sexually transmitted diseases. Philadelphia: Churchill Livingstone, p.855, 1999
- National guideline for the management of chlamydia trachomatis genital tract infection. Clinical Effectiveness Group (Association of Genitourinary Medicine and the Medical Society for the Study of Venereal Diseases). Sex Transm Infect 1999;75(Suppl1):S4–8
- National guideline for the management of epididymoorchitis. Clinical Effectiveness Group (Association of Genitourinary Medicine and the Medical Society for the Study of Venereal Diseases). Sex Transm Infect 1999;75(Suppl1):S51–53
- Rosen P, ed. Emergency medicine concepts and clinical practice, 4th edn. St Louis: Mosby-Year Book Inc, pp.2227–2258, 1998

Guidelines:

1   National guideline for the management of epididymoorchitis. Clinical Effectiveness Group (Association of Genitourinary Medicine and the Medical Society for the Study of Venereal Diseases). Sex Transm Infect 1999;75(Suppl1):S51–53

FAQS
Question 1
What is acute epididymitis? How is it defined?

ANSWER 1
Acute epididymitis is inflammation, pain, and swelling of the epididymis of less than 6 weeks duration.

Question 2
What is chronic epididymitis? How is it defined?

ANSWER 2
Chronic epididymitis develops after recurrent episodes of epididymitis and is associated with scarring and induration of the epididymis.

Question 3
What are the signs and symptoms of acute epididymitis?

ANSWER 3
Rapidly progressive scrotal swelling and pain, which may radiate into the spermatic cord and cause lower abdominal pain. There is often thickening of the scrotal skin of the affected hemiscrotum. Fever can occur along with generalized malaise. Sometimes the epididymis is so swollen and painful as to be indistinguishable from the testis.

Question 4
What are the complications of epididymitis?

ANSWER 4
Infertility, scar tissue, orchitis, abscess, testis atrophy, Fournier's gangrene.

Question 5
What is the most common route of infection of the epididymis?

ANSWER 5
Ascending infection from the urethra, prostate, or urinary bladder.

CONTRIBUTORS
Fred F Ferri, MD, FACP
Philip J Aliotta, MD, MHA, FACS
Anuj K Chopra, MD

ACUTE GLOMERULONEPHRITIS

SUMMARY INFORMATION

DESCRIPTION

- An immunologic response to an infection, most commonly streptococcal
- The majority of patients are children
- Patients typically present with hematuria, edema and hypertension. They may have deranged renal function, which is occasionally permanent
- Therapy is largely supportive, and antibiotics (preferably penicillin) are given to eradicate the infection
- Prognosis is excellent in children, but more guarded in older patients

URGENT ACTION

- Commence antibiotic therapy (preferably penicillin, but erythromycin if there is a history of allergy)
- Immediate referral to nephrologist/pediatrician if there is evidence of compromised renal function, especially in a child

ICD9 CODE
580.9 Acute glomerulonephritis with unspecified pathological lesion in kidney

SYNONYMS
- Bright's disease
- Postinfectious glomerulonephritis
- Acute nephritic syndrome
- Acute post-streptococcal glomerulonephritis

CARDINAL FEATURES
- An immunologic response to an infection, most commonly streptococcal
- Most often associated with Streptococcal pharyngitis and impetigo
- Results in inflammation of the glomeruli leading to damage of the basement membrane, mesangium and capillary endothelium
- Majority of patients are children
- Infection precedes glomerulonephritis by up to 3 weeks
- Typically present with hematuria, edema, hypertension
- May have deranged renal function, which occasionally is permanent
- Therapy is largely supportive, and antibiotics (preferably penicillin) are given to eradicate streptococcal infection
- There is no specific treatment for acute glomerulonephritis
- Prognosis is excellent in children, but more guarded in older patients

CAUSES
Common causes
- Following a Group A beta hemolytic streptococcus infection *(Streptococcus pyogenes)*, which can cause a variety of conditions; most commonly streptococcal pharyngitis or impetigo
- So-called nephritogenic serotypes of group A beta hemolytic streptococcus usually responsible; i.e. groups 1, 4, 11, 12, 49 "Red Lake", 55, 60

Rare causes
May also follow infection with:
- *Streptococcus pneumoniae* (Streptococcal or Pneumococcal pneumonia)
- *Staphylococcus aureus*
- *Streptococcus meningeae* (streptococcal meningitis)
- *Varicella zoster* (chickenpox)
- Hepatitis B

Serious causes
Bacterial endocarditis

Contributory or predisposing factors
Recent infection with nephritogenic strain of *Streptococcus pyogenes* (15% of patients infected with nephritogenic strain develop acute glomerulonephritis).

EPIDEMIOLOGY
Incidence and prevalence
INCIDENCE

0.02 per 1000 new cases per year.

PREVALENCE

Uncertain, as up to 50% of cases may be subclinical.

Demographics
AGE

- Over 50% of cases occur in children less than 13 years of age
- Only 10% of patients are over 40 years of age

GENDER

Male : Female ratio = 60:40.

GENETICS

Currently there is no proven genetic link.

GFOGRAPHY

Incidence declining in the developed world, but is unchanged in developing countries.

DIFFERENTIAL DIAGNOSIS

- The most important differential diagnosis is rapidly progressive glomerulonephritis, associated with multisystem diseases (e.g. SLE), which requires urgent attention to prevent progression to chronic renal failure
- Other common differential diagnoses include IgA nephropathy, hemolytic-uremic syndrome, membranous glomerulonephritis, acute interstitial nephritis, systemic lupus erythematosus, and partial obstruction

Rapidly progressive glomerulonephritis
FEATURES
- Anuria
- Proteinuria
- Hematuria
- Anemia
- Suspect if patient presents with either increased BUN or serum creatinine
- Often associated with multisystem disease. May respond to immunosuppression

Membranous glomerulonephritis
FEATURES
- Commonest in adult men
- Proteinuria (nephrotic range)
- Edema
- Hypertension
- Patient may have history of taking gold, penicillamine, NSAIDs (rare)
- May follow hepatitis B, systemic lupus erythematosus, parasitic infection, malignancy
- Approximately a third develop end stage renal disease over 10–20 years

IgA nephropathy
FEATURES
- Most common glomerulonephritis worldwide
- Most common in second and third decades of life
- More common in males
- 50% present with frank hematuria, often with dysuria
- 40% present with microscopic hematuria and proteinuria
- Often occurs following (or exacerbated by) an upper respiratory tract infection; e.g. tonsillitis, pharyngitis. Fatigue
- Pyrexia
- Hypertension

Hemolytic-uremic syndrome
FEATURES
- Common in children
- May also occur in the elderly, with a high mortality rate
- Typically occurs after gastrointestinal infection with E coli 0157:H7
- Hemolytic anemia
- Anuria in 30% of cases
- Neurological symptoms including headache, visual disturbance, seizures, coma

Acute interstitial nephritis

FEATURES

- Typically antibiotic related, although a range of other drugs implicated; e.g. NSAIDs, diuretics, antiepileptics
- May also occur after a wide range of bacterial and viral infections
- Pyrexia
- Eosinophilia
- Eosinophiluria
- Develop renal failure over a period of days to weeks

Systemic lupus erythematosus
FEATURES

- Chronic multisystem autoimmune inflammatory condition
- Anorexia
- Malaise
- Fever
- Skin lesions
- Mouth ulcers
- Aching muscles and joints
- Painful red eyes
- Headaches
- Psychosis
- Can be fatal

Malignant hypertension
FEATURES

- Over 90% of cases have no identifiable cause
- If idiopathic, age of onset is 20s and 30s.
- 10% of cases have an underlying cause. Some may present in childhood
- More common in men
- Often asymptomatic
- Headache: if severe
- Retinopathy: if severe
- Increased second heart sound
- Other signs and symptoms may depend on an underlying cause, if present

SIGNS & SYMPTOMS
Signs

- Oligo- or anuria
- Proteinuria
- Hypertension: In up to 10% of cases may be severe, with signs and symptoms of encephalopathy (headache, somnolence, confusion, convulsions)
- Pyrexia (uncommon)
- Heart murmur
- Ascites, pleural effusion in severe cases

Symptoms

- Symptoms of preceding streptococcal infection e.g. pharyngitis, respiratory infection, impetigo
- Hematuria: Classically described as 'smoky', but may be dark or tea colored
- Edema of the hands and face in mornings, edema of the ankles and feet in afternoons
- Malaise
- Lethargy
- Anorexia
- Increase in weight

- Pain in the back and joints
- Shortness of breath due to pulmonary edema (rare)

ASSOCIATED DISORDERS
Hypertension.

CONSIDER CONSULT
All patients with hematuria and or proteinuria with or without systemic illness should be referred.

INVESTIGATION OF THE PATIENT
Direct questions to patient
Q Have you recently had a sore throat, skin rash, stomach upset or other illness? If there is no recent history, then poststreptococcal glomerulonephritis is a less likely diagnosis.

Q Are you taking any medications? Many drugs (e.g. gold, penicillamine) may precipitate membranous glomerulonephritis; antibiotics and NSAIDs may cause acute interstitial nephritis.

Q Do you think you are passing any more or less urine than usual? If the patient describes passing less urine than normal, this may indicate impending renal failure. If the patient complains of polyuria, glomerulonephritis is less likely diagnosis. Diabetes mellitus should be considered.

Q Have you ever had this before? Is unusual for acute glomerulonephritis to recur.

Contributory or predisposing factors
Q Any history of predisposing factors? e.g. *Streptococcal pharyngitis*, subacute bacterial endocarditis, impetigo.

Family history
Q Has anyone else in the family been ill recently? If infection with a highly nephritogenic strain, cluster of cases may occur in one household.

Examination
- **Check temperature:** Pyrexia makes the diagnosis of acute glomerulonephritis less likely
- **Check blood pressure:** Many patients are hypertensive
- **Check skin for the lesions of impetigo:** If lesions are present, even without a bacteriological diagnosis, is highly suggestive that the patient has acute glomerulonephritis
- **Examine throat**
- **Auscultate the heart and lungs:** If a murmur is present, especially if not previously documented, consider endocarditis in the diagnosis. Occasionally patients present with pulmonary edema
- **Examine the abdomen;** may be tender

Summary of investigative tests
- Throat swab: Should be taken if patient has history consistent with streptococcal pharyngitis. If available, a rapid antigen test may be performed, but should be followed by cultures for Group A Streptococci
- Skin swab: May be taken if patient suspected of having impetigo, and cultured for Group A streptococci
- Urinalysis (dipstick test): Should be performed in all patients, and will provide rapid confirmation of a variety of abnormalities; including hematuria (if microscopic), and proteinuria
- Urine microscopy: Microscopic examination of urine sediment will confirm the presence or absence of red or white blood cells and casts
- Complete blood count: Should be performed as many patients will be anemic
- Renal function: Should be checked in all patients, as is frequently abnormal
- Serum potassium: This is frequently increased in renal failure, so should be checked in all cases

- Streptozyme test: Is a useful screening test, as it combines several streptococcal antibody assays
- Anti-streptolysin O (ASO) titer: Is an antibody assayed as part of the Streptozyme test, but is a useful test on its own, as a high titer provides good evidence of recent streptococcal infection
- Antibody screen: A wide variety of autoantibodies may be assayed, particularly when the diagnosis is not obvious, but this would normally be performed by a specialist
- Serum C3 and C4 levels: Serial estimation of complement components, particularly C3 and C4, is useful in the diagnosis as they usually are low
- 24-hour urine collection: To examine a variety of parameters, including actual volume produced, and the amount of protein excreted, over a 24-hour period
- Echocardiogram: If the patient has a heart murmur, and endocarditis is suspected
- Renal biopsy: Usually only required if the diagnosis is in doubt. Typically shows a diffuse, proliferative glomerulonephritis. This test would only be performed by a specialist
- Renal imaging: Kidneys in acute nephritis are usually large and lose medullary differentiation. Imaging is useful to rule out obstruction

DIAGNOSTIC DECISION

The development of hematuria and edema in a patient with a recent history of an infective illness (usually streptococcal) indicates a diagnosis of acute glomerulonephritis. Diagnosis usually clinical, but may be guided by laboratory test results

CLINICAL PEARLS

- A delay in referral may result in late dialysis – danger from hyperkalemia, pulmonary edema
- 5% present with nephrotic syndrome
- 3–4% of patients do not recover renal function

THE TESTS
Body fluids
URINALYSIS (DIPSTICK TEST)
Description
Midstream urine specimen.

Advantages/Disadvantages
Advantages:
- Quick and simple to perform at office level
- Provides information about a variety of urinary constituents very quickly

Disadvantages:
- Whether normal or abnormal, does not confirm or refute the diagnosis
- Very nonspecific

Normal
No red or white blood cells, or protein identified.

Abnormal
- Red and/or white blood cells, and/or protein present
- Dipstick tests can be highly sensitive; a false-positive result is possible

Cause of abnormal result
The glomerular membrane, which in the healthy kidney prevents large molecules escaping into the urine can no longer do so.

Drugs, disorders and other factors that may alter results
- If patient is a woman of childbearing age, check that she is not menstruating, as that may lead to a false positive result
- Do not dismiss hematuria as infection. If a patient is treated with antibiotics, then retest after treatment

URINE MICROSCOPY
Description
Centrifuged urine specimen.

Advantages/Disadvantages
Advantage: if dysmorphic red blood cells, or red blood cell or white blood cell casts present, is highly suggestive of acute glomerulonephritis

Disadvantages:
- If normal, does not eliminate acute glomerulonephritis as a diagnosis, because rarely this may present without hematuria.
- Procedure is not standardized, and the degree of urinary sediment concentration may vary. Can therefore be difficult to interpret quantitative reports

Normal
- 0–2 Red blood cells (RBC) per high power field (hpf)
- 0–5 White blood cells (WBC) per high power field (hpf)
- Occasional hyaline cast only

Although these normal results are typical, there is considerable variation; check with local laboratory

Abnormal
- >2 RBC/hpf
- >5 WBC/hpf
- Casts
- Keep in mind the possibility of a false-positive result

Cause of abnormal result
- The glomerular membrane, which in the healthy kidney prevents large molecules escaping into the urine can no longer do so
- Casts are aggregates of protein, blood cells or both. Develop secondary to urinary stasis in renal tubules, the presence of a concentrated urine, and significant proteinuria

Drugs, disorders and other factors that may alter results
If patient is a woman of childbearing age, check that she is not menstruating, as this may lead to a false-positive result.

THROAT SWAB
Description
Throat swab.

Advantages/Disadvantages
- Advantage: if *Streptococcus pyogenes* cultured, the diagnosis of acute glomerulonephritis is highly likely
- Disadvantage: delay whilst waiting for culture results. If negative, doesn't eliminate either recent streptococcal infection or acute glomerulonephritis

Normal
Growth of normal commensals.

Abnormal
- Positive culture for *Streptococcus pyogenes*
- Keep in mind the possibility of a false-positive result

Cause of abnormal result
- Bacteria present
- Keep in mind the possibility of a false positive result. Note that some people are asymptomatic carriers, and therefore culture results must be taken in context with clinical findings

Drugs, disorders and other factors that may alter results
Swab may be contaminated with bacteria from elsewhere, e.g. from person taking swab.

COMPLETE BLOOD COUNT
Description
Cuffed venous blood sample.

Advantages/Disadvantages
Disadvantages:
- Whether normal or abnormal, the result is not diagnostic of acute glomerulonephritis
- As many of the patients are children, they may find venepuncture, especially on a repeated basis, very distressing

Normal
Hemoglobin
Men: 150 +/- 20g/l
Women: 135 +/- 15g/l

Hematocrit
Men: 0.45 +/- 0.05
Women: 0.41 +/- 0.05
Note that reference ranges vary between laboratories, and that ranges for children vary with age. Check with local laboratory

Abnormal
- Anemia or a fall in hematocrit may be seen in acute glomerulonephritis
- Keep in mind the possibility of a false-positive result

Cause of abnormal result
- Systemic illness
- Renal impairment

SKIN LESION SWAB
Description
Because of the relative ease in diagnosing impetigo, skin lesion culture is rarely necessary. If impetigo is suspected, treatment should be instituted before culture results are obtained. Skin lesion culture should only be used in those cases where there is a significant question regarding the diagnosis of impetigo.

Advantages/Disadvantages
Advantage: if *Streptococcus pyogenes* cultured, the diagnosis of acute glomerulonephritis is highly likely

Disadvantages:
- Delay whilst waiting for culture results
- A negative result does not eliminate acute glomerulonephritis

Normal
Growth of normal commensals.

Abnormal
- Positive culture for *Streptococcus pyogenes*
- Keep in mind the possibility of a false-positive result

Cause of abnormal result
Bacteria present.

Drugs, disorders and other factors that may alter results
Swab may be contaminated with bacteria from elsewhere, e.g. from person taking swab.

SERUM BLOOD UREA NITROGEN (BUN) AND CREATININE
Description
Cuffed venous blood sample. Must combine this with measuring serum potassium.

Advantages/Disadvantages
Advantages:
- Will indicate whether renal function is impaired
- Serial measurements may be used to monitor patient's progress

Disadvantage: invasive procedure: children especially may find repeated venepuncture distressing

Normal
- (BUN) urea 3.3 – 6.7mmol/l
- Creatinine 60 – 120micromol/l
Note that reference ranges can vary; check with local laboratory

Abnormal
- (BUN) urea > 6.7mmol/l
- Creatinine >120micromol/l
- Keep in mind the possibility of a false-positive result

Cause of abnormal result
Impaired clearance of nitrogenous waste products from blood.

Drugs, disorders and other factors that may alter results
Renal function can fall to a glomerular filtration rate of 50ml/min before serum creatinine rises above normal range.

SERUM POTASSIUM
Description
Cuffed venous blood sample.

Advantages/Disadvantages
- Advantage: if patient is hyperkalemic, is important to identify this, because of risk to cardiovascular status
- Disadvantage: invasive procedure; children especially may find repeated venepuncture distressing

Normal
3.3–5.0mmol/l.
Note that reference ranges may vary. Check with local laboratory.

Abnormal
- >5.0mmol/l
- Keep in mind the possibility of a false-positive result

Drugs, disorders and other factors that may alter results
- Hemolyzed blood sample
- Significant delay between taking and analyzing blood sample

STREPTOZYME TEST
Description
Cuffed venous blood sample.

Advantages/Disadvantages
Advantage: a useful screening test, as simultaneously tests for several streptococcal antibodies

Disadvantages:
- Some strains of Group A streptococci do not produce streptolysin S or O
- Invasive procedure: children especially may find repeated venepuncture distressing

Normal
Streptococcal antibodies either not detected or if they are, no significant difference (i.e. rise) in titers on serial specimens.

Abnormal
- Rise in antibody titer on serial samples taken 48–72 hours apart
- Keep in mind the possibility of a false-positive result

Cause of abnormal result
Recent streptococcal infection.

Drugs, disorders and other factors that may alter results
After infection, antibodies may persist in blood, still detectable in 20% of patients 12 months after infection. In recent infection, however, rises in titer should be seen.

ANTI-STREPTOLYSIN O (ASO) TITER

Description
Cuffed venous blood sample.

Advantages/Disadvantages
Advantage: if ASO detected, this provides good circumstantial evidence of the diagnosis. A rise in the titer is more important than the actual values obtained

Disadvantages:
- Delay between first and second results
- Actual titer result gives no indication of the duration, severity of illness, or the prognosis
- Invasive procedure: children especially may find repeated venepuncture distressing

Normal
Streptococcal antibodies either not detected or if they are, no significant difference (i.e. rise) in titers on serial specimens.

Abnormal
- Rise in antibody titer on serial samples taken 48 hours apart
- Keep in mind the possibility of a false-positive result

Cause of abnormal result
Recent streptococcal infection.

Drugs, disorders and other factors that may alter results
After infection, antibodies may persist in blood, still detectable in 20% of patients 12 months after infection. In recent infection, however, rises in titer should be seen.

TREATMENT

CONSIDER CONSULT
Refer all children, and adults with hematuria and/or evidence of deteriorating renal function.

IMMEDIATE ACTION
Commence antibiotic treatment with penicillin (or erythromycin, if history of allergy), to eradicate streptococcal infection.

PATIENT AND CAREGIVER ISSUES
Patient or caregiver request
Has there been a recent local epidemic of streptococcal infection?

Health-seeking behavior
Has patient delayed seeing the doctor (e.g. hoping that symptoms would settle on their own)?

MANAGEMENT ISSUES
Goals
- Eradication of streptococcal infection
- Early recognition of the need for referral to a specialist

Management in special circumstances
PATIENT SATISFACTION/LIFESTYLE PRIORITIES
A small proportion of patients are left with permanent renal impairment, which may lead to chronic ill health. This may affect schooling and employment prospects, especially in younger patients.

SUMMARY OF THERAPEUTIC OPTIONS
Choices
There is no specific treatment for acute glomerulonephritis; treatment is largely supportive

- Penicillin G benzathene is the drug of first choice, providing there is no history of allergy, to eradicate the streptococcal infection
- Penicillin V is the second choice, but has the advantage of being given orally
- Erythromycin may be given as an alternative in patients who are allergic to penicillin
- If patients have significant hypertension and/or edema, these conditions may require appropriate therapy
- Dietary measures are very important in all patients

FOLLOW UP
Plan for review
Review every 2–3 days. If there is any doubt regarding the patient's progress, refer to a nephrologist or pediatrician, if this has not been done already. Recovering patients may be reviewed on a weekly basis.

DRUGS AND OTHER THERAPIES: DETAILS
Drugs
PENICILLIN G BENZATHINE
Dose
By IM or slow IV injection or infusion:
- Adults: 1.2g daily in 4 divided doses
- Children: 1 month-12 years: 100mg/kg daily in 4 divided doses

Treat for 10 days.

Efficacy
Preferred therapy for streptococcal infection.

Risks/Benefits
- Use caution in patients allergic to cephalosporins
- Use caution in severe renal failure

Side-effects and adverse reactions
- Gastrointestinal: diarrhea, nausea
- Respiratory: anaphylaxis
- Skin: erythema multiforme, rash, urticaria
- Hematologic: bone marrow suppression, coagulation disorders Renal: interstitial nephritis

Interactions (other drugs)
- Chloramphenicol ■ Macrolide ■ Antibiotics ■ Methotrexate ■ Oral contraceptives
- Tetracyclines

Contraindications
Penicillin hypersensitivity

Acceptability to patient
- Moderate
- Injection may be painful
- Depending on duration of treatment, patient will probably need to be in hospital

Patient and caregiver information
- Purpose of treatment is to control infection and to prevent development of complications
- Does not stop nephritis in patients with established disease

PENICILLIN V
Dose
Given orally:
- Adults: 500 – 750mg 6 hourly
- Children <1yr: 62.5mg 6 hourly
- Children 1–5 years: 125mg 6 hourly
- Children 6–12 years: 250mg 6 hourly

Treat for 10 days.

Efficacy
Good.

Risks/Benefits
- Use caution in patients allergic to cephalosporins
- Use caution in severe renal failure

Side-effects and adverse reactions
- Gastrointestinal: diarrhea, nausea
- Respiratory: anaphylaxis
- Skin: eythema multiforme, rash, urticaria
- Hematologic: bone marrow suppression, coagulation disorders Renal: interstitial nephritis

Interactions (other drugs)
- Chloramphenicol ■ Macrolide ■ Antibiotics ■ Methotrexate ■ Oral contraceptives
- Tetracyclines

Contraindications
Penicillin hypersensitivity

Acceptability to patient
High. Oral preparation preferred by most patients

Follow up plan
Patient should be seen initially every few days.

Patient and caregiver information
Take antibiotic tablets regularly. Finish the course, even if you feel better.

ERYTHROMYCIN
Dose
- Adults and children over 8 years of age 250–500mg every 6 hours orally
- Children < 2 years of age 125mg orally every 6 hours
- Children 2–8 years 250mg orally every 6 hours
- Dose may be doubled in severe infection

Treat for 10 days.

Efficacy
Good, although penicillin preferred

Risks/Benefits
- Caution in hepatic and renal impairment, porphyria
- Prolongs QT interval
- Avoid concomitant administration with terfenadine, astemizole and cisapride

Side-effects and adverse reactions
- Gastrointestinal: anorexia, nausea, diarrhea, abdominal pain
- Skin: rashes, pruritis
- Vaginal candidiasis
- Hearing loss

Interactions (other drugs)
■ Alfentanil ■ Anti-arrhythmic drugs ■ Anti-convulsants ■ Antihistamines (terfenadine, astemizole) ■ Anti viral agents ■ Benzodiazepines ■ Bromocriptine ■ Cisapride ■ Clozapine ■ Colchicine ■ Cyclosporine ■ Ergotamine ■ Felodipine ■ Methylprednisolone ■ Penicillin ■ Quinidine ■ Statins ■ Tacrolimus ■ Theophylline ■ Warfarin ■ Zopiclone

Contraindications
Liver disease

Acceptability to patient
High, as most patients prefer oral treatment.

Follow up plan
Patient should be seen initially every few days.

Patient and caregiver information
Take antibiotic tablets regularly. Finish the course, even if you feel better.

LIFESTYLE
■ Patients with edema and hypertension should take a no-added salt diet until these have resolved
■ High potassium containing foods should be avoided, and protein restricted, to 0.8g/kg/day in patients with impaired renal function
■ Fluid restriction will be required in patients with significant edema

RISKS/BENEFITS
Benefit to patient by reducing load on kidneys.

ACCEPTABILITY TO PATIENT
Some patients may find the diet very restrictive. Children especially may find it difficult to understand why they must adhere to the diet.

PATIENT AND CAREGIVER INFORMATION
Patients (and often their parents) will need to be taught about low protein diets, low potassium diets, and how to restrict fluids, as well as how to make the diet palatable.

PROGNOSIS

Most patients, and children especially, make a full recovery. The prognosis is more guarded in adults. A proportion may develop hypertension, proteinuria, and renal impairment 10–40 years after their original illness. The most common, however, is the development of mild hypertension.

Clinical pearls

Proteinuria and hematuria may persist for up to 2 years after function returns to normal.

Therapeutic failure

Refer patient to nephrologist or pediatrician, if this has not been done already.

COMPLICATIONS

Permanent renal impairment and/or hypertension may occur in a small proportion of patients.

Prevention is not currently possible. Early antibiotic treatment does not influence the subsequent development of acute glomerulonephritis.

MODIFY RISK FACTORS
SCREENING

Screening is not appropriate for acute glomerulonephritis

RESOURCES

ASSOCIATIONS
National Kidney Association
30E 33rd Street,
Suite 1100,
New York, NY 10016
(212) 889-2210

KEY REFERENCES
Brenner BM, Rector FC. The Kidney, 6th edn. Philadelphia: WB Saunders, 2000

CONTRIBUTORS
Randolph L Pearson, MD
Philip J Aliotta, MD, MHA, FACS

HYDROCELE

SUMMARY INFORMATION

DESCRIPTION

- Abnormal fluid accumulation in the scrotum, between the layers of the tunica vaginalis
- In infants, usually the result of incomplete closure of the processus vaginalis; may or may not be associated with inguinal hernia
- In older boys and men, may be idiopathic, but more likely to be secondary to another pathologic process
- May be acute or chronic
- Surgical correction usually not necessary for hydrocele, per se, but may be indicated if symptoms warrant

URGENT ACTION

- If acute presentation, need to rule out testicular torsion or incarcerated/strangulated hernia as primary cause with emergent referral if indicated
- Can attempt manual reduction of incarcerated hernia, but the patient should always be evaluated by a surgical specialist at the same time – a tense hydrocele can compress the blood supply and cause atrophy of the testis

KEY! DON'T MISS!

- Testicular torsion as primary process
- Incarcerated/strangulated hernia as primary process
- Testicular tumor as primary process

ICD9 CODE
603.9 Hydrocele, unspecified

CARDINAL FEATURES
- Abnormal fluid accumulation in the scrotum between the visceral and parietal layers of the tunica vaginalis
- If processus vaginalis closes distally, but not proximally, there is a communication with the peritoneal cavity and it is almost always associated with an indirect inguinal hernia; this is termed a communicating hydrocele or a complete inguinal hernia
- May be unilateral, more commonly on the right hemiscrotum, but often bilateral
- In older boys and men, may be idiopathic, but more likely to be secondary to another pathologic process in the scrotum or adjacent structures
- May present as acute or chronic
- Acute hydroceles may be painful, with erythema and tenderness
- Acute hydrocele of the spermatic cord may become trapped in the inguinal canal and produce testicular ischemia
- Chronic hydroceles are typically painless, but may produce uncomfortable sensation of heaviness
- Transilluminates
- The fluid is clear and yellow
- Not reducible unless there is an associated indirect inguinal hernia
- May appear smaller after period of recumbency
- Scrotal ultrasound with or without dopplers can aid in diagnosis; nuclear scan less useful but may help with difficult diagnoses
- Surgical correction usually not necessary for hydrocele, but may be indicated if symptoms warrant or may be performed in conjunction with other repair, except in some children
- In children, a fluctuating hydrocele size and persistent scrotal swelling after the age of one year suggest a communicating hydrocele, which is an indirect inguinal hernia. This needs to be surgically repaired because of the risk of incarceration and strangulation of abdominal structures when hydroceles/hernias are followed expectantly
- Premature and low-birth-weight infants have a higher incidence of hydroceles and bilateral lesions

CAUSES
Common causes
In infants, usually due to:
- Incomplete closure of the processus vaginalis from the peritoneum
- Residual peritoneal fluid that has yet to be reabsorbed after processus closure (a patent processus vaginalis accompanies the testis during normal descent and normally fuses spontaneously after the testis reaches the scrotum; incomplete obliteration of the patent processus vaginalis can result in simple hydrocele, hydrocele of the cord, communicating hydrocele through a narrow patent processus vaginalis, or a widely patent processus with complete inguinal hernia)

In older boys and men, may be idiopathic, but usually due to abnormal absorption or secretion secondary to another pathologic process such as:
- Trauma
- Ischemia
- Infection
- Testicular tumor
- Increased intra-abdominal pressure

Rare causes

- Infants may sometimes present with hydrocele secondary to intrascrotal or intra-abdominal pathology
- Infant girls may have a hydrocele of the canal of Nuck or meconium hydrocele of the labia
- Filariasis may produce hydrocele in infected boys and men
- Hydrocele may be seen following ipsilateral renal transplantation

Serious causes

- Hydrocele may be secondary to testicular torsion or incarcerated/strangulated hernia
- Hydrocele may be secondary to testicular cancer

Contributory or predisposing factors

- Premature and low-birth-weight infants
- Indirect inguinal hernia
- Primary testicular/intrascrotal pathology
- Trauma
- Surgery
- Increased intra-abdominal pressure
- Lymphatic obstruction
- Ventriculoperitoneal shunt
- Peritoneal dialysis
- Ehlers-Danlos syndrome
- Bladder exstrophy

EPIDEMIOLOGY

Incidence and prevalence

INCIDENCE

- 10–60 per 1000 newborn full-term boys
- 10 per 1000 adult men

Demographics

AGE

More common in infancy, but can occur at any age.

GENDER

Almost exclusively male, but newborn girls can have hydroceles of the canal of Nuck or meconium hydrocele of the labia.

DIFFERENTIAL DIAGNOSIS
Inguinal hernia
The distinguishing features of inguinal hernia are as follows.

FEATURES
- Should be reducible
- Should be able to feel swelling continuous with internal inguinal ring
- Most likely will not transilluminate, but transillumination does NOT rule out a hernia as it may be concurrent with hydrocele
- Complete inguinal hernia sometimes considered synonymous with communicating hydrocele
- Strangulated hernia will be erythematous and tender and is a surgical emergency

Epididymitis
The distinguishing features of epididymitis are as follows.

FEATURES
- Most commonly seen in young men owing to sexually transmitted diseases
- May occur in older men as spread of prostatitis
- May occur in prepubertal boys owing to urinary tract infections
- May have preceding urinary tract symptoms
- Pain gradually rises over period of days
- Almost always associated with fever
- May be able to localize swelling and tenderness to the superior/posterior pole of the testis
- Testis on the affected side will likely be enlarged

Testicular torsion
The distinguishing features of testicular torsion are as follows.

FEATURES
- Rapid onset of severe pain, often associated with nausea and fever
- May have history of similar pain with spontaneous resolution
- Average age 16 years
- Rapid onset of scrotal swelling and erythema
- Bell-clapper deformity may be noted in contralateral testicle
- May lose cremasteric reflex
- Surgical emergency

Trauma
FEATURES
- May have reactive hydrocele
- Hematocele will not transilluminate
- Should be able to elicit history, although patient embarrassment may be a hindrance

Testicular tumor
The distinguishing features of testicular tumor are as follows.

FEATURES
- Can be benign or malignant
- Presentation usually not acute
- Scrotal swelling will usually be diffuse
- Typically painless unless hemorrhage occurs
- Palpation or imaging may detect intratesticular mass

Torsion of testicular appendages
FEATURES

- Signs and symptoms less severe than in testicular torsion, although not always
- May see blue or blue-black dot at superior pole of testis
- Most common in prepubertal boys
- Benign and self-limited
- Cremasteric reflex usually intact

Orchitis
The distinguishing features of orchitis are as follows.

FEATURES

- Usually occurs as a result of the spread of epididymitis, with similar signs and symptoms
- Orchitis due to mumps occurs 7 to 10 days following the parotitis and is usually unilateral; it is more likely to occur in men than boys

Varicocele
The distinguishing features of varicocele are as follows.

FEATURES

- Almost always on the left
- Typical 'bag of worms' appearance when patient is upright; it is smaller when patient is supine
- Usually nontender

Intrascrotal cysts

- Epididymal cysts
- Spermatoceles

FEATURES

- Generally benign
- Will transilluminate
- May be able to localize to superior/posterior aspect of the testis

Acute idiopathic scrotal edema
FEATURES

- Rapid onset of scrotal edema without other associated signs or symptoms
- Scrotum may or may not be erythematous and tender
- Will not transilluminate
- Occurs almost exclusively in prepubertal boys

Vasculitic illnesses
FEATURES

- May have acute or insidious onset
- Scrotal involvement benign and self-limited
- Associated with other hallmarks of disease
- Confined to young children
- More information on Henoch-Schönlein purpura and Kawasaki disease

Increased abdominal pressure

- Ascites
- Lymphatic obstruction
- Ventriculoperitoneal shunting
- Peritoneal dialysis

FEATURES
Should be able to determine on basis of history and physical examination.

Scrotal edema due to fluid overload
FEATURES
- Infants may show edema in the scrotum before it appears elsewhere
- Should not transilluminate
- May have other hallmarks of fluid overload

Groin masses
FEATURES
- Hydrocele of the spermatic cord – acute hydrocele of the spermatic cord may lead to testicular ischemia and should be investigated and treated urgently
- Inguinal hernia – may be able to palpate bowel in hernia
- Inguinal lymphadenopathy – nodes usually multiple
- Lipoma – generally highly mobile
- Saphenous vein varix – may be reducible, softer than hernia, produce bluish discoloration
- Torsion of undescended testis
- Hemoperitoneum

SIGNS & SYMPTOMS
Signs
- Diffuse scrotal swelling
- Not usually reducible unless associated with an inguinal hernia
- May diminish in size following period of recumbency
- Transilluminates
- May be unilateral (more often on the right) or bilateral
- May have generalized bluish discoloration
- Cremasteric reflex should be preserved
- Usually nontender
- Acute hydrocele may be tender and erythematous
- If a secondary or reactive process, may have signs associated with primary pathology (e.g. infection, tumor)

Symptoms
- Typically not painful unless acute onset
- Often has sensation of heaviness
- If a secondary or reactive process, may have preceding symptoms associated with primary pathology

KEY! DON'T MISS!
- Testicular torsion as primary process
- Incarcerated/strangulated hernia as primary process
- Testicular tumor as primary process

CONSIDER CONSULT
- Urgently if any question of testicular torsion
- Urgently if any question of incarcerated/strangulated hernia
- Urgently if acute process with unknown primary pathology
- Urgently if any testicular mass is palpated or imaged
- Urgently if hydrocele is tense because of the risk of compression of blood supply with subsequent testicular atrophy
- Nonurgently if there is an associated inguinal hernia

INVESTIGATION OF THE PATIENT
Direct questions to patient
Q How old is the patient? Infants are more likely than older children and men to have hydrocele as the primary process; for reactive hydroceles, age can help narrow differential diagnosis.

Q When did symptoms first appear? This can be helpful in determining whether hydrocele is primary or secondary process and how quickly work-up needs to proceed.

Q Was the onset acute or gradual? Acute processes need to be investigated urgently.

Q Is there any history of trauma? This can lead to hydrocele or even hematocele.

Q Is the swelling unilateral or bilateral? Primary hydrocele may be either, but if unilateral, it is more common on the right; may help guide work-up.

Q Are there any associated lumps, erythema, or tenderness? These may be indicative of a primary process other than hydrocele and should be investigated urgently.

Q Is there a change in size with position, coughing, Valsalva maneuvers? This is indicative of an inguinal hernia.

Q Is the swelling reduced after a period of recumbency? This is typical of hydrocele.

Q Is it painful? This may be indicative of a primary process other than hydrocele and should be investigated urgently.

Q Have there ever been symptoms like this before? Some 40% of patients with testicular torsion have experienced similar symptoms with spontaneous resolution in the past.

Q Does pain radiate to the back? This can sometimes be associated with hydrocele.

Q Is there a sensation of heaviness? This is typical of hydrocele.

Q Were there any preceding symptoms? These may be a clue to a primary process such as epididymitis.

Q Are there any systemic symptoms? These may be important clues to a primary process other than hydrocele.

Q Are there any pre-existing medical or surgical conditions? Contributory factors.

Q Has the patient been diagnosed with, or exposed to, mumps? Mumps may cause an orchitis that can produce a reactive hydrocele.

Q Has the patient been diagnosed with, or exposed to, any sexually transmitted diseases? This may be a clue to epididymitis or epididymo-orchitis that can produce a reactive hydrocele.

Q Is there a history of urinary tract infections? In children, this is the leading cause of epididymitis.

Q Are there any urinary tract symptoms or urethral discharge? These often accompany epididymitis.

Contributory or predisposing factors
Q Is there a history of premature birth? Premature babies have a higher incidence of inguinal hernia and hydrocele.

Q Is there a known history of indirect inguinal hernia? A complete inguinal hernia will have an associated communicating hydrocele.

Q Is there a known history of undescended testes? This is associated with an increased risk of testicular cancer, regardless of repair status.

Q Is there a known history of primary testicular/intrascrotal pathology? Virtually all intrascrotal conditions can have an associated or reactive hydrocele.

Q Is there a history of scrotal or groin surgery? Hydrocele is a common complication of scrotal surgery (especially varicocelectomy) and can also occur following groin surgery, particularly if there is any lymphatic obstruction.

Q Is there a history of renal transplantation? Ipsilateral hydrocele is a known complication of renal transplantation.

Q Are there any medical problems associated with increased intra-abdominal pressure (e.g. ascites)? Increased intra-abdominal pressure predisposes to hydrocele formation.

Q Is the patient receiving peritoneal dialysis? This predisposes to hydrocele formation.

Q Is there a history of ventriculoperitoneal shunting? This predisposes to hydrocele formation.

Q Is there a history of Ehlers-Danlos syndrome? This syndrome is associated with increased incidence of hydrocele and inguinal hernia.

Q Is there a history of bladder exstrophy? This is associated with increased incidence of hydrocele.

Family history

Q Is there a family history of Ehlers-Danlos syndrome? This syndrome of skin hyperelasticity is associated with increased incidence of hydrocele and inguinal hernia; inheritance is most commonly autosomal dominant but may be recessive.

Examination

- Are vital signs stable? Abnormal vital signs can be important clues to severe pain, systemic illness, widespread infection, or organ damage
- Is the patient febrile? May be indicative of infection or testicular torsion
- Are there any signs of disease in other systems? May provide clues to primary process such as fluid overload, increased abdominal pressure, or vasculitis
- Is swelling diffuse or localized? Hydrocele should be diffuse
- Is swelling unilateral or bilateral? Hydrocele may be either; can help guide work-up
- Is there any erythema? Acute hydrocele may be erythematous, but should raise red flag to investigate further for another primary process such as testicular torsion or epididymitis
- Is there a generalized bluish hue? This is typical of hydrocele, but can also be seen in neonatal testicular torsion
- Is there a blue dot? This can be seen in torsion of testicular appendages
- Is there any evidence of trauma? Trauma may produce reactive hydrocele or even hematocele (will not transilluminate)
- Does the swelling transilluminate? Hydrocele and other cystic lesions should transilluminate
- Does the swelling enlarge if the patient coughs or performs Valsalva maneuvers? This is indicative of inguinal hernia
- Is the swelling reducible? This is indicative of inguinal hernia. Note: in infants and young children, you should not try to examine for inguinal hernia by pressing finger into the inguinal canal, as for adults; instead, can palpate the internal ring through rectal examination, if necessary
- Can you palpate a superior edge to the swelling? The inability to feel a superior edge prior to entering the internal ring is indicative of an inguinal hernia or a hydrocele of the spermatic cord
- Is there any tenderness? Acute hydrocele may be tender, but should raise red flag to investigate further for another primary process such as testicular torsion or epididymitis. If there is a strong suspicion of testicular torsion, do not wait for imaging studies but urgently refer to a urologist or emergency room
- Is pain reduced with elevation of the scrotum? This can occur with epididymitis, but it is NOT a specific sign
- Are the testes and adjacent structures palpable? May or may not be palpable depending on degree of fluid accumulation. If only one side is affected, it is best to examine the unaffected side first. The testis should be palpated between the thumb and first two fingers; the two testes should be equal in size. The epididymis should be distinctly palpable on the superior/posterior pole of the testis, with the spermatic cord running superiorly. Inability to properly palpate the testes and adjacent structures is an indication for imaging studies
- If the testes and adjacent structures are palpable, are there any masses or deformities? If there are, or if there is any doubt, investigate further with imaging studies
- Is the testis enlarged? This can occur with testicular torsion, orchitis, or epididymitis
- Is there a 'bag of worms' appearance when the patient is upright? This is typical of varicocele
- Is there a 'silk glove' feel when the spermatic cord is palpated over the pubic tubercle? This is associated with an inguinal hernia (has also been likened to the feel of few drops of water in a plastic bag)

- **Is one hemiscrotum higher than the other?** While this sign is NOT completely reliable, an affected hemiscrotum that is high-riding is suggestive of testicular torsion
- **If the swelling is unilateral, is there a 'bell-clapper' deformity on the contralateral side?** The lack of normal fixation that predisposes to testicular torsion is often bilateral and results in a transverse, free-hanging testis. It is often easier to evaluate the testis on the unaffected side, particularly if there is tenderness
- **Can you elicit a cremasteric reflex?** Loss of the cremasteric reflex is suggestive of testicular torsion

Summary of investigative tests

- Urinalysis and urine culture: can be abnormal in epididymitis, especially if due to urinary tract infection
- Urethral swab: can be abnormal in epididymitis because of sexually transmitted disease
- Nucleic acid probe
- Ultrasound: can identify anatomical abnormalities, differentiate between testicular and extratesticular pathology, and determine presence of hernia; it is the best radiologic study to evaluate intascrotal processes
- Color flow Doppler: can determine blood flow to testes and epididymes (first choice)
- Nuclear scanning: can determine blood flow to testes and epididymes (second choice)

DIAGNOSTIC DECISION

Diagnostic decision is usually based on history and physical examination, with referral to urologist if there is any doubt as to primary diagnosis. There are no official published guidelines regarding diagnosis, but two protocols that may be helpful are contained within these articles:

- Skoog SJ. Benign and malignant pediatric scrotal masses. Pediatr Clin North Am 1997;44(5):1229–37. Medline
- Kass EJ, Lundak B. The acute scrotum. Pediatr Clin North Am 1997;44(5):1251–66. Medline

CLINICAL PEARLS

In the uncomplicated presentation of hydrocele, physical examination and transillumination are all that is necessary to make the diagnosis, which can then be confirmed with scrotal ultrasonography.

THE TESTS
Body fluids
URINALYSIS AND URINE CULTURE
Description
Midstream urine specimen.

Advantages/Disadvantages
Advantages:
- Fast
- Inexpensive
- Abnormal result aids in diagnosis and treatment

Disadvantage: voided specimens can be contaminated, which could confuse diagnosis and hinder appropriate work-up and treatment

Normal
- Normal urinalysis
- Negative urine culture

Abnormal
- Pyuria indicative of urinary tract infection and epididymitis
- Bactiuria indicative of urinary tract infection and epididymitis
- Positive urine culture indicative of urinary tract infection and epididymitis
- Keep in mind the possibility of a false-positive result, particularly in voided specimens

Cause of abnormal result
- Infection within the genitourinary tract
- Contaminated specimen
- Improper handling of specimen

Drugs, disorders and other factors that may alter results
Voided urine specimens are easily contaminated.

URETHRAL SWAB
Description
Swab of urethra for staining and culture.

Advantages/Disadvantages
Advantages:
- Test can be performed quickly and fairly easily
- Staining can be performed fairly quickly
- Abnormal result can aid in diagnosis and guide treatment
- Gram stain smear of urethral discharge in symptomatic males carries sensitivity and specificity of 95–100%

Disadvantages:
- Procedure can be uncomfortable for patient
- May not get results in time to forestall further work-up

Normal
- Negative stain
- Negative culture

Abnormal
- Positive stain indicative of genital infection and epididymitis
- Positive culture indicative of genital infection and epididymitis
- Keep in mind the possibility of a false-positive result, although this is unlikely

Cause of abnormal result
Sexually transmitted disease in the genital tract.

Tests of function
NUCLEIC ACID PROBE
Description
Nucleic acid amplification test for chlamydia and gonorrhea.

Advantages/Disadvantages
Advantages:
- Simple swab collection
- Sensitivity of 86.5–100% for both chlamydia and gonorrhea depending on test used
- Specificity of 99.7–100%

Disadvantages:

- Result not immediately available for patient who may be unreliable
- Obtaining sample is painful, particularly if patient has symptoms of urethritis

Normal
Negative nucleic acid detection.

Abnormal

- Positive nucleic acid detection
- Keep in mind the possibility of a falsely abnormal result

Cause of abnormal result
Chlamydia or gonorrhea present.

Imaging
ULTRASOUND
Advantages/Disadvantages
Advantages:

- Defines intrascrotal and/or inguinal anatomy and abnormalities
- Can detect presence of bowel in scrotum or inguinal canal
- Can quantitate testicular volume
- Nearly 100% sensitive for detecting testicular masses
- Usually easily obtained in most centers
- Noninvasive
- No known radiation danger

Disadvantages:

- Cannot evaluate blood flow to testis (i.e. cannot be used to rule out testicular torsion); therefore, Doppler is often performed simultaneously to evaluate blood flow to testes/epididymes
- May produce additional discomfort if tender
- Requires expert interpretation
- May not be readily available in some areas
- May be costly
- Results are technician-dependent

Normal

- Testes of equal size bilaterally
- Testes with homogenous echogenicity throughout
- Normal intrascrotal and inguinal anatomy
- No bowel present in scrotum or inguinal canal

Abnormal

- Testes unequal in size
- Mass or calcifications visualized, either intra- or extratesticular
- Abnormal intrascrotal or inguinal anatomy
- Bowel visualized in scrotum and/or inguinal canal
- Keep in mind the possibility of a falsely abnormal result

Cause of abnormal result

- Enlargement of the testis indicative of inflammation or ischemia
- Masses may be benign or malignant; they may have associated calcifications or areas of hemorrhage

- Calcifications of the tunica vaginalis with associated hydrocele suggestive of infection, particularly filariasis
- Abnormal anatomic relationships, including hernias

Drugs, disorders and other factors that may alter results
Large amounts of hydrocele fluid can cause compression and distortion of normal anatomic features.

COLOR FLOW DOPPLER
Advantages/Disadvantages
Advantages:
- Can determine blood flow to testes and epididymes
- Can distinguish intratesticular arteries
- Can distinguish between testicular and scrotal wall blood flow
- Diagnostic accuracy comparable to nuclear scan
- Usually fairly easy to obtain in most centers
- Noninvasive
- No known radiation danger

Disadvantages:
- May produce additional discomfort if tender
- Requires expert interpretation
- May not be readily available in some areas
- May be somewhat costly
- May reveal normal or increased blood flow to testes if testicular torsion early in onset; therefore, a diagnosis or exclusion of testicular torsion should not be made solely on Doppler results

Normal
- Low blood flow to testes
- Prepubertal boys may have minimal or undetectable testicular blood flow
- Testicular blood flow equal bilaterally
- Minimal or undetectable blood flow in the epididymis

Abnormal
- Increased blood flow to testis indicative of inflammation or infection
- Increased blood flow to epididymis indicative of inflammation
- Hypervascularity within a testis may indicate a neoplasm
- Decreased blood flow to a testis is indicative of ischemia
- Keep in mind the possibility of a falsely abnormal result

Cause of abnormal result
- Enlargement of the testis indicative of inflammation or ischemia
- Masses may be benign or malignant; they may have associated calcifications or areas of hemorrhage
- Calcifications of the tunica vaginalis with associated hydrocele suggestive of infection, particularly filariasis
- Abnormal anatomic relationships, including hernias

Drugs, disorders and other factors that may alter results
- The normal low flow state of the testes may make interpretation of results difficult, particularly in prepubertal boys
- Intermittent torsion may make interpretation of results difficult

NUCLEAR SCAN
Advantages/Disadvantages
Advantages:
- Can compare blood flow to testis and epididymis bilaterally
- Diagnostic accuracy comparable to color Dopplers
- Usually fairly easy to obtain in most centers
- Noninvasive
- No known radiation danger

Disadvantages:
- Cannot show anatomical features
- Cannot distinguish intratesticular arteries
- May be difficult to distinguish between testicular and scrotal wall blood flow
- Requires expert interpretation
- Length of time to prepare technetium and perform study may be prohibitive in urgent situation
- May not be readily available in some areas
- May be somewhat costly

Normal
- Low blood flow to testes
- Prepubertal boys may have minimal or undectable testicular blood flow
- Testicular blood flow equal bilaterally
- Minimal or undetectable blood flow in the epididymis

Abnormal
- Increased blood flow to testis indicative of inflammation or infection
- Increased blood flow to epididymis indicative of inflammation
- Decreased blood flow to a testis is indicative of ischemia
- Keep in mind the possibility of a falsely abnormal result

Cause of abnormal result
- Enlargement of the testis indicative of inflammation or ischemia
- Masses may be benign or malignant; they may have associated calcifications or areas of hemorrhage
- Calcifications of the tunica vaginalis with associated hydrocele suggestive of infection, particularly filariasis
- Abnormal anatomic relationships, including hernias

Drugs, disorders and other factors that may alter results
- The normal low flow state of the testes may make interpretation of results difficult, particularly in prepubertal boys
- Hydrocele may interfere with interpretation of results owing to area of photopenia
- Intermittent torsion may make interpretation of results difficult

PATIENT AND CAREGIVER ISSUES
Patient or caregiver request
Any disorder that affects the genital system will cause anxiety and many men find it difficult to voice their concerns about such a private topic. Therefore, it may be helpful to anticipate questions (spoken or unspoken) regarding:

- Will there be any disfigurement? Will it interfere with sexual activity? Will my testicles still function as normal? Will my fertility be impaired? These are major causes for concern for many men
- Is there a way that I can alleviate the discomfort? Patients may want advice about ways of reducing the discomfort while waiting for surgery or as a possible alternative to surgery
- Should I still be going to the gym/playing sports? This will be an important question for some patients
- Do I need surgery? What are the risks of surgery? Many patients will want to discuss these issues with their primary care practitioner as well as with their surgeon

Health-seeking behavior
- Has patient sought help for this problem previously? Patient may have a recurrence of an associated disorder, or require further investigation
- Has embarrassment delayed seeking treatment? Patients may delay treatment if they are embarrassed or nervous about a scrotal examination
- Is embarrassment causing patient to hide information relating to genital trauma or sexually transmitted diseases?
- Has patient been taking pain medication to alleviate discomfort, and if so, which? This is particularly important if surgery is indicated, as need to know if platelet aggregation may be impaired

MANAGEMENT ISSUES
Goals
- Determine whether hydrocele is primary or secondary process
- If secondary process, identify underlying problem
- Determine whether surgical management needed, with referral as indicated
- If conservative management needed, reassurance and teaching as indicated
- Minimize discomfort

Management in special circumstances
Since management is primarily surgical, need to weigh relative risks and benefits of surgery in given patient.

COEXISTING DISEASE
- Since management is primarily surgical, need to consider patient's overall health risk in relation to whether he could tolerate major surgery; if not, may consider a less invasive approach
- If coexisting disease led to onset of hydrocele (e.g., increased abdominal pressure) would want to ligate hydrocele sac to eliminate risk of recurrence, if possible

COEXISTING MEDICATION
Need to consider whether patient has been taking any medication that may:
- Mask pain symptoms
- Mask signs of fever and/or inflammation
- Affect surgical risk (e.g. clotting)

SPECIAL PATIENT GROUPS

- Boys who are found to have a hydrocele secondary to epididymitis owing to urinary tract infection should have their urinary tract investigated as well
- Older men may be suitable for different management options (e.g. sclerosis) if fertility is not an issue to them

PATIENT SATISFACTION/LIFESTYLE PRIORITIES

- Preservation of testicular function is paramount for boys and young men but may be less of a concern to older men who have completed their families
- Physical discomfort and large scrotal size from an otherwise benign hydrocele may warrant repair
- Discomfort with appearance or interference with sexual activity from an otherwise benign hydrocele may warrant repair

SUMMARY OF THERAPEUTIC OPTIONS
Choices

- For congenital noncommunicating hydrocele in infants, conservative management is indicated for the first 1–2 years of life as many close spontaneously; beyond that time surgical repair is usuallly recommended
- For communicating hydrocele in infants, treatment should be elective surgical repair (hydrocelectomy) with possible exploration of contralateral side as well
- For adults with benign hydrocele, hydrocelectomy is not indicated unless there is significant discomfort or impairment of life-satisfaction issues
- For adults with secondary hydrocele who require surgery for the primary problem, surgical correction of the hydrocele can be accomplished simultaneously
- Needle aspiration/decompression may alleviate symptoms; however, hydrocele usually returns
- Sclerosis is a nonsurgical option for older men for whom the possible risk of impaired fertility is acceptable
- Supportive devices may defer need for surgical intervention
- There are no official, published, approved guidelines regarding treatment of hydroceles

Clinical pearls

- Percutaneous drainage of the hydrocele is effective in reducing the hydrocele but uncommonly successful as a permanent therapy
- Infusion of antibiotic (tetracycline powder) can create adhesions and hinder recurrence, but this is neither easy nor particularly successful. When this maneuver fails and surgery is performed, the dissection is much more difficult and recovery more protracted

Never

- Never aspirate hydrocele contents in infants and young children (due to risk of communication with the peritoneal cavity)
- Never perform sclerosis in infants and young children (as may cause a chemical peritonitis)

FOLLOW UP

- For benign hydroceles, re-evaluation at 3-month intervals is the norm
- Postsurgical follow up should be performed by the surgeon, with periodic re-evaluation for recurrence

Plan for review

- For benign hydroceles, periodic re-evaluations should assess whether fluid accumulation is increasing or decreasing; can also check for signs/symptoms of other related pathology such as inguinal hernia
- Postsurgical follow up should assess for signs/symptoms of recurrence
- For congenital hydroceles, follow up provides opportunity to reassure parents and provide appropriate teaching

- For secondary hydroceles, follow up will likely focus more on the primary pathologic process, but also provides opportunity to re-evaluate hydrocele and its impact on patient's life satisfaction
- Boys who are found to have a hydrocele secondary to epididymitis because of urinary tract infection should have their urinary tract investigated as well

Information for patient or caregiver

- Parents of infants with primary hydrocele need to be reassured that the problem is benign and most likely self-limited, and understand the plan for follow up and management
- Older patients with primary hydrocele need reassurance as to the benign nature of the problem and need to understand the plan for follow up and management
- Patients with secondary hydrocele need information regarding the primary problem and how it relates to the etiology and management of the hydrocele

DRUGS AND OTHER THERAPIES: DETAILS
Surgical therapy
HYDROCELECTOMY

- Scrotal approach best for older boys and men with normal ultrasound and clear etiology for hydrocele
- Inguinal approach best for infants and young children as will need high ligation of processus vaginalis
- Inguinal approach best for patients with testicular mass as allows biopsy without risk of seeding
- Excisional techniques are most likely to eliminate hydrocele while minimizing risk of recurrence
- Laparoscopic repair can be used in some cases of communicating hydrocele
- Large and/or longstanding hydroceles can distort intrascrotal anatomy, so extreme caution needed to prevent damage to reproductive tract

Efficacy
- Highly efficacious, although exact data not found
- May recur, although this is largely technique-dependent

Risks/Benefits
Risks:
- Hematoma
- Injury to epididymis or vas deferens
- Wound infection
- Damage to testis
- Recurrence of hydrocele
- General risks of surgery and anesthesia

Benefits:
- Elimination of hydrocele sac
- Ability to inspect intrascrotal structures and to sample tissue and take fluid for analysis
- All but excisional technique are relatively quick with minimal bleeding

Evidence
PDxMD are unable to cite evidence that meets our criteria for evidence.

Acceptability to patient
- Benefits of surgery would have to clearly outweigh the risks in order for this surgery to be acceptable to most patients
- However, most techniques are fairly uncomplicated and should be acceptable to most patients in whom it is indicated

Follow up plan
Usual surgical follow up with re-evaluation at 3 months to assess for recurrence.

Patient and caregiver information
Usual postsurgical care and information.

SCLEROSIS
An irritating agent, usually a tetracycline derivative, is injected into the hydrocele sac.

Risks/Benefits
Risks:
- Obstruction of the epididymis
- Impaired fertility
- Significant pain
- High likelihood of recurrence
- If hydrocele recurs after sclerotherapy, it is more difficult to repair

Benefits:
- Minimally invasive
- Can be utilized in patients for whom the risk of general surgery is unacceptable

Evidence
PDxMD are unable to cite evidence that meets our criteria for evidence.

Acceptability to patient
This approach is most acceptable for patients in whom fertility is no longer an issue and for those with high surgical risks.

Follow up plan
Usual surgical follow up followed by frequent reassessment to look for hydrocele recurrence.

NEEDLE ASPIRATION/DECOMPRESSION
The fluid is drained from the hydrocele with a needle.

Risks/Benefits
Risks:
- Hematoma
- Infection
- Injury to testis, vas deferens, or epididymis
- Subsequent surgery may be more more difficult
- Possibility of recurrence

Benefits:

- Minimally invasive procedure with little discomfort
- May be useful in acute setting

Evidence
PDxMD are unable to cite evidence that meets our criteria for evidence.

Acceptability to patient
Generally good because of minimally invasive nature of the procedure.

Follow up plan
Usual surgical review.

Other therapies
SUPPORTIVE DEVICES
Scrotal supporters.

Efficacy
Subjectively reported to be effective.

Risks/Benefits
Benefit: may alleviate discomfort and defer need for surgical intervention

Evidence
PDxMD are unable to cite evidence that meets our criteria for evidence.

Acceptability to patient
Generally highly acceptable.

Follow up plan
Frequent reassessment of symptoms necessary initially, then can space out if condition is stable.

Patient and caregiver information
Information should be provided regarding the correct use of the device.

EFFICACY OF THERAPIES

- Efficacy of surgical treatment generally very high, although recurrence of hydrocele may occur
- Surgery is usually curative, and after the recovery period patients do well

Evidence
PDxMD are unable to cite evidence which meets our criteria for evidence.

Review period
Frequently postsurgery, then every 3 months appears to be standard.

PROGNOSIS

- For infants with primary hydrocele, the prognosis is excellent: if the disorder is benign, the majority will have spontaneous resolution within 12–24 months; those who undergo surgical repair with high ligation usually do very well with no recurrence
- For older patients with primary hydrocele, the prognosis is also excellent, although would not expect spontaneous resolution; if symptoms warrant treatment, surgical repair generally has excellent results
- For patients with secondary hydrocele, the prognosis is largely dependent on the primary pathologic process; reactive hydroceles should resolve once the primary problem is treated; if surgery is indicated, the majority of patients will do very well; careful surgical technique can minimize risk of hydrocele recurrence

Clinical pearls

- Patients should expect 4–6 weeks for full recovery
- Patients should wear scrotal support to relieve their pain and reduce the inflammation
- Patients should be encouraged to avoid trauma to the scrotum during the recovery period

Therapeutic failure
Reassess need for surgical intervention, with referral to urologist if indicated.

Recurrence
Reassess need for surgical intervention, with referral to urologist if indicated.

Deterioration
Reassess need for surgical Intervention, with referral to urologist if indicated.

COMPLICATIONS
Large, tense, acute hydroceles, particularly of the spermatic cord, may result in testicular ischemia.

CONSIDER CONSULT

- If there is significant recurrence of hydrocele following surgical correction
- If new signs or symptoms develop suggestive of a serious primary disorder

In general, it is very difficult to prevent the development of hydrocele, but there are a few risk factors that can be modified.

RISK FACTORS

- **Scrotal surgery, particularly varicocelectomy:** hydrocele is a common complication following unrelated scrotal surgery
- **Physical activity:** certain activities carry high risk of potential trauma to scrotum, including contact sports, traumatic sexual activity, occupational risks (e.g. straddle injuries from horseback or motorcycle riding), repetitive injuries (e.g. from jackhammer use)
- **Sexual behavior:** sexually transmitted diseases can produce epididymitis with reactive hydrocele
- **Family history:** patients with family history of Ehlers-Danlos syndrome are at higher risk of developing hydrocele

MODIFY RISK FACTORS

For surgeons, use of magnification techniques can help minimize risk of lymphatic obstruction producing postsurgical hydrocele; ligation of the tunica vaginalis can also prevent hydrocele formation.

Lifestyle and wellness
PHYSICAL ACTIVITY
Minimize potential for trauma to scrotum with use of protective devices in high-risk situations.

SEXUAL BEHAVIOR
Minimize potential for transmission of sexually transmitted diseases through patient education regarding prevention.

FAMILY HISTORY
Patients with family history of Ehlers-Danlos syndrome can be alerted to watch for signs of hydrocele formation.

SCREENING

- Screening for hydrocele in the general population is not indicated, as early detection will not significantly change outcome or management in the majority of cases
- Infants with congenital communicating hydrocele (i.e. with associated indirect inguinal hernia) may benefit from exploration of the contralateral side to assess need for bilateral hernia sac ligation, but this is controversial and usually reserved for infants at high risk such as premature infants and those with increased abdominal pressure

SURGICAL EXPLORATION
- If contralateral patent processus vaginalis is found, can electively repair at the same time
- Controversial as exposes patient to longer surgical time and increases risks of surgical complications

Cost/efficacy
- Moderately increases costs of surgery owing to longer surgical time
- 6–20% of patients undergoing repair have been found to have previously unrecognized contralateral patent processus vaginalis

ENDOSCOPY

During correction of congenital communicating hydrocele (i.e. with associated indirect inguinal hernia), some urologists have had success in assessing for patent processus vaginalis on the contralateral side using endoscopy through the ipsilateral internal inguinal ring:

- Less invasive than surgical exploration
- Does not carry risks of surgical complications to the contralateral side
- Sensitivity not known at this time
- This is a relatively new technique and may not be widely available

Cost/efficacy
Data not available.

PREVENT RECURRENCE

- Congenital hydroceles that spontaneously resolve should not recur
- Patients with secondary hydroceles owing to trauma may be able to prevent recurrence by wearing protective devices during high-risk activities
- Patients with secondary hydroceles because of epididymitis may be able to prevent recurrence by preventing reinfection
- Hydroceles that have been surgically corrected have the least chance of recurrence if the surgeon uses magnification techniques to prevent subsequent lymphatic obstruction and if there is high ligation of the sac

Reassess coexisting disease

If there is a coexisting disease (such as increased abdominal pressure), which is predisposed to hydrocele formation, then the same conditions could lead to recurrence unless the sac has been ligated.

ASSOCIATIONS

American Urological Association, Inc.
1120 North Charles Street
Baltimore, MD 21201
Tel: 410-727-1100
http://www.auanet.org

National Kidney and Urologic Diseases Information Clearinghouse
National Institute of Diabetes and Digestive and Kidney Disease
3 Information Way
Bethesda, MD 20892–3580
Fax: 301-907-8906
http://www.niddk.nih.gov/health/kidney/nkudic.htm

KEY REFERENCES

- Behrman. Nelson textbook of pediatrics, 16th edn. W.B. Saunders, 2000
- Goroll. Primary care medicine, 3rd edn. Lippincott-Raven Publishers, 1995
- Horstman WG. Scrotal imaging. Urol Clin North Am 1997;24(3):653–71
- Kaplan GW. Scrotal swelling in children. Pediatr Rev 2000;21:311–4
- Kapur P, Caty MG, Glick PL. Pediatric hernias and hydroceles. Pediatr Clin North Am 1998;45(4):773–89
- Kass EJ, Lundak B. The acute scrotum. Pediatr Clin North Am 1997;44(5):1251–66
- Modarress KJ, Cullen AP et al. Detection of chlamydia trachomatis and neisseria gonorrhoeae in swab specimens by the hybrid capture II and PACE 2 nucleic acid probe tests. Sex Transm Dis 1999;26(5):303–8
- Roberts. Clinical procedures in emergency medicine, 3rd edn. Philadelphia, PA: W.B. Saunders, 1998
- Sabiston. Textbook of surgery, 15th edn. Philadelphia, PA: W.B. Saunders, 1997
- Shalaby-Rana E, Lowe LH, Blask AN, Majd M. Imaging in pediatric urology. Pediatr Clin North Am 1997;44(5):1065–89
- Skoog SJ. Benign and malignant pediatric scrotal masses. Pediatr Clin North Am 1997;44(5):1229–37
- Walsh. Campbell's urology, 7th edn. Philadelphia, PA: W.B. Saunders, 1998

CONTRIBUTORS
Russell C Jones, MD, MPH
Philip J Aliotta, MD, MHA, FACS
Stewart M Polsky, MD

HYPERKALEMIA

SUMMARY INFORMATION

DESCRIPTION

- Defined as a serum potassium of >5.5mEq/L (>5.5mmol/L)
- Artifactual hyperkalemia (spurious hyperkalemia, pseudohyperkalemia) resulting from hemolysis after blood drawing must be excluded; a repeat heparinized sample should be sent immediately to the laboratory for analysis
- Major signs and symptoms are related to adverse effects on skeletal and cardiac muscle
- Severe hyperkalemia of >6.5mEq/L (>6.5mmol/L) is a medical emergency and necessitates immediate treatment
- Initial emergency treatment of severe hyperkalemia is generally intravenous calcium gluconate

URGENT ACTION

- In cases of severe hyperkalemia, urgent treatment is necessary
- ECG monitoring in severe hyperkalemia is essential

KEY! DON'T MISS!

- Asymptomatic hyperkalemia when obvious predisposing factors are present
- Hyperkalemia due to adrenal insufficiency: do not fail to diagnose the hyperpigmented, vomiting, hypotensive patient

ICD9 CODE
276.7 Hyperkalemia

CARDINAL FEATURES

- Hyperkalemia must be reproducible by repeat testing and/or ECG manifestations. To exclude in vitro hemolysis, blood must be collected with short tourniquet time and rapid laboratory analysis of a heparinized sample
- The most important signs and symptoms (cardiac dysrhythmias and muscle weakness) are due to adverse effects of high extracellular/intracellular potassium ratio on cell membranes of cardiac and skeletal muscle
- Tented (peaked) T waves may be present on the 12-lead ECG early in hyperkalemia
- Broad, widened QRS complexes, depressed ST segments, and a prolonged PR interval on the 12-lead ECG may be present in advanced stages
- Initial emergency treatment of severe hyperkalemia (serum potassium >6.5mEq/L and concomitant ECG changes) is intravenous calcium (as gluconate or chloride salt) to antagonize cardiotoxic effects of potassium
- Sudden death from arrhythmia can occur without prompt treatment

CAUSES
Common causes

- Renal failure (acute): reduction in potassium excretion and metabolic acidosis
- Renal failure (chronic): reduction in potassium excretion and metabolic acidosis
- Drug induced (common causes): potassium-sparing diuretics, angiotensin-converting enzyme (ACE) inhibitors, angiotensin II receptor blockers, nonsteroidal anti-inflammatory drugs (NSAIDs)
- Excessive potassium intake in patients with impaired renal function (potassium replacement therapy, high potassium diet)

Rare causes

- Adrenal insufficiency (Addison's disease): deficiency of glucocorticoids and mineralocorticoids
- Tumor lysis syndrome: massive release of potassium from cells
- Rhabdomyolysis: massive release of potassium from cells
- Drug induced (rare causes): suxamethonium, pentamidine therapy, cyclosporine toxicity, digoxin toxicity, trimethoprim
- Hyperkalemic periodic paralysis (congenital, familial)
- Massive blood transfusion
- Intravascular hemolysis
- Type IV renal tubular acidosis, especially in diabetic patients: impaired potassium excretion resulting from aldosterone deficiency or renal tubular resistance to aldosterone
- Diabetic ketoacidosis: impaired insulin-mediated intracellular potassium transport, hyperglycemia, and metabolic acidosis. In most cases of diabetic ketoacidosis, although serum potassium may be high at time of presentation, there is usually total body potassium depletion. After initiation of insulin therapy, potassium replacement is usually required because serum potassium level falls significantly and may result in hypokalemia if not corrected

Serious causes

- Renal failure (acute): treatable, but dire consequences if missed
- Renal failure (chronic): important cause of hyperkalemia and very common
- Diabetic ketoacidosis: hyperkalemia may be fatal if untreated, must not be missed since it responds rapidly to insulin therapy
- Adrenal insufficiency (Addison's disease): deficiency of glucocorticoids and mineralocorticoids; important and easily treatable

Contributory or predisposing factors

- Renal failure: acute or chronic (decreased potassium excretion and metabolic acidosis)
- ACE inhibitors and angiotensin II receptor blockers: decrease aldosterone release and inhibit sodium reabsorption
- Diabetic ketoacidosis: insulin facilitates the passage of potassium into cells; lack of it leads to a rise in extracellular potassium
- Adrenal insufficiency: mineralocorticoid deficiency

EPIDEMIOLOGY

Incidence and prevalence

INCIDENCE

- Overall incidence of hyperkalemia is unknown, but it is a common occurrence in patients with predisposing conditions
- Hyperkalemia can occur in 9–12% of elderly patients receiving ACE inhibitors

FREQUENCY

A small but significant number of patients medicated with NSAIDs will develop hyperkalemia.

Demographics

AGE

More common with increasing age due to increased incidence of etiologic factors such as chronic renal failure and ACE inhibitor use.

GENDER

No difference between males and females in occurrence.

GENETICS

Some genetic causes predispose to hyperkalemia, e.g. the rare hyperkalemic periodic paralysis.

GEOGRAPHY

No variation with geography.

SOCIOECONOMIC STATUS

Increased incidence in lower socioeconomic groups in which monitoring of drug therapies and treatment of diabetes mellitus and hypertension are often inadequate.

DIFFERENTIAL DIAGNOSIS
Spurious hyperkalemia (pseudohyperkalemia)
The main differential diagnosis of true hyperkalemia.

FEATURES
Most common causes include:
- Tight or prolonged tourniquet use
- In vitro hemolysis: more likely when hematologic malignancy coexists
- If severe leukocytosis or thrombocytosis is present, cellular potassium may leak into plasma after blood specimen is drawn

In vitro hemolysis and in vitro leakage from cells can be ameliorated with rapid processing of samples and the use of heparinized vacutainer collectors.

SIGNS & SYMPTOMS
Signs
There are usually no signs of hyperkalemia.

Symptoms
There are often no specific symptoms of hyperkalemia.

ASSOCIATED DISORDERS
- Rheumatoid arthritis and osteoarthritis: often treated with NSAIDs, which can increase risk of hyperkalemia in the elderly
- Disseminated malignancy: often bronchial carcinoma
- Volume depletion: hyperkalemia is more likely to occur when NSAIDs are administered in this setting
- Epilepsy: hyperkalemia may occur with generalized seizures and resultant rhabdomyolysis and potassium leakage from muscle cells
- Organ transplant: as a result of cyclosporine nephrotoxicity
- HIV: pentamidine therapy or trimethoprim therapy may produce hyperkalemia due to inhibition of renal potassium secretion

KEY! DON'T MISS!
- Asymptomatic hyperkalemia when obvious predisposing factors are present
- Hyperkalemia due to adrenal insufficiency: do not fail to diagnose the hyperpigmented, vomiting, hypotensive patient

CONSIDER CONSULT
- Severe hyperkalemia (serum potassium >6.5mEq/L (>6.5mmol/L)): refer immediately for treatment – this condition may be life-threatening
- Serum potassium of 6.0–6.5mEq/L (6.0–6.5mmol/L) and without ECG changes: treat urgently and refer for opinion on further management, e.g. further work-up and withdrawal of predisposing medication (e.g. NSAIDs, ACE inhibitors)
- Serum potassium 5.5–6.0mEq/L (5.5–6.0mmol/L) and no ECG changes: discuss with nephrologist in acute scenario; otherwise do office diagnostic work-up
- Hyperkalemia with characteristic changes on the 12-lead ECG: refer immediately for initiation of therapy

INVESTIGATION OF THE PATIENT

Direct questions to patient

Q **Have you been vomiting or anorexic?** Adrenal insufficiency or renal failure may result in vomiting.

Q **Have you been fainting?** Suggestive of postural hypotension; may be related to volume depletion, adrenal insufficiency, or arrhythmias.

Q **Have you experienced ankle swelling or shortness of breath?** Associated with congestive heart failure or renal failure, leading to renal hypoperfusion and hyperkalemia.

Q **Any history of arthritis?** Hyperkalemia has been linked to the use of NSAIDs.

Q **Are you taking any medication?** Drug history must be reviewed – are there any hyperkalemic drugs (e.g. potassium-sparing diuretics, ACE inhibitors, NSAIDs, etc.)?

Contributory or predisposing factors

Q **Have you suffered from chronic kidney disease?** Associated with chronically raised potassium.

Q **Have you used ACE inhibitors or angiotensin II receptor blockers?** These impair aldosterone release and are a major contributory factor to hyperkalemia.

Q **Do you have diabetes mellitus?** May lead to renal failure or type II renal tubular acidosis, is often associated with ACE inhibitor use, and may also result in diabetic ketoacidosis, causing a rise in extracellular potassium.

Q **Have you suffered from adrenal insufficiency or Addison's disease?** Mineralocorticoid deficiency leads to hyperkalemia.

Family history

Q Do you have a family history of diabetes mellitus?

Q Do you have a family history of Addison's disease?

Q Do you have a family history of hyperkalemic periodic paralysis?

Examination

▓ **Is there fluid overload?** Possibility of renal or cardiac failure

▓ **Check lying and standing blood pressure. Is there hypotension and is there a postural drop?** This could be suggestive of volume depletion or adrenal insufficiency

▓ **Is there peripheral vascular disease or neuropathy?** This may be due to diabetes mellitus

▓ **Is there generalized pigmentation?** Look to see if the armpits or buccal mucosa are spared; if not, there is a possibility of Addison's disease/adrenal insufficiency

▓ **Examination may be normal!**

Summary of investigative tests

▓ Serum electrolytes, urea, creatinine: crucial to diagnosis because they include potassium estimation and evaluation of renal function

▓ Arterial blood gas measurement: useful in patients with suspected acidosis. It can help to assess acid-base status in critically ill patients, especially those with potentially severe or mixed acid-base disorders

▓ 12-lead ECG: looking for cardiac changes secondary to hyperkalemia

▓ Serum calcium, magnesium, glucose, and complete blood count may be useful in selected patients (e.g. complete blood count in suspected spurious hyperkalemia, glucose in suspected diabetic ketoacidosis)

DIAGNOSTIC DECISION

▓ Hyperkalemia is described as serum potassium of >5.5mEq/L (>5.5mmol/L)

▓ Severe hyperkalemia is described as a serum potassium of >6.5mEq/L (>6.5mmol/L)

▓ All patients with hyperkalemia in whom characteristic ECG changes have occurred should be classified as severe even if the serum potassium level is less than 6.5mEq/L (>6.5mmol/L)

- Although severe manifestations of hyperkalemia usually do not occur until the plasma potassium concentration is >7.0mEq/L (>7.0mmol/L) unless the rise has been very rapid, there is substantial variability between patients, since factors such as hypocalcemia and metabolic acidosis can increase the toxicity of excess potassium
- Regardless of the severity of hyperkalemia, if the patient is exhibiting ECG changes or severe muscle weakness, the patient should be treated as having severe hyperkalemia
- Conversely, a patient who has a serum potassium level of 6.5mEq/L (6.5mmol/L) but does not manifest any symptoms or signs of hyperkalemia can be treated with less urgency

CLINICAL PEARLS

- All diabetic patients with established diabetic nephropathy, even those with only moderate renal insufficiency, are vulnerable to hyperkalemia
- The prevalence of type IV renal tubular acidosis is higher in diabetics then in other patients with renal disease, and diabetics have risk factors for other renal insults such as ischemic nephropathy secondary to atherosclerosis of the aorta and renal arteries
- ACE inhibitors, angiotensin II receptor blockers, and NSAIDs should be used with caution in patients older than 75 years and in patients with significant impairment of renal function because of their vulnerability to hyperkalemia
- Hyperglycemia, even without acidosis, may occasionally produce hyperkalemia in diabetic patients as a result of potassium leakage from cells in the presence of insulin deficiency or resistance (glucose-induced hyperkalemia)

THE TESTS
Body fluids
ARTERIAL BLOOD GAS MEASUREMENT
Description
Arterial sample taken in a heparinized syringe, usually from the radial artery. The sample should be put on ice and sent immediately to the laboratory for analysis.

Advantages/Disadvantages
- Advantage: helpful in assessing acid-base status in critically ill patients, especially those with potentially severe or mixed acid-base disorders
- Disadvantage: unpleasant for the patient since taking arterial blood can be painful

Normal
- pH: 7.38–7.42
- pO_2: 80–90mmHg
- pCO_2: 35–45mmHg
- Bicarbonate: 20–30mEq/L (20–30mmol/L)

Abnormal
- Values for pH, pO_2, pCO_2, and bicarbonate that are outside the normal range
- Keep in mind the possibility of a false-positive result due to inappropriate venous sampling

Cause of abnormal result
- The presence of a low pH and decreased serum bicarbonate indicates the presence of a metabolic acidosis. This may be partially compensated by a fall in the pCO_2 achieved by hyperventilation
- Keep in mind the possibility of a false-positive result due to a venous blood sampling error
- Common causes of metabolic acidosis include diabetic ketoacidosis and renal failure

Drugs, disorders and other factors that may alter results
- Type IV renal tubular acidosis typically presents with acidosis in addition to hyperkalemia
- Overdose of commonly available agents such as methanol, ethanol, ethylene glycol, and ecstasy may produce a severe metabolic acidosis

SERUM ELECTROLYTES, BLOOD UREA NITROGEN (BUN), CREATININE
Description
Venous blood sample.

Advantages/Disadvantages
- Advantage: indicates whether renal function is impaired
- Disadvantage: renal function can fall to a glomerular filtration rate of 50mL/min before serum creatinine rises above normal range

Normal
- Sodium: 135–147mEq/L
- Potassium: 3.5–5mEq/L
- BUN: 8–18mg/dL (3–6.5mmol/L)
- Creatinine 0.6–1.2mg/dL (50–110mcmol/L)
- Note that reference ranges can vary; check with local laboratory

Abnormal
- Sodium and potassium outside normal range
- Urea: >18mg/dL (>6.5mmol/L)
- Creatinine: >1.2mg/dL (>110mcmol/L)
- Keep in mind the possibility of a false-positive result

Cause of abnormal result
- Diminished renal function
- Dehydration

Drugs, disorders and other factors that may alter results
- Hemolyzed blood sample
- Significant delay between taking and analyzing blood sample
- Diuretics, steroids, NSAIDs

Other tests
12-LEAD ECG
Advantages/Disadvantages
Advantages:
- Useful in determining the need for immediate referral in hyperkalemia
- Characteristic abnormalities indicate cardiotoxicity and urgent need for referral for further management

Abnormal
- Tall, tented T waves (earliest changes) and widened QRS complexes with bradycardia (late changes) are signs of the cardiac effects of hyperkalemia
- Keep in mind that extracellular calcium abnormalities or changes of ischemic heart disease may produce similar changes and/or potentiate the toxic effects of hyperkalemia

Cause of abnormal result
Cardiac conduction abnormalities caused by the presence of high extracellular/intracellular potassium ratio.

PATIENT AND CAREGIVER ISSUES
Patient or caregiver request
- **Is hyperkalemia life-threatening?** Yes, but with appropriate intervention it can be successfully treated
- **My potassium is raised and my kidneys aren't working properly. What does the future hold?** Unfortunately hyperkalemia due to chronic renal failure is difficult to treat. It entails close compliance with drug therapy and dietary changes

MANAGEMENT ISSUES
Goals
- When potassium is >6.5mEq/L (>6.5mmol/L) or ECG changes of hyperkalemia are present, treatment should be instituted immediately
- When there is moderate hyperkalemia of 6.0–6.5mEq/L (6.0–6.5mmol/L), a cause must be identified and corrected as soon as possible. With appropriate intervention a potassium level of <6.0mEq/L (<6.0mmol/L) should be achieved within the first week
- For mild hyperkalemia in the range 5.5–6.0mEq/L (5.5–6.0mmol/L), predisposing factors should be addressed; regular monitoring must be instituted along with appropriate treatment to control the hyperkalemia

Management in special circumstances
COEXISTING DISEASE
- Where hyperkalemia coexists with worsening chronic renal failure, then opinion from a renal specialist is recommended
- In diabetes mellitus without renal disease, where serum potassium is moderately increased due to poor diabetic control, tightening of diabetic control is often enough to normalize potassium
- Adrenal insufficiency or Addison's disease requires rapid commencement of steroid therapy. This may be the only intervention required to cause a reduction in potassium level

COEXISTING MEDICATION
- If ACE inhibitors for heart failure are discontinued because of hyperkalemia, rebound cardiac failure, which can be severe, may result
- When potassium-sparing diuretics are the cause of hyperkalemia, substitution to a nonpotassium-sparing diuretic is often all that is required, without further addition to therapy

SPECIAL PATIENT GROUPS
- Children with significant hyperkalemia should be referred to a pediatric nephrologist
- When terminal illness coexists with hyperkalemia, the hyperkalemia is often a preterminal event. Treatment options should be extensively discussed with the patient or legal guardian

PATIENT SATISFACTION/LIFESTYLE PRIORITIES
The aged and disabled may have difficulty with frequency of monitoring. Much of this problem can be overcome with the use of home-visiting nurses who can provide monitoring without need for lifestyle adjustments.

SUMMARY OF THERAPEUTIC OPTIONS
Choices
Treatment principles are directed at:
- Antagonism of membrane actions of potassium (calcium)
- Driving extracellular potassium into the cells (insulin and glucose, sodium bicarbonate, and beta-2 adrenergic agonists)
- Removal of potassium from the body (loop/thiazide diuretics, cation-exchange resins, and dialysis)

Note that calcium does not, per se, have any effect on serum potassium level. Moreover, all but diuretics, cation-exchange resins, and dialysis have only temporizing effects on the serum potassium and are reserved for treatment of hyperkalemic emergencies.

In addition to pharmacologic therapy, certain lifestyle measures should be instituted.

Severe hyperkalemia:
- Should be referred to the emergency department or for inpatient management
- First choice: 5–10mL of 10% calcium gluconate intravenously given over 3min (for cardioprotection), plus 50mL of 50% dextrose with 10U of regular insulin given intravenously
- Second choice: sodium bicarbonate intravenously (where acidosis coexists with hyperkalemia in the absence of diabetes mellitus)
- Third choice: nebulized beta-agonist therapy (such as nebulized albuterol)
- Fourth choice: sodium polystyrene sulfonate orally (this is not part of the emergency treatment because potassium removal by binding in the gut begins after 1h and significant removal takes several hours)
- Cessation of precipitating drugs

Moderate and mild hyperkalemia:
Cessation of precipitating drugs, then:
- First choice: oral furosemide if renal function allows
- Second choice: sodium polystyrene sulfonate
- Third choice: sodium bicarbonate orally (useful in chronic renal failure, where acidosis is a problem)

Diabetes mellitus:
- When severe diabetic ketoacidosis is present, patient should be referred for inpatient management

An excellent review is published under the auspices of the National Kidney Foundation containing detailed guidelines [1]

Clinical pearls
When treating severe hyperkalemia, for a patient who has concomitant ECG changes, both intravenous calcium gluconate (or chloride) and insulin/glucose should be administered immediately, virtually simultaneously.

Never
- Initiate therapy for severe hyperkalemia in the office setting
- Attempt to manage Addison's disease or adrenal insufficiency without specialist advice

FOLLOW UP
- Sodium polystyrene sulfonate resins are also effective when given rectally and are very useful in patients with dysfunctional upper gastrointestinal tracts or intestinal obstruction
- Hemodialysis is only occasionally required for hyperkalemia (when above measures fail or the patient has severe renal failure)

Plan for review
- Severe hyperkalemia should be referred to a nephrologist
- Moderate hyperkalemia should be followed with repeat serum electrolytes every 48h initially. If response to therapy does not occur, then referral must take place
- In mild hyperkalemia, monitoring with serum electrolyte determinations should occur at least twice in the first week and thereafter weekly as necessary if response to treatment occurs

- When serum potassium level is mildly raised and precipitating drug therapy is not discontinued, then monthly monitoring of serum electrolytes is necessary

Information for patient or caregiver
- Important to stress the need for regular follow-up
- Crucial message to patients is that hyperkalemia is most often symptomless and that death may occur if they fail to attend for monitoring
- Hyperkalemia is relatively easy to manage if patients comply with regular follow-up

DRUGS AND OTHER THERAPIES: DETAILS
Drugs
CALCIUM GLUCONATE
Dose
- 5–10mL of 10% calcium gluconate intravenously, given slowly at 1.5ml/min, is indicated for treatment of hyperkalemia in the presence of ECG changes
- This can be repeated once if necessary

Efficacy
Effective as a cardioprotective agent in severe hyperkalemia.

Risks/Benefits
Risks:
- Use caution in mild hypercalciuria and renal disease
- Use caution in the elderly

Benefit: any risks of this treatment are outweighed by the benefits of cardioprotection that it affords

Side-effects and adverse reactions
- Burning at injection site, thrombophlebitis
- Gastrointestinal: anorexia, constipation, nausea, vomiting
- Metabolic: hypercalcemia
- Genitourinary: renal dysfunction and failure
- Cardiovascular system: dysrhythmias, hypotension, bradycardia, cardiac arrest

Interactions (other drugs)
- ACE inhibitors ▪ Antibiotics (azithromycin, fluoroquinolone derivatives, tetracyclines)
- Anticonvulsants (gabapentin, phenytoin) ▪ Antifungals ▪ Fexofenadine ▪ Phenothiazines
- Antidysrhythmics (cardiac glycosides, quinidine, calcium channel blockers) ▪ Chloroquine
- Antituberculosis drugs (isoniazid, rifampin) ▪ Bisphosphonates ▪ NSAIDs (aspirin, diflunisal)
- Diuretics, thiazide ▪ Zalcitabine

Contraindications
- Hypercalcemia ▪ Severe hypercalciuria ▪ Ventricular fibrillation ▪ Hyperparathyroidism
- Metatastic calcification ▪ Renal calculi ▪ Digitalis therapy ▪ Sarcoidosis

Follow up plan
Therapy to reduce serum potassium should commence at the earliest opportunity.

Patient and caregiver information
This agent is the first stage in management of severe hyperkalemia and is followed by a number of further treatment steps.

REGULAR INSULIN 10U AND 50% DEXTROSE
Dose
- 10U of regular insulin and 50mL of 50% dextrose as a bolus intravenously, followed by a continuous infusion of 5% dextrose at 100mL/h to prevent late hypoglycemia.
- Give insulin without glucose if hyperkalemia is secondary to hyperglycemia (diabetic ketoacidosis)

Efficacy
Effective in driving extracellular potassium into cells.

Risks/Benefits
Risks:
- Onset of action is faster and of shorter duration with human preparations of insulin
- Renal or hepatic impairment may require dose adjustment

Side-effects and adverse reactions
- Skin: flushing, rash, pruritus, urticaria
- Metabolic: hypoglycemia, decreased ion concentrations (Ca, PO_4, K, Mg), insulin resistance, hyperglycemic rebound reaction
- General: hypersensitivity reactions, anaphylaxis

Interactions (other drugs)
- ACE inhibitors - Anabolic steroids - Beta-blockers - Cigarette smoking - Clonidine - Corticosteroids - Diazoxide - Ethanol - Fibrates - Lithium - Monoamine oxidase inhibitors - Nifedipine - Octreotide - Salicylates - Sex hormones - Thiazides

Contraindications
Hypoglycemia

Acceptability to patient
Acceptable therapy with low incidence of side-effects.

Follow up plan
Serum potassium should be reassessed 1h after intravenous insulin and dextrose therapy, and the infusion should be repeated if serum potassium is still dangerously elevated.

Patient and caregiver information
Frequent blood monitoring of serum potassium is required preinfusion and postinfusion therapy.

SODIUM BICARBONATE INTRAVENOUS PREPARATION
Dose
- Available as 10mL vials of 8.4% sodium bicarbonate
- Three vials dissolved in 1000mL of 5% dextrose to make up a concentration of 150mEq/L (150mmol/L), given at 2–5mEq/kg body weight over 4–8h

Efficacy
- Effective in lowering serum potassium only in the presence of metabolic acidosis
- It takes 3–4h for an effect on serum potassium level to start

Risks/Benefits
Risks:
- Does not have a role to play in the management of diabetic ketoacidosis except in severe acidosis with bicarbonate level <10mmol/L or pH<7.0

- Not of benefit in hyperkalemia related to chronic renal failure because it may precipitate fluid overload
- Use caution in congestive cardiac failure, hypertension, hypocalcemia, and renal failure

Side-effects and adverse reactions
- Confusion, headache, irritability, tremors
- Edema, sodium and water retention, weight gain
- Decreased respiratory effort and hypoventilation

Interactions (other drugs)
- Flecainide: plasma flecainide concentration increased ■ Lithium: plasma lithium concentration decreased ■ Quinidine: plasma quinidine concentration increased ■ Mexiletine: plasma mexiletine concentration increased

Contraindications
- Cirrhosis ■ Toxemia

Acceptability to patient

Generally a treatment of last resort to bring down resistant hyperkalemia; patient acceptability is not a significant consideration in this emergency situation.

Follow up plan

Repeat arterial blood gas and potassium level 1h after cessation of infusion and repeat if necessary.

Patient and caregiver information

Regular repeated potassium and arterial blood gas sampling is necessary.

NEBULIZED ALBUTEROL
Dose
- 5–20mg by inhalation over 10 min
- Use the concentrated form (5mg/mL) of the drug to minimize volume to be inhaled

Efficacy
- Promotes cellular uptake of potassium and may lower serum potassium by 0.5–1.5mEq/L (0.5–1.5mmol/L) for up to 2–4h
- The potassium-lowering effect is additive to that of insulin

Risks/Benefits
Risks:
- Benefit is only short lived and temporary (2–4h)
- Tolerance may occur with prolonged use
- Concomitant use with other sympathomimetics is not recommended; however, inhaled beta-2 agonists can be used cautiously with oral forms
- Use caution in cardiac disease, and hyperglycemia
- Use caution in pregnancy or breast-feeding

Benefit: inhaled solution is less likely to produce side-effects

Side-effects and adverse reactions

- Gastrointestinal: nausea, vomiting, dyspepsia, abdominal pain
- Cardiovascular system: palpitations, sinus tachycardia, hypertension
- Central nervous system: anxiety, tremor, headache, insomnia, dizziness, nightmares, hyperkinesia
- Respiratory: bronchospasm
- Ears, eyes, nose, and throat: cough, throat irritation, epistaxis, hoarseness, congestion
- Skin: rash, urticaria, angioedema
- Musculoskeletal: cramps
- Metabolic: hyperglycemia, hypokalemia
- General: anaphylaxis

Interactions (other drugs)

- Beta-blockers ■ Diuretics ■ Monoamine oxidase inhibitors ■ Sympathomimetics
- Thyroid hormones ■ Tricyclic antidepressants

Contraindications

- Diabetes mellitus ■ Hyperthyroidism ■ Cardiac arrhythmias ■ Ischemic heart disease
- Hypertension ■ Seizures ■ Hypersensitivity to sympathomimetics ■ Children under 2 years

Evidence

Patients in renal failure with hyperkalemia may be effectively treated with albuterol.

- A prospective clinical trial studied the effect of albuterol on potassium metabolism in patients with acute and chronic renal failure. Potassium levels were decreased after administration of albuterol sulfate, and ECG manifestations of hyperkalemia resolved [2] *Level P*

Acceptability to patient

Generally poorly tolerated by patients; there is a short-term bonus in reducing hyperkalemia, but patients often find the tremor and tachycardia that come with high-dose albuterol therapy unacceptable.

Follow up plan

Repeat serum potassium measurement 30min after nebulizer therapy and repeat therapy if necessary.

Patient and caregiver information

Patients should be made aware of the severe side-effects that may be present with this therapy.

SODIUM POLYSTYRENE SULFONATE ORAL PREPARATION

Sodium polystyrene sulfonate is a cation-exchange resin.

Dose

- In severe hyperkalemia with potassium overload: 15–60g made to a 25% solution orally, or 30–50mg in 100ml of aqueous vehicle via a retention enema
- For moderate hyperkalemia: 15g made up to a 25% solution orally up to 4 times per day
- Cleansing enemas should follow retention enemas to minimise local effects on rectal tissue

Efficacy

- May lower serum potassium by 0.5–1mEq/L (0.5–1mmol/L) within 1–2h
- This effect persists for 6–7h

Risks/Benefits

Risks:

- Use caution in patients who need to restrict sodium intake (hypertension, congestive heart failure, edema)
- Use caution in pregnancy

Benefit: offers more long-term benefit than insulin and dextrose or nebulized albuterol

Side-effects and adverse reactions
- Gastrointestinal: nausea, vomiting, anorexia, abdominal pain, gastric irritation, diarrhea, constipation, bowel obstruction, bowel necrosis (after rectal administration)
- Metabolic: hypocalcemia, hypokalemia, sodium retention, hypomagnesemia

Interactions (other drugs)
- Antacids ■ Digoxin ■ Calcium salts (intravenous) ■ Insulin ■ Magnesium hydroxide
- Loop diuretics ■ Sodium bicarbonate (intravenous) ■ Aluminium carbonate

Contraindications
- Hypocalcemia ■ Neonates ■ Bowel obstruction

Acceptability to patient
Generally unpleasant to take in view of gastrointestinal side-effects, and so may be poorly tolerated by some patients.

Follow up plan
- Weekly serum potassium assay if used in the community
- Daily serum potassium assays if used in the inpatient hospital setting

Patient and caregiver information
The importance of attending for repeat blood testing must be stressed to the patient.

FUROSEMIDE
Dose
40–80mg/day by mouth or intravenously in this indication.

Efficacy
- Inhibits renal tubular reabsorption of sodium, chloride, and potassium and facilitates increased renal tubular potassium secretion, thereby increasing renal excretion of potassium
- Where renal function is intact, may lower serum potassium by 1–1.5mEq/L (1.5mmol/L) on average

Risks/Benefits
Risks:
- Potassium redistribution
- Use caution with diabetes mellitus, renal and liver disease, systemic lupus erythematosus, hypertension, gout, and porphyria
- Use caution in pregnancy and nursing mothers

Benefits:
- Reduces fluid congestion
- Causes reduction of total body potassium rather than promoting extracellular to intracellular shift
- Offers a more permanent solution than other therapies that affect potassium redistribution

Side-effects and adverse reactions
- Gastrointestinal: ischemic hepatitis, vomiting, pancreatitis, nausea, diarrhea, anorexia, thirst
- Genitourinary: glycosuria, hyperuricemia, bladder spasm, polyuria
- Hematologic: blood disorders
- Metabolic: hyperglycemia, hyponatremia, hypokalemia, hypomagnesemia, hypochloremia, hypercholesterolemia, hypertriglyceridemia

- Central nervous system: dizziness, headache, paresthesia, fever
- Cardiovascular system: chest pain, hypovolemia, orthostatic hypotension, circulatory collapse
- Eyes, ears, nose, and throat: visual disturbances, tinnitus, hearing impairment
- Skin: erythema multiforme, exfoliative dermatitis, urticaria

Interactions (other drugs)
- ACE inhibitors ▪ Alpha-adrenergic antagonists ▪ Amphotericin ▪ Antibiotics (aminoglycosides, polymixins, vancomycin, cephalosporins) ▪ Antidiabetics ▪ Antidysrhythmics (amiodarone, cardiac glycosides, disopyramide, flecainide, mexiletine, quinidine, sotalol) ▪ Beta-2 adrenergic agonists ▪ Carbenoxolone ▪ Cholestyramine, colestipol ▪ Cisplatin ▪ Clofibrate ▪ Corticosteroids ▪ Diuretics (thiazides, metolazone, acetazolamide) ▪ Lignocaine ▪ Lithium ▪ NSAIDs ▪ Phenobarbital ▪ Phenytoin ▪ Pimozide ▪ SSRIs ▪ Reboxetine ▪ Terbutaline ▪ Tubocurarine

Contraindications
- Renal failure with anuria ▪ Hepatic coma

Acceptability to patient
Generally acceptable to most patients.

Follow up plan
Weekly monitoring of potassium and renal function in the outpatient setting when therapy is initially begun, reducing to monthly once a stable pattern for renal function and serum potassium has been established.

Patient and caregiver information
Must be available for regular follow-up for monitoring of serum electrolytes, urea, creatinine.

SODIUM BICARBONATE (ORAL PREPARATION)
Dose
500–1000mg twice a day, but the precise dose is dependent on the type and severity of the metabolic acidosis being treated.

Efficacy
May aid potassium reduction in chronic renal failure with acidosis when used in the outpatient setting. Use only when serum bicarbonate level <20mEq/L (<20mmol/L).

Risks/Benefits
Risks:
- Does not have a role to play in the management of diabetic ketoacidosis
- Prolonged use not recommended due to hypernatremia
- Use caution in Cushing's syndrome, Bartter's syndrome, and hyperaldosteronism
- Use caution in pregnancy, the elderly, neonates, and children under 2 years of age
- Use caution in cardiac disease (especially congestive cardiac failure), hypertension, respiratory acidosis, hepatic and renal impairment, hypocalemia and patients receiving coricosteroids

Benefits:
- Although fluid overload may be exaccerbated, it is of benefit in reducing some of the manifestations of acidosis in chronic renal failure
- Also has potassium-lowering effect by virtue of reducing level of metabolic acidosis

Side-effects and adverse reactions
- Gastrointestinal: flatulence, bloating, abdominal pain, acid reflux
- Metabolic: metabolic alkalosis, hypernatremia, hyperosmolarity, lactic acidosis, milk-alkali syndrome
- Central nervous system: tetany, tremor, seizures
- Cardiovascular system: peripheral edema

Interactions (other drugs)
- Acetaminophen ■ Benzodiazepines ■ Cefpodoxime ■ Chlorpropamide ■ Corticosteroids ■ Dextroamphetamine ■ Ephedrine, pseudoephedrine ■ Flecainide ■ Iron salts ■ Lithium ■ Ketoconazole ■ Methenamine ■ Methotrexate ■ Quinidine ■ Salicylates ■ Sulfonylureas ■ Sympathomimetics ■ Tetracyclines

Contraindications
- Cirrhosis ■ Toxemia ■ Metabolic alkalosis ■ Respiratory alkalosis

Acceptability to patient
Generally very acceptable to the patient with good tolerability.

Follow up plan
Initially reassessment of fluid balance status, acid-base status, and serum potassium on a weekly basis, reducing to monthly once stable.

Patient and caregiver information
To avoid drug interaction, intake of sodium bicarbonate should be separated from other relevant drugs by 2h if possible.

LIFESTYLE
Dietary changes have a strong benefit in hyperkalemia.

RISKS/BENEFITS
- Risk: the risk of a reduction in dietary potassium is negligible and the potential benefit great compared with a reduction in necessary drug therapy
- Benefit: reduction in dietary intake of potassium is an excellent treatment for chronic hyperkalemia

ACCEPTABILITY TO PATIENT
Generally acceptable, but dietary advice on how to avoid potassium-rich foods is required.

FOLLOW UP PLAN
- Initial visit to a nutritionist for dietary advice is required with 6-monthly follow-up to make sure that eating patterns are maintained
- Serum potassium should be monitored monthly if diet is to be the only initial intervention

PATIENT AND CAREGIVER INFORMATION
Patients should be informed to avoid forbidden foods and that drug therapy may be required if dietary therapy is unsuccessful.

OUTCOMES

EFFICACY OF THERAPIES

- In chronic hyperkalemia, with a normal sequence of events, sodium polystyrene sulfonate, dietary change, and furosemide (if renal function permits) should bring about a fall in serum potassium of 2–3mEq/L (2–3mmol/L) within 1–2 weeks of initiating therapy
- In severe acute hyperkalemia the immediate measures with insulin and dextrose, albuterol nebulizer, and sodium bicarbonate intravenous therapy are only a holding exercise. They buy time and allow for decisions about further management according to underlying pathology of hyperkalemia
- Diabetic ketoacidosis and adrenal failure should preferably be managed by specialist hospital teams to maximize survival

Evidence

- Potassium levels may be reduced and ECG manifestations of hyperkalemia resolved with albuterol sulfate in patients with renal failure and acute hyperkalemia (as found in a prospective clinical trial) [1] *Level P*
- PDxMD are unable to cite evidence that meets our criteria for evidence for other medications used in the management of hyperkalemia

Review period

In acute hyperkalemia:

- Close inpatient observation is preferred
- Measures for rapidly reducing serum potassium levels are only a way to buy time
- Serum potassium should be reviewed after each intervention

In chronic hyperkalemia:

- Once-weekly or twice-weekly review after a therapeutic intervention is recommended
- Monthly review is reasonable once a falling trend for potassium has been established or the potassium level is stable

PROGNOSIS

- Diabetic ketoacidosis and Addison's disease have low mortality rates with appropriate management
- Prognosis in acute renal failure is dependent on its cause and on underlying systemic disease (e.g. cardiovascular disease worsens the prognosis for renal recovery; hyperkalemia and acute renal failure related to glomerulonephritis or vasculitis in the adult patient carry a poor outlook for renal recovery)
- When drugs (e.g. ACE inhibitors) are the cause of the hyperkalemia, the outlook with supportive therapy for a short period is excellent
- Generally, in a hospital critical care setting, the hyperkalemia can be controlled by medical measures and the use of hemodialysis when appropriate. Untreated severe hyperkalemia has an ultimate fatal outcome

- When hyperkalemia coexists with chronic renal failure, once drugs that cause hyperkalemia have been excluded, there is little to be done besides dialysis. There is often a gradual progression to intractable hyperkalemia that fails to respond to simple measures such as loop diuretics and ion exchange resins. At this point a decision about renal replacement therapy has to be made

Clinical pearls
- If a patient with severe hyperkalemia is brought rapidly to a hospital critical care setting, death from hyperkalemia, per se, is usually preventable
- Some patients with severe hyperkalemia (serum potassium >7.0mEq/L) may not show early ECG changes but may still develop rapidly life-threatening cardiotoxicity. Hence emergent effective treatment is essential

Therapeutic failure
If management of hyperkalemia with the drug measures described fails in patients with chronic renal failure then renal replacement therapy with either peritoneal or hemodialysis is indicated.

Recurrence
If hyperkalemia recurs, particularly in the presence of renal impairment, then referral to a nephrologist should be made.

Deterioration
If hyperkalemia deteriorates despite the treatment measures described, then the only option is referral and renal replacement therapy.

Terminal illness
In terminal illness where time is short or the condition carries a particularly poor prognosis, then a decision not to treat hyperkalemia may sometimes be made. Untreated hyperkalemia would eventually result in death from cardiac arrest.

COMPLICATIONS
Sudden death due to cardiac arrest.

CONSIDER CONSULT
Also refer all patients with hyperkalemia and:
- Chronic renal failure
- Acute renal failure

RISK FACTORS

Medication history: A number of drugs may affect renal function and cause increases in serum potassium concentration, most notably the following:

- ACE inhibitors
- Potassium-sparing diuretics
- NSAIDs

These drugs must be discontinued whenever possible.

Diet: is a modifiable risk factor in hyperkalemia, and reducing total dietary intake of potassium is one way to reduce total body potassium. Potassium-rich foods include the following:

- Oranges
- Honeydew melons
- Bananas
- Nuts
- Dried apricots
- Raisins

Specialist dietary advice should be given to hyperkalemic patients in the office setting whenever possible.

MODIFY RISK FACTORS
SCREENING
VENOUS BLOOD SAMPLING FOR SERUM ELECTROLYTES, UREA, CREATININE

- At-risk groups should be screened for raised serum potassium
- All patients beginning a newly prescribed ACE inhibitor should receive blood screening for renal dysfunction and rising potassium within 2 weeks and 6 months after starting a new ACE inhibitor and should be monitored periodically thereafter to look for deterioration in renal function or rising potassium
- All diabetics should be screened periodically with these tests
- All elderly patients should have baseline renal-function testing and electrolytes tested before beginning long-term treatment with an NSAID, and this should be repeated periodically after starting therapy
- All patients with chronic renal failure should be screened regularly to monitor for deteriorating renal function and rising potassium
- All patients on a potassium-sparing diuretic should have these studies performed at 6-monthly intervals

Cost/efficacy
This can be carried out at minimal cost:efficacy ratio – these studies are relatively inexpensive, and a presentation of hyperkalemic acute renal failure is extremely expensive.

PREVENT RECURRENCE
Reassess coexisting disease
- Diabetics with a past history of hyperkalemia, particularly those taking ACE inhibitors, require periodic measurements of serum electrolytes
- Patients with chronic renal failure require periodic studies, as determined in collaboration with the consulting nephrologist

INTERACTION ALERT
- ACE inhibitors
- Angiotensin II receptor blockers
- Spironolactone
- Amiloride
- NSAIDs
- Pentamidine
- Trimethoprim
- Cyclosporine
- Heparin

PATIENT SATISFACTION/LIFESTYLE PRIORITIES
Patient compliance with a low potassium diet is vitally important to the management of hyperkalemia. One of the easiest ways to achieve effective control is via reduced dietary intake.

RESOURCES

ASSOCIATIONS

National Council on Potassium in Clinical Practice
Dr Jay N Cohn, MD
Cardiovascular Division, MMC508
University of Minnesota
420 Delaware St SE
Minneapolis, MN 55455

National Kidney Foundation
30 East 33rd Street
New York, NY 10016
http://www.kidney.org

American Society of Nephrology
2025 M Street NW#800
Washington, DC 20036
http://www.asn-online.org

Diabetes
American Diabetes Association
1701 North Beauregard Street
Alexandria, VA 22311
http://www.diabetes.org

Addison's disease
National Adrenal Diseases Foundation
505 Northern Boulevard
Great Neck, NY 11021
http://www.medhelp.org/nadf

KEY REFERENCES

- Acker CG, Johnson JP, Pavlevsky PM, Greenberg A. Hyperkalemia in hospitalized patients: causes, adequacy of treatment and results of an attempt to improve physician compliance with published therapy guidelines. Arch Intern Med 1998,158:917–924
- Carey C, ed. Washington manual of medical therapeutics, 29th edn. Washington, DC: Lippincott Raven, 1998

Evidence references and guidelines
1   Greenberg A, ed. Primer on kidney diseases. New York: Academic Press, 1998, pp 98–106
2   Montoliu J, Lens XM, Revert L. Potassium-lowering effect of albuterol for hyperkalemia in renal failure. Arch Intern Med 1987,147:713–717

FAQS
Question 1
What are the most common ECG findings in hyperkalemia?

ANSWER 1
Peaked T waves (earliest changes), widened QRS, prolonged PR, and shortened QT.

Question 2
Why is it important to treat hyperkalemia immediately?

ANSWER 2
Hyperkalemia can be life-threatening since it may cause ventricular dysrhythmia leading to cardiac arrest and/or respiratory muscle weakness.

Question 3
What is the most important emergent therapy in severe/symptomatic hyperkalemia?

ANSWER 3
Calcium gluconate intravenous infusion is the most important therapeutic intervention since it acts to stabilize the membrane actions of potassium, thereby helping to prevent ventricular dysrhythmia.

Question 4
For treatment of chronic hyperkalemia, what type of food should be avoided?

ANSWER 4
Fresh meats and fish, most fruits and vegetables, and fluid milk and yogurt are significant sources of potassium. The foods with the most potassium per serving are dried dates, nectarines, peaches, fresh figs, rhubarb, and chicken breast. However, common foods such as potatoes, tomatoes, raisins, prunes, oranges, cantaloupe and honeydew melons, bananas, cooked dried beans, and peanuts are also high in potassium content.

Question 5
What is hyperkalemic periodic paralysis?

ANSWER 5
It is a rare autosomal dominant disorder observed more often in patients of Asian descent. The genetic defect appears to be a mutation in the gene for the skeletal-muscle sodium channel. Stimuli that normally lead to mild hyperkalemia (e.g. exercise) can precipitate episodic weakness or paralysis.

CONTRIBUTORS
Fred F Ferri, MD, FACP
Martin Goldberg, MD, FACP
Dennis Kim, MD

HYPOKALEMIA

DESCRIPTION

- Defined as a serum potassium concentration below 3.5mEq/L (3.5mmol/L)
- Chronic hypokalemia with potassium depletion occurs due to decreased potassium intake and/or increased loss (renal or gastrointestinal)
- Acute hypokalemia results from the transcellular shift of potassium into the cells from the extracellular fluid
- May be successfully treated by the oral or intravenous administration of potassium
- The administration of potassium-sparing drugs and/or correction of the underlying cause or disease process will prevent further episodes

URGENT ACTION

Admit for inpatient management if the following occur:

- Serum potassium concentration is low enough to justify intravenous replacement therapy (i.e. <2.5mEq/L (<2.5mmol/L))
- Cardiac arrhythmias or QRS abnormalities on 12-lead ECG
- Rapid ventricular response
- Severe muscular weakness or paralysis
- Severe myopathy

KEY! DON'T MISS!

- The ECG in hypokalemic patients should be reviewed for T-wave flattening and the presence of U waves
- Diminished or absent deep tendon reflexes are characteristic of significant hypokalemia

ICD9 CODE
276.8 Hypokalemia

SYNONYMS
Hypopotassemia.

CARDINAL FEATURES
- A serum potassium concentration less than 3.5mEq/L (3.5mmol/L); 98% of intracellular potassium constitutes a major body ion
- Total body potassium 50mEq/kg
- Chronic hypokalemia with potassium depletion occurring along with decreased potassium intake and/or increased loss of potassium through renal or gastrointestinal routes
- Acute hypokalemia is the result of potassium shift into cells from the extracellular fluid
- Hypokalemia can cause ECG changes including T-wave flattening and U waves
- Hypokalemia may be successfully treated by administering potassium either orally or intravenously
- The use of potassium-sparing drugs and correction of underlying cause or disease process will prevent further episodes of hypokalemia

CAUSES
Common causes
Medications:
- Drugs, particularly thiazide and loop diuretics, aminoglycosides, amphotericin B, beta-2 agonists, and adrenal steroids
- Chronic laxative abuse

Gastrointestinal:
- Vomiting, which in some eating disorders may be self-induced, causes loss of hydrochloric acid, metabolic alkalosis, and a low urinary chloride level
- Gastric outlet obstruction, which may be caused by peptic ulcers in adults or by pyloric stenosis in infants and children, produces a similar metabolic pattern to vomiting
- Gastric suction, which also produces a similar metabolic pattern to vomiting
- Diarrhea can cause hypokalemia and metabolic acidosis

Renal:
- Renal tubular acidosis
- Secondary hyperaldosteronism, which can occur in conditions such as congestive heart failure, hypertension, cirrhosis, and nephrotic syndrome
- Magnesium deficiency associated with alcoholism, and the use of cisplatin, gentamicin, or levodopa, can cause refractory hypokalemia

Other causes:
- Alcohol abuse causes hypokalemia through a combination of poor diet, vomiting, and renal loss of potassium
- Poor dietary intake

Rare causes
Renal:
- Primary hyperaldosteronism caused by single adrenal adenoma (Conn's syndrome) and bilateral adrenal hyperplasia

- Cushing's syndrome due to Cushing's disease or adrenal Cushing's (cortisol producing adenoma)
- Renal tubular acidosis, which may be distal (severe hypokalemia) or proximal (milder hypokalemia)

Other causes:
- Cushing's syndrome due to ectopic secretion of adrenocorticotropic hormone from a small cell carcinoma of the lung
- Sodium glycyrrhizinate ingestion from chewing tobacco and excessive licorice consumption (usually in laxatives) owing to a genetic defect in the adrenal gland and which results in high desoxycorticosterone acetate levels, low aldosterone and decreased renin production

Serious causes
- Diabetic ketoacidosis can mask hypokalemia until insulin and fluids are administered which leads to a rapid influx of potassium into cells
- Vitamin B_{12} therapy for megaloblastic anemia produces new red blood cells which results in an intracellular influx of potassium leading to severe and potentially lethal hypokalemia

Contributory or predisposing factors
- Hypertension – diuretic treatment, hyperaldosteronism
- Congestive heart failure – diuretic treatment aggravated by secondary hyperaldosteronism
- Gastrointestinal disorders – vomiting, gastric suction, diarrhea
- Diabetes – especially when poorly controlled
- Eating disorders – self-induced vomiting, abuse of laxatives or diuretics, very low calorie diets
- Hypomagnesemia
- Alcoholism – low dietary intake, magnesium depletion
- Renal diseases – renal tubular acidosis, interstitial nephritis
- Family history – familial hypokalemic periodic paralysis is an autosomal dominant disorder and therefore occurs in multiple members of the same family

EPIDEMIOLOGY
Incidence and prevalence
Exact figures are not available, but hypokalemia is relatively common.

Demographics
AGE
- Can occur at any age but uncommon in children
- The elderly are at risk because of poor dietary intake or the use of diuretics

GENDER
Affects males and females equally.

RACE
No racial variance.

GENETICS
Hypokalemia is associated with some rare genetic disorders, namely:
- Familial (hypokalemic) periodic paralysis
- Congenital adrenogenital syndromes
- Liddle's syndrome
- Familial interstitial nephritis
- Glucocorticoid-remediable aldosteronism

SOCIOECONOMIC STATUS
Poverty may be associated with malnutrition leading to hypokalemia.

DIFFERENTIAL DIAGNOSIS
Spurious hypokalemia or pseudohypokalemia
Low potassium due to a leukocytosis which causes an intracellular influx in vitro.

FEATURES
- Rare condition
- Metabolically active white blood cells extract potassium when blood with a high white-cell count (>100,000/mm^3) is allowed to stand at room temperature
- Most likely to occur in patients with leukemia

Cushing's Syndrome
Clinical abnormalities due to excess glucocorticoids lead to hypokalemia. The main features of Cushing's syndrome are:

FEATURES
- Hypertension and edema
- Central obesity and facial rounding
- Skin fragility, ecchymoses, acne, and skin striae
- Hypogonadism, menstrual irregularities
- Muscle wasting and proximal myopathy
- Psychosis and emotional lability
- May result from excess adrenal cortisol production or chronic glucocorticoid therapy

Hypocalcemia
Defined as >9mg/dL calcium, occurs commonly in critically ill patients, especially patients with Gram-negative bacterial sepsis. The main features of hypocalcemia are:

FEATURES
- Muscle cramps and tetany
- Convulsions, stridor, and dyspnea
- Diplopia and the development of cataracts
- Urinary frequency
- If chronic, mental retardation and stunted growth in children
- Chovostek's and Trousseau's signs readily elicited
- Multiple causes including endocrine, sepsis, malnutrition, and renal disease
- Serum calcium must be correlated with serum albumin

SIGNS & SYMPTOMS
Signs
Neuromuscular signs:
- Mild skeletal muscle fatigue
- Diminished deep tendon reflexes
- Abdominal distention with reduced or absent bowel sounds leading to ileus
- Paralysis involving limbs and occasionally trunk and respiratory muscles
- Hypoventilation leading to respiratory failure
- Fasciculations

Cardiac abnormalities:
- Hypotension
- Atrioventricular block
- Supraventricular arrhythmias
- Ventricular tachyarrhythmias
- Cardiac arrest

Symptoms

Neuromuscular symptoms:

- Skeletal muscle weakness exacerbated by exertion
- Abdominal pain and bloating
- Constipation
- Paralysis of arms and legs
- Breathing difficulties

Renal symptoms:

- Urinary frequency
- Nocturia
- Excessive thirst

Cardiovascular symptoms:

- Palpitations

ASSOCIATED DISORDERS

- Hypertension – if treated with diuretics or secondary to hyperaldosteronism
- Diabetes is associated with hypokalemia especially during treatment for diabetic ketoacidosis
- Congestive heart failure – can lead to hypokalemia due to use of diuretics
- Asthma – treatment with beta-2 agonists can lead to hypokalemia

KEY! DON'T MISS!

- The ECG in hypokalemic patients should be reviewed for T-wave flattening and the presence of U waves
- Diminished or absent deep tendon reflexes are characteristic of significant hypokalemia

CONSIDER CONSULT

- Persistent hypokalemia with no identified cause
- If hypokalemia is severe (<2.5mEq/L, <2.5mmol/L)
- When hypokalemia is associated with cardiac arrhythmias, rapid ventricular rate or QRS abnormalities on ECG
- If the cause of paralysis or cardiovascular symptoms is unknown
- If there is suspicion of an adrenal, pituitary, or other tumor that may suggest an endocrine cause of hypokalemia (e.g. Cushing's disease, cortisol tumor, Conn's syndrome, ectopic ACTH production, small cell carcinoma)

INVESTIGATION OF THE PATIENT

Direct questions to patient

The patient's history is important in determining the possible cause of the hypokalemia.

Q **Have you had any vomiting or diarrhea recently?** Self-induced vomiting and abuse of laxatives should be ruled out.

Q **Are you taking any medication?** Include prescribed (diuretics) and over-the-counter preparations as well as herbal and homeopathic remedies.

Q **Have you experienced episodes of extreme muscle weakness or paralysis?** There may be a history of such attacks in patients with familial hypokalemic periodic paralysis.

Q **Have you experienced any muscle weakness, fatigue, palpitations, increased frequency and volume of urination, thirst, increased fluid consumption or constipation?** These can be symptoms of hypokalemia, but mild to moderate hypokalemia may not produce any noticeable symptoms at all.

Q **Do you suffer from any of the following: hypertension, congestive heart failure, diabetes, asthma, kidney disease?** All may be associated with hypokalemia either through a direct pathophysiologic mechanism or indirectly through the action of the drugs used to treat these diseases.

Q **What is your average alcohol consumption?** Hypokalemia secondary to alcoholism is due to a combination of poor diet, vomiting, and renal loss.

Q **Do you eat fruit, vegetables and fish as part of your diet?** Citrus fruits, apples, bananas, and apricots all contain significant amounts of potassium. Most green vegetables, lima beans, tomatoes, and potatoes are also good sources. Potassium-rich fish include salmon, cod, flounder, and sardines.

Contributory or predisposing factors

Q **Is there a history of diuretic or laxative abuse, congestive heart failure, vomiting, diarrhea, diabetes, eating disorders, alcoholism, genetic disease, renal disease, mineralocorticoid excess, glucocorticoid excess, or leukemia?** These disorders may be associated with hypokalemia either by way of a direct pathophysiologic mechanism or indirectly through the action of the drugs used to treat the disorders.

Q **Is the patient taking diuretics, beta-2 agonists, penicillin antibiotics, aminoglycosides, amphotericin B, or any other drug associated with hypokalemia?** These can cause hypokalemia.

Q **Is the patient consuming excessive amounts of licorice, laxatives or chewing tobacco products?** These can cause hypokalemia.

Q **Has the patient been using herbal medicines?** There are a number of reports in the literature of hypokalemia resulting from a variety of self-administered herbal medicines.

Family history

Q **Is there a family history of intermittent episodes of paralysis?** Familial hypokalemic periodic paralysis is an autosomal dominant disorder and therefore occurs in multiple members of the same family.

Q **Is there a family history of any rare genetic disorders such as Bartter's syndrome, Liddle's syndrome, or glucocorticoid-remediable aldosteronism?** These disorders can cause hypokalemia.

Examination

Examination will not lead to the diagnosis of hypokalemia, but the signs will arouse suspicion and may identify the cause.

- **Physical appearance:** look for a Cushingoid appearance or signs of poor dietary intake or weight loss which can cause hypokalemia
- **Cardiovascular examination:** check pulse (for arrhythmia) and blood pressure (for hypotension)
- **Oral examination:** chronic self-induced vomiting in bulimia may produce characteristic acid damage to the dentition
- **Abdominal examination:** look for signs of paralytic ileus and/or a loaded colon
- **Neurologic examination:** muscle weakness, hypotonia, paralysis, and diminished deep tendon reflexes occur with hypokalemia
- **Check for hyperglycemia:** urine glucose level and finger-prick blood glucose level are raised in hypokalemia

Summary of investigative tests

The diagnosis of hypokalemia can be made on the basis of a simple blood test; it is often an incidental finding during routine investigation and management of a variety of disorders.

- Serum potassium – is the primary test used to diagnose hypokalemia
- Urinary potassium and urinary chloride levels – in the presence of hypokalemia can help determine the cause of the hypokalemia
- Plasma aldosterone – if the hypokalemia is unrelated to diuretic therapy and is associated with hypertension and high serum sodium, then an elevated aldosterone level may indicate hyperaldosteronism
- Plasma renin – if hypokalemia is associated with hypertension and normal or high serum sodium levels then a low renin level may indicate hyperaldosteronism

- Serum magnesium – magnesium deficiency can cause hypokalemia and must be corrected if potassium replacement is to be effective
- Plasma glucose – hypokalemia is associated with hyperglycemia in cases of poorly controlled diabetes and plasma glucose should be checked, especially in patients not already known to be diabetic
- Renal function (urea, creatinine and routine urinalysis) – should be checked to identify any underlying renal disease as a potential cause of the hypokalemia
- ECG – is essential in patients with pre-existing cardiovascular disease and patients receiving digoxin therapy. It cannot be used alone to diagnose hypokalemia
- CT scan of adrenal glands – should be ordered by the primary care physician only after consultation with a specialist, because adrenal lesions are rare causes of hypokalemia and the procedure is expensive and inconvenient. The scan may identify adrenal hyperplasia or an adrenal adenoma
- Radionuclide scanning of adrenal glands – may distinguish between a single adenoma that is secreting excess aldosterone or diffuse hyperplasia of the adrenal gland. The scan should generally only be ordered by the primary care physician after consultation with a specialist, because adrenal lesions are rare causes of hypokalemia and the procedure is expensive and inconvenient

DIAGNOSTIC DECISION

- The diagnosis of hypokalemia is based on results of serum potassium tests
- Chronic hypokalemia indicates total body potassium depletion
- Acute hypokalemia usually results from shifts of potassium from the extracellular fluid into the cells
- Determining the cause of the hypokalemia requires additional investigations
- The first aim is to check for gastrointestinal and renal losses
- The diagnosis of hypokalemia cannot be based on symptoms because similar symptoms can occur in a number of other disorders and are not specific to hypokalemia

Guidelines:
A guideline was published under the auspices of the National Kidney Foundation and containing an excellent summary of guidelines for the diagnosis and management of hypokalemia and potassium depletion [1]

CLINICAL PEARLS

- >90% of hypokalemic patients have one or more of the following underlying causes: diuretics, vomiting, diarrhea, inadequate dietary intake of potassium
- In patients with hypertension and/or congestive heart failure, the major cause of hypokalemia is potassium depletion due to the use of diuretics
- Primary hyperaldosteronism is very uncommon; therefore prior consultation with an expert is strongly recommended before proceeding with expensive and complex diagnostic procedures such as CT scans and nuclear imaging

THE TESTS
Body fluids
SERUM POTASSIUM
Description
Cuffed venous blood sample. Avoid causing hemolysis in the sample as this may result in a falsely high serum potassium.

Advantages/Disadvantages
- Advantage: this test is diagnostic, provided care is taken in avoiding sources of false-positive and false-negative results.

Normal
3.5–5.0mEq/L (3.5–5.0mmol/L).

Abnormal
- A serum potassium of <3.5mEq/L (<3.5mmol/L) indicates hypokalemia
- Beware of falsely abnormal results

Drugs, disorders and other factors that may alter results
- False-positive results may arise from pseudohypokalemia
- Hemolysis in the blood sample prior to processing can result in falsely high serum potassium levels

URINARY POTASSIUM
Description
Spot urine sample, which can be taken at any time of day.

Advantages/Disadvantages
Advantages:
- Easy to collect
- May differentiate between gastrointestinal and renal losses

Disadvantage: results ranging from 20–40mEq/L (20–40mmol/L) can be nondiagnostic

Abnormal
Levels of <20mEq/L (<20mmol/L) or >40mEq/L (>40mmol/L) in the presence of hypokalemia are useful in helping to determine the cause.

Cause of abnormal result
Urinary potassium <20mEq/L (<20mmol/L) suggests:
- Extrarenal losses (diarrhea, sweating, vomiting)
- Poor potassium intake or severe chronic potassium depletion from any cause

Urinary potassium >40mEq/L (>40mmol/L) in the presence of hypokalemia indicates:
- Renal losses from renal tubular defect
- Drug effects
- Mineralocorticoid deficiency or resistance
- Hypomagnesemia

PLASMA ALDOSTERONE LEVEL
Description
- A cuffed venous blood sample
- Two samples are required – one taken after the patient has remained in a supine position for 30min and the other after 2h of normal erect activity
- The specimens may require special transportation and handling
- The test is performed by measuring plasma renin levels
- The test is not routine and should generally only be performed and interpreted in consultation with a neurologist or endocrinologist

Advantages/Disadvantages

Advantage: useful to exclude hyperaldosteronism as a cause of hypokalemia

Disadvantages:

- Inconvenient for the patient, especially if two samples are required
- Taken alone the test does not distinguish between primary and secondary hyperaldosteronism
- The test requires prior cessation of diuretic therapy
- A specialist's interpretation is required

Normal

- Supine plasma aldosterone: 50–150ng/L (100–500pmol/L)
- Erect plasma aldosterone: 200–750ng/L (200–900pmol/L)

Abnormal

- Supine plasma aldosterone: >150ng/L (>500pmol/L)
- Erect plasma aldosterone: >750ng/L (>900pmol/L)
- False-positive results can occur

Cause of abnormal result

- Primary or secondary hyperaldosteronism
- Hypovolemia
- Sodium depletion

Drugs, disorders and other factors that may alter results

- Diuretics increase aldosterone levels
- Aldosterone is also elevated in Bartter's syndrome

PLASMA RENIN LEVEL

Description

- Cuffed venous blood sample
- Two samples are required – one taken after the patient has remained in a supine position for 30min, the other after 2h of normal erect activity
- The specimens may require special handling and transportation
- The test is performed along with plasma aldosterone level testing to differentiate the type of hyperaldosteronism

Advantages/Disadvantages

Advantages:

- Aids in the diagnosis of hyperaldosteronism
- Aids in diagnosing the type of hyperaldosteronism, i.e. it is lowered in primary and raised in secondary hyperaldosteronism

Disadvantage:

- Inconvenient for the patient, especially because two samples are required

Normal

- Supine plasma renin: 48–119mcg/L per h (1.1–2.7pmol/mL per h)
- Erect plasma renin: 132–190mcg/L per h (2.8–4.5pmol/mL per h)

Abnormal

- Hyporeninemia: supine plasma renin <48mcg/L/h (<1.1pmol/mL/h) and/or erect plasma renin <132mcg/L/h (<2.8pmol/mL/h)

- Hyperreninemia: supine plasma renin >119mcg/L/h (>2.7pmol/mL/h) and/or erect plasma renin >190mcg/L/h (>4.5pmol/mL/h)
- Keep in mind the possibility of a false-positive result

Cause of abnormal result
- Hyporeninemia in association with hyperaldosteronism suggests primary hyperaldosteronism
- Hyperreninemia in association with hyperaldosteronism suggests secondary hyperaldosteronism or Bartter's syndrome

Drugs, disorders and other factors that may alter results
Hyperreninemia may be caused by the administration of antihypertensive medications such as diuretics.

SERUM MAGNESIUM
Description
Cuffed venous blood sample.

Normal
Plasma magnesium: 1.5–2.1mEq/L (0.75–1.05mmol/L).

Abnormal
Magnesium deficiency: plasma magnesium <1.5mEq/L (<0.75mmol/L).

Cause of abnormal result
- Hypomagnesemia
- False-positive result for hypomagnesemia may occur

Drugs, disorders and other factors that may alter results
The following can cause hypomagnesemia:
- Alcoholism
- Starvation
- Use of loop diuretics
- Malabsorption syndrome
- Treatment with gentamicin, amphotericin B, or cisplatin

URINARY CHLORIDE
Description
A spot urine collection.

Advantages/Disadvantages
Advantage: easy to collect

Disadvantages:
- Frequently difficult to interpret
- Variable and affected by diet and diuretics
- Requires discontinuation of diuretic therapy >24h before testing

Normal
40–100mEq/L (40–100mmol/L).

Abnormal
Value <40mEq/L (<40mmol/L).

Cause of abnormal result

- Value <20mEq/L (<20mmol/L) with hypokalemia suggests gastrointestinal loss of potassium
- Value >50mEq/L (>50mmol/L) with hypokalemia suggests hyperaldosteronism, Bartter's syndrome or losses resulting from diuretic therapy

Drugs, disorders and other factors that may alter results
Urine chloride concentration is variable depending on many factors including dietary salt intake and the effects of diuretics.

PLASMA GLUCOSE
Description

- The sample must be clearly defined as 'fasting' or 'random'
- 'Fasting' is defined as no consumption of food or drink other than water for >8h before testing

Advantages/Disadvantages
Advantages:

- Easy to perform
- Inexpensive
- Universally available
- May help diagnose the cause of hypokalemia, which can be associated with hyperglycemia in patients with diabetes mellitus

Disadvantages:

- Random blood glucose testing is rarely helpful; a fasting sample is needed to confirm the glucose level
- Fasting of >8h is required

Normal

- Normal fasting plasma glucose: 70–110mg/dl (3.9–6.1mmol/l)
- Random (postprandial) glucose: <140mg/dL (7.8mmol/L)

Abnormal
Values outside the normal reference range.

Cause of abnormal result
Hypoglycemia or hyperglycemia.

Drugs, disorders and other factors that may alter results
Hyperglycemia can be caused by the following:

- Diabetes mellitus
- Gestational diabetes
- Cushing's syndrome
- Acromegaly
- Pheochromocytoma
- Hormones: glucagon, glucocorticoids, growth hormone, epinephrine, estrogen and progesterone (oral contraceptives), thyroid preparations
- Drugs: thiazide diuretics, furosemide, acetazolamide, diazoxide, beta-blockers, alpha-agonists, calcium-channel blockers, phenytoin, phenobarbital sodium, nicotinic acid, cyclophosphamide, l-asparaginase, epinephrine-like drugs (decongestants and diet pills), nonsteroidal anti-inflammatory agents, nicotine, caffeine, sugar-containing syrups, fish oils

Hypoglycemia can be caused by the following:

- Hypoglycemic medications: insulin, metformin, rosiglitazone and sulfonylureas
- Exercise
- Malnutrition
- Insulinoma

Tests of function
RENAL FUNCTION
Description
Cuffed venous blood sample to determine renal electrolytes.

Normal
The normal ranges may vary among laboratories, but typically normal ranges are:

- Blood urea nitrogen: 15–40mg/dL (2.5–6.7mmol/L)
- Serum creatinine: 0.7–1.7mg/dL (70–150mcmol/L)

Abnormal

- Generally only values above the upper limit of normal are considered abnormal
- It is common to find healthy individuals with values below the lower limit of the normal range
- Keep in mind the possibility of a falsely abnormal result

Cause of abnormal result
Elevated values may indicate renal impairment.

Drugs, disorders and other factors that may alter results

- Extracellular volume depletion can cause abnormal results without concomitant renal disease
- Urea is more influenced by factors other than intrinsic renal disease than is creatinine. Urea/creatinine ratio (normally between 10:1 and 15:1) is increased by high protein intake, acute volume depletion, dehydration, acute urinary tract obstruction; it is decreased by a low-protein diet, intestinal malabsorption and hepatic failure
- Serum creatinine is increased by a high-meat diet, independent of changes in renal function

Imaging
CT SCAN OF ADRENAL GLANDS
Description
This test should be prescribed and performed by a specialist.

Advantages/Disadvantages
Advantage: very sensitive in identifying a single adenoma of the adrenal gland or detecting diffuse hyperplasia of the glands

Disadvantages:

- Exposes patient to radiation and therefore MRI scanning may be preferred
- Some patients may require sedation to make the procedure tolerable, owing to other physical or psychological factors
- The test is expensive and must be conducted at a hospital center
- Must be interpreted by a radiology specialist
- Technical issues may make it impossible to obtain images clear enough to confirm the diagnosis

Abnormal
- Appearance of an adrenal adenoma or diffuse adrenal hyperplasia
- Falsely abnormal results can occur

RADIONUCLIDE SCANNING OF ADRENALS USING LABELED CHOLESTEROL
Description
This test should only be prescribed and performed by a specialist.

Advantages/Disadvantages
Advantage: may clearly distinguish between a single adenoma secreting excess aldosterone and diffuse hyperplasia

Disadvantages:
- Requires intravenous radiolabeled cholesterol and exposure to X-rays on more than one occasion over a period of approximately 7 days
- Results may be inconclusive

Abnormal
Actively secreting adrenal adenoma identified on X-ray as an area of increased uptake of radiolabeled cholesterol.

Other tests
ECG
Advantages/Disadvantages
Advantages:
- Rapid interpretation of arrhythmias
- Can help in diagnosing hypokalemia-flattened T waves with U-wave formation

Disadvantage: ECG on its own is not diagnostic of hypokalemia

Abnormal
- Mild hypokalemia: flattened T waves, slight ST segment depression and U waves >1mm
- Moderate hypokalemia: increased P wave amplitude, longer PR interval and widening of the QRS complex
- Severe hypokalemia: atrioventricular block, supraventricular and ventricular tachyarrhythmias, including ventricular fibrillation

Cause of abnormal result
Hypokalemia.

Drugs, disorders and other factors that may alter results
The ECG characteristic of hypokalemia may result from other cardiovascular diseases or digoxin therapy.

TREATMENT

CONSIDER CONSULT

- If intravenous potassium replacement is indicated (potassium <2.5mEq/L; <2.5mmol/L)
- If the patient's general condition requires close monitoring (e.g. ECG)
- If the underlying cause of the hypokalemia indicates the need for a specialist, for example to perform a surgical procedure (e.g. adrenalectomy)
- If an eating disorder is suspected to be the cause of the hypokalemia

IMMEDIATE ACTION

Immediate potassium replacement is indicated in the presence of:

- ECG abnormalities
- Paralysis, especially involving the respiratory muscles

PATIENT AND CAREGIVER ISSUES
Patient or caregiver request

- Patients receiving specific medication may identify themselves as being at risk of hypokalemia from information obtained in the media, from their pharmacist or from the drug information literature supplied with their medication. They may ask about preventive measures
- Patients with a family history of disorders such as familial hypokalemic periodic paralysis, Liddle's syndrome or glucocorticoid-remediable aldosteronism may seek genetic testing and serum potassium testing

MANAGEMENT ISSUES
Goals

- Restore serum potassium level to normal without producing hyperkalemia
- Identify and correct the cause of the hypokalemia
- Prevent recurrence through treatment and follow-up

Management in special circumstances

Special management may be required in patients who:

- Have coexisting disease
- Are receiving essential medication for coexisting disease
- Have an underlying cause of the hypokalemia that cannot be corrected

COEXISTING DISEASE

- Avoid the use of treatments for coexisting disease that are known to potentiate hypokalemia
- Treat the coexisting disease appropriately (e.g. surgical removal of an adrenal adenoma)
- Monitor potassium levels closely in patients with a coexisting disease associated with hypokalemia

COEXISTING MEDICATION

- Prescribed and over-the-counter medications are major causes of hypokalemia
- The elderly are at particular risk of hypokalemia owing to polypharmacy
- Consider alternative drugs that do not cause hypokalemia when treating coexisting disease
- Caution patients about over-the-counter preparations and herbal/homeopathic medications that may cause hypokalemia

SUMMARY OF THERAPEUTIC OPTIONS
Choices

- Treatment choices for hypokalemia depend on the severity of the problem and its underlying cause
- Potassium levels between 3.0 and 3.5 mEq/L may not need correcting if the patient is asymptomatic

- It is generally agreed that a serum potassium level below 3.0 mEq/L requires treatment
- The first choice in the management of hypokalemia is to eliminate the cause
- Oral potassium chloride salts are first-line therapy in most cases of hypokalemia because they are easy to administer, safe, inexpensive and readily absorbed from the gastrointestinal tract
- Potassium-sparing diuretics (such as spironolactone, amiloride, and triamterene) alone, or in combination with other diuretics, are used in patients with hyperaldosteronism, congestive heart failure or nephrotic syndrome
- Infusions of intravenous potassium salts should only be used when serum potassium has fallen rapidly to <2.5mEq/L and when there are complications, including cardiac arrhythmias or paralysis, or if oral treatment is unfeasible (e.g. vomiting)
- Magnesium is a treatment that should only be used in cases of hypokalemia associated with proven magnesium deficiency
- Hypokalemic periodic paralysis can be avoided with the use of acetazolamide
- Adrenalectomy is indicated for an adrenal adenoma that causes hypertension and hypokalemia. It is unsuitable for adrenal hyperplasia
- Lifestyle measures including dietary sources of potassium are not likely to be useful in treating and preventing hypokalemia

Guidelines:
New guidelines for potassium replacement in clinical practice: a contemporary review by the National Council on Potassium in Clinical Practice [2]

Never
- Never inject potassium salts directly into a vein as this may precipitate cardiac arrest
- Do not use magnesium to treat hypokalemia without first confirming the presence of magnesium deficiency
- Do not begin treatment with potassium salts if pseudohypokalemia is suspected
- Do not administer potassium to patients with diabetic ketoacidosis until the serum potassium has actually started falling

FOLLOW UP
Plan for review
- Check serum potassium levels regularly after commencing treatment
- Patients receiving oral potassium supplements, potassium-containing diuretics or potassium-sparing diuretics should have their serum potassium levels checked every 3–6 months
- In mild hypokalemia recheck serum potassium every 2–4 weeks until levels are stable; then, if on diuretic therapy, recheck every 3–6 months
- Check serum potassium more frequently when altering diuretic therapy
- Patients with moderate to severe hypokalemia who are treated with oral potassium salts should have serum potassium checked daily until satisfactory levels are reached. They should then be checked every 2–4 weeks
- During intravenous administration of potassium the serum level and ECG must be monitored continuously
- Patients receiving potassium-sparing drugs should have their serum potassium level checked every 3–6 months

Information for patient or caregiver
- Maintain an adequate dietary intake of potassium (e.g. bananas, tomatoes, peaches) and reduce salt intake

Emphasize importance of:
- Report for regular serum potassium checks
- Comply with medication to prevent recurrence

DRUGS AND OTHER THERAPIES: DETAILS
Drugs
ORAL POTASSIUM SALTS

- These are available as potassium chloride, potassium bicarbonate, potassium citrate, and potassium gluconate
- Potassium chloride is the most commonly used form
- Oral potassium salts can be administered in tablet or capsule (including extended-release and effervescent forms), liquid, or powder form

Dose
- Adults: 40–120 mEq/day in 2–3 divided doses
- Children: 1–2 mEq/kg/day in 1–2 divided doses
- May need to be adjusted in presence of concomitant disease (e.g. renal impairment), or if the patient is taking other medication (e.g. angiotensin-converting enzyme (ACE) inhibitors)

Efficacy
Serum potassium should start to rise within 72h of initiation of therapy

Risks/Benefits
Risks:
- Use with caution in the following cases: in renal disease and impairment, adrenal insufficiency, acute dehydration or diarrhea, cardiac arrhythmias, patients with severe burns, heat or muscle cramps
- Use with caution in the elderly

Benefits:
- Relatively rapid correction of potassium deficit in most cases of uncomplicated hypokalemia
- Usually safe
- Easy to administer
- Rapidly absorbed from the gastrointestinal tract

Side-effects and adverse reactions
- Gastrointestinal: nausea, vomiting, abdominal pain, diarrhea, gastrointestinal bleeding, esophageal/small bowel ulceration
- Metabolic: hyperkalemia
- Cardiovascular system: ECG changes, arrhythmias, hypotension, atrioventricular block, cardiac arrest
- Central nervous system: paresthesia, confusion, shock
- Musculoskeletal: weakness

Interactions (other drugs)
- ACE inhibitors ■ Amphotericin B ■ Angiotensin II receptor antagonists ■ Antimuscarinics
- Beta-blockers ■ Cyclosporine ■ Diuretics (potassium-sparing, loop, thiazide) ■ Heparin
- H1 antagonists ■ Loperamide ■ Opiate agonists ■ NSAIDs ■ Tricyclic antidepressants
- Phenothiazines ■ Sodium polystyrene sulfonate ■ Penicillins

Contraindications
- Gastrointestinal obstruction ■ Sodium polystyrene sulfonate ■ Esophageal obstruction
- Hyperkalemia ■ Severe renal impairment ■ Oliguria, anuria, azotemia ■ Severe hemolytic reactions

Acceptability to patient

■ Tablet and powder preparations are acceptable but more likely to cause gastrointestinal ulceration

■ The liquid form has an unpleasant acrid taste which can be minimized by mixing it with fruit juice

Follow up plan

Patients should be informed that regular follow-up is needed to monitor serum potassium.

Patient and caregiver information

Patients need to:

■ Take medication regularly

■ Tell the prescriber of any changes in other medications

■ Keep the prescriber aware of any new concomitant disease

■ Report any side-effects

INTRAVENOUS POTASSIUM SALTS

Available as potassium chloride and potassium acetate for infusion. These should only be used in cases where oral preparations are contraindicated:

■ Persistent vomiting

■ Emergency situations such as when hypokalemia is associated with cardiac arrhythmias

Dose

Potassium for injection must be diluted to a maximum of 40mEq/L prior to administration.

■ Adult infusion rate: 10mEq/h (should not exceed 60mEq/h)

■ In children: do not exceed 0.02mEq/kg per min

Efficacy

Very effective.

Risks/Benefits

Risks:

■ Use caution in patients with cardiac disease, renal impairment, systemic acidosis

■ Use caution in patients receiving concurrent treatment with potassium-sparing diuretics

Benefits:

■ Rapid correction of hypokalemia

■ Rapid resolution of symptoms – including cardiac arrhythmias and paralysis

Side-effects and adverse reactions

■ Gastrointestinal: nausea, vomiting, diarrhea, abdominal pain

■ Cardiovascular system: cardiac depression, cardiac arrest, changes in the ECG, dysrhythmias, bradycardia

■ Metabolic: hyperkalemia, metabolic acidosis

Interactions (other drugs)

■ ACE inhibitors ■ Aluminum-containing antacids ■ Angiotensin II receptor antagonists ■ Cardiac glycosides ■ Cyclosporine ■ Potassium-sparing diuretics ■ Quinidine ■ Heparin ■ Disopyramide ■ Hypoglycemics

Contraindications

■ Aluminum toxicity ■ Heart failure ■ Severe renal disease ■ Hyperkalemia ■ Dehydration ■ Peptic ulcer disease ■ Always dilute – adding concentrated potassium solution intravenously is fatal

Follow up plan
- Close monitoring of serum potassium levels is required and the rate of infusion should be reduced gradually as serum potassium rises
- Once serum potassium has reached a satisfactory level the intravenous potassium should be replaced with an oral equivalent

Patient and caregiver information
Patients need to:
- Report for regular serum potassium monitoring
- Take oral medication regularly
- Tell prescriber of any changes in concomitant medication
- Keep prescriber aware of any new concomitant disease and report any side-effects

SPIRONOLACTONE
- Potassium-sparing diuretic
- Used for the treatment or prevention of hypokalemia associated with hyperaldosteronism, other diuretics, or congestive heart failure

Dose
- Adults: 25–100mg/day orally either as a single dose or 2–4 divided doses
- In hyperaldosteronism the dose may need to be as high as 200–300mg/day

Efficacy
Serum potassium levels should respond within 48h.

Risks/Benefits
Risks:
- Spironolactone is a potassium-sparing diuretic; therefore use with caution when given with potassium supplements and hyponatremia
- Use caution in patients with renal and hepatic impairment; diabetes, acidosis, and dehydration; menstrual problems and gynecomastia
- Use with caution in pregnant women and the elderly

Benefits:
- Can be used prophylactically to prevent hypokalemia
- Supplants the need for a separate diuretic and potassium supplement

Side-effects and adverse reactions
- Gastrointestinal: nausea, vomiting, diarrhea, bleeding, abdominal pain
- Metabolic: hyperkalemia, hyponatremia, acidosis
- Central nervous system: headache, drowsiness
- Genitourinary: menstrual irregularities, gynecomastia, hirsutism, impotence
- Cardiovascular system: hypotension, bradycardia
- Skin: rashes, pruritus

Interactions (other drugs)
- Angiotensin-converting enzyme (ACE) inhibitors ■ Ammonium chloride ■ Anticoagulants ■ Angiotensin II receptor antagonists ■ Cardiac glycosides ■ Carbenoxolone ■ Lithium ■ Cyclosporine, tacrolimus ■ Disopyramide ■ Mitotane ■ Potassium ■ Salicylates

Contraindications
- Severe renal disease ■ Anuria ■ ACE inhibitors and angiotensin receptor antagonists in antikaliuretic therapy ■ Hyperkalemia

Acceptability to patient
The side-effect profile of spironolactone may be intolerable to some patients.

Follow up plan
Regular monitoring of renal function and serum potassium is required.

Patient and caregiver information
Patients need to:
- Take medication regularly
- Keep prescriber aware of any changes in concomitant medication
- Avoid taking licorice extract
- Keep prescriber aware of any new concomitant disease and report any side-effects
- Notify prescriber if pregnancy occurs during therapy because the medication may cause congenital abnormalities

AMILORIDE
- Potassium-sparing diuretic available in tablet form
- A combination product containing amiloride and hydrochlorothiazide is also available
- Only used alone in cases of persistent hypokalemia
- Generally used in cases where hypokalemia is secondary to the use of another diuretic which has not been discontinued

Dose
Adults: 5mg once daily increasing to 10mg in severe hypokalemia.

Efficacy
Serum potassium levels should respond within 48h.

Risks/Benefits
Risks:
- Use caution in children and the elderly; pregnancy and breast-feeding
- Use caution in patients with hyponatremia, hepatic disease, diabetes mellitus, and cardiopulmonary disease

Side-effects and adverse reactions
- Gastrointestinal: nausea, vomiting, anorexia, abdominal pain, constipation, jaundice
- Metabolic: hyperkalemia, hyponatremia, hypochloremia, metabolic acidosis
- Cardiovascular system: sinus bradycardia, ECG changes, angina, orthostatic hypotension, arrhythmias, palpitations
- Genitourinary: polyuria, dysuria, bladder spasms, impotence, libido decrease, azotemia
- Central nervous system: headache, dizziness, encephalopathy, paresthesias
- Hematologic: blood cell disorders (rare)
- Respiratory: cough, dyspnea
- Musculoskeletal: cramps, weakness, fatigue
- Ears, eyes, nose, and throat: visual disturbances

Interactions (other drugs)
- ACE inhibitors - Amoxicillin - Angiotensin II receptor antagonists - Antihypertensives - Beta-blockers - Cyclosporine - Digoxin - Diuretics (potassium-sparing, loop, thiazide) - Dofetilide - Heparin - Lithium - NSAIDs - Penicillin G - Potassium salts - Quinidine

Contraindications
- Renal disease/failure - Diabetic neuropathy - Anuria - Hyperkalemia - Cyclosporine - Spironolactone, triamterene - Antikaliuretic therapy

Evidence
Amiloride may be effective in correcting thiazide-induced hypokalemia.
- A small randomized crossover trial assessed the efficacy of potassium chloride, amiloride, and triamterene in hypokalemic patients receiving thiazide diuretics for heart failure. Amiloride was as effective as triamterene in maintaining potassium levels, and superior to potassium chloride (N.B. Amiloride and triamterene were given in a randomized crossover manner, followed by open administration of potassium chloride) [3] *Level P*

Acceptability to patient
Generally well tolerated with minimal side-effects.

Follow up plan
Monitor serum potassium and renal function regularly.

Patient and caregiver information
Patients need to:
- Take medication regularly
- Tell prescriber of any alterations to other medication
- Keep prescriber aware of development of any new concomitant disease and report any side-effects
- Notify prescriber if they become pregnant during therapy

TRIAMTERENE
- Potassium-sparing diuretic available in capsule form
- Available as a combination product of 25mg hydrochlorthiazide and 50mg triamterene

Dose
Adult oral dose: 50mg twice daily to a maximum of 100mg twice daily.

Efficacy
Serum potassium levels should respond within 48h.

Risks/Benefits
Risks:
- Use caution in patients with diabetes mellitus, pre-existing hyponatremia, cardiac disease, hepatic disease, gout, hyperuricemia, or nephrolithiasis
- Use with caution in the elderly

Benefit: combines diuretic properties with potassium conservation, without the need to add supplemental potassium

Side-effects and adverse reactions
- Gastrointestinal: nausea, vomiting, diarrhea, jaundice, dry mouth
- Metabolic: hyperkalemia, hypomagnesemia (with thiazide diuretics), hyponatremia
- Genitourinary: polyuria, interstitial nephritis, azotemia, nephrolithiasis
- Hematologic: megaloblastic anemia (with alcoholic patients), thrombocytopenia, agranulocytosis (both rare)
- Central nervous system: headache, weakness, dizziness, fatigue
- Musculoskeletal: muscle cramps
- Skin: rash, photosensitivity

Interactions (other drugs)

■ Amantadine ■ Amiloride ■ Antidiabetic agents ■ Antihypertensive agents (ACE inhibitors, angiotensin-II receptor antagonists, diuretics) ■ Cyclosporine ■ Dofetilide ■ NSAIDs ■ Heparin ■ Lithium ■ Potassium salts ■ Potassium-containing medications ■ Spironolactone

Contraindications

■ Hyperkalemia ■ Renal disease ■ Anuria ■ Diabetic nephropathy ■ Spironolactone ■ Pregnancy and breast-feeding ■ Amiloride

Evidence

Triamterene may be effective in correcting thiazide-induced hypokalemia.

■ A small randomized crossover trial assessed the efficacy of potassium chloride, amiloride and triamterene in hypokalemic patients receiving thiazide diuretics for heart failure. Triamterene was as effective as amiloride in maintaining potassium levels, and superior to potassium chloride (N.B. Amiloride and triamterene were given in a randomized crossover manner, followed by open administration of potassium chloride) [3] *Level P*

Acceptability to patient

Generally well tolerated.

Follow up plan

Need to monitor serum potassium levels and renal function regularly.

Patient and caregiver information

Patients need to:

■ Take medication regularly
■ Tell prescriber of any changes in concomitant medication
■ Keep prescriber aware of any new concomitant disease and report any side-effects
■ Report immediately if patient becomes pregnant during therapy

MAGNESIUM

■ This is an off-label indication
■ If serum potassium fails to rise in response to oral or intravenous potassium supplements within 4–5 days then concomitant magnesium depletion may be present
■ Magnesium sulfate is available for intravenous or intramuscular injection in 50% or 10% solutions

Dose

■ If serum magnesium level is <1mEq/L give 2ml of 50% magnesium sulfate intramuscularly: on day 1, twice; on day 2, twice; on day 3, once
■ Alternatively, magnesium sulfate may be administered orally in water at a dose of 3g every 6h for four doses

Risks/Benefits

Risks:

■ Use caution in patients with renal and hepatic impairment, or dehydration
■ Use caution in the elderly and debilitated

Benefit: restoring the serum magnesium level to normal should correct the hypokalemia

Side-effects and adverse reactions

■ Gastrointestinal: nausea, vomiting, diarrhea, abdominal pain
■ Metabolic: hypermagnesemia, magnesium toxicity

- Central nervous system: flushing, muscle paralysis, hypothermia, central nervous system depression
- Cardiovascular system: circulatory collapse, cardiac depression, cardiac arrest, hypotension
- Respiratory: respiratory depression
- Skin: sweating

Interactions (other drugs)
- Allopurinol ▪ Antacids, iron salts, calcium salts ▪ Antibiotics (cephalosporins, fluoroquinolones, tetracyclines) ▪ Aspirin ▪ Atenolol ▪ Cardiac glycosides ▪ Cellulose sodium phosphate, edetate disodium, etidronate, vitamin D analogs ▪ Central nervous system depressants (barbiturates, opiate agonists, H1 blockers, antidepressants, benzodiazepines, general and local anesthetics, phenothiazines, ethanol) ▪ Diuretics ▪ Glipizide, glyburide ▪ Isoniazid ▪ Ketoconazole ▪ Nifedipine ▪ Penicillamine ▪ Quinidine ▪ Succinylcholine ▪ Sodium polystyrene sulfonate

Contraindications
- Atrioventricular block ▪ Cardiac disease ▪ Gastrointestinal obstruction ▪ Hypermagnesemia

Follow up plan
- Regular checks of serum magnesium and potassium
- Correction of any concomitant disease that might contribute to recurrence of hypomagnesemia

Surgical therapy
ADRENALECTOMY
- Indicated for hypokalemia secondary to an adrenal adenoma
- Hypokalemia must be corrected prior to surgery

Efficacy
Removal of the adenoma will resolve the hypokalemia.

Risks/Benefits
Risks:
- Those of any surgical procedure requiring a general anesthetic
- Advanced age and concomitant disease can cause complications

Benefit: complete resolution of hypokalemia if this is the only cause of hypokalemia

Evidence
Two small, retrospective studies have shown that patients with hypokalemia in association with an aldosterone-producing adrenal adenoma become normokalemic following adrenalectomy [4,5]
Level S

Acceptability to patient
- Surgery may not be acceptable to all patients
- Need to weigh benefits against risks for each individual

Follow up plan
Will still need to monitor serum potassium regularly, especially in the presence of concomitant adrenal hyperplasia.

Patient and caregiver information
- Will need to provide specific information, such as what surgery involves, the expected recovery time, and the likely outcome
- Full informed consent is required prior to surgery

LIFESTYLE

Ensure adequate dietary intake of potassium-rich foods including bananas, tomatoes, and peaches.

RISKS/BENEFITS

Risks:

- Diet alone is unlikely to be sufficient in all but the mildest cases
- Condition may worsen if too great a reliance is placed on lifestyle factors

Benefit: may avoid or reduce the need for potassium supplements in patients with mild hypokalemia

ACCEPTABILITY TO PATIENT

Generally well tolerated and acceptable.

FOLLOW UP PLAN

- Need to monitor serum potassium regularly
- Drug therapy may be needed if the patient does not repond or if the condition worsens

PATIENT AND CAREGIVER INFORMATION

- Potassium is present in many common foods
- A balanced diet should be sufficient to prevent hypokalemia unless there are other underlying causes
- A list of potassium-rich foods, including bananas, tomatoes, and peaches

EFFICACY OF THERAPIES

- Drug treatment, both oral and intravenous, will lead to resolution of the problem within 24–72h
- Surgery for hyperaldosteronism caused by an adrenal adenoma will resolve hypokalemia

Evidence

- PDxMD is unable to cite evidence meeting its criteria for evidence for most treatments of hypokalemia
- The efficacy of oral and intravenous potassium supplements is easily demonstrated by simple monitoring of serum potassium levels after treatment is initiated
- There is some evidence that triamterene and amiloride are effective in maintaining potassium levels in patients with thiazide-induced hypokalemia [3] *Level P*

Review period

12 months.

PROGNOSIS

- Most cases of hypokalemia will resolve soon after commencing treatment
- Recurrences are common depending on the cause of the hypokalemia

Therapeutic failure

- Failure of oral therapy suggests noncompliance, possible misdiagnosis, worsening of an underlying cause, or interaction with concomitant medication
- Poor compliance may be resolved by changing to alternative preparation
- Refer to a specialist for further investigations if the patient is refractory to treatment

Recurrence

- Recurrence is unlikely if drug therapy is continued
- Serum potassium needs to be monitored regularly

Deterioration

- If oral and/or intravenous potassium supplements are ineffective within 3–4 days and hypokalemia persists, then check serum magnesium
- If the patient develops cardiac arrhythmia or paralysis, immediate hospital admission is indicated for intravenous therapy

COMPLICATIONS

- Hyperkalemia – can result from replacement therapy particularly when using potassium-sparing diuretics
- Hyperkalemia can be avoided with careful monitoring and following recommended dosage regimens
- Intravenous potassium replacement can lead to cardiac arrhythmias
- Intravenous potassium administration can lead to phlebitis

CONSIDER CONSULT

- If a new cause for the hypokalemia is discovered that requires the intervention of a specialist (e.g. surgery for adrenal adenoma)

PREVENTION

Prevention of hypokalemia is based on identifying at-risk individuals and reducing their risks or providing prophylactic therapy and monitoring.

RISK FACTORS

- **Drugs:** Prescribed, over-the-counter, and herbal/homeopathic medications are associated with hypokalemia
- **Alcohol:** Excessive alcohol can be associated with hypokalemia owing to a number of mechanisms
- **Eating disorders:** Particularly where self-induced vomiting is a feature
- **Coexisting disease:** Either directly or through drug treatment (e.g. for diabetes, hypertension)
- **Genetics:** Patients with a family history of hypokalemic periodic paralysis
- **Diet:** Can be potassium-deficient or high in foodstuffs such as licorice

MODIFY RISK FACTORS

Identify patients at risk of developing hypokalemia as a result of:

- Concurrent medication
- Concurrent disease
- Genetic disease

Lifestyle and wellness

ALCOHOL AND DRUGS

Consume alcohol in moderation only.

DIET

- Advise regarding potassium-rich diet
- In patients with eating disorders discourage self-induced vomiting and, if necessary, refer for further management
- Discourage eating large quantities of licorice

FAMILY HISTORY

Identify individuals with a family history of hypokalemia including:

- Familial (hypokalemic) periodic paralysis
- Congenital adrenogenital syndromes
- Liddle's syndrome
- Bartter's syndrome
- Familial interstitial nephritis
- Glucocorticoid-remediable aldosteronism

DRUG HISTORY
- Discontinue, adjust doses, or replace drugs where possible
- Discourage the use of over-the-counter, herbal, or homeopathic medications

CHEMOPROPHYLAXIS
If diuretics are essential, consider giving prophylactic potassium supplements or using a potassium-sparing diuretic.

Cost/efficacy
Generally highly effective in preventing hypokalemia for little extra cost.

SCREENING
- Regular monitoring of serum potassium levels in patients known to be at-risk including patients taking diuretics
- Monitoring promotes early identification and treatment of hypokalemia

PREVENT RECURRENCE
- Monitor regularly and use oral potassium supplements in patients at-risk, including those on diuretics
- Compliance with medication and advice should be optimal to prevent recurrence

Reassess coexisting disease
- Altering coexisting medication may precipitate a recurrence (e.g. if a potassium-sparing diuretic is replaced by a thiazide or loop diuretic)
- Reassess when resuming treatment with medication known to cause hypokalemia

INTERACTION ALERT
- Thiazide and loop diuretics
- Penicillin antibiotics
- Aminoglycosides
- Amphotericin B
- Beta-2 agonists
- Theophylline
- Laxatives
- Steroids

RESOURCES

ASSOCIATIONS

National Council on Potassium in Clinical Practice
Dr Jay N Cohn MD
Cardiovascular Division
MMC508
University of Minnesota
420 Delaware St SE
Minneapolis
MN 55455

KEY REFERENCES

- Allon M. Disorders of potassium metabolism. In: Primer on renal diseases, 2nd edn. New York: Academic press, 1998
- Cohn et al. New guidelines for potassium replacement in clinical practice: a contemporary review by the National Council on potassium in clinical practice. Arch Intern Med 2000;160:2429–2436
- Fulop M. Algorithms for diagnosing some electrolyte disorders. Am J Emerg Med 1998;16:76–84
- Mandal AK. Hypokalemia and hyperkalemia. Med Clin North Am 1997,81:611–639

Evidence References

1 Allon M. Disorders of potassium metabolism. In Greenberg A, ed. Primer on Renal Diseases, 2nd edn. New York: Academic Press, 1998

2 Cohn JN, Kowey PR, Whelton PK, Prisant LM. New guidelines for potassium replacement in clinical practice: a contemporary review by the National Council on Potassium in Clinical Practice. Arch Intern Med 2000;160:2429–2436. Medline

3 Kohvakka, A. Maintenance of potassium balance during long-term diuretic therapy in chronic heart failure patients with thiazide-induced hypokalemia: comparison of potassium supplementation with potassium chloride and potassium-sparing agents, amiloride and triamterene. Int J Clin Pharmacol Ther Toxicol 1988;26:273–7. Medline

4 Quarmby CJ, Burch VC, Dent DM, Opie LH. Conn's syndrome due to adrenocortical adenoma – a rare but rewarding cause of curable hypertension. S Afr Med J 1995;85:1353–6

5 Lo CY, Tam PC, Kung AW, Lam KS, Wong J. Primary aldosteronism. Results of surgical treatment. Ann Surg 1996;224:125–30. Medline

CONTRIBUTORS

Gordon H Baustian, MD
Martin Goldberg, MD, FACP
David W Toth, MD

HYPONATREMIA

DESCRIPTION

Hyponatremia is defined as a sodium concentration in the plasma (or serum) of less than 135mEq/L (135mmol/L). It is the result of an accumulation of total body water greater than the body's accumulation of electrolytes (sodium + potassium). Classification is traditionally according to volume status:

- Hypovolemic hyponatremia (sodium depletion in excess of water depletion)
- Euvolemic hyponatremia (normal body sodium with increase in total body water)
- Hypervolemic hyponatremia (increase in total body sodium with greater increase in total body water)

But hyponatremia must also be evaluated with regard to changes in body fluid tonicity (effective osmolality), since signs and symptoms are directly caused by hypotonicity. Thus, at any volume status, hyponatremia must be further subclassified into:

- Hypotonic hyponatremia
- Isotonic hyponatremia
- Hypertonic hyponatremia

Consequently, clinical features of hyponatremia occur with hypotonic hyponatremia, mainly due to cell swelling and disturbances in the function of the central nervous and cardiovascular systems.

URGENT ACTION

Consider urgent referral for inhospital stabilization in patients with acute hypotonic hyponatremia and:

- Plasma sodium concentrations of less than 120mEq/L (120mmol/L) (high risk of seizures, coma, respiratory arrest)
- Existing severe and/or rapidly developing central nervous system signs (confusion, hyperactive or pathologic deep tendon reflexes, seizures, cranial nerve palsies), regardless of plasma levels

BACKGROUND

ICD9 CODE
276.1 Hyponatremia.

CARDINAL FEATURES
- Hyponatremia is generally due to excessive accumulation of total body water relative to body sodium content
- Hyponatremia can occur with low body sodium (hypovolemic), normal body sodium (euvolemic), or high body sodium (hypervolemic) content
- Signs and symptoms are related to hypotonicity (low effective osmolality), which produces cell swelling, particularly in the brain. Signs and symptoms include headache, nausea, vomiting, confusion, and seizures
- Only hypotonic hyponatremia is of clinical significance regarding the necessity for treatment and its urgency
- Chronic hypotonic hyponatremia with gradual development results in adaptation with minimal or late symptomatology
- Acute hypotonic hyponatremia with rapid fall in plasma sodium concentration is typically associated with symptoms and signs

CAUSES
Common causes
- Sampling error (either laboratory error, or blood was drawn through a heparin lock and was diluted)
- Isotonic or hypertonic hyponatremia: excess of other osmotically active substances in plasma (e.g. glucose or mannitol). In this situation there are no signs or symptoms directly related to hyponatremia because hypotonicity is not present. Serum sodium will rise when the nonsodium solutes are removed from the extracellular fluid by excretion or metabolism. Therapy for the hyponatremia per se is not indicated
- Factitious (pseudo-) hyponatremia: in this situation the laboratory has provided an erroneous value for plasma sodium because large amounts of lipid or protein occupy a high fraction of the plasma volume. This is a less common problem now since most laboratories measure sodium with ion-selective electrodes
- Severe hyperlipidemia
- Severe paraproteinemia

Common causes of hypotonic hyponatremia:
Cardiovascular:
- Congestive heart failure (advanced stages; hypervolemic)

Respiratory:
- Cystic fibrosis (hypovolemic; also see SIADH)

Renal:
- Salt-losing renal disease (hypovolemic; usually diseases of the renal medulla – interstitial nephritis, obstructive nephropathy)
- Acute renal failure (hypervolemic)
- Chronic renal failure (hypervolemic)
- Nephrotic syndrome (hypervolemic)

Gastrointestinal:
- Severe diarrhea and vomiting (hypovolemic)
- Liver cirrhosis (hypervolemic)
- Acute abdomen (hypovolemic; due to sequestration into third space – peritonitis, pancreatitis, bowel obstruction)
- Gastric suction (hypovolemic)
- Protein-losing enteropathy (hypovolemic; rare)

Endocrine:
- Syndrome of inappropriate antidiuretic hormone secretion (SIADH) (euvolemic), including carcinomas (particularly bronchogenic and pancreatic, but SIADH has been reported with many other solid tumors and hematologic malignancies), pulmonary disorders (bacterial, viral and fungal pneumonias; lung abscess; active tuberculosis and many other less common disorders), and central nervous system disorders (encephalitis and meningitis (all etiologies); head trauma; brain abscess; strokes; schizophrenia and almost any disease that causes diffuse anatomic, physiological, or metabolic abnormalities of the brain)
- Hypothyroidism (euvolemic or hypovolemic)
- Addison's disease (hypovolemic)
- Glucocorticoid insufficiency (euvolemic; sudden withdrawal of therapeutic glucocorticoids, hypopituitarism)

Infectious diseases:
- AIDS (multifactorial causes)

Iatrogenic:
- Repeated tap of serous cavities (hypovolemic; ascites, pleural effusions)
- Prolonged nasogastric suction

Drugs (this list is not exhaustive – always check all patient medication):
- Diuretics (hypovolemic; particularly thiazide diuretics, less commonly loop diuretics)

Drugs causing euvolemic hyponatremia resembling SIADH:
- Carbamazepine
- Narcotics
- Barbiturates
- Vincristine
- Desmopressin
- Clofibrate
- Cyclophosphamide
- Chlorpropramide
- Ecstasy

Neurological and psychiatric:
- Stress (euvolemic; trauma, pain + high fluid intake – the elderly are more susceptible)
- Psychogenic polydipsia (euvolemic; hyponatremia is rare in the presence of normal kidney function except when subject is ingesting a low-protein, low-sodium diet)
- Neuropsychiatric disorders (euvolemic; particularly schizophrenia; see also under SIADH)

Environmental:
- Excessive sweating (hypovolemic)

Pediatric:
- Prematurity (euvolemic)
- Oral rehydration with tap water (hypovolemic, e.g. in gastroenteritis)
- And others listed above

Contributory or predisposing factors
- Extremes of age
- Debilitating disease
- Malnutrition
- Alcoholism
- Pulmonary disease
- Central nervous system disorders (infectious, vascular, metabolic, traumatic)
- Carcinomas and other malignancies

EPIDEMIOLOGY
Incidence and prevalence
In hospitalized adults (with a serum sodium concentration <130mEq/L):
- Incidence is 0.97%
- Prevalence is 2.48%

see: Anderson RJ. Hospital-associated hyponatremia. Kidney Int 1986;29:1237

FREQUENCY
- More common in hospitalized patients
- An estimated 7% of healthy elderly have serum sodium concentrations of 137mEq/L (137mmol/L) or less, rising to 15% of elderly in chronic care facilities

DIFFERENTIAL DIAGNOSIS
Hypovolemic hypotonic hyponatremia
FEATURES
- Characterized by volume loss due to underlying disorder
- Causes include nonrenal loss of electrolyte-containing fluid (diuretics, severe diarrhea and vomiting, third space losses in acute abdomen, excessive sweating), salt-losing renal diseases (interstitial nephritis, obstructive nephropathy) and mineralocorticoid deficiencies, including Addison's disease (characterized by hyperpigmentation, nausea/vomiting, fatigability, hypotension, anorexia/weight loss, and hypoglycemia)

Euvolemic hypotonic hyponatremia
FEATURES
- Very common; most hyponatremic states that cause differential diagnostic problems fall into this category
- Characterized by clinically normal volume status (total body water is usually slightly elevated, which may cause subtle clinical signs of fluid overload; however, frank edema is not a feature)
- Causes include SIADH, drugs, hypothyroidism, glucocorticoid insufficiency, polydipsia in patients on starvation diets

Hypervolemic hypotonic hyponatremia
FEATURES
- Characterized by clinical fluid overload with edema; hypotonic hyponatremia occurs in advanced stages of the underlying disorder
- Causes include congestive cardiac failure, liver cirrhosis with ascites, nephrotic syndrome, protein-losing enteropathy
- In the above conditions, hyponatremia is a marker indicating a poor prognosis for the primary cardiac, hepatic, or renal disease. This prognosis is not directly attributable to the hyponatremia

SIGNS & SYMPTOMS
Signs
Important: clinical manifestations of hypotonic hyponatremia depend mainly on the rate of fall in plasma sodium concentration and, to a lesser extent, the absolute level of the hypotonicity. This is because, in chronic hypotonic hyponatremia, the cells of the brain slowly adapt by inactivating osmotically active substances to protect against cell swelling. Thus, patients with chronic hypotonic hyponatremia often have minimal manifestations of hypotonicity even when serum sodium level is as low as 120mEq/L (sometimes much lower), whereas patients with acute hypotonic hyponatremia may exhibit major signs and symptoms at higher levels of hypotonicity and serum sodium levels.

Hypotonic hyponatremia with values above 120mEq/L (120mmol/L) is often asymptomatic, unless acute. Physical signs are caused by increases in cell volume due to osmotic forces. Effects are seen in the central nervous system and the cardiovascular system and often overlay signs of underlying disease.

Central nervous system signs:
- Signs are dependent on degree of cerebral edema, which is more marked in acute hyponatremia. In chronic hyponatremia, signs are usually mild to absent until serum sodium concentration is <120mEq/L
- Mild hypotonic hyponatremia: patients typically have no specific signs; if decrease in serum sodium is acute, patients may manifest impairment of mentation, subtle reflex abnormalities

- Moderate hypotonic hyponatremia: chronic hypotonic hyponatremia may show no signs; if hyponatremia is acute, there may be signs of raised intracranial pressure (headache, vomiting), cranial nerve palsies
- Severe hypotonic hyponatremia: if hyponatremia is acute, there may be seizures, coma, respiratory arrest. In chronic severe hypotonic hyponatremia, the above manifestations are variably present

Cardiovascular signs:
- Hypovolemic hypotonic hyponatremia: volume depletion causes orthostatic hypotension, tachycardia, poor skin turgor
- Hypervolemic hypotonic hyponatremia: manifestations of underlying edematous disorder
- Euvolemic hypotonic hyponatremia: no specific cardiovascular signs

Symptoms
Symptoms are nonspecific, related to changes in total body water and its effects on the cardiovascular and central nervous systems. They are frequently difficult to distinguish from those caused by the underlying disease. Symptoms are also dependent on the time it took to become hyponatremic (e.g. more acute being more severe, subacute or chronic being less severe, or even absent).
- Anorexia
- Agitation, confusion, headaches, dizziness
- Lethargy
- Nausea and vomiting
- Muscle cramps
- Neurological deficits

CONSIDER CONSULT
Although laboratory values are important, clinical state and speed of change in the patient's condition should guide decision to refer.
- All patients with recent development of hypotonic hyponatremia (serum sodium <130mEq/L) without symptoms should be referred to a specialist in the outpatient setting to help with diagnostic evaluation and management
- Consider urgent referral for inhospital consultation, management, and stabilization in patients with hypotonic hyponatremia and: newly discovered plasma sodium <120mEq/L (<120mmol/) (risk of seizures and coma high); severe existing and/or rapidly progressive central nervous system signs, regardless of plasma level; acute onset of hypotonic hyponatremia with decrease in plasma sodium 10mEq/L or more; postoperative development of hypotonic hyponatremia in menstruating women, who represent a higher risk in terms of potential morbidity and mortality

There is a hyponatremia admission proforma available from the American Association for Family Physicians.

INVESTIGATION OF THE PATIENT
Direct questions to patient
Even when the cause is obvious (e.g. severe diarrhea and vomiting), a full history is mandatory to elicit possible contributing factors.

Q **Do you take any medications?** Check all drugs for possible side-effects on water balance and inquire about illicit drug use (opiates and barbiturates).

Q **Are you drinking more than usual?** Psychogenic polydipsia may go unnoticed in confused or elderly. Increased thirst may point to recent onset of diabetes.

Q **Are you passing more (or less) urine recently?**

Q **Do you get breathless?**

Q **Can you lie flat?**

Q Do your ankles swell up?
Q Do you get dizzy spells?
Q Do you feel more lethargic recently? Acute hypotonic hyponatremia, hypothyroidism,
   Addison's disease.
Q Do you get muscle cramps?
Q How much do you smoke (and for how long)?
Q Have you lost weight recently?
Q How is your appetite?
Q Have you had any stomach pains recently?
Q Do you have a cough (productive or nonproductive)? Could suggest pneumonia, COPD,
   congestive heart failure.

The most common causes of a new presentation of SIADH in primary care practice and which
may not be immediately obvious are drugs, bronchogenic carcinoma, carcinoma of the pancreas,
and cerebral vascular disease.

Examination
Due to the multiple causes of hyponatremia and the interrelation of signs caused by hypotonic
hyponatremia and underlying disease, full clinical examination is mandatory, both for diagnosis
and to monitor therapy.

- Assess for hypovolemia (reduced skin turgor, lying/standing blood pressure and pulse,
  lowered jugular venous pressure, absence of axillary sweat) and hypervolemia (raised jugular
  venous pressure, pitting edema, pulmonary edema)
- Assess fluid intake/output and total body water balance
- Full neurological examination (assessment of mental state, reflexes, muscle weaknesses,
  cranial nerve abnormalities, gross and fine motor co-ordination). This is required to assess
  central nervous system symptoms that may be caused by the changes in total body water
  associated with the hyponatremia or by the underlying disease
- Look for signs of hypothyroidism (coarse features, dry skin, weight gain, goiter)
- Look for signs of Addison's disease (typical pigmentation, orthostatic hypotension)
- Examine for evidence of lymph node metastases. To assess possible SIADH due to
  malignancy
- Examine for abdominal mass and scleral jaundice
- Examine for signs of ascites (fluid wave, shifting dullness)

Summary of investigative tests
- Blood biochemistry, including serum electrolytes, glucose, creatinine, and blood urea nitrogen
  are important in monitoring overall fluid balance, identifying possible hyperglycemia and may
  help identify possible renal causes
- Plasma and urine osmolality can help determine differential diagnosis if the underlying cause is
  not evident
- Urine sodium concentration is useful in distinguishing renal from extrarenal sodium losses

DIAGNOSTIC DECISION
- Signs and symptoms which may indicate hyponatremia include headache, nausea, vomiting,
  confusion, and seizures
- Diagnosis requires measurement of the plasma sodium level. Sodium concentration of less
  than 135mEq/L (135mmol/L) defines hyponatremia
- Assessment of hydration status and measurement of urine osmolality, serum osmolality or
  tonicity, and urine sodium will help determine the cause of hyponatremia

Guidelines
The American Academy of Family Physicians has published diagnostic information on
hyponatremia [1]

CLINICAL PEARLS

- Assessing tonicity (effective osmolality) using serum sodium concentration and blood glucose level is more helpful diagnostically than a measured serum osmolality in most cases
- Most common cause of glucocorticoid insufficiency with hyponatremia is rapid tapering of glucocorticoids (e.g. prednisone) when used in the treatment of chronic conditions such as asthma, rheumatoid arthritis, and nephrotic syndrome
- Euvolemic hypotonic hyponatremia is common postoperatively, and is related to the stimulation of ADH secretion by the trauma of surgery and to the administration of general anesthetics and various analgesic and sedative medications. Particularly at risk in this setting are menstruating women and frail elderly patients

THE TESTS
Body fluids
BLOOD BIOCHEMISTRY
Description
Cuffed venous sample in heparinized container.
- Serum electrolytes
- Glucose
- Creatinine
- Urea nitrogen

Advantages/Disadvantages
Advantages:
- Simple and reliable test, giving information on renal function and concomitant status of electrolytes
- Also indicates presence of hyperglycemia

Normal
Laboratory dependent.

Cause of abnormal result
- Dependent on the underlying disease process
- The blood urea nitrogen to creatinine ratio may be greater than 20 in prerenal volume depletion states
- Serum bicarbonate may be elevated in volume depletion
- Serum chloride may be lowered in disorders of sodium depletion
- Serum glucose may be elevated

SERUM AND PLASMA OSMOLALITY
Description
Cuffed venous sample and midstream urine.

Advantages/Disadvantages
- Advantage: simple and reliable tests, most useful in the diagnosis of SIADH

Normal
- Serum plasma osmolality: 285–295mOsmol/kg
- Urine osmolality: 50–1400mOsmol/kg; evaluating normality requires evaluation of state of hydration

Cause of abnormal result
- Serum osmolality is normal in factitious hyponatremia and in isotonic hyponatremia (e.g. in the presence of hyperglycemia)
- Serum osmolality is elevated in hypertonic hyponatremia

- Serum osmolality is low in all other states of hyponatremia (i.e. hypotonic hyponatremia)
- Urine osmolality is greater than 150mOsmol/kg (i.e. inappropriately concentrated) in hypotonic hyponatremia with SIADH

URINE SODIUM CONCENTRATION
Description
Midstream urine sample.

Advantages/Disadvantages
- Advantage: simple and often diagnostically helpful

Cause of abnormal result
- Urine sodium less than 20mEq/L (in the presence of hypotonic hyponatremia) is indicative of extrarenal losses of sodium (e.g. diarrhea, vomiting, burns)
- Urine sodium greater than 40mEq/L (in the presence of hypotonic hyponatremia) is indicative of pathologic renal sodium loss (diuretics, aldosterone deficiency) if the patient is hypovolemic, but if the patient is euvolemic, it is compatible with SIADH

TREATMENT

CONSIDER CONSULT
Patients should be referred if:
- They develop central nervous symptoms and signs despite treatment
- There is uncertainty over diagnosis of underlying disease

IMMEDIATE ACTION
- Severe hypovolemic hypotonic hyponatremia with predominantly hemodynamic manifestations (hypotension, tachycardia, azotemia) due to excessive fluid loss should be treated with infusion of normal saline (0.9%) titrated against blood pressure and urine output
- Seizures should be managed according to standard seizure protocols
- If severe hypotonic hyponatremia is associated with coma or status epilepticus, consider infusion of hypertonic (3%) saline (250mL at a rate of 1–2mL/kg/h). If volume overload is a risk, a loop diuretic can be added. The aim is to raise plasma sodium concentration by no more than 1mEq/L/h and not more than 12mEq/L/day. But beware: too rapid correction of hyponatremia causes abrupt fluid shifts, which may lead to worsening of cerebral edema and central pontine myelinolysis (a progressive demyelination appearing several days after treatment, characterized by spastic quadriparesis, bulbar palsy, and mutism). Treatment with hypertonic saline generally requires a critical care hospital setting; it should not be undertaken unless infusion rate can be strictly controlled and hourly monitoring of plasma sodium is available (or will be after transport to hospital)

MANAGEMENT ISSUES
Goals
- Avoid deterioration of central nervous symptoms due to overzealous correction
- Asymptomatic patient
- Plasma sodium levels above 125mEq/L (125mmol/L)
- Identification and correction of underlying disorder and/or removal of offending drugs

Management in special circumstances
COEXISTING DISEASE
- Correct hypothyroidism or glucocorticoid insufficiency, if present
- Treat congestive heart failure and cirrhosis, if the underlying causes
- Treat oncologic, pulmonary, or central nervous system causes of SIADH if possible
- Discontinue, if possible, all potentially causative drugs

SPECIAL PATIENT GROUPS
SIADH may not respond adequately to fluid restriction alone, or severe fluid restriction may not be acceptable to patient. In these circumstances, consider demeclocycline (600–1200mg/day) unless contraindicated (liver disease and renal failure). This causes a nephrogenic diabetes insipidus that will cause the kidneys to lose more free water. This drug should probably be reserved for use only in patients with signs/symptoms of hypotonicity. It would be prudent to consult a specialist or one who is familiar with outcomes of this treatment before undertaking this.

SUMMARY OF THERAPEUTIC OPTIONS
Choices
- First choice: fluid restriction in asymptomatic, symptomatic or mildly symptomatic patients with euvolemic or hypervolemic hypotonic hyponatremia. In euvolemic hyponatremia, restrict fluid to less than 1L/day; in hypervolemic hyponatremia: restrict both fluid and sodium. Monitor body weight, fluid intake/output, and serum electrolytes while doing this

- Second choice: in patients where fluid restriction is not sufficient or not acceptable to patient, and patient manifests symptoms and/or signs of hypotonicity, consider demeclocycline in a dose of 600–1200mg/day. Demeclocycline is contraindicated in patients with liver or renal failure and may cause photosensitivity, nausea, and azotemia. Since this drug, in effect, causes nephrogenic diabetes insipidus, one should consult a specialist or someone who is familiar with this treatment modality before undertaking this

Also:
- Treat mineralocorticoid deficiency, if present. In such patients, fludrocortisone can be used to replace mineralocorticoids
- Review all medication and adjust if possible (e.g. exchange thiazide diuretic for loop diuretic)
- Treat underlying disorder. In hypovolemic hyponatremia, treatment of the underlying disorder with intravenous normal saline (0.9%) usually will correct hyponatremia

Guidelines
The American Academy of Family Physicans has published information on hyponatremia [1]

Never
- When correcting hypotonic hyponatremia of any cause, never raise serum sodium more than 1mEq/L/h and never more than 12mEq/L/day
- The above applies especially to the use of hypertonic saline infusions, which should only be used for patients with acute, symptomatic hypotonic hyponatremia in a critical care setting

FOLLOW UP
- In asymptomatic or mildly symptomatic hyponatremia treated conservatively, check sodium levels after a few days
- When treatment with intravenous normal saline is required, check levels frequently according to clinical response of underlying condition

DRUGS AND OTHER THERAPIES: DETAILS
Drugs
DEMECLOCYCLINE
Dose
600–1200mg/day.

Efficacy
Demeclocycline acts by inhibiting the action of ADH on the kidney, thus enhancing the excretion of free water. In the above dose range, this drug was shown, in a group of patients with hypotonic hyponatremia due to SIADH, to restore serum sodium levels to normal in 5–14 days, permitting liberalization of water intake.

Risks/Benefits
Risks:
- Use caution in renal and hepatic impairment
- Photosensitivty reactions are common
- Reversible nephrogenic diabetes insipidus has been reported
- Do not use out of date democlocyline

Benefits:
- Correction of the hyponatremia
- Since side-effects and adverse reactions are finite (see below), the risk/benefit ratio is favorable primarily in patients with symptomatic and/or severe chronic hypotonic hyponatremia without hepatic or renal disease

Side-effects and adverse reactions
- Cardiovascular system: pericarditis
- Central nervous system: pseudotumor cerebri, paresthesias
- Eyes, eyes, nose, and throat: tooth discoloration, enamel hypoplasia
- Gastrointestinal: nausea, vomiting, diarrhea, anorexia, dysphagia, esophageal irritation, hepatotoxicity, pancreatitis, pseudomembranous colitis
- Genitourinary: nephrotoxicity, nephrogenic diabetes insipidus, polyuria, polydipsia
- Hematologic: blood dyscrasias
- Skin: photosensitivity, rash, pruritus, urticaria, exfoliative dermatitis

Interactions (other drugs)
- ACE inhibitors ▪ Angiotensin II antagonists ▪ Antacids ▪ Anticoagulants ▪ Barbiturates ▪ Bismuth ▪ Carbamazepine ▪ Cephalosporins ▪ Cholestyramine ▪ Colestipol ▪ Desmopressin ▪ Digoxin ▪ Food ▪ Iron ▪ Methoxyflurane ▪ Oral contraceptives ▪ Penicillins ▪ Phenytoin ▪ Sodium bicarbonate ▪ Vitamin A ▪ Warfarin ▪ Zinc

Contraindications
- Breast-feeding ▪ Avoid use in children under 8 years ▪ Severe renal impairment ▪ Pregnancy

Evidence
A prospective trial of only 10 patients (no control group) examined the efficacy of demeclocycline and lithium in patients with SIADH, who remained hyponatremic after water restriction. Sodium levels returned to normal within 5–14 days for patients treated with demeclocycline, allowing unrestricted water intake. Three patients were treated with lithium, which did not alter sodium levels, and adverse effects were noted [2] *This study does not meet the criteria for category P*

Acceptability to patient
Generally well tolerated.

Follow up plan
Monitor serum electrolyte and volume status at regular intervals, according to progress and activity of underlying disease.

FLUDROCORTISONE
Dose
Usual dose is 0.05–0.15mg/day.

Risks/Benefits
Risks:
- Use extreme caution in cardiac disease, congestive heart failure, hypertension, recent MI, and in renal disease
- Use caution in children and the elderly, in patients with psychosis, seizure disorders or myasthenia gravis
- Use caution in ulcerative colitis, peptic ulcer, or esophagitis
- Use caution in trauma, severe illness, or surgery
- Do not withdraw abruptly

Benefits:
- Risk/benefit ratio is favorable when this drug is used as an effective mineralocorticoid in adrenal insufficiency
- This drug has no benefit in other causes of hyponatremia

Side-effects and adverse reactions
- Cardiovascular system: hypertension, edema, CHF, ECG changes
- Central nervous system: dizziness, headache
- Gastrointestinal: nausea, vomiting, anorexia
- Metabolic: fluid imbalance, hypokalemia, metabolic alkalosis, hypernatremia
- Musculoskeletal: cramps, weakness
- Skin: bruising, sweating, hives, rash

Interactions (other drugs)
- Amphotericin B ▪ Androgens ▪ Barbiturates ▪ Cardiac glycosides ▪ Diuretics (loop and thiazide) ▪ Dofeltilide ▪ Nondepolarising neuromuscular blockers ▪ NSAIDs ▪ Phenytoin ▪ Rifampin

Contraindications
- Systemic fungal infections ▪ Avoid in pregnancy and breast–feeding

Follow up plan
Should have serum electrolytes and blood pressure monitored regularly.

Patient and caregiver information
- Do not abruptly discontinue medication
- Report any dizziness, headache, edema

EFFICACY OF THERAPIES

Asymptomatic or mildly symptomatic hyponatremia usually responds to conservative measures within days.

Evidence

PDxMD are unable to cite evidence which meets our criteria for evidence.

Although there are no published controlled studies on the efficacy of fluid restriction in the treatment and prevention of hyponatremia, there is a wealth of time-honored clinical experience, numerous clinical publications, and firm physiological principles supporting the use of this treatment to produce negative free water balance and correction of hyponatremia.

PROGNOSIS

Excellent for asymptomatic and mildly symptomatic disease. However, mortality in patients with severe central nervous systems can be as high as 80%.

Clinical pearls

Prognosis for ultimate patient survival is poor with hypervolemic hypotonic hyponatremia, but this is primarily because of the severity and irreversibility of the underlying cardiac, hepatic, or renal disease rather than the hyponatremia per se.

PREVENTION

Hyponatremia is not specifically preventable in the general population.

KEY REFERENCES

▣ Berl T, Robertson GL. Pathophysiology of water metabolism. In: Brenner BM, ed. The kidney, 6th edn. Philadelphia: WB Saunders, 2000

▣ Fried LF, Palevsky PM. Hyponatremia and hypernatremia. Med Clin North Am 1997;3:585–609

▣ Goldberg M, Hyponatremia. Med Clin North Am 1981;65:251–69

▣ Halterman R, Berl T. Therapy of dysnatremic disorders. In: Brady H, Wilcox C, eds. Therapy in nephrology and hypertension. Philadelphia: WB Saunders, 1999

▣ Kugler JP, Hustead T. Hyponatremia and hypernatremia in the elderly. Am Fam Physician 2000;12:3623–30

▣ Martinez FJ, Lash RW. Endocrinologic and metabolic complications in the intensive care unit. Clin Chest Med 1999;2:401–21

▣ Verbalis JG. Hyponatremia and hypoosmolar disorders. In: Greenberg A, ed. Primer on kidney diseases, 2nd edn. New York: Academic Press, 1998

Evidence and guidelines

1 The American Academy of Family Physicans has published information on hyponatremia. Kugler JP, Hunstead T. Hyponatremia and hypernatremia in the elderly. Am Fam Physician 2000;15;61(12):3623–30

2 Forrest JN, Cox M, Hong C, et al. Superiority of demeclocycline over lithium in the treatment of chronic syndrome of inappropriate secretion of antidiuretic hormone. N Eng J Med 1978;298:173–7. Medline

FAQS

Question 1

How does one treat diabetic patients who develop hyponatremia in association with an elevated blood glucose level?

ANSWER 1

In this situation the decrease in serum sodium is due to the movement of water from cells due to the osmotic effects of the elevated glucose in the extracellular fluid. The patient has isotonic or hypertonic hyponatremia. Since hypotonicity is not present, no specific treatment of the hyponatremia is indicated. When the hyperglycemia is corrected with appropriate treatment, the serum sodium will automatically increase.

Question 2

In the treatment of euvolemic hypotonic hyponatremia due to SIADH, why doesn't the administration of isotonic saline infusions effectively correct the hyponatremia?

ANSWER 2

This is because these patients are euvolemic or slightly hypervolemic. Therefore any therapy which provides volume expansion such as saline produces a rapid increase in renal sodium excretion, thereby preventing correction of the hyponatremia. That is why fluid restriction is the key to correcting the hyponatremia in patients with chronic euvolemic or hypervolemic hyponatremia.

Question 3

Are there any new drugs being developed which are effective in reversing the effects of antidiuretic hormone, which appears to be important in causing and maintaining hyponatremia in the euvolemic and hypervolemic types?

ANSWER 3

It is true that ADH plays a major role in perpetuating hyponatremia due to water retention in these patients. There is currently under investigation in several research laboratories a new class of agents known as vasopressin V2 receptor antagonists. Studies have already shown that these drugs are effective orally and can antagonize ADH in patients with SIADH, congestive heart failure, and hepatic cirrhosis, thereby increasing excretion of free water. They are not ready for commercial release, but their future potential as therapeutic agents in certain patients with chronic hyponatremia is exciting.

CONTRIBUTORS

Fred F Ferri, MD, FACP
Martin Goldberg, MD, FACP
David W Toth, MD

HYPOSPADIAS

DESCRIPTION

- A congenital defect of the penis
- The anterior urethra is incompletely developed, and the meatus is proximal and ventral to its normal location
- As the urethral meatus moves proximally, there is an increased chance of chordee – a curvature of the penis during erection that is secondary to shortening of its ventral side

URGENT ACTION

Because the prepuce or foreskin is sometimes used when hypospadias is repaired, it is important that the child not be circumcised.

KEY! DON'T MISS!

- Hypospadias is usually evident when the external genitalia are inspected during a routine newborn nursery admission examination
- Do not circumcise a baby with hypospadias

ICD9 CODE
752.61 Hypospadias

CARDINAL FEATURES
- The urethral meatus may be visible on the inferior or ventral surface of the glans penis, in the balanopenile furrow, or anywhere along the penile shaft
- Less commonly, the meatus is at the base of the penile shaft in front of the scrotum, on the scrotum itself, or even behind the scrotum or behind the genital swellings
- Skin distal to the meatus usually has a V-shaped defect that has been called the urethral delta. The edges of the delta merge into the divided prepuce

CAUSES
Common causes
The cause of hypospadias is unknown.

Contributory or predisposing factors
- Deficiencies of fetal testosterone or dihydrotestosterone may play a role in the etiology of hypospadias, especially if the testes are fully descended
- Some investigators believe that the disorder is caused by abnormal stimulation of the fetus by maternal human chorionic gonadotropin
- On occasion, a leak of amniotic fluid causes a fetal foot to compress the perineum. It has been suggested that hypospadias may arise from this mechanism, especially when there are other perineal defects
- Maternal oral contraceptive use has not been shown to be associated with hypospadias

EPIDEMIOLOGY
Demographics
AGE

Hypospadias is a congenital disorder that is present at birth.

GENDER

Males only.

RACE

More common in Caucasians than in African-Americans.

GENETICS
- The disorder is 8.5 times more common in monozygotic twins
- 8% of hypospadias patients have fathers who also had hypospadias
- Approximately one in eight male (14%) siblings of hypospadias patients also have hypospadias

SIGNS & SYMPTOMS
Signs
Hypospadias is classified according to the location of the ectopic urethral meatus:
- Approximately 50% of cases are classified as anterior – the meatus is on the inferior surface of the glans penis, in the balanopenile furrow, or somewhere on the distal third of the penile shaft
- Approximately 20% of cases are classified as middle – the meatus is on the middle third of the penile shaft
- The remaining 30% of cases are classified as posterior – the meatus is on the proximal third of the penile shaft, at the base of the shaft in front of the scrotum, on the scrotum itself, or behind the scrotum

ASSOCIATED DISORDERS
- Chordee: an abnormal ventral curvature of the penis during erection is often associated with hypospadias
- Cryptorchidism: found in 9.3% of hypospadias patients
- Dorsal hood: a condition in which the prepuce is deficient ventrally. Thought to be produced by the inhibition of 5-alpha reductase by maternal exposure to estrogen-like compounds
- Inguinal hernia: found with and without hydrocele in 9% of hypospadias patients

KEY! DON'T MISS!
- Hypospadias is usually evident when the external genitalia are inspected during a routine newborn nursery admission examination
- Do not circumcise a baby with hypospadias

CONSIDER CONSULT
All patients with hypospadias require referral to a urologist trained in the surgical management of this disorder

INVESTIGATION OF THE PATIENT
Direct questions to patient
Hypospadias is usually evident when the external genitalia are inspected during a routine newborn nursery admission examination.

Family history
Q **Did the father have hypospadias?** 8% of hypospadias patients have fathers who also had hypospadias.
Q **Does a sibling have hypospadias?** Approximately one in eight male siblings (14%) of hypospadias patients also have hypospadias.

Examination
- **Palpation of undescended testis:** 9.3% of hypospadias patients also have cryptorchidism
- **Check for inguinal hernia with and without hydrocele:** 9% of hypospadias patients

DIAGNOSTIC DECISION
- The diagnosis is evident when the genitalia are inspected
- Mild anterior hypospadias may not be appreciated unless the foreskin is retracted

CLINICAL PEARLS
Presumed males with any degree of hypospadias in whom one or both gonads are not palpable should be evaluated for an intersex state.

IMMEDIATE ACTION

Circumcision should not be performed before pediatric urology consultation has been obtained.

PATIENT AND CAREGIVER ISSUES
Patient or caregiver request

- As is the case with other congenital defects, parents may feel guilty that some action or inaction on their part may have caused the defect
- Since the cause of hypospadias is unknown, parents should be reassured that they have not caused the problem

MANAGEMENT ISSUES
Goals

- Restoring the urethral meatus to its normal location allows the patient to urinate while standing
- Restoring normal appearance and function of the penis will avoid psychological distress in cases of severe hypospadias where the child cannot stand to urinate
- Correcting chordee is important for normal sexual function

SUMMARY OF THERAPEUTIC OPTIONS
Choices

- This congenital defect can only be treated by surgical therapy
- Preoperative medical management with androgens has been reported to enhance surgical repair
- There is no single, universally acceptable technique for hypospadias repair
- The nature of the surgical repair depends on the location of the urethral defect, and various procedures are available
- Most anterior cases are repaired with a meatoplasty and glanuloplasty (MAGPI)
- Orthoplasty may be required for correction of chordee
- Expert opinion suggests that the optimal age at the time of repair is 6–15 months

Therapies are directed at the level of the hypospadias.
Anterior hypospadias:
- MAGPI technique
- Glans approximation procedure (GAP)
- Heineke-Mikulicz meatoplasty with GAP
- Megameatus intact prepuce (MIP)

Middle hypospadias:
- Mathieu perimeatal based flap
- Onlay island flap
- Modified Thiersch-Duplay technique
- Tubularized incised plate urethroplasty (Snodgrass technique)

Posterior hypospadias:
- One stage – transverse preputial island flap; Onlay island flap
- Two stage – orthoplasty followed 6 months later by Thiersch-Duplay

MAGPI is appropriate for glanular hypospadias without chordee. Following degloving of the penis, a deep vertical incision is made on the glanular groove and closed horizontally. While advancing the ventral glanular edge, the sides are reapproximated, creating a lumen, and the penile skin is closed.

For more proximal hypospadias, flap-based repairs are indicated. In distal lesions a Mathieu procedure may be performed in which a perimeatal flap of penile skin is advanced distally to cover the defect. More proximal lesions require more extensive flaps/advancements in one- or two-stage procedures.

Clinical pearls

- While controversial, the use of androgens in children with hypospadias has been associated with an increase in penile length, a decrease in the severity of the hypospadias, and a decrease in the severity of the chordee
- Controversy continues with the ongoing debate among reconstructive urologic surgeons over the use of urethral stents and fistula formation in the correction of hypospadias

Never

Never circumcise a baby with hypospadias – consult a board-certified urologist before circumcising the child.

EFFICACY OF THERAPIES

In general, surgery is highly efficacious in correcting hypospadias and its associated chordee.

PROGNOSIS
Clinical pearls

- The use of bladder mucosa has been reported for primary repair of severe hypospadias in patients who present with a paucity of preputial skin. The complication of protruding mucosa at the meatus results in a significant reoperation rate for revision of the neomeatus
- Buccal mucosa can also be used. It has the benefit of requiring less tissue due to the fact that, when compared with bladder mucosa, buccal mucosa shrinks less
- Evaluation for penile curvature by injection of the corpora cavernosa: artificial erection is a crucial step in hypospadias repair and is performed after degloving the penis and resecting the fibrotic corpus spongiosum when present. Techniques used to correct chordee/penile curvature include the Nesbit procedure, tunica vaginalis graft, penile disassembly, and coporoplasty

Therapeutic failure

The complications of hypospadias repair may be categorized as:

- Intraoperative complications – excessive bleeding, inadvertent urethrostomy
- Early complications – urinary retention, erections causing disruptions of the sutures
- Late complications – urethral fistulae from infection and tissue ischemia, urethral stricture, meatal stenosis, persistent chordee, urethral diverticula, urethral redundancy, hairy urethra, sexual dysfunction, breakdown of repair

For reoperative hypospadias repair after a failed Mathieu, failed Onlay flap, and some tubularized procedures, the Snodgrass technique has proven to be an ideal procedure.

PREVENTION

No preventive strategies exist because the precise cause of hypospadias is unknown.

RESOURCES

ASSOCIATIONS
Hypospadias Association of America
4950 S. Yosemite Street
Box F2–156
Greenwood Village, Colorado 80111
www.hypospadias.net/

Parents with kids with hypospadias – online club
http://clubs.yahoo.com/clubs/mumswithhypospadiaskids

Online information on male anatomy and health problems including hypospadias (over 18 only)
http://www.the-penis.com

KEY REFERENCES

- Duckett JW, Baskin LS. Hypospadias. In Gillenwalter JY, Grayhack JT, Howards SS, Dukett JW, eds. Adult and pediatric urology, 3d edn. St Louis: Mosby, 1996, p2549–89
- Belman AB. Hypospadias update. Urology 1997;49:166–72
- Zaontz MR, Packer MG. Abnormalities of the external genitalia. Pediatr Clin N Amer 1997;44:1267–97
- Stephens FD, Smith ED, Hutson JM. Congenital anomalies of the urinary and genital tracts. Oxford: Isis Medical Media, 1996, p80–90, 383
- American Academy of Pediatrics. Timing of elective surgery on the genitalia of male children with particular reference to the risks, benefits, and psychological effects of surgery and anesthesia. Pediatrics 1996;97:590–4
- Borer JG, Retik AB. Current trends in hypospadias repair. Urol Clin North Am 1999;26:1:15–37

FAQS
Question 1
What is hypospadias?

ANSWER 1
Any condition where the meatus or opening of the urethra is in any place on the undersurface of the penis except for the tip.

Question 2
What is epispadias?

ANSWER 2
When the meatus is found to open on the dorsal side of the penis.

Question 3
What is a hypospadias cripple?

ANSWER 3
Though presently not commonly seen due to refinements in procedures, it represents an older male child who has been subjected to numerous operative attempts at correcting the hypospadias but who continues to have a urethral defect.

Question 4

What is the optimal age for correction of the hypospadias?

ANSWER 4

The ideal age is between 6 and 15 months.

Question 5

Do all children with hooded foreskins have hypospadias?

ANSWER 5

No. Some children are born with a normal penis with redundant hooded foreskin. Other penile deformities should be ruled out, such as atretic urethra and chordee.

CONTRIBUTORS

Randolph L Pearson, MD
Philip J Aliotta, MD, MHA, FACS
Anuj K Chopra, MD

IMPOTENCE

SUMMARY INFORMATION

DESCRIPTION

- Impotence is defined as the persistent inability to achieve or maintain penile erection sufficient for sexual intercourse
- There are multiple causes (some reversible)
- Treatment is aimed at the cause

URGENT ACTION

Immediate action is only required if it is the presenting feature of a more serious disorder such as uncontrolled diabetes mellitus or a spinal lesion.

KEY! DON'T MISS!

Associated or underlying serious disease presenting as impotence (classically with diabetes mellitus).

CODES
DSM-IV
DSM-IV code 302.72 Male erectile disorder.

ICD9 code
- F52.2 Male erectile disorder
- ICD-9CM 302.72 Psychosexual
- ICD-9CM 607.84 Organic
- ICD-9CM 997.99 Organic postprostatectomy

SYNONYMS
- Male erectile disorder (ED)
- Sexual dysfunction (nonspecific)
- 'Withered Yang' (Chinese medicine)

CARDINAL FEATURES
- Characterized by penile erections not sufficiently rigid to allow successful penetration of vaginal or other orifices
- Erectile dysfunction can cause marked distress and interpersonal difficulty
- Affects males only

CAUSES
Common causes
- Psychosomatic: primary or secondary
- Endocrine: diabetes mellitus
- Vascular: arterial insufficiency
- Local trauma
- Medications: antihypertensives, antidepressants, antipsychotics, histamine blockers, nicotine, alcohol, and others
- Neurogenic: stroke, multiple sclerosis, temporal lobe epilepsy, peripheral neuropathy, autonomic or sensory neuropathy
- Prostatectomy
- Multifactorial causes (several causes in combination)

Rare causes
- Endocrine: hypothalamic-pituitary-testicular axis dysfunction, hyperthyroidism, hypothyroidism, hyperprolactinemia, Cushing's syndrome
- Vascular: venous leakage, arteriovenous malformation
- Spinal cord trauma or tumor
- Neurotransmitter deficiency
- Systemic illness: renal failure, chronic obstructive pulmonary disease, cirrhosis of the liver
- Myotonic dystrophy
- Peyronie's disease
- Idiopathic reaction to drug

Serious causes
- Diabetes mellitus
- Hypothalamic-pituitary-testicular axis dysfunction
- Thyroid: hyperthyroidism, hypothyroidism
- Hyperprolactinemia
- Cushing's syndrome

- Peripheral neuropathy, autonomic or sensory neuropathy
- Spinal cord trauma or tumor
- Central nervous system: stroke, multiple sclerosis, temporal lobe epilepsy
- Neurotransmitter deficiency
- Renal failure
- Chronic obstructive pulmonary disease
- Cirrhosis of the liver
- Myotonic dystrophy

Contributory or predisposing factors

- Alcohol
- Drugs, legal and illicit (anabolic steroids, heroin, and marijuana)

EPIDEMIOLOGY
Incidence and prevalence
INCIDENCE
Overall probability of some degree of erectile dysfunction 52%.

PREVALENCE
Rises markedly with age.

FREQUENCY
- Erectile dysfunction is a vastly under-reported problem
- In the US, between the ages of 40 and 70 the probability of complete erectile dysfunction triples from 5% to 15%
- Greater than 70% of erectile dysfunction is thought to remain undiagnosed in the US

Demographics
AGE
- Rises markodly with age (US figures)
- 2% of men in their 40s
- 25% of men in their 60s
- 89% of men in their 80s

GENDER
Occurs only in men.

RACE
Mostly equal between races.

GEOGRAPHY
Worldwide.

SOCIOECONOMIC STATUS
- Less prevalent among married men
- Less prevalent in higher-educated groups

Data from the National Health and Social Life Survey published early in 1999 report that a higher educational level seems to decrease the risk of sexual dysfunction. In the same survey, married men were found to have less sexual dysfunction than their unmarried counterparts.

DIFFERENTIAL DIAGNOSIS

- Impotence is a clinical syndrome or symptom and can, therefore, cause diagnostic confusion itself
- The differential diagnosis lies in the causes of the impotence, which may be psychosomatic or organic

SIGNS & SYMPTOMS
Signs
General examination:

- Signs of vascular disease (hypertension, ischemic ulcers)
- Signs of neurologic disease (hemiparesis following stroke, impaired gait of multiple sclerosis)
- Signs of major hormonal dysfunction (hypothyroid facies, hyperthyroid eye signs, lack of facial hair and gynecomastia in hypopituitarism)

Genital examination:

- Presence of penile plaques (suggestive of Peyronie's disease)
- Size, position, and consistency of testes (small, malpositioned, or atrophic testes suggest hypogonadism)

Symptoms
General:

- Symptoms of organic underlying causative disease (lethargy, weight change, thirst, impaired urinary stream)
- Symptoms of underlying psychosomatic problem (depressive symptoms, relationship difficulties)

Specific:

- Erections either absent, poor quality, not sustained, or in combination
- Patient may have noticed anatomical anomalies (Peyronie's plaques, lack of normal gonad size/position/consistency)

ASSOCIATED DISORDERS
General stress levels may be raised, may be cause or effect.

KEY! DON'T MISS!
Associated or underlying serious disease presenting as impotence (classically with diabetes mellitus).

CONSIDER CONSULT

- Refer if there is a possible organic cause of impotence, unless PCP is very confident and experienced with the suspected conditions
- If PCP's initial evaluation rules out organic causes of impotence, referral may still be indicated in psychosomatic cases, if not straightforward

INVESTIGATION OF THE PATIENT
Direct questions to patient
It is important for the dialogue to be conducted in a nonthreatening, comfortable manner. Some physicians like to introduce the patient to the subject by prior reassuring mail contact, if possible, and some may include a questionnaire to be filled in before the first personal interview. Standardized questionnaires are available. Interview of the partner contributes greatly.

Q **What do you mean by the problem?** Is it failure to achieve or maintain an erection?

Q **For how long have you had the problem?** Long-standing problems may prove more intractable.

Q **Did the problem come on suddenly?** Slow onset occurs with age and causes that have a gradual effect, while rapid onset may indicate a specific event, psychologic or physical.

Q **Has the problem occurred before?** Recurrence is a feature of psychosomatic impotence.

Q **Do you wake up in the morning with an erection?** The sudden onset of erectile dysfunction, with normal morning erections points toward psychosomatic impotence.

Q **Do you still feel the desire for sexual intercourse?** A poor relationship points toward psychosomatic impotence.

Q **When you get an erection, is it normal? Is it rigid enough for penetration and can you sustain it long enough for coitus?** Full, normal erection that is not sustained points toward psychosomatic impotence.

Q **Do you have normal erections with masturbation and other partners?** If the answer is positive, the cause is almost certainly psychosomatic.

Q **Have you noticed any change in your sexual organs?** Secondary sexual characteristics decrease in hypogonadism (hypopituitarism), and the penis curves in Peyronie's disease.

Q **Are there any emotional problems at present or problems with your partner?** Emotion plays an important part in the sexual drive, and the problem is likely to be psychosomatic in origin.

Q **Are you generally well?** Any concurrent disease can decrease libido.

Q **Do you suffer with heart or circulation problems, diabetes, liver or kidney problems?** All can contribute to impotence, as can some medications used to treat them.

Q **Have you had any abdominal or pelvic surgery?** Could point to an underlying disease or postoperative vascular or neurologic complications. There could be a functional problem such as retrograde ejaculation after prostatectomy.

Q **Is your weight steady and your appetite normal?** Changes can suggest the presence of unsuspected diabetes or thyroid disease.

Q **Do you suffer with excessive fatigue?** Hormone imbalances and chronic disease could be the cause of this symptom.

Q **Do you suffer from excessive thirst?** This occurs in diabetes mellitus and also diabetes insipidus, which can occur with pituitary adenomas.

Q **Do you still shave as regularly as before?** If not, may suggest hypopituitarism or hyperprolactinemia.

Q **Has there been any change in sensation or strength in your limbs?** Could point to a neurologic disorder or be a manifestation of hypogonadism.

Q **Have you had any headaches, breast enlargement, visual disturbances, or discharge from your nipples (galactorrhea)?** These symptoms may point to hyperprolactinemia.

Q **Are you experiencing any mood disturbances?** Depression and other mental illness can dispose to psychosomatic ED. Some of the drugs used in treatment may also be implicated. Erectile dysfunction can be an underlying symptom of depression and does not, by itself, cause depression.

Q **What medication are you taking (including over-the-counter)?** Many classes of medication directly cause ED.

Contributory or predisposing factors

Q **Are you a smoker?** Smoking impairs circulation and creates other secondary problems such as COPD, which may contribute to erectile dysfunction.

Q **How much alcohol do you consume?** Excessive consumption points to alcohol as a source of erectile dysfunction.

Q **What recreational drugs do you take?** Several narcotics, steroids, testosterone, and marijuana use can cause erectile dysfunction.

Family history
Q Does anyone in your family suffer from diabetes/thyroid disease/circulatory disease?
Q Is there a family history of malignancies, specifically prostate cancer or colorectal cancer?

Examination
General examination – signs of underlying disease:
- Are there signs of anemia, renal or liver disease? (Pallor, sallowness, tremor, telangiectasia)
- Are there signs of vascular disease? (Hypertension, ischemic ulcers, absent peripheral pulses)
- Are there signs of neurologic disease? (Hemiparesis following stroke, impaired gait)
- Are there signs of major hormonal dysfunction? (Hypothyroid facies, hyperthyroid eye signs, lack of facial hair and gynecomastia in hypopituitarism)
- Is the abdominal examination normal? (Renal, hepatic or other masses, surgical scars)

Genital examination:
- Is digital rectal examination normal? Prostatic evaluation is essential (hypertrophy and postprostatectomy states are significant)
- Is the penis normal? Presence of penile plaques is suggestive of Peyronie's disease
- Are the bulbocavernosus and cremasteric reflexes normal? Absence suggests neurologic impairment (bulbocavernosus reflex is elicited by squeezing the glans penis and noting anal sphincter constriction)
- Is the examination of the external genitalia normal? Check size, position, and consistency of testes (small, malpositioned, or atrophic testes suggest hypogonadism)
- Is the penile vibratory sensation normal? This may be conducted in the office if there is access to biothesiometry

Summary of investigative tests
The tests are tailored to the individual, and relate to the history and physical examination. However, the minimum expected will be:
- Random or fasting blood glucose
- Free and total testosterone – request in patients >50 years of age, or in those <50 years if there are indicators of hypogonadism (decreased libido, bilateral testicular atrophy, reduced amount of body hair)
- Prolactin levels – should be drawn in the presence of low libido, loss of hair, visual problems, headaches, and gynecomastia. Refer if these levels are abnormal
- Thyroid screen – thyroid-stimulating hormone (TSH) may suffice initially

If appropriate, the patient will need to be screened for any undiagnosed medical disease that may underlie the erectile dysfunction.

DIAGNOSTIC DECISION
Impotence is a clinical syndrome or symptom and is diagnosed on the history.

Guidelines
- The American Academy of Neurology has produced guidelines for the evaluation of patients with impotence secondary to neurogenic causes [1]
- The American Academy of Family Physicians has published information on diagnosis and treatment of impotence [2]

CLINICAL PEARLS

- Attempt to make discussions about erectile function easy and present them in a relaxed fashion
- Encourage a warm, open, and nonjudgmental atmosphere
- Do not be afraid or intimidated by the topic of human sexuality. Find a way to introduce the topic as part of your day-to-day patient evaluation protocol
- Be reassuring and easygoing about the topic of erectile dysfunction
- Be optimistic about resolving the problem
- A male patient that has multiple nebulous complaints, frequent office visits, and is evasive in answers may be depressed or may be suffering from ED

THE TESTS
Body fluids
THYROID-STIMULATING HORMONE
Description

- Venous blood sample
- Primary test used in the diagnosis of thyroid dysfunction
- As thyroid disease can be subtle, especially in elderly men, it is important to screen for this
- In one study evaluating endocrine dysfunction as a cause of erectile dysfunction, 6% were found to have hypothyroidism
- This is a good screening test to determine thyroid status

Advantages/Disadvantages
Advantages:

- Relatively readily available test, simple to perform
- Current assays are very sensitive

Normal
? 11mcU/ml

Abnormal

- <2mcU/mL or >11mcU/mL
- Keep in mind the possibility of a false-positive result

Cause of abnormal result

- Raised TSH levels occur in primary hypothyroidism and other diseases
- Abnormally low TSH levels occur in hyperthyroidism

Drugs, disorders and other factors that may alter results
Many factors can cause raised TSH levels, including:

- Insufficient dose of euthyroid therapy
- Recovery from severe nonthyroid illness
- Addison's disease
- Lithium, amiodarone, amphetamines
- Blood sample taken in the evening, the peak of the normal diurnal variation in TSH levels

Many factors can cause lowered TSH levels, including:

- Excessive hypothyroid therapy
- Severe nonthyroid illness
- Active thyroiditis
- Pituitary insufficiency, Cushing's syndrome
- Hyperthyroidism

FREE AND TOTAL TESTOSTERONE

Description
- Venous blood sample
- Indicated in patients >50 years of age, or in those <50 years if there are indicators of hypogonadism (decreased libido, bilateral testicular atrophy, reduced amount of body hair)
- The test should be performed in the early morning and may need to be repeated anywhere from 1 to 3 times in order to confirm abnormally low levels
- The absence of libido and other findings makes this blood test worthwhile
- In the absence of these symptoms, the cost utility of ordering these tests is questionable

Advantages/Disadvantages
Advantage:
- Sample easy to obtain

Disadvantages:
- May be difficult to get test at local laboratory
- Expensive
- May need repeat testing to confirm results

Normal
Serum plasma levels 280–1100ng/dL.

Abnormal
<280ng/dL or >1100ng/dL.

Cause of abnormal result
- Elevated in some testicular tumors
- Decreased in hypogonadism and hyperprolactinemia

Drugs, disorders and other factors that may alter results
Anabolic steroid use (e.g. athletes).

RANDOM OR FASTING BLOOD GLUCOSE

Description
Pinprick finger test or venous blood sample.

Advantages/Disadvantages
Advantages:
- Inexpensive
- Easy to perform
- Widely available
- Clear guidelines for interpretation

Normal
- Random glucose: <11.1mmol/L (200mg/dL)
- Fasting glucose: <7.5mmol/L (135mg/dL)

Abnormal
- Random glucose: >11.1mmol/L (200mg/dL)
- Fasting glucose: >7.5mmol/L (135mg/dL)

Cause of abnormal result

- Diabetes mellitus
- Impaired glucose tolerance
- Other endocrine abnormalities such as acromegaly

Drugs, disorders and other factors that may alter results

- Hormones: glucagon, glucocorticoids, growth hormone, epinephrine, thyroid preparations
- Drugs: thiazide diuretics, furosemide, acetazolamide, diazoxide, alpha-agonists, calcium channel blockers, phenytoin, phenobarbital sodium, nicotinic acid, cyclophosphamide, 1-asparaginase, epinephrine-like drugs (decongestants and diet pills), NSAIDs, nicotine, caffeine, sugar-containing syrups, fish oils

PROLACTIN LEVEL

Description

- Venous blood sample
- Prolactin levels should be drawn in the presence of low libido, loss of hair, visual problems, headaches, and gynecomastia
- Referral is required if these levels are abnormal

Advantages/Disadvantages

Advantage:

- Sample easy to obtain, but at least three levels should be taken

Disadvantages:

- May be difficult to get test at local laboratory
- Expensive
- Results can be difficult to interpret

Normal

<400mU/L.

Abnormal

400–600mU/L is mildly elevated. Levels >2000–3000mU/L suggest prolactinoma.

Cause of abnormal result

- Mildly elevated levels may be due to normal physiologic events such as sleeping, stress, or postcoitus
- Many drugs can also raise prolactin levels
- Some chronic medical conditions such as renal or liver failure can raise serum prolactin
- Higher prolactin levels may be due to more serious causes such as tumor in the hypothalamic/pituitary axis and require immediate referral to a specialist for evaluation

Drugs, disorders and other factors that may alter results

- Several different physiologic or pathologic states can cause elevated prolactin levels
- Many drugs can also raise prolactin, e.g. cimetidine, metoclopramide, or methyldopa

CONSIDER CONSULT
- Refer when there is an underlying medical condition that the PCP is unable to treat. Treatment of an underlying chronic disease such as diabetes or atherosclerosis does not guarantee the return of erectile function
- Refer when there is endocrine dysfunction for a thorough investigation as to the cause as well as treatment
- Refer when there is a neurologic disorder for full evaluation and treatment
- If medication is thought to be a causal factor and specialist evaluation is needed in changing the drugs
- Counseling for substance abuse
- When specialist psychologic input is required
- For surgical management (corrective or implants)

IMMEDIATE ACTION
Immediate referral mandatory if serious, life-threatening underlying disease detected.

PATIENT AND CAREGIVER ISSUES
Forensic and legal issues
Impotence may be cited in divorce actions, hence the importance of correct diagnosis and treatment, plus careful explanation of the condition to the patient and his partner.

Impact on career, dependants, family, friends
Impotence places enormous strain on many sexual relationships, whatever the cause of the dysfunction.

Patient or caregiver request
- Do I have a sexually transmitted disease? There may be misunderstanding linking impotence and STDs
- Am I sterile, and will I be so after treatment? There is no effect on the patient's ability to father a child other than mechanical
- Will I get ejaculation with treatment? Yes, unless it was absent before as in postprostatectomy patients

Health-seeking behavior
- What other remedies have you tried? With what result?
- Have you made any other changes? Diet, weight loss, exercise may help
- Have you sought counseling? Patients may realize many impotence problems are psychosomatic and seek counseling help directly

MANAGEMENT ISSUES
Goals
- Proper diagnosis of the cause of the patient's impotence
- Restoration of sexual function using appropriate treatment
- Good patient understanding of the condition

Management in special circumstances
Many underlying or coexisting diseases limit the options available to treat impotence, and may also modify the achievable goals in the condition.

COEXISTING DISEASE
- Diabetes and vascular disease create major high-priority medical problems and may force the problem of impotence to be overlooked or put to one side

- Any severe chronic illness may significantly limit what can be achieved in treating ED
- Some diseases are relative contraindications to the use of first-choice drugs, e.g. sickle cell anemia, leukemia, multiple myeloma (which all predispose to priapism); plus renal insufficiency, hepatic dysfunction, and bleeding disorders

COEXISTING MEDICATION

As well as some drugs being implicated in causing ED, certain drugs necessary to treat other coexisting diseases may restrict ED treatment options (e.g. the use of nitrates to treat angina precludes the use of sildenafil).

SPECIAL PATIENT GROUPS

Elderly men may simply want reassurance that there is no other serious problem. If they do want treatment, caution must be used with all of the drug therapies available.

PATIENT SATISFACTION/LIFESTYLE PRIORITIES

The patient's own goals must be discovered in order to plan the treatment effectively. If the patient (and physician) expects full return to normal sexual function, this must be the goal for treatment.

SUMMARY OF THERAPEUTIC OPTIONS
Choices

- Pharmocotherapeutic agents, e.g. sildenafil
- Intracavernosal alprostadil
- Transurethral alprostadil
- Physical: pelvic floor muscle exercises
- Nonpharmocologic: vacuum-constriction erection devices
- Psychologic or psychiatric – these are specially areas of treatment. It is not in the scope of this article to detail all the possible therapies that could be employed by a psychotherapist, psychologist, psychiatrist, or trained sex therapist
- Surgical: penile prosthesis, penile revascularization – these are performed by a specialist
- Alternative therapies, e.g. Chinese medicine
- Reducing alcohol consumption may significantly reduce ED

Guidelines

- The American Urological Association, 1996. The treatment of organic erectile dysfunction [3]
- The American Academy of Family Physicians has published information on diagnosis and treatment of impotence [2]

Clinical pearls

- Presently, the treatment of choice for erectile dysfunction is oral therapy with sildenafil
- Referral to a urologist should occur when the patient fails on sildenafil therapy

Never

Never commence sildenafil without establishing that the patient does not take nitrates.

FOLLOW UP

- Follow-up should be offered with all treatment strategies for ED
- It is especially necessary with the drug therapies to monitor effectiveness and side-effects

Plan for review

With drug therapies, ideally the patient should return to report after his first dose, but at the least he should be seen at weekly intervals until the treatment goals have been achieved, and both patient and PCP are happy to reduce appointment frequency.

Information for patient or caregiver

- The common and frequently temporary nature of ED should be explained to the patient, ideally with his partner
- When drug therapies are prescribed, it is important that their possible side-effects are fully discussed

DRUGS AND OTHER THERAPIES: DETAILS
Drugs
SILDENAFIL

- Absorbed rapidly; peak plasma levels within 1h
- Is effective in men with erectile dysfunction of organic, psychosomatic, or combined causes
- Do not prescribe to patients on nitrates because of the potential for severe hypotension and cardiac compromise

Dose

- Initially prescribe 50mg to be taken 1h before the anticipated intercourse
- The dose can be increased to 100mg if needed
- For men over 65 years, a 25mg tablet is available and is recommended as the starting dose
- 25mg starting dose is recommended in patients with hepatic or renal dysfunction

Efficacy
Erection appropriate for intercourse was attained in:

- 72% of men on 25mg
- 80% of men on 50mg
- 85% of men on 100mg

Risks/Benefits
Risks:

- Use caution with elderly
- Use caution with hepatic dysfunction
- Use caution with renal insufficiency
- Use caution with cardiac disease
- Use caution with penile deformity
- Use caution with predisposition to priapism
- Use caution in bleeding disorders
- Use caution with peptic ulcer disease
- Use caution with retinitis pigmentosa
- Avoid simultaneous use of cytochrome P450 inhibitors
- Should not be prescribed more than once a day or in combination with other drugs for erectile dysfunction
- Should never be prescribed with nitrate therapy and nitrates should not be given within 24h of taking sildenafil

Benefits:

- Relatively quick acting (about 1h)
- Effective
- Oral administration
- Does not interrupt intercourse
- Well tolerated

Side-effects and adverse reactions

- Cardiovascular system: cardiac arrest, angina, AV block, migraine, syncope, tachycardia, palpitations, hypotension, myocardial ischemia, cerebral thrombosis, heart failure, abnormal electrocardiogram, cardiomyopathy

- Central nervous system: headache, abnormal vision, photosensitivity, ataxia, hypertonia, neuralgia, neuropathy, parasthesia, tremor, vertigo, depression, insomnia, somnolence, abnormal dreams, hypoesthesia
- Ears, eyes, nose and throat: dizziness, mydriasis, tinnitus, eye pain, ear pain
- Hematologic: anemia, leukopenia
- Gastrointestinal: dyspepsia, diarrhea, vomiting, gastritis, esophagitis, stomatitis, abnormal liver function tests
- Genitourinary: urinary tract infection, nocturia, frequency, incontinence, abnormal ejaculation, breast enlargement, anorgasmy
- Metabolic: hyperglycemia, hypoglycemia, hyperuricemia, hypernatremia, thirst, edema, gout, unstable diabetes
- Musculoskeletal: arthritis, arthrosis, synovitis, myalgia, tendon rupture, tenosynovitis, bone pain, myasthenia
- Respiratory: asthma, dyspnea, laryngitis, cough, pharyngitis, sinusitis, bronchitis, sputum increased, cough
- Skin: flushing, urticaria, pruritus, dermatitis, herpes simplex, sweating, skin ulcer

Interactions (other drugs)
- Cimetidine (increased sildenafil levels) ▪ Cytochrome P450 inhibitors (may reduce sildenafil clearance) ▪ Erythromycin ▪ Itraconazole (increased sildenafil levels) ▪ Ketoconazole (increased sildenafil levels) ▪ Nitrates (cardiac arrest, death) (increased sildenafil levels) ▪ Rifampin (decreased sildenafil levels)

Contraindications
- Concurrent treatment with nitrates ▪ Hypotension ▪ Recent stroke or myocardial infarction ▪ Hereditary degenerative retinal disorders

Evidence
Oral sildenafil is an effective and safe treatment for impotence.
- Two sequential blinded RCTs examined the use of sildenafil versus placebo in the management of impotence. Increasing doses of medication caused improved erectile function, and sildenafil was significantly more effective than placebo [4] *Level P*
- A blinded RCT compared sildenafil with placebo for the treatment of erectile dysfunction in diabetic men. 56% of patients in the treatment group compared with 10% in the placebo group reported improved erectile function at 12 weeks. Adverse effects (headache, dyspepsia, sinus congestion) were more common in the treatment group [5] *Level P*

Acceptability to patient
- Well accepted in general
- Side-effects are often overridden by the desire for intercourse
- A small proportion of patients report an alteration in color perception
- Occasional priapism, which may be serious

Follow up plan
Evaluate dose-responsiveness and efficacy after initial administration and counsel on avoidance of nitrates.

Patient and caregiver information
- Limit use of sildenafil to one dose in any 24-h period
- If priapism occurs, report immediately to PCP or emergency room
- Avoid the use of nitrates and other ED drugs

INTRACAVERNOSAL ALPROSTADIL

When injected direct into the corpus cavernosum, alprostadil (prostaglandin-E1) acts on the arteriolar smooth muscle cells, inducing an erection within several minutes.

Dose
- Usually between 5 and 40mcg per injection
- Patients usually start at 2.5mcg and titrate up in 5mcg increments for effect
- Maximum dose: 60mcg
- No more than three injections per week is recommended with a minimum period of 24h between injections
- Initial dosing and required adjustments should be carried out in the physician's office

Efficacy
- Success rates of between 67% and 85% are reported
- In a study of patients on this therapy, 56% discontinue therapy within one year and 68% within 2 years

Risks/Benefits
Risks:
- Prolonged erection and priapism may occur
- A risk of penile fibrosis
- Bleeding after injection may occur in patients taking anticoagulants

Benefits:
- Self-administered
- Quick response

Side-effects and adverse reactions
- Cardiovascular system: bradycardia, congestive heart failure, edema, hypotension, tachycardia, ventricular fibrillation
- Central nervous system: cerebral bleeding, fever, hyperextension of the neck, hyperirritability, hypothermia, seizures
- Gastrointestinal: diarrhea, hyperbilirubinemia, regurgitation
- Genitourinary: injection site hematoma, penile fibrosis, penile pain, prolonged erection
- Hematologic: bleeding, disseminated intravascular coagulation, thrombocytopenia
- Metabolic: hyperkalemia, hypoglycemia, hypokalemia
- Musculoskeletal: cortical proliferation of the long bones
- Respiratory: apnea, bradypnea, hypercapnia, tachypnea, wheezing
- Skin: flushing

Interactions (other drugs)
Antihypertensives (may cause hypotension).

Contraindications
- Known hypersensitivity to alprostadil ▪ Penile implants ▪ Where sexual activity is inadvisable

Evidence
Alprostadil monotherapy is the preferred initial therapy for patients beginning vasoactive drug injection [3] Level C.

Acceptability to patient
- The major problems lie in the complication of prolonged erection and priapism, which deter use
- Many patients find it unacceptable to administer an injection into their penis

Follow up plan
- Evaluate dose responsiveness and efficacy after initial administration
- Continue counseling on correct usage of intracavernosal alprostadil

Patient and caregiver information
If priapism occurs, report immediately to PCP or emergency room.

TRANSURETHRAL ALPROSTADIL
- A better tolerated mode of delivery than its injectable counterpart with the same significant improvement
- The drug is thought to diffuse into the corpus spongiosum

Dose
- Initially 125–250mcg. Pellets are available up to strength of 1000mcg
- Can be used twice in a 24-h period, unlike other therapies

Efficacy
In one large study 65% of patients reported success.

Risks/Benefits
Risks:
- Prolonged erection and priapism may occur
- Hypotension and syncope are risks

Benefits:
- Self-administered
- Quick acting

Side-effects and adverse reactions
- Cardiovascular system: bradycardia, congestive heart failure, edema, hypotension, tachycardia, ventricular fibrillation
- Central nervous system: cerebral bleeding, fever, hyperextension of the neck, hyperirritability, hypothermia, seizures
- Gastrointestinal: diarrhea, hyperbilirubinemia, regurgitation
- Genitourinary: penile pain, urethral burning, urethral bleeding, testicular pain, prolonged erection
- Hematologic: bleeding, disseminated intravascular coagulation, thrombocytopenia
- Metabolic: hyperkalemia, hypoglycemia, hypokalemia
- Musculoskeletal: cortical proliferation of the long bones
- Respiratory: apnea, bradypnea, hypercapnia, tachypnea, wheezing
- Skin: flushing

Interactions (other drugs)
Antihypertensives (may cause hypotension).

Contraindications
- Known hypersensitivity to alprostadil ■ Where sexual activity is inadvisable ■ Abnormal penile anatomy, including urethral stricture, balanitis, severe hypospadias and curvature, urethritis ■ Sickle cell anemia or trait ■ Thrombocytopenia ■ Multiple myeloma ■ Polycythemia ■ Susceptibility to venous thrombosis

Evidence
There is some evidence for the use of transurethral alprostadil in the management of impotence.

- A double-blind RCT compared transurethral alprostadil with placebo in the management of chronic organic erectile dysfunction. 64.9% of patients in the treatment group had satisfactory intercourse at least once, compared with 18.6% in the placebo group. Efficacy of alprostadil was similar regardless of age and cause of erectile dysfunction [6] *Level P*
- A prospective trial compared intraurethral liposomal alprostadil with intracavernosal injection of alprostadil in patients with erectile dysfunction secondary to organic or psychosomatic causes. Patients with organic ED were not effectively treated with intraurethral alprostadil; however, psychosomatic ED patients may derive some benefit. Duplex ultrasound of the deep penile artery showed reduced blood flow with intraurethral compared with intracavernosal application [7] *Level P*

Acceptability to patient
- More acceptable to some patients than injections
- Some patients may find urethral application too uncomfortable
- Can be used twice in a 24-h period

Follow up plan
- A physician must administer the first dose
- Evaluate dose-responsiveness and efficacy after initial administration
- Self-administration can only be approved after adequate training in the technique

Patient and caregiver information
- If priapism occurs, report immediately to PCP or emergency room
- Should not be used during sexual intercourse if the partner is pregnant

Physical therapy
PELVIC FLOOR MUSCLE EXERCISES
This simple course of exercises (also used in postpartum women to prevent pelvic prolapse) can easily be tried alone or in conjunction with other therapies for ED.

Efficacy
There is limited evidence that pelvic floor muscle exercises are an effective treatment, particularly as an alternative to surgery.

Risks/Benefits
Benefits:
- Easy to learn
- Noninvasive
- No risk of side-effects

Acceptability to patient
Usually acceptable, unless exercises are physically difficult for patient to perform, e.g. after stroke.

Follow up plan
Minimum trial of 6 weeks is recommended before evaluating response.

Patient and caregiver information
To be effective, the exercises must be done at least twice daily.

Complementary therapy
Many different types of complementary therapy are available, few with much real success.

CHINESE MEDICINE
This is a complex range of therapies, too extensive for the scope of this article.

Efficacy
Some claims for effectiveness have been partly confirmed.

Risks/Benefits
Difficult to quantify.

Acceptability to patient
Depends on patient's view of Chinese medicine.

Follow up plan
Conducted by Chinese medicine practitioner.

Other therapies
VACUUM-CONSTRICTION DEVICES
These devices have been available under many names for a great number of years.

Efficacy
- Relatively efficient at causing a mechanical erection
- One study reported 92% of patients achieved erection

Risks/Benefits
Risks:
- Simple to use
- Noninvasive
- Priapism can occur, albeit not true priapism

Evidence
Vacuum constriction devices may be a safe alternative treatment for impotence in coloctcd patients.
- A prospective trial (not controlled) examined the efficacy of a vacuum-constriction device for patients with erectile dysfunction. 32 of 35 men achieved an erection sufficient for intercourse. Follow-up over 8 to 22 months revealed that 24 of 30 patients used the device regularly, with satisfaction [8] *This study does not meet the criteria for level P*
- A retrospective study of patients using a vacuum-constriction device for impotence found that 92% of users achieved an erection sufficient for intercourse [9] *Level S*

Acceptability to patient
- May be difficult to learn to use
- May be intrusive and prevent successful intercourse

Follow up plan
Follow-up should be after initial teaching of the technique, followed by adequate time to try it out.

Patient and caregiver information
The best way of ensuring maximum effectiveness is to integrate the use of the device into sexual foreplay as a prelude to intercourse.

LIFESTYLE
Reducing alcohol consumption from high levels may significantly reduce ED.

RISKS/BENEFITS
Rapid detoxification of heavily dependent alcoholics may result in fits and withdrawal symptoms.

ACCEPTABILITY TO PATIENT
ED may be a significant trigger to helping the alcoholic patient decide to stop drinking.

FOLLOW UP PLAN
Depends on the patient.

PATIENT AND CAREGIVER INFORMATION
Patient will need high degree of support (also Alcoholics Anonymous).

EFFICACY OF THERAPIES

- Outcomes of therapy depend on the underlying cause to some degree, linked with the severity and duration of ED for each patient
- Patients suitable for and willing to try sildenafil have a high degree of satisfaction with their rapid improvement
- Many patients benefit from counseling and physical exercises, even if their problem is not primarily psychosomatic or due to muscle weakness

Evidence

- Increasing doses of sildenafil improve erectile function [4] *Level P*
- Sildenafil is effective in improving erectile function after 12 weeks of treatment in diabetic men [5] *Level P*
- There is evidence that transurethral alprostadil is effective in the management of chronic organic erectile dysfunction. Efficacy of alprostadil is similar regardless of patient age and cause of erectile dysfunction [6] *Level P*

Review period

Depends on therapy selected.

PROGNOSIS

- The prognosis for ED can be highly variable
- Depending on the cause, ED can resolve, improve on therapy, or continue unchanged

Clinical pearls

- 25mg of sildenafil rarely works sufficiently, except in the young patient suffering from psychosomatic erectile dysfunction. Start most patients on a dose of 50mg of sildenafil and titrate the dose according to patient response
- For the most effectiveness from transurethral alprostadil, have the male patient apply the product and massage the urethra in the standing position
- Patients can use transurethral alprostadil in conjunction with a vacuum device, placing the ring on prior to using transurethral alprostadil. The ring maintains the blood flow in the cavernosal tissues, enhancing the erection

Therapeutic failure

- Assess for noncompliance with chosen therapy (e.g. side-effects)
- Reassess for occult underlying cause
- Assess other therapeutic options (see summary of Therapeutic Options)

Recurrence

- Recurrence may be due to therapeutic failure (may be noncompliance) or the development/recurrence of an underlying cause
- Often requires referral to appropriate specialist (depending on cause)

COMPLICATIONS

Priapism due to therapy or concurrent underlying disease.

CONSIDER CONSULT

- Failure of PCP-initiated therapy (drug and nonpharmacologic)

PREVENTION

Prevention is not possible, not least because ED is so common that it can be regarded as part of the aging process.

RISK FACTORS
- Alcohol
- **Drugs**, legal and illicit (anabolic steroids, heroin, and marijuana)

MODIFY RISK FACTORS
Lifestyle and wellness
TOBACCO
Smoking contributes to vascular disease and hence to ED.

ALCOHOL AND DRUGS
Alcohol and drugs (anabolic steroids, heroin, and marijuana) can all directly cause ED.

SEXUAL BEHAVIOR
Psychosexual problems often involve ED.

DRUG HISTORY
Antihypertensives, antidepressants, antipsychotics, and histamine blockers can all cause ED.

RESOURCES

ASSOCIATIONS

Impotence Information Center
P.O. Box 9
Minneapolis, MN 55440
Tel: 1-800-843-4315

KEY REFERENCES

- Chun J, Carson C. Physician-patient dialogue and clinical evaluation of erectile dysfunction. Urol Clin North Am 2001;28:249–58
- Engelhardt PF, Plas E, Hübner WA, Pflüger H. Comparison of intraurethral liposomal and intracavernosal prostaglandin-E1 in the management of erectile dysfunction. Br J Urol 1998;81:441–4
- Feldman HA, Goldstein I, Hatzichchristou DG et al. ED and its medical and psychological correlates: results of the Massachusetts male aging study. J Urol 1994;151:54–61
- Goldstein I, Lue TF, Padma-Nathan H et al. Oral sildenafil in the treatment of erectile dysfunction: Sildenafil Study Group. N Engl J Med 1998;338:1397–404
- Padma-Nathan H, Hellstrom WJ, Keiser FE et al. Treatment of men with erectile dysfunction with transurethral alprostadil: Medicated Urethral System for Erection (MUSE) Study Group. N Engl J Med 1997;336:1–7
- Rendell MS, Raifer J, Wicker PA, Smith MD. Sildenafil for the treatment of erectile dysfunction in men with diabetes a randomised controlled trial: Sildenafil Diabetes Study Group. JAMA 1999;822:421–6
- Sundaram CP, Thomas W, Pryor LE et al. Long term followup of patients receiving injection therapy for erectile dysfunction. Urology 1997;48:932–5
- Viera AJ, Clenney TL, Shenenberger DW, Green GF. Newer pharmacologic alternatives for erectile dysfunction. Am Fam Physician 1999;60:1159–66, 1169, 1172

Evidence references

1. The American Academy of Neurology has produced guidelines for the evaluation of patients with impotence secondary to neurogenic causes. Assessment: neurological evaluation of male sexual dysfunction. Therapeutics and Technology Assessment Subcommittee. Neurology 1995;45:2287–92
2. The American Academy of Family Physicians has published information on diagnosis and treatment of impotence. Viera AJ, Clenney TL, Shenenberger DW, Green GF. Newer pharmacologic alternatives for erectile dysfunction, 1999
3. The American Urological Association, 1996. The treatment of organic erectile dysfunction. Erectile dysfunction Clinical Guidelines Panel Members and Consultants. Also available at the National Guideline Clearinghouse
4. Goldstein I, Lue TF, Padma-Nathan H, Rosen RC, Steers WD, Wicker PA. Oral sildenafil in the treatment of erectile dysfunction: Sildenafil Study Group. N Engl J Med 1998:338;1397–404 Medline
5. Rendell MS, Rajfer J, Wicker PA, Smith MD. Sildenafil for the treatment of erectile dysfunction in men with diabetes: a randomised controlled trial. Sildenafil Diabetes Study Group. JAMA 1999:281:421–6 Medline
6. Padma-Nathan H, Hellstrom WJ, Kaiser FE, et al. Treatment of men with erectile dysfunction with transurethral alprostadil. Medicated Urethral System for Erection (MUSE) Study Group. N Engl J Med 1997;336:1–7 Medline
7. Engelhardt PF, Plas E, Hübner WA, Pflüger H. Comparison of intraurethral liposomal and intracavernosal prostaglandin-E1 in the management of erectile dysfunction. Br J Urol 1998;81:441–4 Medline
8. Nadig PW, Ware JC, Blumoff R. Noninvasive device to produce and maintain an erection-like state. Urology 1986;27:126–31 Medline
9. Witherington R. Vacuum-constriction device for management of erectile impotence. J Urol 1989;141:320–2 Medline

FAQS

Question 1
What is erectile dysfunction?

ANSWER 1
Erectile dysfunction is the persistent inability to obtain or maintain a penile erection for the mutual satisfaction of both partners.

Question 2
What are the organic causes of erectile dysfunction?

ANSWER 2
There are many organic causes of erectile dysfunction, including inflammatory (prostatitis), mechanical (Peyronie's disease), postoperative (radical prostatectomy), vascular (atherosclerosis), trauma (pelvic surgery or fracture), neurogenic (MS), drugs (antihypertensives, recreational), endocrine (DM, hypogonadism), cancer (prostate cancer, colorectal cancer), and systemic (renal failure).

Question 3
What are the tests for erectile dysfunction?

ANSWER 3
Sexual history, history of comorbid factors, psychologic assessment, physical examination, and blood studies.

Question 4
What are some of the tests that a urologist will do?

ANSWER 4
Nocturnal penile tumescence studies, duplex ultrasonography, cavernosometry, arteriogram of pelvic and penile vessels.

Question 5
What are the treatments for erectile dysfunction?

ANSWER 5
Sex therapy, medical management, vacuum devices, oral pharmacotherapy, injection therapy, intraurethral therapy, penile prosthesis, arterial revascularization, and penile venous ligation.

CONTRIBUTORS
Martin L Kabongo, MD, PhD
Philip J Aliotta, MD, MHA, FACS

Impotence – RESOURCES

313

KIDNEY STONES (NEPHROLITHIASIS)

SUMMARY INFORMATION

DESCRIPTION
- Severe, colicky flank pain
- Hematuria (gross or microscopic)
- Nausea and vomiting
- Dysuria, urinary frequency and/or urgency

URGENT ACTION
Urologic referral should be considered for fever and chills suggestive of obstruction or pyelonephritis; concurrent pregnancy; history of recurrent calculi, especially if they required intervention; history of renal failure or single kidney.

KEY! DON'T MISS!
- Fever and chills, indicative of concomitant infection
- Symptoms which may be referable to a more serious, potentially lethal condition, including abdominal aneurysm; bowel obstruction; appendicitis

ICD9 CODE
592. Calculus of kidney and ureter (renal stone, kidney stone, urolithiasis, ureteric stone)
592.0 Calculus of kidney; nephrolithiasis; renal calculus or stone; staghorn calculus; kidney stone
592.1 Calculus of ureter; ureteric stone; ureterolithiasis
592.9 Urinary calculus, unspecified

SYNONYMS
Nephrolithiasis; urolithiasis; urinary lithiasis; ureterolithiasis; urinary or renal calculi; staghorn calculus; kidney or urinary stones; renal colic

CARDINAL FEATURES
- Excruciating colicky flank pain of sudden onset
- A restless, writhing patient, unable to decrease pain with a change in position
- Hematuria
- Dysuria, urinary frequency and/or urgency
- Nausea, vomiting

CAUSES
Common causes
- Idiopathic hypercalciuria may be due to absorptive, renal, or resorptive causes
- Hypercalcemia: often associated with primary hyperparathyroidism, malignancy; granulomatous disease (including sarcoidosis, tuberculosis, histoplasmosis, coccidioidomycosis, leprosy, or silicosis); hyperthyroidism; glucocorticoid administration; pheochromocytoma; prolonged immobilization
- Hyperoxaluria: due to a genetic primary hyperoxaluria; enteric hyperoxaluria secondary to malabsorption syndromes, including short bowel syndrome;Crohn's disease; or may be idiopathic. Hyperuricosuria: may occur concomitantly with gout symptoms; may reflect excess purine intake in the diet; may be associated with myeloproliferative disorders (especially in children)
- Hypocitraturia: may be anomalous or due to metabolic abnormalities such as acidosis
- Hypomagnesuria: often due to malabsorption secondary to inflammatory bowel disease
- Renal tubular acidosis
- Cystinuria
- Chronic urinary tract infection with urease-producing bacteria (including *Proteus mirabilis* and *Ureaplasma urealyticum*)
- Patients on chemotherapy for malignancy are at increased risk for developing uric acid stones

Rare causes
- Adenine phosphoribosyltransferase deficiency
- Xanthinuria: may be an autosomal recessive trait, resulting in decreased xanthine oxidase production; may follow allopurinol treatment in patients with Lesch-Nyhan syndrome
- Administration of triamterene, a potassium-sparing diuretic
- Excessive ingestion of antacids containing silicates

Contributory or predisposing factors
- Decreased fluid intake
- Increased fluid losses, as occurs in hot, dry climates
- Increased intake of animal protein, sodium, oxalate-containing foodstuffs in diet

EPIDEMIOLOGY
Incidence and prevalence
INCIDENCE
0.7–2.1 per 1000

PREVALENCE
- 30% of the population has kidney stones
- Approximately 50% of this population will experience symptoms from their stone disease

FREQUENCY
10% of population of United States will suffer from nephrolithiasis at some time in their lives.

Demographics
AGE
Peak incidence between 20 and 40 years of age.

GENDER
3 males: 1 female

RACE
- Increased incidence in Whites and Asians
- Decreased incidence in Native Americans, Africans and African-Americans, and native-born Israelis; people from Middle East

GENETICS
Some studies have suggested polygenic defect with partial penetrance; other studies weigh more heavily towards influence of diet rather than familial tendencies.

GEOGRAPHY
Increased incidence found in mountainous, desert, and tropical regions suggesting dehydration and decreased fluid intake. In the United States, the southeast has a particularly high incidence, and is therefore dubbed the 'stone belt'.

SOCIOECONOMIC STATUS
- Increased risk linked to higher socioeconomic status, believed to be linked to increased dietary consumption of animal protein
- Sedentary occupations at increased risk

DIFFERENTIAL DIAGNOSIS
Abdominal aneurysm
FEATURES
- Pain in lower back, abdomen, flank, groin
- May note hematuria
- Pulsatile abdominal mass is diagnostic, but only present in under 50% of cases
- Important to consider and rule out, due to potentially lethal nature of this disorder

Acute appendicitis
FEATURES
- May begin with anorexia and periumbilical pain
- Migration of pain to right lower quadrant
- Nausea, vomiting
- Appendiceal rupture may lead to peritoneal signs, including abdominal rigidity, and guarding

Mechanical back pain
FEATURES
- Low back pain
- Radiculopathy
- Paresthesias
- Point tenderness
- Stiffness

Bowel obstruction
FEATURES
- Crampy abdominal pain, may be constant or colicky in nature
- Nausea, vomiting
- Constipation, absent flatus

SIGNS & SYMPTOMS
Signs
- A restless, writhing patient, unable to decrease pain by changing position
- Frequent flank/costovertebral angle tenderness demonstrated
- May be tachycardic or bradycardic
- May be hypertensive
- Benign abdominal exam
- May note hypoactive bowel sounds, indicative of associated ileus

Symptoms
- Severe colicky flank pain, may include radiation of pain into the groin, labia, penis, testicles, thigh
- Hematuria
- Nausea, vomiting, diarrhea
- Dysuria, urinary frequency and/or urgency

KEY! DON'T MISS!
- Fever and chills, indicative of concomitant infection
- Symptoms which may be referable to a more serious, potentially lethal condition, including abdominal aneurysm; bowel obstruction; appendicitis

CONSIDER CONSULT

- Fever, chills
- Ureteral obstruction
- Persistent nausea and/or emesis, preventing oral fluid intake or oral medications
- Intractable pain
- History of renal failure, previous renal transplant, single functional kidney
- Invasive procedures performed for previous stones

INVESTIGATION OF THE PATIENT
Direct questions to patient

Q **What is the pain like? Does it seem to come and go? Does it travel anywhere? Is it improved or worsened by position, or any other maneuvers?** Pain is usually very intense, may have colicky characteristics, may radiate, isn't usually improved or worsened by position or other palliative attempts.

Q **Do you have any urinary symptoms?** May note urinary urgency, frequency, hematuria.

Q **Have you had any stomach upset?** Nausea, vomiting, diarrhea, symptoms of ileus may accompany passage of urinary calculi.

Q **Have you had this before?** May have past history of kidney stones, with similar presentation.

Q **Do you have any other medical conditions?** May have history of gout, bowel disease/malabsorption syndromes, hyperthyroidism, hyperparathyroidism, sarcoidosis, malignancy.

Q **What medications/vitamins do you take?** Increased risk of kidney stones with corticosteroids, thiazide diuretics, triamterene, antibiotics, excess ingestion of vitamins D or A, excess ingestion of antacids (especially in conjunction with large quantities of milk), estrogen preparations or tamoxifen (especially in the presence of bony metastases secondary to breast cancer).

Contributory or predisposing factors

Q **How often do you eat meat? How much meat do you eat? Do you add salt to your food at the table? Describe your general diet.**

Q **Do you have a sense of how much water you drink daily? What is your water source?**

Q **Do you exercise?** Stone formers may have a history of exercising to the point of dehydration, resulting in supersaturated urine.

Family history

Q **Have any other members of your family had kidney stones?** Some research has indicated a familial tendency to nephrolithiasis.

Q **Do you live with anyone who has had kidney stones?** Some research has indicated that diet tendencies within a household may increase the chance of nephrolithiasis, even among non-blood relatives.

Q **Does anyone in your family have gout? Bowel disease? Thyroid disease? Parathyroid disease/hyperparathyroidism? Sarcoidosis?**

Examination

- **Check pulse, blood pressure, respiration.** Patients in acute pain are often tachycardic and tachypneic; patients with renal obstruction secondary to urinary calculi may be hypertensive
- **Take temperature.** Fever unusual in nephrolithiasis, unless infection is also present
- **Auscultate abdomen, listening for bowel sounds.** Ileus may accompany a passing urinary calculus
- **Palpate abdomen, noting guarding, rigidity, any masses.** A passing urinary calculus does not usually produce guarding or rigidity, as would acute abdominal pain; a pulsatile mass indicates the presence of an abdominal aneurysm; while ileus can occur with renal calculi, presence would indicate importance of ruling out bowel obstruction
- **Percuss costovertebral angle.** Often can elicit pain response in either a passing renal calculus or even more commonly in pyelonephritis

Summary of investigative tests
- Urinalysis (dip + microscopy)
- Urine culture, if indicated by suspicion of infection
- Blood tests usually yield little in acute syndrome
- Plain abdominal film, kidney, ureter and bladder (KUB): note that this test has a low sensitivity and specificity for identifying stones, more helpful in order to follow progress of already-diagnosed radio-opaque stone
- Renal ultrasonography: color Doppler methods are most accurate
- Spiral computed tomography: spiral CT is becoming more popular, superceding IVP as a way of verifying stones and ruling out other disorders
- Intravenous pyelogram: note chance of allergic/anaphylactic reaction to iodine-containing contrast dyes
- Calculus analysis of any stones or fragments collected
- Twenty-four hour urine collection (performed after acute episode has resolved): check volume, urine pH, and levels of calcium, phosphorus, sodium, uric acid, oxalate, citrate, creatinine

DIAGNOSTIC DECISION
- Presence of stone indicated by blood in urine
- Severe pain, with quality and intensity evocative of renal colic
- Stone may be radiodense or radiolucent; indication of stone on radiologic examination may be based on direct visualization of calculus, or indirect extrapolation, based on presence of hydroureter and hydronephrosis
- After presence of urinary calculus has been confirmed, attention turns towards evaluating cause of calculus formation; this may require a consultation with a urologist

CLINICAL PEARLS
- Pain may actually radiate into the genitalia, or present in an atypical fashion, testicular pain
- X-ray findings of hydroureter and hydronephrosis without an identifiable stone, may be seen in patients who have passed a calculus
- Look for crystalluria in the urine. The type of crystals present may be a key to stone diagnosis

THE TESTS
Body fluids
URINALYSIS
Description
Clean-catch, midstream urine specimen for dipstick analysis with microscopy.

Advantages/Disadvantages
Generally simple for patient to provide sample.

Normal
- pH 4.6–8.0
- Specific gravity 1.001–1.035
- Negative for red blood cells, leukocytes, protein, glucose, bilirubin, ketones, nitrites, urobilinogen on dip
- No microorganisms, casts, crystals, red blood cells, white blood cells, squamous and/or transitional epithelial cells on microscopy

Abnormal
- pH outside normal range
- Specific gravity outside normal range
- Presence of red blood cells, leukocytes, protein, glucose, bilirubin, ketones, nitrites, urobilinogen on dipstick

321

- Presence of significant numbers of microorganisms, casts, crystals, red blood cells, white blood cells, squamous and/or transitional epithelial cells on microscopy
- Keep in mind the possibility of a false-positive result

Cause of abnormal result
- Abnormalities may result from presence of renal calculus, infection, contamination of sample, kidney damage, diabetes, dehydration
- High pH (over 7.0) may indicate renal tubular acidosis or the presence of urea-splitting microorganisms with resultant struvite stones
- low pH (under 5.0) may indicate uric acid stone formation

Drugs, disorders and other factors that may alter results
- Many medications can affect results, therefore a complete drug history must be obtained prior to interpreting results of urinalysis, e.g. rifampin turns urine orange
- Dilute urine alters specific gravity/osmolarity and increases risk of false negative results
- Old urine or urine exposed to air will have a falsely elevated pH due to diffusional loss of CO_2

URINE CULTURE WITH ANTIBIOTIC SENSITIVITIES
Description
Clean-catch, midstream urine specimen.

Advantages/Disadvantages
Usually easy for patients to provide specimen; can utilize quick, in-and-out, sterile straight-catheter specimen if necessary.

Normal
No microorganisms present.

Abnormal
- Presence of significant bacterial growth
- Particular significance if urease-splitting organisms are identified (may be source of struvite calculi)
- Keep in mind the possibility of a false-positive result

Cause of abnormal result
- True bacterial infection
- Accidental specimen contamination

BLOOD TESTS
Description
Blood sample, for measurement of electrolytes, calcium, uric acid, creatinine, blood urea nitrogen (BUN), and phosphate.

Advantages/Disadvantages
- Relatively easy collection
- Multiple vacuum tubes can be collected simultaneously to perform battery of blood tests

Normal
Serum sodium: 135–147mEq/l (135–147mmol/l)
Serum potassium: 3–5mEq/l (3–5mmol/l)
Serum chloride: 95–105mEq/l (95–105mmol/l)
Serum carbon dioxide: 24–30mEq/l (24–30mmol/l)
Serum calcium: 8.8–10.3mg/dl (2.2–2.58mmol/l)
Serum uric acid: 2–7mg/dl (50–110mcmol/l)

Serum creatinine: 0.6–1.2mg/dl (120–420mcmol/l)
Blood urea nitrogen: (BUN) 8–18mg/dl (3–6.5mcmol/l)
Serum phosphate: 2.5–5mg/dl (0.8–1.6mmol/l)

Abnormal
- Values outside the normal range
- Keep in mind the possibility of a false-positive result

Cause of abnormal result
- Metabolic abnormalities which are the underlying cause of nephrolithiasis
- Altered renal function

Drugs, disorders and other factors that may alter results
- Calcium level should be corrected according to albumin concentration
- Dehydration and IV hydration can make interpretation of results difficult
- Drugs to control gout may affect serum uric acid levels
- Family history should be obtained regarding electrolyte abnormalities such as familial hypocalciuric hypercalcemia

24-HOUR URINE COLLECTION
Description
24 hours-worth of urine, collected in a single jug, and refrigerated throughout test (results are most useful when correlated with results of accompanying blood sample).

Advantages/Disadvantages
- Collection is simple, although patient must schedule activities so as not to be away from refrigerated jug when need to urinate arises
- Patient must also attempt to keep to normal schedule of eating and drinking, rather than pushing fluids during time-frame of urine collection

Normal
- Creatinine: 15–25 mg/kg
- Calcium: <200 mg/day
- Citrate: <320 mg/day
- Cystine: <200 mg/day
- Oxalate: <44 mg/day
- Uric acid: <600 mg/day

Abnormal
- Values outside the normal range
- Keep in mind the possibility of a false-positive result

Cause of abnormal result
- Dietary excess
- Over-hydration
- Metabolic abnormality, such as hypercalciuria, hyperuricosuria, hypocitraturia, hypomagnesuria, cystinuria
- Renal abnormality, such as renal tubular acidosis

Drugs, disorders and other factors that may alter results
Many drugs can affect urine contents, therefore a careful drug history must be attained, i.e. administration of vitamin D to prevent osteoporosis or to treat hyperparathyroidism may induce hypercalciuria.

Imaging

PLAIN ABDOMINAL FILM, KIDNEY, URETER AND BLADDER (KUB)

Advantages/Disadvantages

- Simple, quick, noninvasive
- Yields low specificity and sensitivity for identifying renal calculi
- Most useful for tracking previously identified radio-opaque calculi

Normal

- No stones present
- Keep in mind relatively high rate of false-negatives

Abnormal

- Stones present
- Keep in mind the possibility of imaging artifacts

Cause of abnormal result

- Renal calculus formation
- Passage of renal calculus

RENAL ULTRASONOGRAPHY

Advantages/Disadvantages

- Noninvasive
- Can be performed on pregnant patients
- May demonstrate hydronephrosis, hydroureter
- If hydronephrosis and/or hydroureter are absent, and calculus is relatively small, test may yield a false negative

Normal

Normal anatomy, no stone visualized.

Abnormal

- Presence of hydronephrosis, hydroureter
- Visualization of calculus
- Keep in mind the possibility of imaging artifacts

Cause of abnormal result

- Renal calculus formation
- Passage of renal calculus
- Renal obstruction

Drugs, disorders and other factors that may alter results

- Ultrasound scanning is most commonly performed by a radiographer and is a very operator-dependent test
- An experienced operator is less likely to produce a false negative result

SPIRAL OR HELICAL COMPUTED TOMOGRAPHY

Advantages/Disadvantages

- Noninvasive and quick
- Low exposure to radiation
- Can rule out other serious disease (abdominal aneurysm, bowel disease, pancreatitis, appendicitis, biliary tract disease)
- Can detect radiolucent stones that are not visible on KUB film
- Does not reveal information relating to renal function or degree of obstruction

Normal
Normal anatomy.

Abnormal
- Presence of renal calculus
- Keep in mind the possibility of imaging artifacts

Cause of abnormal result
Renal calculus, passage of calculus.

INTRAVENOUS PYELOGRAM
Advantages/Disadvantages
- Gives excellent and accurate information regarding presence of renal calculi, passage of calculi into ureter, renal function, presence/degree of renal obstruction
- Requires intravenous administration of dye, with patient discomfort
- Iodine-sensitive patients at risk of nephrotoxicity secondary to the contrast dye, or allergic or anaphylactic reaction
- Significant degree of exposure to radiation

Normal
Normal anatomy, normal function.

Abnormal
- Presence of renal calculi; passing calculus; delayed passage of dye into ureter; hydronephrosis; hydroureter; perirenal extravasation of contrast dye
- Keep in mind the possibility of imaging artifacts

Cause of abnormal result
Presence of calculus or ureteral obstruction.

Drugs, disorders and other factors that may alter results
- In females the right ureter at the level of L4–5 may appear compressed due to the passage of the ovarian vein
- Dilation of the middle third of the ureters is a normal finding due to compression by the iliac vessels
- Bladder shape can be altered in women superiorly by the uterus while the bladder base may be altered in men by a hypertrophic prostate.

Special tests
CALCULUS ANALYSIS
Description
Analysis of passed calculus.

Advantages/Disadvantages
Gives information regarding the chemical composition of a calculus which has been passed.

Abnormal
May reveal calcium oxalate calculi; uric acid calculi; struvite calculi; cystine calculi; dihydroxyadenine calculi, xanthine calculi, triamterene calculi; calculi containing proteinaceous or fungal material.

Cause of abnormal result
Tendency to calculus formation.

TREATMENT

CONSIDER CONSULT

- When passing a calculus is complicated by renal obstruction
- If the patient has had multiple calculi
- When the patient is pregnant
- If the patient is under 16

IMMEDIATE ACTION

- Consider immediate administration of medications for pain control
- Consider imaging to rule out obstruction and hydronephrosis

PATIENT AND CAREGIVER ISSUES
Patient or caregiver request

- **Am I more susceptible to kidney stones in the future?** Stones are likely to recur. After passing the first stone, the likelihood of forming a second stone after 1 year is 14%, 35% within 5 years and 52% within 10 years
- **Is there any way I can prevent recurrence?** The risk of recurrence can be decreased by reducing risk factors

MANAGEMENT ISSUES
Goals

- Relieve pain
- Ensure any complications, including infection and obstruction, are identified and treated
- Reduce the risk of recurrence

Management in special circumstances

SPECIAL PATIENT GROUPS

Pregnant patients and children with symptoms suggestive of acute obstruction may be referred to a urologist

PATIENT SATISFACTION/LIFESTYLE PRIORITIES

Inform patient that many medications used to control pain have significant side-effects which interfere with alertness

SUMMARY OF THERAPEUTIC OPTIONS
Choices

- NSAIDs are being increasingly utilized for pain control, particularly IV ketorolac
- IV narcotic analgesics for pain control
- Pushing fluids (orally if tolerated by patient; intravenously if not) has both proponents and opponents; proponents stating that increasing fluid intake can "push" the calculus through the urinary system; opponents stating that increased fluid intake may result in increased pain in patients with obstruction secondary to calculus. There is no evidence that forced diuresis enhances the passing of the stone
- If infection is present, treat with appropriate antibiotics based on antibiotic sensitivities found on urine culture
- In patients with struvite stones, especially staghorn calculi, removal of the stones (by extracorporeal shock wave lithotripsy, percutaneous nephrolithotomy or ureteroscopy) is indicated, with antibiotic flush of the kidneys
- Advise all patients on lifestyle measures relating to hydration and diet
- Supplementation with magnesium and vitamin B6 may be effective in preventing kidney stone recurrences
- A number of other therapeutic options are available for recurrences

Guidelines
The American Urological Association, Inc. (AUA) has produced guidelines [1]
According to the guidelines:

- Patients with calculi bearing high probability of spontaneous passage: provide adequate pain relief, await passage of calculus
- Patients with calculi bearing low probability of spontaneous passage: provide information regarding risks/benefits of various intervention strategies
- Patients with calculus < 1 cm, located in proximal ureter: recommend extracorporeal shock wave lithotripsy
- Patients with calculus > 1 cm, located in proximal ureter: recommend extracorporeal shock wave lithotripsy, percutaneous nephrolithotomy, or ureteroscopy
- Patients with calculus located in distal ureter: recommend extracorporeal shock wave lithotripsy or ureteroscopy

Never
Never dismiss a patient that has an obstructed ureter, fever, raised white cell count and a urinalysis that reveals bacterial content. These individuals can develop severe sepsis with shock and multiorgan systems failure. They should immediately be brought to the attention of the urologist.

FOLLOW UP
Plan for review
- Patients with complicated calculi (infection, obstruction, intractable pain, patients with poor renal function or single kidney) should be referred to a urologist
- Recovered calculi should be sent for analysis
- 24-hour urine collection should be undertaken to begin metabolic assessment in patients with repeated calculi

Information for patient or caregiver
Until results of 24-hour urine collection and other metabolic workups are available:

- Patients should be instructed to increase their fluid intake considerably (ideally to around 4 pints per day)
- The patient should be advised to drink half a pint of fluid just before bedtime to dilute urine during sleep
- Reasonable dietary intake of sodium, animal protein, and oxalate should be discussed

DRUGS AND OTHER THERAPIES: DETAILS
Drugs
KETOROLAC
Dose
30mg IM, loading dose; follow with 15–30mg every 6 hours as required. Maximum dose recommended is 120mg/day.

Efficacy
- Thought to be equal in efficacy to 100mg of meperidine
- Theoretically is thought to relieve ureteral muscle spasm

Risks/Benefits
Risks:
- More expensive than many opiate analgesics
- Poor choice for people with one kidney, chronic renal insufficiency, may exacerbate renal failure
- Use caution in renal or hepatic disease

- Use caution in the elderly
- Use caution in diabetes mellitus
- Use caution in immunosuppression
- Use caution in congestive heart failure

Benefit: Compared to opiate analgesics, ketorolac causes less nausea and sedation, doesn't depress respiration, and isn't a drug of abuse

Side-effects and adverse reactions
- Gastrointestinal: abdominal pain, nausea, vomiting, diarrhea, constipation, dyspepsia, peptic ulcer, gastrointestinal bleeding, perforation, elevated hepatic enzymes
- Central nervous system: headache, dizziness, drowsiness, seizures
- Hematologic: purpura, thrombocytopenia, anemia, agranulocytosis, leukopenia, neutropenia
- Genitourinary: uremia, hematuria, proteinuria, acute renal failure
- Cardiovascular system: edema
- Ears, eyes, nose and throat: (ophthamlic) blurred vision, ocular irritation and inflammation, iritis
- Skin: rashes, urticaria, maculopapular rash, sweating, pruritus

Interactions (other drugs)
- ACE inhibitors ▪ Alcohol ▪ Alendronate ▪ Anticoagulants ▪ Antineoplastic agents ▪ Beta blockers ▪ Cidofovir ▪ Corticosteroids ▪ Cyclosporine ▪ Diuretics ▪ Lithium ▪ Methotrexate ▪ NSAIDs ▪ Platelet inhibitors ▪ Probenecid ▪ Salicylates ▪ Thrombolytic agents

Contraindications
- Renal impairment or dehydration ▪ History of, or active, gastrointestinal disease, bleeding, perforation, peptic ulcer or ulcerative colitis ▪ Concurrent NSAIDs ▪ Probenecid ▪ Cidofovir ▪ Epidural/intrathecal administration ▪ Cerebrovascular disease or bleeding ▪ Should not be used as a prophylactic analgesic before surgery, during surgery or during labor ▪ Pregnancy and breastfeeding

Acceptability to patient
Currently only administered IV or IM; efficacy of oral dosing not established; therefore ketorolac tends to be given only in physician's office, or when patient is hospitalized.

NARCOTIC ANALGESICS
Dose
- Morphine: 4–15mg every 4 hours as needed, SC/IM; 5–30mg every 4 hours as needed, orally
- Meperidine: 50–150mg every 3–4 hours as needed, PO/IM/IV/SC
- Acetaminophen and Hydrocodone: 5–10mg every 4–6 hours as needed, orally

Efficacy
Proven efficacious.

Risks/Benefits
Risks:
- Significant risks of nausea, sedation, respiratory depression
- Known potential for abuse/addiction
- Use caution in the elderly and children under 18 years old
- Use caution in hepatic and renal disease
- Use caution in hypothryoidism and Addison's disease
- Use caution in abdominal disorders
- Use caution in prostatic hypertrophy

Benefit: Low cost

Side-effects and adverse reactions
- Gastrointestinal: constipation, nausea, vomiting, abdominal pain, biliary spasm
- Central nervous system: drowsiness, sedation, headache, vertigo, hallucinations, dysphoria, euphoria, mood changes, dependence, anxiety, restlessness
- Ears, eyes, nose and throat: dry mouth, miosis, blurred vision
- Cardiovascular system: bradycardia, tachycardia, palpitations, hypotension, hypertension, syncope
- Genitourinary: urinary difficulties, decreased libido
- Skin: rashes, pruritis, urticaria, sweating, flushing
- Respiratory: respiratory depression

Interactions (other drugs)
- Alcohol ▪ Anticoagulants ▪ Antidepressants (tricyclic) ▪ Antihistamines ▪ Antihypertensives ▪ Antipsychotics ▪ Anxiolytics and Hypnotics ▪ Cimetidine ▪ Ciprofloxacin ▪ Domperidone ▪ Esmolol ▪ MAOIs ▪ Metoclopramide ▪ Mexiletine ▪ Moclobemide ▪ Opiate antagonists ▪ Rifamycins ▪ Ritonavir

Contraindications
- Heart failure secondary to chronic lung disease ▪ Cardiac arrhythmias ▪ Brain tumor ▪ Acute alcoholism ▪ MAOI therapy (within 14 days) ▪ Delerium tremens ▪ Hemorrhage ▪ Convulsive states ▪ Respiratory depression ▪ Acute asthma attack ▪ Paralytic ileus ▪ Head injury or raised intracranial pressure ▪ Injection in pheochromocytoma

Patient and caregiver information
Patient should be made aware that they will not become addicted to opiates when they are used for analgesia in the acute setting for a limited period of time.

ALLOPURINOL
Dose
200–300mg, orally, once daily for prevention of recurrence in patients with uric acid stones.

Efficacy
Excellent; always brings down uric acid.

Risks/Benefits
Risks:
- Hypersensitivity, rash, elevated liver function test results (all rare)
- Ensure adequate fluid intake during treatment
- Caution in hepatic and renal impairment

Benefit: new stone formation reduced or eliminated

Side-effects and adverse reactions
- Gastrointestinal: nausea, abdominal pain, peptic ulceration, cholestatic jaundice, diarrhea, liver failure
- Genitourinary: renal failure
- Skin: rashes, alopecia, Stevens-Johnson syndrome
- Central nervous system: drowsiness, headache
- Musculoskeletal: athralgia, myopathy

Interactions (other drugs)
- ACE inhibitors ■ Antacids ■ Azathioprine ■ Cyclophosphamide ■ Mercaptopurine
- Oral anticoagulants ■ Theophylline

Contraindications
Relative contraindication is concurrent acute gout.

Acceptability to patient
High: great advantage is once-daily dose and rarity of side-effects.

HYDROCHLOROTHIAZIDE
Thiazides have been shown to reduce stone formation rates.

Dose
12.5–50mg once daily for prevention of recurrence of stones in hypercalciuric patients.

Risks/Benefits
- In patients with an underlying metabolic disorder such as primary hyperparathyroidism, thiazides may produce hypercalciuria
- Other drugs can alter effectiveness i.e., excess vitamin D therapy and thiazides can produce hypercalciuria
- May exacerbate systemic lupus erythematosus
- Use caution in renal and hepatic disease
- Use caution in the elderly, pregnancy and breastfeeding
- May aggravate diabetes or gout
- May cause hypokalemia
- Use caution in serum electrolyte imbalances
- Use caution in sulfonamide and carbonic anydrase inhibitor hypersensitivity

Side-effects and adverse reactions
- Gastrointestinal: nausea, vomiting, diarrhea, constipation, abdominal pain
- Metabolic: hypokalemia, hypomagnesemia, hyponatremia, hypercalcemia, hypochloremic alkalosis, hyperuricaemia, hyperglycemia, and altered plasma lipid concentration
- Cardiovascular system: postural hypotension
- Central nervous system: headache, dizziness, vertigo, weakness
- Hematologic: agranulocytosis, aplastic anemia, pancytopenia, hemolytic anemia, leukopenia, and thrombocytopenia
- Genitourinary: urinary problems, impotence
- Skin: rashes, urticaria, Steven-Johnson's syndrome, exfoliative dermatitis, photosensitivity

Interactions (other drugs)
- ACE inhibitors ■ Allopurinol ■ Anesthetics ■ Anticholinergics ■ Antineoplastics
- Anticoagulants ■ Antidiabetics ■ Antigout ■ Calcium salts ■ Cardiac glycosides
- Cholestyramine, colestipol ■ Corticosteroids ■ Diazoxide ■ Disopyramide ■ Fluconazole
- Lithium ■ Loop diuretics ■ Methotrexate ■ Nondepolarizing muscular blockers
- NSAIDs ■ Vitamin D

Contraindications
- Anuria ■ Severe renal or hepatic impairment ■ Refractory hyponatremia, hypokalemia, hypercalcemia ■ Addison's disease

Acceptability to patient
- Side-effects may be troublesome
- Patient will need biochemical follow-up

Follow up plan
- Serum calcium and other electrolyte levels should be monitored for two months after initiating thiazide therapy
- If a patient requires medication to control stone disease they should be under the care of a urologist

Patient and caregiver information
- Take with food or milk
- May cause sensitivity to sunlight

CELLULOSE SODIUM PHOSPHATE
Dose
15g per day, divided between each meal, then 10g per day when calcium excretion <150mg in 24 hours, for the prevention of recurrence of stones in patients with absorptive hypercalciuria.

Efficacy
Significantly reduces urinary calcium excretion.

Risks/Benefits
- May increase oxaluria
- May increase risk of osteoporosis
- Use caution in congestive heart failure
- Use caution in ascites
- Use caution in liver impairment
- Use caution in pregnancy
- Use caution in the elderly

Side-effects and adverse reactions
- Gastrointestinal: nausea, vomiting, diarrhea, dyspepsia
- Metabolic: magnesium deficiency
- Genitourinary: hypomagnesuria, hyperoxaluria, hyperphosphaturia

Interactions (other drugs)
No known interactions.

Contraindications
- Hypomagnesemia, hypocalcemia ▪ Hyperparathyroidism ▪ Children under 16 years old
- Osteoporosis, osteomalacia, osteitis ▪ Hyperoxaluria ▪ Severe renal impairment

Patient and caregiver information
The powder should be suspended in water, soft drink or fruit juice and taken within 30 minutes of a meal.

TIOPRONIN
Dose
800–1000mg/day, divided into three doses at least 1 hour before or 2 hours after meals, for the prevention of recurrence of cystine stones.

Risks/Benefits
Risks:
- Dosage regime is complex
- Use caution in Goodpasture's syndrome
- Use caution in children
- Use caution in patients who have shown toxicity to d-penicillamine

Benefit: significant reduction in urinary cystine

Side-effects and adverse reactions
- Gastrointestinal: nausea, vomiting, diarrhea, abdominal pain and bloating, jaundice
- Genitourinary: hematuria, proteinuria, nephrotic syndrome
- Metabolic: vitamin B6 deficiency
- Skin: rash, lupus erythematous-like reaction, pruritis, wrinkling, friability
- Hematologic: increased bleeding, anemia, leukopenia, thrombocytopenia, eosinophilia
- Ears, eyes, nose and throat: taste and smell disturbances
- Respiratory: dyspnea, bronchiolitis
- Central nervous system: myasthenic syndrome
- Hypersensitivity: adenopathy, fever, chills, dyspnea, myalgia, drug fever

Interactions (other drugs)
No known interactions.

Contraindications
- Thrombocytopenia or aplastic anemia on this treatment ■ History of agranulocytosis
- Pregnancy and breast feeding

Follow up plan
If patient is taking a medication to control their stone disease they should be under the care of a physician.

Patient and caregiver information
Review the dosage regime carefully.

Surgical therapy
EXTRACORPOREAL SHOCKWAVE LITHOTRIPSY (ESWL)
Efficacy
Efficacious as a sole therapy for about 70% of stones.

Risks/Benefits
- May require multiple primary treatments for adequate fragmentation
- May require ancillary treatment.
- Contraindicated for pregnant patients; patients with certain bleeding tendencies; obese patients weighing >300 lbs.; impacted stones; cystine stones; distal ureteral obstruction
- Minimally invasive and can often be performed without anesthesia or under intravenous sedation

Evidence
- Shock wave lithotripsy is recommended as a first line therapy for most patients with stones 1cm or less in the proximal ureter [1] *Level C*
- Shock wave lithotripsy is an acceptable treatment option for patients with stones greater than 1cm in the proximal ureter [1] *Level C*
- Shock wave lithotripsy is effective for the management of distal urethral stones [1] *Level C*

Acceptability to patient
High patient satisfaction, minimally invasive with few side-effects.

Follow up plan
Must follow up to ensure that stone fragments have been passed, no obstruction has supervened.

Patient and caregiver information
- Patient may note blood in the urine for several days following ESWL and bruising/tenderness of back and/or abdomen
- Fragmented bits of calculi may continue to cause pain as they pass

- A ureteral stent may be required to drain the kidney past inflammation
- The patient should be aware of signs of infection

URETEROSCOPY
Efficacy
A higher success rate than lithotripsy. Particularly efficacious for stones impacted below the iliac crest.

Risks/Benefits
- Requires anesthesia or heavy sedation
- Good success rate
- Low risk of requiring multiple or ancillary treatments
- A stent may need to be placed for up to a week post operatively

Evidence
- Uteroscopy is an acceptable treatment option for patients with stones greater than 1cm in the proximal ureter. Uteroscopy may be less appropriate for larger stones [1] *Level C*
- Uteroscopy is an acceptable alternative option to lithotripsy (when lithotripsy is inappropriate or fails), in patients with stones less than or equal to1cm in the proximal ureter [1] *Level C*
- Uteroscopy is an effective treatment option for distal ureteric stones [1] *Level C*

Acceptability to patient
May require general anesthesia which carries its own risks.

Follow up plan
Requires careful surveillance for post-procedure urinary infections.

Patient and caregiver information
Patient will require information regarding how to self-monitor for development of infection.

PERCUTANEOUS NEPHROLITHOTOMY
Efficacy
Proven efficacious.

Risks/Benefits
- Requires anesthesia, heavy sedation
- Removes stone fragments, rather than awaiting passage
- Safest procedure when intervention is required in a pregnant patient
- Can remove stones that are greater than 2cm diameter that are not amenable to ESWL
- Can remove stones of different chemical composition, ie cystine, calcium oxalate.

Evidence
- Percutaneous nephrolithotomy is an acceptable alternative option to lithotripsy (when lithotripsy is inappropriate or fails), in patients with stones less than or equal to1cm in the proximal ureter [1] *Level C*
- Percutaneous nephrolithotomy is also an acceptable treatment option for patients with stones greater than 1cm in the proximal ureter [1] *Level C*

Acceptability to patient
May require placement of a nephrostomy tube.

Follow up plan
This is an invasive procedure that will require hospitalization in the immediate post operative period.

Patient and caregiver information
- Education regarding nephrostomy tube
- How to self-monitor for development of infection

Complementary therapy
MAGNESIUM AND VITAMIN B6
Efficacy
Magnesium increases the solubility of calcium oxalate, thereby inhibiting precipitation of calcium phosphate and calcium oxalate as stones. A low urinary magnesium:calcium ratio is an independent risk factor for stone formation. Supplementation with magnesium has been shown to be effective in preventing kidney stone recurrences. Adding vitamin B6 provides even greater benefit. Patients with recurrent oxalate stones show chemical evidence of insufficient B6 activity, and supplementation returns these levels to normal within 3 months.

Risks/Benefits
Certain forms of magnesium can cause gastrointestinal irritation and diarrhea. Very high dose vitamin B6 (>150–200mg/day over many months) has been reported to cause peripheral neuropathy.

Acceptability to patient
Both magnesium and vitamin B6 in the doses recommended are affordable and well tolerated.

Follow up plan
Standard patient care.

Patient and caregiver information
- Vitamin B6 25mg/day
- Magnesium 600mg/day
- Magnesium citrate and oxide tend to cause diarrhea; magnesium gluconate or chelate tend to be better tolerated.

LIFESTYLE

- Need to increase hydration to around 4 pints of fluid daily
- Recommend half a pint of fluid before bedtime, to keep urine from becoming overly-concentrated during sleep
- May need to decrease dietary intake of animal protein, oxalate-containing foodstuffs, sodium
- Contrary to previous practices, dietary calcium should not be restricted in the vast majority of nephrolithiasis patients
- Increasing fiber in the diet may be help prevent calculus formation
- Variable intake for different individuals, drink enough water to produce 3 litres of urine per day
- Reduction of alcohol consumption, dietary fat, and vitamin D enriched food may also reduce calculus formation

RISKS/BENEFITS

Increased hydration and improved diet will bring all-round health benefits.

ACCEPTABILITY TO PATIENT

Lifestyle changes, including dietary changes, are some of the hardest for patients to maintain; support will be needed to encourage adherence to increase fluid intake and decreased animal protein, oxalate, and/or sodium intake.

FOLLOW UP PLAN

Repeat 24-hour urine studies after sufficient time on altered diet/fluid intake schedule, to verify that these interventions are having desired effect on urine composition.

PATIENT AND CAREGIVER INFORMATION

Patients may need to be taught how to monitor their own fluid balance in order to produce approximately 3 litres of urine. This will require consuming a variable amount of fluid depending on the individual and other fluid losses.

EFFICACY OF THERAPIES

Stones can be removed endoscopically with greater than a 95% certainty.

Evidence

PDxMD are unable to cite evidence which meets our criteria for evidence.

PROGNOSIS

Most renal calculi (about 80–85%) pass spontaneously within a few days. Those that don't, or those which are complicated by obstruction, infection, intractable pain, or large stone size may require surgical intervention.

Therapeutic failure

Patients with recurrent stones should be referred to a urologist.

Recurrence

- Recurrence rates are considerable: 14% within 1 year of first calculus episode; 35% within 5 years; 52% within 10 years
- In recurrent calculi, more extensive metabolic workup may indicate the need for metabolic intervention based on the type of calculus formed
- Patients with recurrent calculi should be referred to a urologist
- Patients identified as having uric acid stones may require treatment with uric acid-lowering agents, including allopurinol
- Patients identified as being hypercalciuric may benefit from diuretic administration (particularly hydrochlorothiazide)
- Patients identified with absorptive hypercalciuria may benefit from cellulose sodium phosphate
- Patients with cystine stones may require administration of tiopronin
- Patients with struvite stones may require prophylactic antibiotic administration with or without adjunctive acetohydroxamic acid treatment
- Patients with underlying disorders (sarcoidosis or other granulomatous conditions, thyroid disease, parathyroid disease, inflammatory bowel disease, malignancy) will benefit from careful treatment of the underlying condition

COMPLICATIONS

- Obstruction
- Infection
- Hematuria

CONSIDER CONSULT

- Complications necessitate referral to a urologist

RISK FACTORS
Inadequate hydration: this causes concentrated urine, the most important cause of urinary stones.

MODIFY RISK FACTORS
Lifestyle and wellness
DIET
2–4 pints of fluid per day is recommended

PHYSICAL ACTIVITY
It is important to avoid exercise-induced dehydration

PREVENT RECURRENCE
- The key factor in preventing recurrence is adequate hydration
- Dietary modification can be of benefit.
- Specific metabolic interventions are effective in reducing new stone formation

RESOURCES

ASSOCIATIONS
National Institute of Diabetes and Digestive and Kidney Diseases (NIDDK)
National Institutes of Health
31 Center Drive
MSC 2560
Bethesda
MD 20892–2560
USA
http://www.niddk.nih.gov/

KEY REFERENCES
- Craig, Sandy. "Renal Calculi," from emedicine at http://www.emedicine.com.
- Curhan, Gary C. Concise Review: Calcium Intake and the Risk of Kidney Stones. In: Harrison's Principles of Internal Medicine, edited by Anthony S. Fauci. New York: McGraw-Hill, 1998.
- Goldfarb, David S, Coe FL. Prevention of Recurrent Nephrolithiasis. In: American Family Physician, November 15, 1999.
- Graber, Mark A, Viviana Martinez-Bianchi. Genitorurinary and Renal Disease: Urolithiasis. In: University of Iowa Family Practice Handbook. http://www.vh.org.
- Kidney Stones in Adults. National Institute of Diabetes and Digestive and Kidney Diseases at National Institutes of Health. http://www.niddk.nih.gov.
- Menon, Mani et al. Urinary Lithiasis. In Walsh: Campbell's Urology. Philadelphia: W.B. Saunders Company, 1998.
- National Guideline Clearinghouse, Brief Summary: The Management of Ureteral Calculi from American Urological Association.
- National Guideline Clearinghouse, Complete Summary: The Management of Ureteral Calculi from American Urological Association.
- Segura JW, Preminger GM, Assimos DG, Dretler SP, Kahn RI, Lingeman JE, Macaluso JN Jr. Special communication. Ureteral Stones Clinical Guidelines Panel summary report on the management of ureteral calculi. J Urol 1997 Nov;158(5):1915–21.
- Special Medical Reports: American Urological Association Recommends Observation for the Majority of Cases of Ureteral Calculi. In American Family Physician, February 15, 1998.

Guidelines
1 The American Urological Association, Inc. (AUA) has produced guidelines. The management of ureteral calculi. Ureteral Stones Clinical Guidelines Panel Members and Consultants, 1997. Available at the National Guidelines Clearing house

FAQS
Question 1
How do stones form?

ANSWER 1
Multiple factors are involved in stone formation. Some of the most common are:
- Urinary supersaturation
- Reduced urinary stone inhibitors
- The presence of urinary proteins

Question 2
What are the most common stones?

ANSWER 2
Calcium stones, followed by infection stones, uric acid stones, and cystine stones.

Question 3
What are the indications for stone surgery?

ANSWER 3
Surgery for stone removal is indicated when:
- There is persistent pain
- Recurrent, gross hematuria
- Obstruction with progressive renal damage
- Recurrent urinary tract infection

Question 4
Is there a stone that can be dissolved with medication?

ANSWER 4
Pure uric acid stones are dissolved with oral alkalinization, potassium citrate, sodium bicarbonate with the goal to bring the urinary pH between 6.5–7.0.

Question 5
What stones resist therapy with extracorporeal shock wave lithotripsy?

ANSWER 5
Cystine stones

CONTRIBUTORS
Martin L Kabongo, MD, PhD
Jane L Murray, MD
Philip J Aliotta, MD, MHA, FACS
Vitaly Raykhman, MD

NEPHRITIC SYNDROME

SUMMARY INFORMATION

DESCRIPTION

- Denotes the clinical syndrome of active glomerulonephritis of hematuria, red blood cell casts, and dystrophic red blood cells in the urine sediment and minimal-to-moderate proteinuria
- Due to a variety of known and unknown etiologies
- In severe cases may be associated with decreased glomerular filtration rate, salt and water retention, and hypertension
- Related to inflammation in the glomeruli, which may be focal or diffuse and, in some cases, immune complex deposition in the glomeruli or antiglomerular basement membrane antibodies, which can be triggered by a number of diseases
- Therapy is generally supportive, but specific therapies are available for a limited subset of patients
- Prognosis depends on etiology and degree of renal damage

URGENT ACTION

- Assess for acute renal failure
- Assess for hypertensive urgency or emergency and treat as indicated
- Assess electrocardiogram for changes related to hyperkalemia, pericardial tamponade, or arrhythmia and treat as indicated
- Assess for pulmonary edema and treat as indicated
- Assess indications for dialysis, with urgent referral if present: intractable uremic symptoms; refractory fluid overload; refractory hyperkalemia; refractory severe acidosis; encephalopathy or seizures; creatinine clearance or glomerular filtration rate <10–15mL/min

KEY! DON'T MISS!

These signs or symptoms require urgent action:

- Hypertensive urgency or emergency
- ECG changes related to hyperkalemia, pericarditis, or arrhythmia
- Pulmonary edema
- Indications for dialysis: intractable uremic symptoms, refractory fluid overload, refractory hyperkalemia, encephalopathy or seizures, creatinine clearance or glomerular filtration rate <10–15mL/min

BACKGROUND

ICD9 CODE

- 580.9 Glomerulonephritis, acute
- 583.4 Glomerulonephritis, rapidly progressive, necrotizing
- 582.9 Glomerulonephritis, chronic

SYNONYMS

- Active nephritis
- Acute nephritis
- Rapidly progressing glomerulonephritis (RPGN)

CARDINAL FEATURES

- Denotes the clinical syndrome of active glomerulonephritis due to a variety of known and unknown etiologies
- Characterized by gross or microscopic hematuria with urine sediment containing rbc casts and/or dysmorphic red blood cells and mild-to-moderate proteinuria ($<3.5g/24h$ ($40mg/m^2/h$ in children))
- In severe cases, associated with decreased glomerular filtration rate, hypertension, and signs of fluid overload
- Related to inflammation and, in some cases, immune complex deposition in the glomeruli or antiglomerular basement membrane antibodies that can be triggered by a number of diseases
- Inflammatory and proliferative changes in glomeruli may be focal or diffuse
- Course can be transient (as when related to infection), indolent (as in thin basement membrane disease), or rapidly progressive (as in certain autoimmune or pauci immune disorders)
- Therapy is generally supportive, but specific therapies are available for a limited subset of patients
- Prognosis depends on etiology and degree of renal damage and, in some cases, timeliness of therapy

CAUSES

Common causes

Idiopathic:

- Idiopathic glomerulonephritis
- Immunoglobulin A (IgA) nephropathy
- Membranoproliferative glomerulonephritis types I and II

Hereditary:

- Alport's disease
- Thin basement membrane disease

Immune response to bacterial infection:

- Group A beta-hemolytic *Streptococcus*
- Bacterial endocarditis
- Chronic bacteremia (e.g. shunts, visceral abscesses)
- Sepsis
- *Staphylococcus* species
- *Pneumococcus* species
- *Klebsiella* pneumonia

Immune response to viral infection:

- Hepatitis B
- Hepatitis C

- Varicella
- Coxsackie virus
- Epstein-Barr virus
- Rubeola
- Mumps

Drug induced:
- Gold
- Penicillamine

Other causes:
- Systemic lupus erythematosus (SLE)
- Cryoglobulinemia
- Vasculitis
- Henoch-Schönlein purpura
- Wegener's granulomatosis
- Polyarteritis nodosa (microscopic)

Rapidly progressive (crescentic) glomerulonephritis (RPGN):
- Pauci-immune RPGN
- Immune complex RPGN
- Antiglomerular basement membrane (GBM) antibody disease
- Goodpasture's syndrome (glomerulonephritis with lung hemorrhage and anti-GBM antibodies)
- Idiopathic
- Churg-Strauss Disease (RPGN with asthma and eosinophilia)

Rare causes
- Typhoid fever
- Syphilis
- Malaria
- Toxoplasmosis
- Schistosomiasis

Serious causes
RPGN of any etiology can be fulminant with progression to end-stage renal disease in 80% of untreated patients within 6 months.

Contributory or predisposing factors
Slight hereditary and environmental predisposition has been reported in cases of acute glomerulonephritis.

EPIDEMIOLOGY

Incidence and prevalence

Variable and depends on specific etiologies.

PREVALENCE
0.04/1000 people.

Demographics

AGE
- All age groups can be affected
- More than half of patients are under 13 years old
- Causative disorders may show an age difference (e.g. poststreptococcal glomerulonephritis, IgA nephropathy, and Henoch-Schönlein purpura are more commonly seen in children and adolescents)

GENDER
Generally, no gender predilection except:
- In Alport's disease is typically more severe and progressive in males compared with females
- Some causative disorders may show a gender difference (e.g. IgA nephropathy, Henoch-Schönlein purpura, and Goodpasture's syndrome are more commonly seen in males)

RACE
- Generally, no racial predilection
- Causative disorders may show a racial difference (for example, IgA nephropathy is rarely seen in African-Americans and is a common form of nephritis in people of Asian descent)

GENETICS
Genetic predisposition is seen with Alport's disease, thin basement membrane disease, and systemic lupus erythematosus.

GEOGRAPHY
- Generally, no geographic predilection in idiopathic cases but outbreaks have occurred in areas of high altitude
- Causative disorders may show a geographic difference (e.g. IgA nephropathy is two to four times more common in southern Europe and Australia than in the US, and six to eight times more common in Asia)

SOCIOECONOMIC STATUS
Poststreptococcal glomerulonephritis is more common in lower socioeconomic groups.

DIFFERENTIAL DIAGNOSIS

Prerenal (hypovolemic) acute renal failure

Prerenal (hypovolemic) acute renal failure results from inadequate perfusion of the kidneys due to decreased effective circulating arterial volume (although total plasma volume may be increased).

FEATURES

- History of hypovolemia or hypotension
- Oliguria
- Urine sediment may contain only hyaline casts; no red blood cell (RBC) casts or dysmorphic RBCs
- Blood urea nitrogen (BUN):creatinine ratio over 20:1
- Fractional excretion of sodium below 1% (note: acute glomerulonephritis and radiocontrast-induced renal failure may also produce fractional excretion under 1% but are not prerenal conditions)
- Urine osmolality above 500mOsm/kg unless renal failure is severe (i.e. if serum creatinine over 3.0mg/dL)
- Early reperfusion improves renal function
- Responsible for approx. 70% of acute renal failure

Acute tubular necrosis

Syndrome accounting for approx. 70% of renal failure patients.

FEATURES

- History of renal insult, e.g. severe prolonged hypovolemia, sepsis, nephrotoxin
- Oliguria may or may not be manifest
- Urine sediment: muddy brown casts, epithelial cells; no RBC casts or dystrophic RBCs
- BUN/creatinine ratio below 20:1
- Fractional excretion of sodium above 1%
- Urine osmolality 250–350mOsm/kg

Acute interstitial nephritis

May be drug related (more common in adults), infection related (e.g. streptococcal infection; more common in children), or idiopathic.

FEATURES

- History of prior exposure to a potentially causative drug in adults
- Absence of RBC casts or dystrophic RBCs
- Eosinophiles may be observed in urine sediment using Wright or Hansel stain
- Renal biopsy showing mononuclear interstitial infiltration required for definitive diagnosis

Postrenal obstruction

Urinary tract obstruction involving both kidneys, ureters, or bladder outlet.

FEATURES

- Poor or no urinary flow; also may be intermittent if obstruction is partial, as with bladder or ureteric stones
- Dysuria
- Hematuria without RBC casts or dysmorphic RBCs
- Flank, back, or groin pain
- BUN:creatinine ratio above 20:1
- Catheterization can be diagnostic and therapeutic
- Causes approx. 5% of acute renal failure
- Renal ultrasound is the best diagnostic tool

Nephrotic syndrome

Nephrotic syndrome comprises a group of diseases featuring abnormal glomerular permeability to albumin. Many disorders that cause nephritic syndrome can also cause nephrotic syndrome – some syndromes may start nephritic but progress to nephrotic, or they can have mixed nephritic and nephrotic features.

FEATURES
- Proteinuria 3.5g/24h (40mg/m^2/h in children)
- Hypoalbuminemia
- Hyperlipidemia
- Edema
- Oval fat bodies in the urine are characteristic
- No RBC casts or dysmorphic RBCs in urine sediment. Presence of these in face of other signs of nephrotic syndrome would indicate a mixed nephritic and nephrotic picture
- Predisposed to deep vein thrombosis and to infections, especially in children; most common are viral infections and *Escherichia coli* peritonitis in children who have ascites as manifestation of nephrotic syndrome

SIGNS & SYMPTOMS
Signs
- Signs of nephritic syndrome are variable depending on etiology, severity of glomerular damage, and manifestations of any causative systemic disorder
- Many patients with isolated hematuria and RBC casts with minimal-to-moderate proteinuria are totally asymptomatic
- Patients with diffuse proliferative or rapid progressive glomerulonephritis are symptomatic
- There may also be signs related to a causative systemic disorder

Signs common to all patients with nephritic syndrome:
- Gross or microscopic hematuria
- Urine sediment containing RBC casts and/or dysmorphic erythrocytes and/or hemepigmented coarsely granular casts (blood casts)
- Mild-to-moderate proteinuria (<3.0g/24h in adults; 40mg/m^2/h in children)

Additional signs in severe glomerulonephritis with diffuse glomerular involvement:
- Hypertension
- Decreased glomerular filtration rate
- Salt and water retention, often out of proportion to degree of decreased glomerular filtration rate
- Decreased urine output

Other nonspecific signs of renal failure may be seen in severe progressive glomerulonephritis:
- Fluid overload (peripheral and/or pulmonary edema)
- Encephalopathy with classic flapping tremors or asterixis
- Seizures
- Muscle weakness
- Breath smells of urine
- Muscle myoclonus or fasciculations
- Tachypnea
- Tachycardia
- Hyperkalemia
- Electrocardiographic (ECG) changes related to hyperkalemia, pericarditis, or arrhythmia

Symptoms

- Symptoms of nephritic syndrome are variable depending on etiology, severity of glomerular damage, and manifestations of any causative systemic disorder
- Many patients with isolated hematuria and RBC casts with minimal-to-moderate proteinuria are totally asymptomatic
- Patients with diffuse proliferative or rapid progressive glomerulonephritis are symptomatic
- Symptoms are generally nonspecific and related to the degree of renal failure in severe rapidly progressive cases
- Typically no specific symptoms are present except urine discoloration (cola-colored) if gross hematuria occurs in patients with isolated hematuria and minimal-to-moderate proteinuria
- There may also be symptoms related to a causative systemic disorder (e.g. systemic lupus erythematosis)

In severe cases progressing to renal failure and uremia one or more of the following symptoms may be present:
- Lethargy
- Nausea and vomiting, especially early in the morning
- Malaise
- Weakness
- Anorexia
- Altered taste in mouth
- Muscle cramps
- Swollen ankles
- Shortness of breath
- Sleep disturbance with disruption of normal sleep pattern
- Subtle mental slowing and personality changes progressing to lethargy and coma in end-stage renal disease
- Decreased urine output

ASSOCIATED DISORDERS

Disorders that commonly cause nephritic syndrome may coexist.

KEY! DON'T MISS!

These signs or symptoms require urgent action:
- Hypertensive urgency or emergency
- ECG changes related to hyperkalemia, pericarditis, or arrhythmia
- Pulmonary edema
- Indications for dialysis: intractable uremic symptoms, refractory fluid overload, refractory hyperkalemia, encephalopathy or seizures, creatinine clearance or glomerular filtration rate <10–15mL/min

CONSIDER CONSULT

- Referral to a nephrologist is indicated whenever diagnosis of nephritic syndrome is made or suspected in order to determine if sophisticated diagnostic techniques (e.g. renal biopsy) are needed and to develop a therapeutic plan
- Referral to a nephrologist is indicated whenever doubt exists as to the diagnosis or etiology of acute renal failure

INVESTIGATION OF THE PATIENT
Direct questions to patient

Q **Have you or your family noticed bloody urine or dark (cola-colored) urine?** This is more specific for nephritic syndrome.

Q **Is there a recent history of sore throat or skin infection?** This may indicate beta-hemolytic *Streptococcus* infection.

Q **Do you have any symptoms that may indicate renal failure, including reduced urine output, malaise, and anorexia?** Other nonspecific symptoms of renal failure include lethargy, nausea and vomiting, weakness, joint pains, back pain, muscle cramps, shortness of breath, swollen ankles, face or abdomen, altered mental status, seizures, muscle weakness, muscle myoclonus or fasciculations, tachypnea, tachycardia, and pallor.

Q **When did symptoms start?** Nephritic syndrome with gross hematuria is sometimes sudden in onset. Symptoms of renal failure are gradual in onset.

Q **Have the symptoms (of renal failure) been stable or getting worse?** Can help in assessing prognosis.

Q **Are there any other signs or symptoms?** Can help in differential diagnosis and in diagnosing causative disorder.

Q **Has there been any diagnosis of, or exposure to, infectious diseases?** Can help in differential diagnosis and in diagnosing causative disorder.

Q **Has there been any exposure to drugs or toxins?** Can help in differential diagnosis and in diagnosing causative disorder.

Q **Is there a history of volume depletion, ineffective circulation, or reduced blood pressure?** If short-term, suggests prerenal azotemia; if long-term, suggests acute tubular necrosis.

Q **Is there a history of urologic problems?** May suggest postrenal obstruction.

Q **What is the patient's past medical history?** Can help in differential diagnosis, diagnosing causative disorder, and in determining prognosis and response to treatment.

Contributory or predisposing factors

- Recent history of throat or skin infection with nephritogenic strain of beta-hemolytic *Streptococcus*
- History of other bacterial or viral infections

Family history

Q **Is there a family history of kidney, vascular, or autoimmune disease?** Can help in differential diagnosis and in diagnosing causative disorders such as lupus, thin basement membrane disease, hepatitis C, and Alport's disease.

Examination

- **Complete physical examination:** necessary to assess the degree of renal failure, help differentiate the type of renal disorder, and seek signs of a causative disorder
- **Check vital signs:** look for tachypnea, tachycardia, and hypertension
- **Examine the retina** for signs of hypertension, diabetes, lupus, and endocarditis
- **Examine the neck:** are there any signs of jugular venous distension?
- **Auscultate the heart and lungs** for murmur, arrhythmia, or congestion
- **Palpate the abdomen** for tenderness or distension (as in ascites)
- **Examine the genitourinary system** for signs of infection, obstruction, or hematuria
- **Check extremities** for signs of edema or arthritis
- **Examine the skin** for pallor, rash, purpura, uremic rash, scratch marks due to itching
- **Check neurologic function** for altered mental status, muscle weakness, myoclonus, fasciculations, or single or multiple nerve neuropathies

Summary of investigative tests

- Urinalysis, complete blood count, serum chemistries including electrolytes, and BUN are useful to evaluate the severity of the nephritic syndrome
- Abdominal radiograph and renal ultrasound are useful in most patients with nephritic syndrome or acute renal insufficiency to evaluate renal size and echogenicity and to rule out hydronephrosis
- Specific tests normally recommended by the specialist can be useful in diagnosing the causative condition. These include: serum complements (C3, C4), anti-streptolysin O, anti-hyaluronidase titers, antinuclear antibody (ANA), antidouble-stranded DNA, erythrocyte sedimentation rate, serum protein electrophoresis, antineutrophilic cytoplasmic antibody, serum immunoglobulins, urinary immunoglobulins, and electrophoresis, and others as required

- Renal biopsy (performed by an experienced consultant) is indicated when precise diagnosis is unclear, the renal disease is severe or progressive and potentially amenable to therapy
- ECG can detect cardiac abnormalities that might be found with nephritic syndrome in patients who have severe or progressive form of renal disease with renal failure

DIAGNOSTIC DECISION

- Diagnosis is based on the constellation of historic and physical findings and laboratory values consistent with the nephritic syndrome, most particularly RBC casts and dystrophic RBCs in urine sediment
- Renal biopsy may be necessary for definitive diagnosis, especially in adults in whom the renal disease is severe or progressive and potentially amenable to therapy

CLINICAL PEARLS

- Microscopic examination of the urine sediment by a physician is most important in the diagnosis of the nephritic syndrome (critical in the recognition of RBC casts and dystrophic RBCs). Even technicians in the best clinical laboratories do not have the experience or the time to identify these elements consistently. If the PCP is inexperienced in the identification, he or she should make sure a freshly voided specimen is available for the consulting nephrologist
- Nephritic syndrome may occur in patients in whom the kidney is the sole target of the immunologic insult, or the kidney may be just one of several organs involved in the process, as with Goodpasture's syndrome, systemic lupus erythematosis, and the vasculitides
- It is important to remember that a significant proportion of adults and children with the nephritic syndrome are asymptomatic with microscopic hematuria and mild proteinuria as the sole manifestation (perhaps with intermittent episodes of gross hematuria). In these patients a period of observation may be in order after the initial workup
- In certain asymptomatic patients, a renal biopsy may be indicated at some point to rule out a progressive disorder such as IgA nephropathy. Hence, close collaboration with a nephrologist is indicated even with these patients who appear to have a 'benign' disorder

THE TESTS
Body fluids
URINALYSIS
Description

- Voided or catheterized urine specimen for analysis of chemical, cellular, and structural components
- Need a freshly voided 'spot' specimen for dipstick, and sample is spun down to allow microscopic examination of sediment
- 24h urine collection is also obtained for protein, creatinine (creatinine clearance: urine creatinine concentration multiplied by urine volume divided by plasma creatinine level), and any other special studies recommended by the consultants

Advantages/Disadvantages
Advantages:

- Findings of RBC casts and dystrophic RBCs are crucial in determining diagnosis
- Sample is generally easy to obtain
- Testing is inexpensive and readily available
- Results are available quickly

Disadvantages:

- Sample may be difficult to obtain for some patients
- Catheterization is invasive and may be painful or traumatic for some patients
- Samples are easily contaminated, which may produce misleading results
- 24h specimens may be collected improperly
- Visual observation of dipstick results is subject to observer's skill and interpretation

Normal
- Specific gravity: 1.005–1.030
- Protein: below 150mg/24h (dipstick negative to trace)
- Red blood cells: 0–5/high-power field
- White blood cells: 0–5/high-power field
- Casts: 0–4 hyaline/low-power field
- Creatinine clearance: 75–140mL/min
- Fractional excretion of sodium ((urine sodium divided by plasma sodium) x (plasma creatinine divided by urine creatinine) x 100%); normal values depend on patient's sodium balance and type of pathophysiologic insult
- Osmolality: 50–1200 mOsm/kg (50–1200mmol/kg)

Abnormal
Values higher or lower than the above reference ranges; abnormalities typically found in nephritis syndrome include:
- Protein: 150–300mg/24h ($40mg/m^2/h$ in children)
- Dipstick positive for protein (mainly sensitive to albumin)
- RBCs: over 5/high-power field, dysmorphic
- WBCs: over 5/high-power field
- Renal tubular cells
- Oval fat bodies present if patient has nephrotic syndrome in addition to nephritic syndrome
- Casts: RBC casts, WBC casts, hemepigmented granular casts, fine and coarsely granular casts, and epithelial cell casts (typical of acute tubular necrosis)
- Creatinine clearance: <75mL/min
- Fractional excretion of sodium: >1% in acute tubular necrosis and may be <1% in acute glomerulonephritis
- Osmolarity: >500mOsm/kg (500mmol/kg) in presence of hyponatremia is abnormal

Cause of abnormal result
Protein:
- Increased albumin: renal glomerular disease, severe hypertension
- 350mg/24h ($40mg/m^2/h$ in children) or greater: nephrotic syndrome
- Nonalbumin protein increased in multiple myeloma, light chain disease

RBCs:
- Increased: nephritic syndrome, urinary tract inflammation/trauma/calculi/neoplasms, disorders of hemostasis
- Dysmorphic: nephritic syndrome

WBCs:
- Increased: urinary tract infection or inflammation (including inflammation of nephritic syndrome)

Oval fat bodies:
- Heavy proteinuria

Eosinophiles:
- Present: suggestive of allergic interstitial nephritis

Squamous epithelial cells:
- Present: contamination

Casts:
- RBC or hemepigmented coarsely granular: nephritic syndrome most likely
- WBC: interstitial nephritis, pyelonephritis; occasionally seen in acute glomerulonephritis and rapid progressive glomerulonephritis

- Renal tubular epithelial cell: typical of acute tubular necrosis
- Granular: nonspecific for renal parenchymal disease
- Hyaline: nonspecific
- Fatty: heavy proteinuria
- Waxy: end-stage renal disease

Creatinine clearance:
- Increased: pregnancy, exercise
- Decreased: renal insufficiency

Fractional excretion of sodium:
- Increased: acute tubular necrosis, chronic renal failure
- Decreased: prerenal failure; acute glomerulonephritis

Drugs, disorders and other factors that may alter results
Unless drugs and disorders trigger an immune reaction involving the kidneys, they do not influence RBC casts, dysmorphic red cells, and proteinuria that characterize nephritic syndrome.

COMPLETE BLOOD COUNT
Description
Arterial or venous blood specimen for analysis of hematologic components.

Advantages/Disadvantages
Advantages:
- Specimen is usually easily obtained from patients
- Testing is inexpensive and widely available
- Results are usually available quickly
- Can provide information on several factors simultaneously

Disadvantages:
- Obtaining specimen may be difficult and painful for some patients
- Findings are nonspecific

Normal
Hemoglobin:
- Men: 13.6–17.7g/dL (136–172g/L)
- Women: 12–15g/dL (120–150g/L)
- Boys 12–18 years: 13.0–16.0g/dL (130–160g/L)
- Girls 12–18 years: 12.0–16.0g/dL (120–160g/L)
- 6–12 years: 11.5–15.5g/dL (115–155g/L)
- 2–6 years: 11.5–13.5g/dL (115–135g/L)
- Under 2 years: variable; see age-specific indices

Hematocrit:
- Men: 39–49% (0.39–0.49)
- Women: 33–43% (0.33–0.43)
- Boys 12–18 years: 36–50% (0.36–0.50)
- Girls 12–18 years: 37–45% (0.37–0.45)
- 6–12 years: 35–45% (0.35–0.45)
- 2–6 years: 34–40% (0.34–0.40)
- Under 2 years: variable; see age-specific indices

Mean corpuscular volume:
- Adults: 76–100mcm^3 (76–100fL)
- 2–18 years: 75–108mcm^3 (75–108fL)
- Under 2 years: variable; see age-specific indices

Leukocytes:
- Adults: 3200–9800/mm^3 (3.2–9.8x10^9/L)
- 6–18 years: 4500–13,500/mm^3 (4.5–13.5x10^9/L)
- 2–6 years: 5000–15,500/mm^3 (5.0–15.5x10^9/L)
- Under 2 years: variable; see age specific indices

Platelets:
- Adults: 130–400x10^3/mm^3 (130–400x10^9/L)
- 6 months-18 years: 150–300x10^3/mm^3 (150–300x10^9/L)
- Under 6 months: variable; see age-specific indices

Abnormal
- Values higher or lower than the above reference ranges
- Aside from the urinary abnormalities, the abnormalities typically found in nephritic syndrome are nonspecific findings of renal failure and/or reflect associated or causative disorders
- If the nephritic syndrome is associated with an etiology that produces renal failure, then anemia with decreased hemoglobin, decreased hematocrit, normal or decreased mean corpuscular volume, normal or increased leukocytes, normal or decreased platelets may be present
- Other findings may help with differential diagnosis or with diagnosis and management of causative disorder

Cause of abnormal result
Hemoglobin:
- Decreased: renal failure with decreased erythropoietin production, blood loss

Hematocrit:
- Decreased: renal failure with decreased erythropoietin production, blood loss

Leukocytes:
- Increased: infections, vasculitides
- Decreased: certain infections (especially viral); drug hypersensitivity reactions with suppressed bone marrow

Platelets:
- Increased: acute reactant, infections
- Decreased: renal failure, drugs, immune disorders with marrow suppression (e.g. systemic lupus erythermatosus)

Drugs, disorders and other factors that may alter results
Multiple drugs and disorders can affect the complete blood count and complicate interpretation.

SERUM CHEMISTRIES
Description
Arterial or venous blood specimen for analysis of chemical components.

Advantages/Disadvantages
Advantages:
- Specimen is usually easily obtained from patients
- Testing is inexpensive and widely available
- Results are usually available quickly
- Can provide information on several factors simultaneously

Disadvantages:
- Obtaining specimen can be difficult and painful for some patients
- Findings are nonspecific

Normal
- Sodium: 135–145mEq/L (135–145mmol/L)
- Potassium: 3.5–5.0mEq/L (3.5–5.0mmol/L)
- Bicarbonate: venous – 22–30mEq/L (22–30mmol/L); arterial – 20–28mEq/L (20–28mmol/L)
- Chloride: 95–105mEq/L (95–105mmol/L)
- BUN: adults – 8–18mg/dL (3–6.5mmol/L); children – 5–20mg/dL (2–7mmol/L)
- Creatinine: men – 0.6–1.2mg/dL (53–106mcmol/L); women – 0.5–1.1mg/dL (44–97mcmol/L); 12–18 years – 0.5–1.0 mg/dL (44–88mcmol/L); 2–12 years – 0.3–0.7mg/dL (27–62mcmol/L); 6 months-2 years – 0.2–0.4mg/dL (18–35mcmol/L); under 6 months – 0.3–1.0mg/dL (27–88mcmol/L)
- Calcium: 8.8–10.3mg/dL (2.2–2.58mmol/L)
- Magnesium: adults – 1.8–3.0mg/dL (0.75–1.2mmol/L); children – 1.8–2.4mg/dL (0.75–1.0mmol/L)
- Phosphate: adults – 2.5–5.0 mg/dL (0.8–1.6mmol/L); children – 3.5–6.8mg/dL (1.13–2.20mmol/L)

Abnormal
- Values higher or lower than the above reference ranges
- Abnormal values, when found in nephritic syndrome are nonspecific and are caused by renal failure, such as decreased sodium, increased potassium, decreased bicarbonate, increased chloride, increased BUN, increased creatinine, decreased calcium, increased magnesium, increased phosphate
- Other findings may help with the diagnosis and management of causative disorders

Cause of abnormal result
Sodium:
- Increased: dehydration
- Decreased: positive free water balance greater than positive sodium balance

Potassium:
- Increased: renal failure, iatrogenic, specimen hemolysis (pseudohyperkalemia)
- Decreased: decreased intake, excess loss, iatrogenic (excessive response to diuretic therapy)

Bicarbonate:
- Increased: metabolic alkalosis
- Decreased: metabolic acidosis

Chloride:
- Parallels changes in serum sodium levels except in chronic nephritis with severe tubular damage when hyperchloremic acidosis may develop

BUN:
- Increased: hypovolemia, dehydration, increased protein catabolism, drugs, gastrointestinal bleeding, renal failure
- Decreased: severe liver disease, malnutrition, low protein diet, late pregnancy

Creatinine:
- Increased: renal failure, rhabdomyolysis (increases release into circulation), drugs that block tubular secretion (cimetidine, trimethoprim, stilbamidine), ketonemia (interferes with creatinine assay)
- Decreased: decreased muscle mass, pregnancy

Calcium:
- Increased: secondary hyperparathyroidism in patients in whom nephritic syndrome progresses to renal failure
- Decreased: vitamin D deficiency associated with renal failure, hypoalbuminemia which lowers protein-bound calcium

Magnesium:
- Increased: oliguric renal failure, excess intake, specimen hemolysis
- Decreased: severe malnutrition, hypoalbuminemia (decreases protein bound magnesium)

Phosphate:
- Increased: in patients in whom nephritic syndrome progresses to renal failure, severe muscle trauma excess intake
- Decreased: nutritional deficiency, phosphorus binders used to treat renal failure

Drugs, disorders and other factors that may alter results
Multiple drugs and disorders can impact on the biochemical profile and complicate interpretation.

SPECIFIC TESTS
Description
Arterial or venous blood or other body fluid specimen for analysis of specific diagnostic markers as indicated by the individual presentation and/or as recommended by the consultants.

Advantages/Disadvantages
Advantages:
- Samples are usually easy to obtain from most patients
- Tests are generally inexpensive and widely available
- Can help establish diagnosis of causative disorder

Disadvantages:
- Obtaining sample can be difficult and painful for some patients
- Some tests may need to be sent to outside laboratories
- Results may not be quick
- Results may be nonspecific
- Results may not help in diagnosing renal disorder

Normal
Culture:
- Throat: normal flora
- Skin: normal flora
- Sputum: normal flora
- Urine: sterile
- Blood: sterile

Other tests:

- Antistreptolysin O (ASO) titer: <160 Todd units
- Antihyaluronidase titer: undetectable
- Antideoxyribonuclease B titer: undetectable
- Complement (C3, C4, CH_{50}) levels: C3: 70–160mg/dL (0.7–1.6g/L); C4: 20–40mg/dL (0.2–0.4g/L); CH_{50}: 75–160 U/mL (75–160 U/mL)
- Antinuclear antibody (ANA): below 1:20
- Anti-double stranded DNA: undetectable
- Cryoglobulins: undetectable
- Rheumatoid factor: below 1:20
- Antineutrophil cytoplasmic antibody (ANCA): p-ANCA: undetectable; c-ANCA: undetectable
- Antiglomerular basement membrane antibody (anti-GBM Ab): undetectable

Immunoglobulins (Ig):

- IgA – adults: 50–350mg/dL (0.5–3.5g/L); 12–16 years: 50–232mg/dL (0.5–2.3g/L); 6–12 years: 40–270mg/dL (0.4–2.7g/L); 2–6 years: 40–190mg/dL (0.4–1.9g/L); under 2 years: variable – see age-specific indices
- IgG – adults: 800–1500mg/dL (8–15g/L); 12–16 years: 700–1550mg/dL (7–15.5g/L); 6–12 years: 700–1650mg/dL (7.0–16.5g/L); 2–6 years: 500–1300mg/dL (5.0–13g/L); under 2 years: variable – see age-specific indices

Abnormal

- Cultures: positive
- Antibodies: present
- Complement (C3, C4, CH_{50}) levels: decreased
- Cryoglobulins: present
- Rheumatoid factor: present
- IgA: increased
- IgG: increased
- Hepatitis B and C: positive

Cause of abnormal result

- Culture: positive in cases of ongoing infection
- ASO titer: elevated following 80% pharyngeal streptococcal infections. Level should be detectable at time of presentation. Magnitude of titer has no prognostic significance
- Antihyaluronidase titer: elevated following skin streptococcal infection. Level should be detectable at time of presentation. Magnitude of titer has no prognostic significance
- Antideoxyribonuclease B titer: elevated following skin streptococcal infection. Level should be detectable at time of presentation. Magnitude of titer has no prognostic significance
- Complement (C3, C4, CH_{50}) levels: low – poststreptococcal glomerulonephritis (PSGN), membranoproliferative glomerulonephritis (MPGN) I and II, systemic lupus erythematosus, endocarditis, chronic bacteremia, cryoglobulinemia. Levels will be low during active disease. Levels return to normal 6–8 weeks following most cases of PSGN. Levels remain low in MPGN
- Complement (C3, C4, CH_{50}) levels: normal – IgA nephropathy, idiopathic rapidly progressive glomerulonephritis, anti-GBM disease, polyarteritis nodosa, Wegener's granulomatosis, Henoch-Schönlein purpura, Goodpasture's syndrome
- Anti-double stranded DNA: highly suggestive of systemic lupus erythematosus
- ANA: nonspecifically positive in a variety of immune-related conditions; not diagnostic or pathognomonic
- Cryoglobulins: cryoglobulinemia, often in association with another disorder (e.g. PSGN, hepatitis C)
- Rheumatoid factor: elevated in 43% cases PSGN and over 80% cases of MPGN with cryoglobulinemia

- IgA: elevated in 50% cases IgA nephropathy; elevated in 50% cases Henoch-Schönlein purpura nephritis. Levels have no prognostic significance
- IgG: elevated in over 90% cases PSGN
- ANCA (some overlap exists): p-ANCA – pauci-immune rapidly progressive glomerulonephritis; c-ANCA – Wegener's granulomatosis
- Positive serologies: HIV, hepatitis B or C
- Anti-GBM antibody: Goodpasture's syndrome or idiopathic anti-GBM disease

Drugs, disorders and other factors that may alter results
Some of the markers listed above are nonspecific and could be affected by a number of different disorders; however, specific markers would not be affected by drugs or other disorders.

Biopsy
RENAL BIOPSY
Description
- Obtaining a sample of renal parenchyma for pathologic analysis; to be performed only by experienced specialist when indicated to aid in diagnosis and the development of a therapeutic plan
- Usual indication is for a suspected glomerular lesion
- Adults with nephritic syndrome are more likely to require biopsy to establish diagnosis than children
- May also be indicated for unexplained acute renal failure
- Percutaneous needle biopsy favored in most cases
- Open surgical approach may be used in patients with a single functioning kidney or with a bleeding disorder

Advantages/Disadvantages
Advantage:
- Provides definitive diagnosis of renal lesion

Disadvantages:
- Invasive procedure with risk of complications including hematuria, renal hematoma, vascular laceration, development of arteriovenous fistula, laceration of other abdominal organs
- Requires expert to perform procedure
- Requires expert interpretation
- Procedure can be expensive

Normal
Normal histology.

Abnormal
Pathologic abnormalities vary with etiology and severity of the renal insult. Abnormalities that may be found in nephritic syndrome include:
- Thin glomerular basement membrane with no other proliferative or exudative changes found in thin basement membrane disease
- Enlarged and hypercellular glomeruli distributed in a focal or diffuse manner
- Diffuse or focal proliferation of mesangial and endothelial cells
- Exudate of neutrophils, monocytes, and eosinophils
- Obstruction of Bowman's space
- Occlusion of capillary lumina
- Fibroepithelial glomerular crescents in severe cases
- Severity of glomerular proliferative changes and interstitial fibrosis are directly related to prognosis

- Hypocomplementemic glomerulonephritis
- Immunofluorescence: coarsely granular capillary loop subepithelial deposits of IgG and C3
- Electron microscopy: subepithelial electron-dense humps; glomerulonephritis due to endocarditis or chronic bacteremia has lesions tending to be more focal and segmental

IgA nephropathy and Henoch-Schönlein purpura nephritis:
- Light microscopy: immunofluorescence shows deposits of IgA plus equal or lesser amounts of IgG in mesangium
- Electron microscopy: mesangial electron-dense deposits

Rapidly progressive glomerulonephritis (RPGN):
- Diffuse glomerular crescent formation
- Pauci-immune RPGN: negative immunofluorescence and electron microscopy

Immune complex RPGN:
- Granular deposits of IgG and/or IgM, possibly with complement, in mesangium and subendothelial space of GBM
- Anti-GBM antibody disease:
- Linear capillary loop deposits of IgG and C3 along GBM

Cause of abnormal result
- Pathogenesis is variable depending on etiology and not completely understood
- Alport's disease and thin basement membrane disease are hereditary and familial
- Primarily immune mediated: subepithelial immune complexes can form *in situ* or can be deposited preformed; subendothelial and mesangial immune complexes most likely form *in situ*; immune complexes form in reaction to endogenous or exogenous antigens; immune complexes activate cellular and humoral mediators that are toxic to glomeruli
- Coagulation factors also contribute: fibrin deposits at sites of glomerular injury form nidus for crescent formation; platelet activation causes release of substances harmful to glomeruli
- Exogenous toxins may play a role: can cause direct insult to glomerulus; can induce immune complexes; most often produce membranous glomerulonephritis and nephrotic syndrome

Drugs, disorders and other factors that may alter results
Drugs and other disorders would affect biopsy results if they also produced renal damage or if they modify the glomerular inflammatory reaction. For example:
- Some penicillins and nonsteroidal anti-inflammatory drugs may cause an acute interstitial nephritis
- Adrenal cortical steroids may reduce the degree of glomerular inflammation if administered prebiopsy

Imaging
ABDOMINAL RADIOGRAPH
Description
- Plain films of abdomen
- Encompasses kidneys, ureters, and bladder

Advantages/Disadvantages
Advantages:
- Noninvasive and well tolerated by most patients
- Inexpensive and widely available in most settings
- Can show kidney size and shape
- Can show radio-opaque renal calculi
- No exposure to potentially injurious contrast material
- Basic interpretation does not usually require a specialist

Disadvantages:
- Exposes patient to low-level radiation, particularly to reproductive organs
- Results are nonspecific and nondiagnostic regarding nephritic syndrome

Normal
Kidney shadow is usually about 12cm in adults, or approximately the length of 3.5 vertebrae.

Abnormal
- Small kidneys indicative of chronic renal disease
- Presence of renal calculi

Cause of abnormal result
- Small kidneys: chronic renal failure
- Radio-opaque renal calculi: calcium, struvite, or cystine

RENAL ULTRASOUND
Description
- Ultrasound examination of kidneys and adjacent structures
- May be combined with doppler imaging of renal blood flow
- Usually first choice for imaging kidneys

Advantages/Disadvantages
Advantages:
- Noninvasive and well tolerated by most patients
- Relatively inexpensive and readily available in most areas
- No known radiation risk
- No exposure to potentially injurious contrast
- Can show size and anatomy of kidneys and collecting systems
- Can rule in or rule out hydronephrosis
- Can show radio-opaque and radiolucent renal calculi in kidney
- When combined with doppler, can also assess renal blood flow

Disadvantages:
- Results are often nonspecific
- Usually requires expert interpretation

Normal
Kidney size is usually about 11–12cm in adults, or approximately the length of 3.5 vertebrae.

Abnormal
- Small kidneys indicative of chronic renal disease
- Dilated collecting system (hydronephrosis)
- Masses
- Cysts
- Calculi
- Abnormal renal arterial or venous blood flow

Cause of abnormal result
- Small kidneys: chronic renal failure
- Masses: solid tumor
- Cysts: polycystic kidney disease
- Dilated collecting system (hydronephrosis): obstruction
- Calculi: radio-opaque or radiolucent renal calculi
- Abnormal blood flow: vasculopathy

Drugs, disorders and other factors that may alter results
Ultrasound examination of abdomen is poorly visualized in patients with large amounts of adipose tissue in abdominal wall and omentum.

Other tests
ELECTROCARDIOGRAM
Description
Graphic recording of electric potentials of the heart as measured from electrodes on chest and limbs.

Advantages/Disadvantages
Advantages:
- Noninvasive
- Inexpensive and readily available in most areas
- Quickly delivers information about possibly life-threatening conditions
- Basic interpretation does not usually require a specialist

Disadvantage:
- Body habitus and technical factors can interfere with reading

Normal
No abnormalities observed.

Abnormal
Abnormalities that might be found with nephritic syndrome in patients who have severe or progressive form of renal disease with renal failure include:
- Hyperkalemia (sequentially): peaked T waves, prolongation of PR interval, widening of QRS complex, sine wave pattern in relation to increasing potassium
- Pericarditis: diffuse ST segment elevation with an upward concave appearance, PR segment depression
- Pericardial effusion: diminished voltage, electrical alternans (alternating QRS, and sometimes P and T wave, voltage or morphology with every other beat)
- Arrhythmias

Cause of abnormal result
- Hyperkalemia (sequentially): peaked T waves, prolongation of PR interval, widening of QRS complex, sine wave pattern in relation to increasing potassium
- Pericarditis: diffuse ST segment elevation with an upward concave appearance, PR segment depression
- Pericardial effusion: diminished voltage, electrical alternans (alternating QRS, and sometimes P and T wave, voltage or morphology with every other beat)
- Arrhythmias

Drugs, disorders and other factors that may alter results
- Pre-existing cardiac conditions and drugs used in their treatment (such as digoxin, quinidine) can complicate ECG interpretation
- Body habitus and technical factors can affect the recording

TREATMENT

CONSIDER CONSULT
- Referral to a nephrologist is indicated to assist in diagnosis and management of any renal disease that is not mild and self-limited

IMMEDIATE ACTION
These signs or symptoms require urgent action:
- Hypertensive emergency
- Electrocardiographic changes related to hyperkalemia, pericarditis, or arrhythmia
- Pulmonary edema
- Indications for dialysis: intractable uremic symptoms, refractory fluid overload, refractory hyperkalemia, encephalopathy or seizures, creatinine clearance, or glomerular filtration rate <10–15mL/min

PATIENT AND CAREGIVER ISSUES
Forensic and legal issues
- While every attempt should be made to obtain informed consent, it may be necessary to initiate life-saving treatment, including dialysis, in some cases of life-threatening emergencies when the patient is unable to give consent
- Although regulations may vary, in most instances two physicians should document in the patient's chart what the indications for emergency treatment are and why they are unable to obtain informed consent

Impact on career, dependants, family, friends
- In many cases, nephritic syndrome is transient and/or asymptomatic with normal renal function and should not cause much interruption to the patient's life
- Cases that progress to chronic renal failure have a significant impact on patients' lifestyle, particularly as they approach end stage and become dependent on dialysis

Patient or caregiver request
- **Could this disease have been prevented?** Not usually, except in certain unusual situations where prophylactic antibiotics or very early administration of appropriate antibiotics could have prevented infection with immunogenic organisms; or if knowledge of a patient's prior sensitivity to a drug (e.g. a sulfonamide) might have prevented its use in a situation where drug hypersensitivity caused a vasculitis
- **Is this disease contagious?** No
- **How long will it last?** Depends on the etiology and severity of the renal insult. Some cases of acute glomerulonephritis may be treatable with steroids and immunosuppressive agents
- **What are the long-term consequences?** Prognosis and likely response to therapy depends on the etiology and prognosis of any causative systemic disorder including systemic lupus erythematosus, hepatitis B and C, endocarditis, and vasculitis. Permanent dialysis is required to sustain life in patients with end-stage renal disease
- **Will it recur?** Recurrence is possible but uncommon

Health-seeking behavior
- **Has the patient sought help for this problem before?** Patient may be progressing to chronic disease
- **What medicines or herbs has the patient taken?** Over-the-counter remedies may mask or exacerbate certain symptoms and signs

MANAGEMENT ISSUES
Goals
- Treat presenting manifestations
- Prevent progression of disease and complications of renal failure
- Restore normal renal function, if possible
- Treat causative disorder

Management in special circumstances
Treatment of rapidly progressive glomerulonephritis needs to be aggressive with frequent monitoring and follow up, as prognosis is poorer in this category.

COEXISTING DISEASE
Patients with any of the following pre-existing diseases would be more vulnerable to exacerbation due to renal insult:
- Renal disease
- Hypertension
- Congestive heart failure
- Liver failure

COEXISTING MEDICATION
- Medication must be carefully monitored and doses adjusted for the glomerular filtration rate
- Potentially nephrotoxic medications should be avoided as much as possible
- Medications containing salt, potassium, magnesium, or phosphorus should be avoided as much as possible

SPECIAL PATIENT GROUPS
Children tend to recover from nephritic syndrome more quickly and more completely than adults.

PATIENT SATISFACTION/LIFESTYLE PRIORITIES
In those patients with nephritic syndrome with progressive renal disease, dietary restrictions and adherence to prescribed drug regimens and dialysis may conflict with a patient's lifestyle priorities.

SUMMARY OF THERAPEUTIC OPTIONS
Choices
Treatment is aimed at:
- Preventing progression to chronic renal failure
- Controlling manifestations of renal failure with antihypertensives in those patients with progressive renal disease. In patients with significant proteinuria, angiotensin-converting enzyme (ACE) inhibitors may play a special role and should be considered. In addition to their antihypertensive effects they can inhibit proteinuria, which may slow the rate of progression of the renal disease
- Treat hypertensive emergencies appropriately in critical care unit, using intravenous rapid-acting medications such as nitroprusside or nitroglycerin as indicated
- Control fluid overload and cardiac disease as indicated with use of diuretics and other cardiotonic drugs as recommended by the consultants. The most commonly used diuretic is furosemide
- Thiazide diuretics (e.g. hydrochlorothiazide) are second-line therapy but require caution due to greater renal metabolism
- Corrective therapies for metabolic imbalances, supportive care, and dialysis
- Anti-infectives may be used if causative disorder is an infection, e.g. penicillin, erythromycin ethyl succinate, or erythromycin estolate for nephritic syndrome caused by group A beta-hemolytic streptococcal infection

There are specific treatments only for limited subsets of nephritic syndrome:

- Autoimmune disease may be treated with immunosuppressants, such as steroids and cyclophosphamide
- Rapidly progressive glomerulonephritis may be treated with immunosuppressants and plasmapheresis

Clinical pearls

- Use of ACE inhibitors such as enalapril, lisinopril, or captopril have been shown in many studies to reduce proteinuria in a variety of chronic renal diseases with and without a nephritic component. Studies suggest that prognosis for the rate of progression is adversely affected by the magnitude of the proteinuria. It has been suggested in a few studies that the action of ACE inhibitors to slow rate of progression may, at least partially, be due to its effect on reducing the proteinuria. Therefore, if 24h protein excretion is 1.5g, then it is strongly suggested that ACE inhibitors be added to the therapeutic regimen
- Nephritic syndrome with systemic lupus eythematosus in adults may represent either mild (e.g. focal) renal disease, which requires no specific therapy and typically improves with successful treatment of the systemic manifestations of systemic lupus erythematosus. If the nephritis is associated with diffuse proliferative changes on renal biopsy, aggressive therapy with steroids and cyclophosphamide is often used to reverse or ameliorate the renal disease
- Nephritic syndrome or mixed nephritic/nephrotic syndrome associated with Wegener's granulomatosis typically responds dramatically to cyclophosphamide

Never

- Never administer immunosuppressive therapy without the recommendation of a consultant experienced in the treatment of autoimmune disease and without a renal biopsy showing a potentially treatable condition
- Never administer intravenous fluids before checking patient's fluid and electrolyte status
- Never treat a potentially life-threatening metabolic imbalance with only short-term, protective treatment; instead concomitant use of definitive therapy is essential
- Never treat a metabolic imbalance without assessing the results afterwards

FOLLOW UP

- Regular and frequent laboratory measurements
- Check compliance with medications
- Advise patients on how to avoid infections and malnutrition

Plan for review

- Frequent reassessment is indicated during ongoing treatment
- If infection-related glomerulonephritis remits, no specific follow up is indicated
- If autoimmune-related glomerulonephritis remits, periodic follow up to check for recurrence is indicated in collaboration with the consulting nephrologist
- If chronic renal dysfunction persists, periodic follow up to monitor status is indicated

Information for patient or caregiver

- Fluid, diet, and medication limitations must be observed closely to prevent serious morbidity
- Any medications the patient is taking should be continued until told otherwise by the physician or provider
- Before starting any new medications or dietary supplements they should be reviewed by the provider and/or pharmacist to ensure safety

DRUGS AND OTHER THERAPIES: DETAILS
Drugs
ANGIOTENSIN-CONVERTING ENZYME (ACE) INHIBITORS
ACE inhibitors such as ramipril, enalapril, captopril.

Dose

Enalapril (adult):

- Initial dose in patients not on diuretics is 5mg once a day
- Dosage should be adjusted according to blood pressure response
- The usual dosage range is 10–40mg/day administered in a single dose or two divided doses
- In patients who are currently being treated with a diuretic, symptomatic hypotension occasionally may occur following the initial dose of enalapril maleate. The diuretic should, if possible, be discontinued for 2–3 days before beginning therapy with enalapril maleate to reduce the likelihood of hypotension. If the patient's blood pressure is not controlled with enalapril maleate alone, diuretic therapy may be resumed
- For patients with creatinine clearance of 30mL/min (serum creatinine is 3mg/dL), the first dose is 2.5mg once daily
- The dosage may be titrated upward until blood pressure is controlled or to a maximum of 40mg/day

Lisinopril (adult):

- In patients with uncomplicated essential hypertension not on diuretic therapy, the recommended initial dose is 10mg once a day
- Dosage should be adjusted according to blood pressure response
- The usual dosage range is 20–40mg/day administered in a single daily dose
- In hypertensive patients who are currently being treated with a diuretic, symptomatic hypotension may occur occasionally following the initial dose of lisinopril. The diuretic should be discontinued, if possible, for 2–3 days before beginning therapy with lisinopril to reduce the likelihood of hypotension. The dosage of lisinopril should be adjusted according to blood pressure response. If the patient's blood pressure is not controlled with lisinopril alone, diuretic therapy may be resumed as described above

Efficacy

ACE inhibitor agents have been shown to be highly efficacious antihypertensives and may reduce proteinuria.

Risks/Benefits

Risks

Enalapril:

- Use caution in renal impairment, hyperkalemia, neutropenia
- Use caution in hypotension and aortic stenosis

Lisinopril:

- Lisinopril should be discontinued as soon as pregnancy is detected
- Risk of anaphylactoid reaction
- Risk of hyperkalemia
- Use caution in patients with obstruction in the outflow tract of the left ventricle
- Use caution with renal impairment
- Use caution with nursing mothers

Benefits:

- Protective against proteinuria
- May retard rate of progression of chronic renal disease with proteinuria

Side-effects and adverse reactions

Enalapril:

- Gastrointestinal: nausea, vomiting, diarrhea, constipation, abdominal pain
- Cardiovascular system: orthostatic hypotension and syncope, angina, palpitations, sinus tachycardia

- Hematologic: neutropenia, agranulocytosis, aplastic and hemolytic anemia, pancytopenia, thrombocytopenia
- Central nervous system: headache, dizziness, fatigue
- Genitourinary: renal damage, impotence
- Metabolic: hyperkalemia, hypornatremia
- Respiratory: cough
- Skin: angioedema, maculopapular rash

Lisinopril:
- Cardiovascular system: hypertension, hypotension
- Central nervous system: fatigue, asthenia, headache dizziness, paresthesia
- Gastrointestinal: diarrhea, nausea, vomiting, dyspepsia
- Genitourinary: impotence, decreased libido
- Musculoskeletal: muscle cramps
- Respiratory: cough, upper respiratory infection
- Skin: rash

Interactions (other drugs)
Enalapril:
- Allopurinol ■ Antihypertensives (loop and potassium-sparing diuretics, prazosin, terazosin, doxazosin) ■ Azathioprine ■ Heparin ■ Insulin ■ Iron ■ Lithium ■ Nonsteroidal anti-inflammatory drugs (NSAIDs) ■ Potassium ■ Sodium ■ Trimethoprim

Lisinopril:
- Diuretics ■ Lithium ■ NSAIDs

Contraindications
Enalapril:
- Hypersensitivity to enalapril ■ Pregnancy ■ Angioedema ■ Renal artery stenosis
- Hypotension ■ Safety and efficacy in pediatric patients have not been established

Lisinopril:
- Hypersensitivity to lisinopril ■ Safety and efficacy in pediatric patients have not been established ■ Patients with a history of angioedema related to previous treatment with an ACE inhibitor and in patients with hereditary or idiopathic angioedema

Acceptability to patient
- Antihypertensive therapy is usually very acceptable to patients during a hypertensive urgency or emergency
- Long-term therapy may be more troublesome due to medication side-effects

Follow up plan
During maintenance antihypertensive therapy, follow up every 3–4 months should suffice.

Patient and caregiver information
- Explain importance of blood pressure control
- Discuss side-effect profile
- Describe what follow up to expect
- Describe signs/symptoms of therapeutic failure and what to do if therapy is failing

FUROSEMIDE
Loop diuretics (e.g. furosemide) are treatment of choice for fluid overload in nephritic syndrome.

Dose
Adult:

- Pulmonary edema: 40mg intravenously given over several minutes; repeat in one hour as needed; increase to 80mg as needed
- Intravenously: 20–40mg increased by 20mg every 2h as needed
- By mouth: 20–80mg/day each morning; increase by 20–40mg every 6h as needed to maximum 400mg/day (estimate oral dose as twice intravenous dose)

Child:

- Intravenously or by mouth: 1–2mg/kg/dose every 6–12h as needed to maximum 6mg/kg/day

Efficacy
Loop diuretics are highly efficacious in treatment of fluid overload.

Risks/Benefits
Risks:

- Excessive diuresis may cause dehydration and blood volume reduction with circulatory collapse and possibly vascular thrombosis and embolism, particularly in elderly patients
- Use caution with diabetes mellitus, porphyria
- Use caution with renal and liver disease
- Use caution with systemic lupus erythematosis
- Use caution with pregnancy and nursing mothers
- Use caution with hypertension and gout

Benefits:

- Rapid onset of action of furosemide and other loop diuretics
- Controls hypertension as well as fluid overload
- Cause renal potassium wasting

Side-effects and adverse reactions

- Cardiovascular system: chest pain, circulatory collapse, orthostatic hypotension
- Central nervous system: dizziness, headache, paresthesia, fever
- Eyes, ears, nose, and throat: visual disturbances, ototoxicity, tinnitus, hearing impairment, thirst
- Gastrointestinal: ischemic hepatitis, vomiting, pancreatitis, nausea, diarrhea, anorexia
- Genitourinary: glycosuria, hyperuricemia, bladder spasm, polyuria
- Hematologic: blood disorders
- Metabolic: hyperglycemia, hyponatremia, hypokalemia, hypomagnesemia, hypovolemia, hypochloremia, hypercholesterolemia, hypertriglyceridemia
- Skin: erythema multiforme, exfoliative dermatitis, urticaria

Interactions (other drugs)

- ACE inhibitors - Alpha-adrenergic antagonists - Amphotericin - Antibiotics (aminoglycosides, polymixins, vancomycin, cephalosporins) - Antidiabetics - Antidysrhythmics (amiodarone, cardiac glycosides, disopyramide, flecainide, mexelitine, quinidine, sotalol) - Beta-2 adrenergic agonists - Carbenoxolone - Cholestyramine, colestipol - Cisplatin - Clofibrate - Corticosteroids - Diuretics (thiazides, metolazone, acetazolamide) - Lignocaine - Lithium - NSAIDs - Phenobarbital - Phenytoin - Pimozide - Reboxetine - Selective serotonin reuptake inhibitors - Terbutaline - Tubocurarine

Contraindications

- Allergic reactions (rare) - Renal failure with anuria - Hepatic coma

Acceptability to patient

- Diuretics are usually acceptable to patients, especially in acute setting
- Long-term use may be less acceptable, especially to older patients, due to urinary frequency

Follow up plan
- In acute setting, near-constant monitoring of patient's urine output is needed
- Patient's electrolyte balance should be monitored closely while dosage is being established
- For maintenance therapy, follow up every 3–4 months should suffice

Patient and caregiver information
- Explain importance of treating pulmonary edema and volume overload
- Discuss side-effect profile
- Explain what follow up to expect
- Describe signs/symptoms of therapeutic failure and what to do if therapy is failing

HYDROCHLOROTHIAZIDE
Thiazide diuretics (e.g. hydrochlorothiazide) are second-line therapy but require caution due to greater renal metabolism.

Dose
Adult:
- 12.5–50mg/day orally; can go up to maximum 200mg/day but little therapeutic benefit vs metabolic imbalances

Child:
- Under 6 months: 1–3.3mg/kg/day orally divided twice daily
- Over 6 months: 2mg/kg/day orally divided twice daily

Efficacy
Thiazides are less effective than loop diuretics when creatinine clearance falls below 40–50mL/min and should not be used as single drug under these circumstances.

Risks/Benefits
Risks:
- Use caution in renal and hepatic disease
- Use caution in the elderly, pregnancy and breast-feeding
- May aggravate diabetes or gout
- May cause hypokalemia
- Use caution in serum electrolyte imbalances
- Use caution in sulfonamide and carbonic anydrase inhibitor hypersensitivity

Benefits:
- Rapid onset of action of furosemide and other loop diuretics
- Controls hypertension as well as fluid overload

Side-effects and adverse reactions
- Cardiovascular system: postural hypotension
- Central nervous system: headache, dizziness, vertigo, weakness
- Gastrointestinal: nausea, vomiting, diarrhea, constipation, abdominal pain
- Genitourinary: urinary problems, impotence
- Hematologic: agranulocytosis, aplastic anemia, pancytopenia, hemolytic anemia, leukopenia, and thrombocytopenia
- Hypersensitivity: anaphylactic reactions, necrotizing angiitis (vasculitis and cutaneous vasculitis), respiratory distress including pneumonitis and pulmonary edema, photosensitivity, fever, urticaria, rash, purpura
- Metabolic: hypokalemia, hypomagnesemia, hyponatremia, hypercalcemia, hypochloremic alkalosis, hyperuricaemia, hyperglycemia, and altered plasma lipid concentration
- Skin: rashes, urticaria, Stevens-Johnson syndrome, exfoliative dermatitis, photosensitivity
- Other: acute interstitial nephritis (rare)

Interactions (other drugs)
- ACE inhibitors ■ Allopurinol ■ Anesthetics ■ Anticholinergics ■ Anticoagulants
- Antidiabetics ■ Antigout ■ Antineoplastics ■ Calcium salts ■ Cardiac glycosides
- Cholestyramine, colestipol ■ Corticosteroids ■ Diazoxide ■ Disopyramide ■ Fluconazole
- Lithium ■ Loop diuretics ■ Methotrexate ■ Nondepolarizing muscular blockers ■ NSAIDs
- Vitamin D

Contraindications
- Anuria ■ Severe renal or hepatic impairment ■ Refractory hyponatremia, hypokalemia, hypercalcemia ■ Addison's disease

Acceptability to patient
- Diuretics are usually acceptable to patients, especially in acute setting
- Long-term use may be less acceptable, especially to older patients, due to urinary frequency

Follow up plan
- In acute setting, near constant monitoring of patient's urine output is needed
- Patient's electrolyte balance should be monitored closely while dosage is being established
- For maintenance therapy, follow up every 3–4 months should suffice

Patient and caregiver information
- Explain importance of treating pulmonary edema and volume overload
- Discuss side-effect profile
- Explain what follow up to expect
- Describe signs/symptoms of therapeutic failure and what to do if therapy is failing

ANTI-INFECTIVES
- If causative disorder is an active infection, treatment for that infection should be instituted
- Many infections can cause nephritic syndrome, but the most common in children is group A beta-hemolytic *Streptococcus*, for which there are clear guidelines for therapy
- In adults, however, proven bacterial infections are responsible for only a minority of cases of nephritic syndrome
- Note that treatment of group A beta-hemolytic *Streptococcus* prior to onset of poststreptococcal glomerulonephritis does not prevent its development

Dose
Pharyngitis (adult):
- Oral: penicillin V 250mg three or four times daily
- Intramuscular: one dose of benzathine penicillin G 1.2×10^6 units
- Penicillin allergic: erythromycin ethyl succinate 40mg/kg/day divided two or three times daily for 10 days, or erythromycin estolate 15–0mg/kg/day divided four times daily

Pharyngitis (child):
- Oral: penicillin V 15–50mg/kg/day in divided doses for 10 days
- Intramuscular: one dose of benzathine penicillin G 5.0×10^5 units
- Penicillin allergic: erythromycin ethyl succinate 40mg/kg/day divided two or three times daily for 10 days, or erythromycin estolate 20–40mg/kg/day divided two or three times daily for 10 days

Moderate-to-severe infection (adult):
- Oral: penicillin V 125–250mg three to four times daily for 10 days
- Intramuscular: benzathine penicillin G 1.2×10^6 units/day as needed
- Penicillin allergic: erythromycin ethyl succinate 400–800mg two to four times daily as needed or erythromycin estolate 250–500mg two to four times daily as needed

Moderate-to-severe infection (child):

- Oral: penicillin V 15–50mg/kg/day divided four times daily for 10 days
- Intramuscular: over 27kg – benzathine penicillin G 9.0×10^6 units/day; below 27kg – benzathine penicillin G 5.0×10^5 units/kg in single dose
- Penicillin allergic: erythromycin ethyl succinate 30–50mg/kg/day divided three or four times daily as needed or erythromycin estolate 30–50mg/kg/day divided two or three times daily

Efficacy

These therapies are highly effective treatments for group A beta-hemolytic *Streptococcus* infection.

Risks/Benefits

Risks

Penicillin V:

- Use caution in patients allergic to cephalosporins
- Use caution in severe renal failure

Benzathine penicillin G:

- Use caution in patients allergic to cephalosporins
- Use caution in asthma, severe renal failure
- Prolonged use may result in overgrowth of nonsusceptible organisms

Erythromycin ethylsuccinate:

- Risk of hepatic dysfunction
- Risk of pseudomembranous colitis
- May aggravate weakness in patients with myasthenia gravis
- Use caution with impaired hepatic function
- Use caution with nursing mothers
- Prolonged or repeated use of erythromycin may result in an overgrowth of nonsusceptible bacteria or fungi

Erythromycin estolate:

- Risk of hepatic dysfunction with or without jaundice
- If malaise, nausea, vomiting, abdominal colic, and fever occur, treatment should be discontinued promptly
- Risk of cholestatic hepatitis
- Use caution with impaired hepatic function
- Use caution in nursing mothers

Benefits:

- Oral therapies have rapid onset of action
- Intramuscular therapies have slow onset of action but sustained release, enabling single-dose therapy for uncomplicated infections

Side-effects and adverse reactions

Penicillin V:

- Central nervous system: seizures, depression, anxiety, fever
- Gastrointestinal: diarrhea, nausea, vomiting, abdominal pain, antibiotic-associated colitis
- Hematologic: bone marrow suppression, coagulation disorders
- Renal: interstitial nephritis
- Respiratory: anaphylaxis
- Skin: erythema multiforme, rash, urticaria

Benzathine penicillin G:

- Cardiovascular system: cardiac arrest, hypotension, tachycardia, palpitations, pulmonary hypertension, pulmonary embolism, vasodilatation, vasovagal reaction, cerebrovascular accident, syncope
- Central nervous system: tremors, dizziness, somnolence, anxiety, transverse myelitis, seizures, coma, tinnitus, fever, fatigue, asthenia, pain, headache
- Ears, eyes, nose, and throat: blurred vision, blindness
- Gastrointestinal: pseudomembranous colitis
- Hematologic: hemolytic anemia, leukopenia, thrombocytopenia
- Genitourinary: nephropathy, hematuria, proteinuria, renal failure, impotence, priapism
- Hemic: lymphadenopathy
- Metabolic: elevates blood urea nitrogen, creatinine, and serum aspartate aminotransferase
- Musculoskeletal: joint disorder, periostitis, myoglobinura, rhabdomyelysis, worsening of arthritis
- Skin: pruritus, diaphoresis, edema at injection site

Erythromycin ethylsuccinate:

- Gastrointestinal: nausea, vomiting, abdominal pain, diarrhea, anorexia
- Other: hepatitis, hepatic dysfunction, and/or abnormal liver function test results

Erythromycin estolate:

- Gastrointestinal: nausea, vomiting, abdominal pain, diarrhea, anorexia
- Ears: tinnitus and/or hearing loss
- Other: hepatitis, hepatic dysfunction, and/or abnormal liver function test results

Interactions (other drugs)
Penicillin V:

- Chloramphenicol ■ Macrolide antibiotics ■ Methotrexate ■ Oral contraceptives
- Probenecid ■ Tetracyclines

Benzathine penicillin G:

- Tetracycline (may antagonize penicillin action) ■ Probenecid (increases serum penicillin)
- Estrogens (contraceptive effect may be reduced) ■ Methotrexate (excretion reduced
- Warfarin (international normalized ratio may be altered) ■ Typhoid vaccine (inactivated by antibiotics)

Erythromycin ethylsuccinate:

- Alfentanil ■ Astemizole (discontinued drug) ■ Bromocriptine ■ Cisapride (discontinued drug) ■ Cyclosporine ■ Digoxin ■ Disopyramide ■ Ergotamine or dihydroergotamine ■ Lovastatin ■ Oral anticoagulants ■ Tacrolimus ■ Theophylline ■ Terfenadine (discontinued drug) ■ Triazolam and midazolam ■ Valproate

Erythromycin estolate:

- Alfentanil ■ Astemizole (discontinued drug) ■ Bromocriptine ■ Clindamycin ■ Cisapride (discintinued drug) ■ Cyclosporine ■ Digoxin ■ Disopyramide ■ Ergotamine or dihydroergotamine ■ Lincomycin ■ Lovastatin ■ Oral anticoagulants ■ Probenecid ■ Tacrolimus ■ Terfenadine (discontinued drug) ■ Theophylline ■ Triazolam and midazolam ■ Valproate

Contraindications
Penicillin V:

- Hypersensitivity to cephalosporins

Benzathine penicillin G:

- Penicillin hypersensitivity ■ Nonintramuscular use

Erythromycin ethylsuccinate:
- Known hypersensitivity to erythormycin ethylsuccinate - Patients taking terfenadine, astemizole, or cisapride (these have been discontinued) - Pregnancy category C

Erythromycin estolate:
- Hypersensitivity to erythromycin estolate - Pre-existing liver disease - Pregnancy category B
- Concurrent use of terfenadine or astemizole (these are discontinued drugs)

Acceptability to patient
Anti-infective therapy is generally well accepted by patients, although side-effects and frequency of dosing may limit acceptability in some.

Follow up plan
Clinical course should be monitored closely during therapy; repeat cultures after therapy are not usually indicated.

Patient and caregiver information
- Explain that therapy prevents renal failure and carditis
- Discuss side-effect profile
- Explain what follow up to expect
- Describe signs/symptoms of therapeutic failure and what to do if therapy is failing

IMMUNOSUPPRESSANTS
- Immunosuppressants are standard therapy in limited circumstances to be used only with the recommendation by and under supervision of a consultant nephrologist. In the following examples (list is far from complete), commonly used drugs are listed, but good clinical trials providing strong evidence for their efficacy are meager in most cases:
- Rapidly progressive glomerulonephritis: steroids plus cyclophosphamide
- Antineutrophil cytoplasmic antibody (ANCA) positive glomerulonephritis: steroids plus cyclophosphamide
- Systemic lupus erythematosus glomerulonephritis: steroids and sometimes cyclophosphamide in diffuse proliferative type
- Wegener's granulomatosis: good evidence for efficacy of cyclophosphamide
- Microscopic polyarteritis nodosa: steroids plus cyclophosphamide sometimes
- Antiglomerular basement membrane glomerulonephritis: steroids plus cyclophosphamide plus plasmaphoresis

Dose
Doses for these extremely potent and potentially toxic drugs are not given here because their use is outside the realm of the PCP, and the regimens are frequently undergoing modification.

Efficacy
Rapidly progressive glomerulonephritis:
- Efficacy is best when therapy is instituted early in course, when serum creatinine is below 5mg/dL (400mcmol/L)
- One study suggested that steroid therapy may decrease serum creatinine or delay dialysis over 3 years in 50% patients, but this conclusion requires further observations

ANCA-positive glomerulonephritis:
- Efficacy and optimal duration of therapy not yet fully established

Systemic lupus erythematosus glomerulonephritis:
- Steroid therapy has variable efficacy in controlling clinical signs of nephritic syndrome
- Cyclophosphamide therapy has an additive effect to steroids in controlling disease activity in diffuse proliferative lupus nephritis and may inhibit progression of renal failure

Risks/Benefits
Risks:
- Use caution when administering with radiation therapy
- May increase susceptibility to infection

Benefits:
- May control disease activity in some situations
- May delay or prevent progression of renal failure
- In some instances, therapy can be given on a monthly basis

Side-effects and adverse reactions
Cyclophosphamide:
- Cardiovascular system: cardiotoxicity (at high doses)
- Central nervous system: dizziness, headache
- Gastrointestinal: nausea, vomiting, diarrhea
- Genitourinary: amenorrhea, azoospermia, ovarian fibrosis, sterility, hematuria, hemorrhagic cystitis, neoplasms
- Hematologic: leukopenia, myelosuppression, panycytopenia, thrombocytopenia
- Metabolic: bone marrow supression
- Respiratory: fibrosis
- Skin: alopecia, dermatitis
- Other: teratogenicity

Steroids:
- Cardiovascular system: hypertension
- Hematologic: azotemia
- Metabolic: fluid overload
- Musculoskeletal: osteoporosis
- Other: precipitation of diabetes

Interactions (other drugs)
Cyclophosphamide:
- Allopurinol (increased cyclophosphamide toxicity) ▪ Clozapine (may cause agranulocytosis) ▪ Cyclophosphamide (causes a marked and persistent inhibition of cholinesterase activity and potentiates the effect of succinylcholine chloride) ▪ Digoxin (decreased digoxin absorption from tablet form) ▪ General anesthesia (if a patient has been treated with cyclophosphamide within 10 days the anesthesiologist should be alerted) ▪ Pentostatin (increased toxicity with high-dose cyclophosphamide) ▪ Phenytoin (reduced absorption of phenytoin) ▪ Phenobarbital (increases the metabolism rate and leukopenic activity of cyclophosphamide) ▪ Succinylcholine (prolonged neuromuscular blockade) ▪ Warfarin (inhibits hypoprothrombinemic response to warfarin)

Contraindications
▪ Hypersensitivity to cyclophosphamide or steroid ▪ Serious infections, including chicken pox and herpes zoster ▪ Myelosuppression ▪ Sustained serum creatinine level of 6.0mg/dL.

Acceptability to patient
Considerable side-effects of immunosuppressant therapy may limit acceptability to some patients, although monthly dosing can increase adherence.

Follow up plan
Close follow up of renal function and monitoring for side-effects is required throughout therapy with immunosuppressants.

Patient and caregiver information
- Explain that therapy may be in some cases best chance of remission
- Discuss side-effect profile
- Explain what follow up to expect
- Describe signs/symptoms of therapeutic failure and what to do if therapy is failing

Other therapies
PLASMAPHERESIS
- To be performed only by, or under the direct supervision of, an experienced nephrologist in those unusual cases where this form of therapy is indicated
- Removal of whole blood to remove plasma (and proteins), followed by reinfusion of cellular elements resuspended in plasma substitute
- Removes free antibody, immune complexes, and inflammatory mediators
- Indicated as an adjunct to drug therapy for rapidly progressive glomerulonephritis associated with circulating antiglomerular basement membrane antibodies or certain circulating immune complexes

Indications for use include:
- Antiglomerular basement membrane antibody disease: 4L (or approximate body fluid volume) exchanges daily for 14 days
- Pauci-immune or immune-complex rapidly progressive glomerulonephritis : 3–4L (or approximate body fluid volume) exchanges daily for 4–6 days

Efficacy
- Specific data unknown
- Relapse common in first few months
- Efficacy reduced in patients who are oliguric, on dialysis, have creatinine level over 6.5mg/dL (572mcmol/L)

Risks/Benefits
Risks:
- Invasive procedure with risk of infection
- Volume shifts carry risk of hypotensive event

Benefits:
- May prevent or delay progression of renal failure
- Relatively few side-effects

Acceptability to patient
May not be acceptable to patients whose religious beliefs prohibit return of blood that has been taken from the body (e.g. Jehovah's Witnesses).

Follow up plan
Close monitoring of vital signs, metabolic status, glomerular filtration rate, and antiglomerular basement membrane antibody is necessary throughout treatment with plasmapheresis.

Patient and caregiver information
- Explain what to expect before, during, and after the procedure
- Discuss side-effect profile (low blood pressure, risk of infections)
- Describe signs/symptoms of therapeutic failure and what to do if therapy is failing

EFFICACY OF THERAPIES

- Majority of therapies for nephritic syndrome are supportive in nature and are generally successful, but the ultimate outcome depends primarily on the etiology and severity of renal disease in an individual patient
- Those subsets of nephritic syndrome that have a specific treatment do not have well defined efficacy rates

Review period

- Patients successfully treated for autoimmune-related glomerulonephritis should be followed up periodically to check for recurrence
- Persistent chronic renal dysfunction in any patient, requires periodic follow up to monitor status

PROGNOSIS

- Prognosis is variable depending on causative disorder and severity of renal lesions (focal glomerular lesions have a better prognosis than diffuse lesions)
- Prognosis is excellent for patients with isolated hematuria (gross or microscopic) associated with thin basement membrane nephropathy
- Prognosis is inversely related to degree of glomerular crescent formation
- Prognosis is inversely related to degree of interstitial fibrosis on renal biopsy

Poststreptococcal glomerulonephritis (PSGN):

- Usually resolves spontaneously in children
- 2–5% of adults can have persistent abnormalities, but progression to end-stage renal disease is rare
- Negative prognostic factors include mature age at disease onset, oliguria lasting more than a week, nephrotic syndrome with glomerular crescents (in adults, 30% will progress to end-stage renal disease)

Other infection-related glomerulonephritis:

- Severity of renal damage related to duration of infection
- If infection is eliminated before much renal damage occurred, prognosis is good
- If extensive renal damage has occurred prior to treatment of infection, it may be irreversible
- In cases involving visceral abscesses, antibiotic therapy is effective in restoring renal function in only 50%

Rapidly progressive glomerulonephritis (idiopathic):

- 80% untreated patients will progress to end-stage renal disease within 6 months
- One study suggested that 50% of patients will respond to therapy and can delay dialysis for more than 3 years, but this outcome requires further study and confirmation

Rapidly progressive glomerulonephritis (other causes):

- Therapy may improve prognosis, but response rates vary
- Therapy of antiglomerular basement membrane antibody disease increases short-term survival from 10–50%
- Prognosis is worse in patients older than 60 years with oliguric renal failure
- Prognosis is worse in patients in whom >75% glomeruli have crescent formation

Immunoglobulin A (IgA) nephropathy:

- 20% of patients will develop renal insufficiency and hypertension within 10–15 years
- 25% of patients will progress to end-stage renal disease within 20 years
- Negative prognostic factors include disease onset beyond childhood, hypertension, persistent marked proteinuria, lack of recurrent gross hematuria, increased serum creatinine level, high levels of glomerular sclerosis, and crescent formation

Clinical pearls

Rate of progression to end stage renal disease is adversely affected by:

- Presence of large proteinuria (over 1.0g/24h)
- Lack of control of hypertension
- Age
- Presence of interstitial fibrosis on renal biopsy
- Percentage of glomeruli with fibroepithelial crescents on renal biopsy

Therapeutic failure

- In most cases of nephritic syndrome caused by infection, alternative anti-infective agents can be used
- Steroids do not have a convincing role in the therapy of nephritic syndrome, and one must weigh the potential benefits of their use vs the morbidity and mortality from complications when considering the dose and duration of steroid therapy

Recurrence

Recurrence rates are unclear and depend on the specific etiologies.

Deterioration

Deterioration may be accelerated by uncontrolled hypertension.

Terminal illness

- Dialysis can produce a long survival period
- Renal transplantation is an option, but some forms of nephritic syndrome may recur in the transplanted kidney (e.g. membranoproliferative glomerulonephritis)

COMPLICATIONS

- Acute renal failure and its complications
- Chronic renal failure and its complications

CONSIDER CONSULT

- Referral back to a nephrologist is indicated if disorder is not responding to therapy or if patient continues to deteriorate

PREVENTION

- There are no real measures that would effectively prevent onset of nephritic syndrome
- Treatment of group A beta-hemolytic *Streptococcus* prior to onset of glomerulonephritis does not reduce the risk of developing glomerulonephritis
- In theory, reducing the risk of contracting an infectious disease may help prevent the onset of infection-related glomerulonephritis

RISK FACTORS

No known risk factors common to all forms of renal disease associated with the nephritic syndrome.

MODIFY RISK FACTORS

Blood pressure control, good hygiene, and a low-protein diet may reduce risk for nephritic syndrome.

Lifestyle and wellness

ALCOHOL AND DRUGS
It makes clinical sense to avoid alcohol.

SCREENING

Since the onset of nephritic syndrome is usually sudden, and since asymptomatic patients are likely not to require treatment, screening for early detection is not warranted.

PREVENT RECURRENCE

There is no known way to prevent recurrence of nephritic syndrome.

ASSOCIATIONS

National Kidney and Urologic Diseases Information Clearinghouse
3 Information Way
Bethesda, MD 20892–3580
Tel: 1-800-891-5390 or (301) 654-4415
Fax: (301) 907-8906
E mail: nkudic@info.niddk.nih.gov
http://www.niddk.nih.gov/health/kidney/nkudic.htm

American Society of Nephrology
2025 M Street, NW
Suite 800
Washington, DC 20036
Tel: (202) 367-1190
Fax: (202) 367-2190
E-mail: asn@dc.sba.com
Website: http://www.asn-online.org

American Society of Pediatric Nephrology
Rainbow Babies and Children's Hospital
11100 Euclid Avenue
Mail code 6003
Cleveland, OH 44106–6003
Tel: (216) 844-3884
Fax: (216) 844-1479
http://www.aspneph.com

National Kidney Foundation (NKF)
30 East 33rd Street
New York, NY 10016
Tel: 1-800-622-9010 or (212) 889-2210
http://www.kidney.org

American Association of Kidney Patients
100 South Ashley Drive, Suite 280
Tampa, FL 33602
Tel: 1-800-749-2257 or (813) 223-7099
Fax: (813) 223-0001
E-mail: AAKPnat@aol.com
http://www.aakp.org

KEY REFERENCES

- Jennette JC, Falk RJ. Glomerular clinicopathologic syndromes. In: Greenberg A, ed. Primer on kidney diseases. New York: Academic Press, 2001, p124–143
- Klahr S, Levey AS, Beck GJ, et al. The effects of dietary protein restriction and blood pressure control on the progression of chronic renal disease. N Engl J Med 1994;330:877–84
- Bison AL, Gerber MA, Gwaltney JM Jr, et al. Diagnosis and management of group A streptococcal pharyngitis: a practice guideline. Clin Infect Dis 1997;27:574–83
- Glockner WM, Sieberth HG, Wichmann HE, et al. Plasma exchange and immunosuppressive therapy in rapidly progressive glomerulonephritis. Clin Nephrol 1988;29:1–8
- Gourley MF, Austin HA 3rd, Scott D, et al. Methylprednisolone and cyclophosphamide, alone or in combination, in patients with lupus nephritis. Ann Intern Med 1996;125:549–57
- Hattori M, Ito K, Konomoto T, et al. Plasmapheresis as sole therapy for rapidly progressing Henoch-Schönlein purpura nephritis in children. Am J Kidney Dis 1999;33:427–33

FAQS

Question 1

Besides a renal biopsy, what is the best way to confirm the diagnosis of nephritic syndrome?

ANSWER 1

Nephritic syndrome implies the clinical features associated with inflammation of the renal glomeruli. The hallmark of glomerulitis is leakage of red blood cells (RBCs) from the blood into the renal tubules. During passage through the tubules, the RBCs are modified in at least two ways: they become distorted and are excreted as dystrophic RBCs, and they become incorporated into casts and excreted as RBC casts or hemepigmented blood casts. The discovery of these elements in the urine sediment by microscopy provides strong confirmation of the diagnosis of nephritic syndrome.

Question 2

How significant prognostically is recurrent gross hematuria in a patient in whom RBC casts are found in the urine sediment?

ANSWER 2

The combination of hematuria and RBC casts certainly supports the diagnosis of nephritis (nephritic syndrome). In fact, the discovery of these casts in a patient with hematuria precludes the necessity to proceed with an invasive urologic workup for the hematuria. The findings in this patient do not predict a negative prognosis in regard to developing progressive renal disease. More important clinical factors that have been demonstrated to influence an unfavorable prognosis are the magnitude of concomitant proteinuria, the presence of uncontrollable hypertension, and an elevated serum creatinine. In fact, studies in patients with immunoglobulin A (IgA) nephropathy have suggested that the most favorable outcomes occurred in patients with gross hematuria.

Question 3

Under what circumstances does mixed nephritic/nephrotic syndrome occur?

ANSWER 3

Nephritic syndrome implies hematuria with RBC casts, and nephrotic syndrome implies excretion of protein (albumin) is 3.5g/24h. Both of these abnormalities are due to pathologic changes in the glomeruli leading to abnormal leakage of RBCs and albumin into the renal tubules and, ultimately, into the final urine. Therefore, any condition that causes severe diffuse glomerulonephritis will manifest both hematuria and heavy proteinuria regardless of the etiology. Mixed nephritic/nephrotic syndrome may occur with a severe form of acute poststreptococcal glomerulonephritis, diffuse lupus glomerulonephritis, membranoproliferative glomerulonephritis, progressive IgA nephropathy, and rapidly progressive glomerulonephritis.

CONTRIBUTORS

Fred F Ferri, MD, FACP
Martin Goldberg, MD, FACP
Ankush Gulati, MD

NEPHROTIC SYNDROME

SUMMARY INFORMATION

DESCRIPTION

- Consists of clinical and laboratory abnormalities common to a variety of primary and secondary kidney diseases, each characterized by increased permeability of the glomerular capillary wall to circulating plasma proteins, particularly albumin
- Presents with edema, hypoalbuminemia, and massive proteinuria (>3g/24h)
- Hyperlipidemia, lipiduria, and hypercoagulability are typically also present
- Most common primary cause in children is minimal change glomerulopathy, and in adults, membranous glomerulopathy
- A significant proportion of adults who show signs of nephrotic syndrome have a related systemic disease, e.g. diabetic glomerulosclerosis, amyloidosis, lupus erythematosus

URGENT ACTION

- Urgent referral/admission of patients with acute renal failure or rapidly deteriorating renal function
- Urgent referral/admission of patients with nephrotic crisis, e.g. massive edema, anorexia, vomiting, pleural effusions, muscle wasting
- Urgent admission for acute hypovolemia with hypotension due to severe hypoalbuminuria

KEY! DON'T MISS!

Rapidly deteriorating renal function.

ICD9 CODE
581.9 Nephrotic syndrome

SYNONYMS
For minimal change glomerulopathy:
- Minimal change nephropathy
- Minimal change disease
- Lipoid nephrosis
- Nil disease

For membranous glomerulopathy:
- Membranous glomerulonephritis

For membranoproliferative glomerulonephritis:
- Mesangiocapillary glomerulonephritis (type I membranoproliferative glomerulonephritis)
- Dense deposit disease (type II membranoproliferative glomerulonephritis)

CARDINAL FEATURES
- Nephrotic syndrome with proteinuria, hypoalbuminemia, and edema results from either a primary glomerular disorder (idiopathic nephrotic syndrome) or is a manifestation of systemic disease (in 30–50% of cases)
- Renal biopsy in idiopathic nephrotic syndrome in adults usually shows one of four pathologic entities: membranous glomerulonephropathy (30–40% of idiopathic cases); focal segmental glomerulosclerosis (20–30%); minimal change disease (10–15%); membranoproliferative glomerulonephritis (10–20%)
- Minimal change disease accounts for >80% of all cases of nephrotic syndrome in children <10 years of age but only 10–15% of primary cases in adults
- Most common associated multisystem diseases are diabetes mellitus (by far the most common), systemic lupus erythematosus and other collagen vascular diseases, and primary or secondary amyloidosis
- Proteinuria in nephrotic syndrome is due to increased permeability of the glomerular basement membrane to albumin and arises in response to alterations in both the size and charge barriers of the glomerular filtration apparatus. Albumin is the predominant protein excreted
- Hypoalbuminemia appears to be due to a failure to enhance hepatic synthesis sufficiently to compensate for increased urinary loss
- Edema: as a consequence of proteinuria and a fall in serum albumin concentration, plasma oncotic pressure falls. This causes fluid to move from the vascular to the interstitial fluid compartment, initiating a series of pathophysiologic events resulting in renal sodium retention and generalized edema. Edema may be massive, widely distributed, and may vary with posture. Facial and upper limb edema are characteristic and particularly obvious after recumbency. Transudative ascites and pleural effusions are often seen
- Hyperlipidemia and lipiduria: increase in serum cholesterol and phospholipids, and lipiduria are typically components of the nephrotic syndrome. This is due to increased hepatic synthesis which may be triggered by the fall in plasma oncotic pressure
- Other metabolic derangements: many patients with nephrotic syndrome have a hypercoagulable state, possibly due to urinary loss of antithrombin III, decreased activity of proteins S and C. Loss of vitamin D-binding globulin may result in vitamin D deficiency, hypocalcemia, osteomalacia, and secondary hyperparathyroidism. Loss of immunoglobulins may result in impaired immunity and increased rates of infections. Depletion of transferrin may result in iron-deficiency anemia

CAUSES
Common causes

Most commonly nephrotic syndrome is primary or idiopathic.

Minimal change glomerulopathy:

- Accounts for 80% of cases of nephrotic syndrome in children under 10 years, approx. 50% of cases in older children, and 10–15% of adult cases
- No cause is found in most patients. Immunologically mediated, related to abnormal T cell function rather than immune complex deposition
- Patients usually present with full-blown pure nephrotic syndrome
- Hypertension and/or microscopic hematuria are uncommon, but one of these may occur in 20–30% of patients
- Renal impairment and even acute renal failure occurs rarely
- Severe edema, ascites, and pleural effusions may occur
- Spontaneous remission may rarely occur but it is seldom justified to leave patient untreated as persistent nephrotic syndrome carries significant morbidity and mortality
- Risk of relapse decreases with time and relapse is often precipitated by minor upper respiratory tract infection

Focal segmental glomerulosclerosis (FSGS):

- Important entity associated with primary nephrotic syndrome in adults and children; forms part of a spectrum with minimal change at benign end and steroid-resistant FSGS at the other
- Incidence appears to be increasing, particularly in African-American males
- Primary FSGS accounts for 10–15% of cases of nephrotic syndrome in children and as many as 35% of adult cases
- May be idiopathic or secondary to a systemic disease such as reflux nephropathy, HIV, or heroin-associated nephropathy
- Poor prognosis with high rate of progression to end-stage renal disease (>80% untreated cases)
- Presents with proteinuria, often full blown nephrotic syndrome, impaired or deteriorating renal function, and hypertension in 30–50%. Proteinuria is unselective
- Spontaneous remission is rare
- Secondary FSGS is the final result of many different causes of glomerular injury: late-stage focal glomerulonephritis, renal dysplasia, reflux nephropathy, surgical loss of renal mass, sickle cell disease, obesity, cyanotic heart disease, heroin abuse, HIV nephropathy, aging. Prognosis determined by underlying condition

Membranous nephropathy:

- Most common clinicopathologic entity associated with idiopathic nephrotic syndrome in adults
- May be primary or secondary to a wide range of diseases. Pathogenesis unknown and treatment is controversial
- 80% present with nephrotic syndrome, the remainder with lesser degrees of proteinuria. Occasional patient may present with acute renal failure as complication of nephrotic syndrome
- Up to 50% are hypertensive at presentation

Membranoproliferative glomerulonephritis:

- Group of immune complex diseases – type I (mesangiocapillary glomerulonephritis), type II (dense deposit disease) – with characteristic histologic appearances that may be primary or caused by another disease (e.g. hepatitis C, cryoglobulinemia)
- Both types usually present with mixed nephrotic and nephritic syndrome; urine sediment contains nephritic components such as hematuria and red blood cell casts as well as evidence of lipiduria (oval fat bodies) associated with nephrotic range proteinuria

- Hypertension is common
- Up to 30% of patients present with rapidly deteriorating renal function
- Slow progression to end-stage renal disease is the usual course
- Spontaneous remission is rare

Secondary causes:
- Diabetic glomerulosclerosis due to both type 1 and type 2 diabetes mellitus is the most common systemic disease causing nephrotic syndrome
- Systemic lupus erythematosus with renal involvement may occasionally present with nephrotic syndrome and the morphology on renal biopsy of membranous glomerulopathy
- Amyloid causes proteinuria, nephrotic syndrome, and progressive renal failure
- Myeloma may present initially with nephrotic syndrome associated with secondary amyloid

Rare causes
- Syphilis
- Sickle cell disease
- Malignancies (carcinomas and lymphomas)
- Reflux nephropathy
- Nonsteroidal anti-inflammatory drugs (NSAIDs)

Contributory or predisposing factors
Minimal change disease:
- History of atopic diseases is often present
- Although usually idiopathic, may also be caused by mercury or lead exposure, Hodgkin's disease, and other malignancies, drugs such as NSAIDs, sulfasalazine and derivatives, food allergies, infectious mononucleosis, and HIV infection

FSCS:
- 20–30% of patients have underlying disease
- Infection: hepatitis B, malaria, schistomasiasis, many others
- Malignancy – may be occult at presentation: carcinomas at many sites, lymphomas, leukemias
- Autoimmune diseases: systemic lupus erythematosus and variants, Hashimoto's thyroiditis, myasthenia gravis
- Sarcoidosis
- Drugs and toxins: gold, penicillamine, captopril

Membranous nephropathy:
- Tumors (15% of cases, proportion increases with age)
- Drugs: especially gold and penicillamine
- Infection: hepatitis B, syphilis, malaria
- Systemic lupus erythematosus
- Sickle cell disease

Mesangiocapillary glomerulonephritis:
- Systemic lupus erythematosus
- Mixed essential cryoglobulinemia
- Cryoglobulinemia secondary to chronic infection, including hepatitis C, subacute bacterial endocarditis (SBE), HIV
- Homozygous sickle cell
- Intravenous drug abuse
- Partial lipodystrophy
- Malignancies and chronic lymphatic leukemia

EPIDEMIOLOGY
Incidence and prevalence
INCIDENCE
- Children: 2/100,000/year
- Adults: 3–4/100,000/year

Demographics
AGE

Minimal change disease accounts for >80% of all cases of nephrotic syndrome in children <10 years of age and only 10–15% of primary cases in adults.

GENDER

Minimal change disease: boys affected twice as frequently as girls but gender ratio is equal in adults.

RACE

FSGS is predominant cause of nephrotic syndrome in African-Americans.

GENETICS
- Familial renal diseases may cause nephrotic syndrome, e.g. Alport's syndrome, nail-patella syndrome, congenital nephrotic syndrome
- Reflux nephropathy has a strong familial component and may cause renal failure with nephrotic syndrome

DIFFERENTIAL DIAGNOSIS

Important to differentiate from nephritic syndrome which manifests hematuria, red blood cell casts, and proteinuria which may or may not be in the nephrotic range (>3.0g/24h). Membranoproliferative glomerulonephritis often manifests nephrotic syndrome but there is almost always a concomitant nephritic syndrome.

Edematous states

Cirrhosis:
- In decompensated cirrhosis with hypoalbuminemia, there may be pitting edema
- Other signs of liver disease such as palmar erythema, gynecomastia, testicular atrophy, xanthelasmata, spider naevi, signs of portal hypertension (ascites, abnormal abdominal veins, varices, splenomegaly), jaundice, and hepatic encephalopathy

Congestive heart failure:
- Peripheral pitting edema and pleural effusions
- Other cardiopulmonary signs of heart failure can be elicited
- Nephrotic range proteinuria is absent

SIGNS & SYMPTOMS

Signs

- Hypertension: severe hypertension is unusual in minimal change disease; often accompanies nephrotic syndrome and some degree of renal insufficiency in focal segmental glomerulosclerosis (FSGS)
- Edema, which may be severe. Facial edema that is most marked in the morning is characteristic, particularly in children
- Ascites
- Pleural effusions
- Signs of underlying disorder in secondary nephrotic syndrome

Symptoms

- Asymptomatic with incidental detection of proteinuria
- Severe peripheral edema
- Abdominal fullness
- Weight gain
- Symptoms of contributory disease in secondary nephrotic syndrome

ASSOCIATED DISORDERS

- Most common multisystem diseases found in conjunction with nephrotic syndrome are diabetes mellitus, systemic lupus erythematosus and other collagen vascular diseases, and primary or secondary amyloidosis
- Other multisystem disorders include cryoglobulinemia and sarcoid
- Infection: chronic hepatitis C infection may be the most common infectious condition associated with nephrotic/nephritic syndrome and membranoproliferative glomerulonephritis*; HIV infection can cause a glomerular lesion resembling FSGS which usually leads to nephrotic syndrome and can cause rapidly progressive renal failure; post-streptococcal nephritis*, endocarditis, syphilis, hepatitis B, malaria
- Neoplasms: carcinomas produce features typical of membranous glomerulonephropathy implicating an immune response to tumor antigens; lymphomas and leukemias are more often associated with minimal change disease; multiple myeloma is associated with nephrotic syndrome due to amyloidosis
- Unilateral renal artery stenosis, malignant hypertension

- Hereditary disorders: Alport's syndrome*, sickle cell disease, nail-patella syndrome, congenital nephrotic syndrome
- Pre-eclampsia
- Renal transplant rejection
- Reflux nephropathy
- Conditions marked with an asterisk (*) typically manifest both nephrotic and nephritic syndrome

KEY! DON'T MISS!
Rapidly deteriorating renal function.

CONSIDER CONSULT

- After infection has been excluded, all patients with proteinuria should be referred to a nephrologist to develop a plan for diagnosis, including possible renal biopsy

INVESTIGATION OF THE PATIENT
Direct questions to patient
Q **How old are you?** About 90% of cases of nephrotic syndrome in children under 10 years are due to minimal change disease. Membranous nephropathy is most common in adults. Males with membraneous nephropathy and aged over 50 have a poorer prognosis.

Q **What ethnic origin are you?** Homozygous sickle cell disease is associated with nephrotic syndrome. FSGS is the predominant lesion in idiopathic nephrotic syndrome in African-Americans.

Q **Are you well?** Patient may be asymptomatic and proteinuria is detected incidentally.

Q **Have you noticed any weight change?** Weight gain may occur with fluid retention.

Q **Have you noticed any swelling anywhere?** Severe peripheral edema may occur. Facial edema, most marked in the morning, is particularly characteristic in children. Ascites may lead to a feeling of abdominal fullness.

Q **Have you noticed any breathlessness?** Exertional dyspnea may occur with pleural effusion. Pulmonary edema may occur at very low serum albumin levels.

Q **Have you experienced recent upper respiratory tract symptoms, other infectious symptoms, polyuria/polydipsia, or joint problems?** Such a symptom review may elicit symptoms due to possible underlying disorders.

Contributory or predisposing factors
Q **Do you have any history of kidney disease?** For example, vesical reflux, amyloidosis.

Q **Have you had any urologic surgery in the past?** For example, for reflux, removal of part of kidney.

Q **Are you known to have high blood pressure?** May be a presenting symptom of renal disease. Unilateral renal artery stenosis and malignant hypertension may be associated with nephrotic syndrome.

Q **Do you have any history of other systemic diseases?** Diabetes mellitus, collagen vascular diseases, chronic infections, malignancy, and amyloidosis may be associated with nephrotic syndrome.

Q **Have you taken any medications recently?** Analgesics, NSAIDs, gold, penicillamine, aminoglycosides, cisplatin, and captopril are all implicated in nephrotic syndrome.

Q **Have you been exposed to any organic solvents or heavy metals?** Organic solvents may increase risk of glomerulonephritis. Heavy metals such as cadmium and lead are nephrotoxic.

Q **Do you smoke?** Diabetics who smoke are more likely to have renal disease than those who do not.

Q **Have you ever injected drugs?** Most important risk factor for hepatitis C infection. Drug users are at increased risk for other blood-borne infections, e.g. hepatitis B, HIV.

Q **Have you been on any foreign travels?** Protozoal and helminthic infections may be implicated in nephrotic syndrome.

Family history

Q Is there any family history of kidney disease? Familial renal diseases may cause nephrotic syndrome, e.g. Alport's syndrome, nail-patella syndrome, congenital nephrotic syndrome. Reflux nephropathy has a strong familial component and may cause renal failure with nephrotic syndrome.

Examination

- **General examination:** may show nonspecific signs associated with renal insufficiency: white nails, pallor, increased skin pigmentation
- **Blood pressure:** hypertension may be present, especially in FSGS
- **Assessment of fluid overload:** pitting edema, particularly in dependent areas, jugular vein pressure and blood pressure lying and standing. Facial edema is also characteristic in nephrotic syndrome in children
- **Chest examination:** may show signs consistent with pleural effusion
- **Abdominal examination:** may show ascites

Summary of investigative tests

Tests likely to be performed by the PCP and which confirm presence of nephrotic syndrome:
- Urinalysis
- 24h urine collection for proteinuria

Renal function and metabolic disturbance should be assessed by:
- Blood urea nitrogen (BUN), creatinine, creatinine clearance
- Complete blood count
- Biochemical profile: serum electrolytes, serum albumin, total protein cholesterol
- Chest X-ray may be useful

Tests likely to be performed by specialist, and which can identify underlying cause:
- Hepatitis serology: positive in hepatitis B and C infection
- Antinuclear antibodies, double-stranded DNA: usually present in lupus nephritis
- C3, C4, CH50: low C3 and C4 complement occur in systemic lupus erythematosus, postinfectious glomerulonephritis, membranoproliferative glomerulonephritis
- Serum and urine electrophoresis and immunoglobulin levels: may show abnormal paraproteins in amyloidosis, multiple myeloma
- Renal biopsy: often required for definitive diagnosis, prognosis, and development of an appropriate plan of therapy. Can usually be performed as outpatient if patient can be monitored for at least 8–12h as major bleeding generally occurs within that time
- Consider other investigations for underlying malignancy, e.g. ultrasound, computed tomography scan

DIAGNOSTIC DECISION

- Nephrotic syndrome is a clinical diagnosis confirmed by the finding of protein excretion of >3g/24h on laboratory investigation
- In most cases renal biopsy is needed to make a definitive diagnosis (except children, diabetics, patients with obvious end-stage renal disease), e.g. glomerulonephritis, amyloidosis
- Associated disorders may require further appropriate investigation

CLINICAL PEARLS

- In general, patients with obvious diabetic nephropathy do not require renal biopsy since biopsy confirmation will not alter course of therapy
- Urinalysis is critical in evaluation of patients with nephrotic syndrome. Aside from heavy proteinuria, nephrotic patients excrete oval fat bodies observed on microscopic examination of urine sediment. If, however, a nephritic urine sediment is also observed (dystrophic red blood cells and red blood cell casts), then this suggests a more complicated and difficult to treat type of renal disease, e.g. severe glomerulonephritis or membranoproliferative glomerulonephritis

THE TESTS
Body fluids
URINALYSIS

Description

- Observation of urine
- Dipstick testing for blood, protein
- Microscopy for oval fat bodies (manifestation of lipiduria), pyuria, hematuria, epithelial cells, casts

Advantages/Disadvantages

- Advantage: simple, noninvasive, readily available in the office; useful in classifying type of renal disease
- Disadvantage: not diagnostic of cause of nephrotic syndrome

Normal

- Urine is yellow in color
- Urine is usually crystal clear
- Dipstick test is negative for protein, blood
- Pyuria, oval fat bodies are not present
- Hyaline casts and a few epithelial cells are normal
- Granular, white cells, red cells, and waxy casts are not normally present

Abnormal

- Urine may be frothy due to high protein content
- Red or smoky urine is usually due to hematuria. May change color on standing with porphyria or on levodopa
- Cloudy urine may be due to pyuria, crystalluria, or (rarely) chyluria
- Dipstick is positive for protein and/or blood
- Presence of pus cells, large numbers of epithelial cells, red cells, and all casts except hyaline
- May be oval fat bodies, fatty casts or doubly refractile lipoid bodies under polarized light

Cause of abnormal result

- Dipstick test is sensitive to albumin but not other urinary proteins, e.g. light chains. A protein concentration of around 300mg/L is required for color change on stick. Highly concentrated normal urine may cause a 1+ reaction. Strongly positive tests nearly always indicate renal disease
- Presence of hematuria suggests nephritic syndrome but in minimal change disease and primary FSGS moderate microscopic hematuria may be present, although red blood cell casts are absent. Deformed red cells are strongly suggestive of glomerular bleeding
- Pus cells are usually due to inflammation (infection or nephritis); eosinophils are present in acute interstitial nephritis
- Epithelial cells are shed in increased numbers in acute tubular necrosis
- Granular casts are abnormal but do not indicate specific site. White cell casts are diagnostic of acute pyelonephritis; red cell casts indicate glomerular hematuria; waxy casts indicate chronic renal disease

Drugs, disorders and other factors that may alter results

- Bacterial urine infection may cause a positive dipstick test for protein
- Bence Jones protein may not be detected by dipsticks
- Myoglobinuria, contamination with iodine or hypochlorite, and bacterial peroxidase may also give positive dipstick test for 'blood', since this test really tests for iron-containing pigment (hemoglobin or myoglobin)

24-HOUR URINE COLLECTION FOR PROTEINURIA
Description
- Urinary protein:creatinine ratio (random urine sample)
- Electrophoresis allows qualitative assessment of which proteins are present

Advantages/Disadvantages
- Advantage: same collection can be used to assess creatinine clearance
- Disadvantage: accurate 24h urine collection is difficult to obtain

Normal
Proteinuria < 150mg/24h in urine.

Abnormal
- Proteinuria >300mg/24h is pathologic
- Nephrotic range proteinuria is >3g/24h
- Protein >30mg/113.1mg (1mmol) creatinine is pathologic
- Presence of monoclonal light chains. Also detects polyclonal light chains and tubular proteins

Cause of abnormal result
Increased permeability of glomerular basement membrane to proteins.

Drugs, disorders and other factors that may alter results
- Increased proteinuria may be functional and occurs as a result of fever, exercise, congestive heart failure, and upright posture, but seldom >1g/24h
- Tubular disease leads to decreased absorption of low molecular-weight proteins and, to lesser extent, of albumin
- Overflow from massively increased protein filtration may occur, e.g. Bence Jones protein overproduction

RENAL FUNCTION
Description
- BUN: serum sample. Product of protein catabolism in liver, eliminated mainly by glomerular filtration. Blood concentration reflects balance between production and removal of urea
- Creatinine: serum sample. Produced at a constant rate from muscle and is excreted by a combination of glomerular filtration and proximal tubular secretion in the kidney
- Creatinine clearance: requires 24h urine collection

Advantages/Disadvantages
Disadvantages:
- Accurate 24h urine collection may be difficult
- Alone, BUN is not a good guide to renal excretory function
- Serum creatinine is a better marker for gross renal function but not for early impairment. Does not normally rise above normal range until clearance has fallen by 50%

Normal
- BUN: 8–18mg/dL (2.9–6.4mmol/L)
- Creatinine: 0.6–1.2mg/dL (53.0–106.1mcmol/L), but this varies with body's muscle mass and gender
- Creatinine clearance: 75–124mL/min

Abnormal
- Minimal change disease: creatinine clearance may be mildly decreased
- FSGS: reduced glomerular filtration rate is not unusual on presentation, since this is more likely to be a progressive disease

Cause of abnormal result
Renal insufficiency.

Drugs, disorders and other factors that may alter results
- Urea production is increased by steroids, catabolic stress, and gastrointestinal bleeding and decreased by advanced liver disease
- Urea removal is decreased by congestive cardiac failure, hypovolemia, and chronic diuretic treatment
- Apart from renal dysfunction, serum creatinine may be elevated in rhabdomyolysis and falsely increased in ketonemia; it may be decreased in low muscle mass, pregnancy, and prolonged debilitation
- Creatinine clearance is elevated in pregnancy and exercise, and decreased in renal insufficiency and by some drugs

BIOCHEMICAL PROFILE
Description
- Serum electrolytes
- Serum albumin
- Total protein
- Cholesterol

Advantages/Disadvantages
Disadvantage: not specifically diagnostic for underlying cause, reflects pathologic processes in nephrotic syndrome.

Normal
- Albumin: 4–6g/dL (40–60g/L)
- Total protein: 6–8g/dL (60–80g/L)
- Cholesterol: varies with age, but generally <201.mg/dL (<5.2mmol/L)
- Sodium: 135–145mEq/L (135–145mmol/L)
- Potassium: 3.6–5.0mEq/L (3.6–5.0mmol/L)
- Chloride: 97–105mEq/L (97–105mmol/L)
- Bicarbonate: 23–27mEq/L (23–27mmol/L)

Abnormal
Values outside normal range.

Cause of abnormal result
- Hypoalbuminemia appears to be due to a failure to enhance hepatic synthesis sufficiently to compensate for increased urinary loss
- Hypercholesterolemia is characteristically a component of the nephrotic syndrome due to hepatic overproduction
- In severe cases of nephrotic syndrome, hyponatremia due to impaired water excretion may occur
- Hypokalemia may be a complication of diuretic therapy
- When renal failure occurs, metabolic acidosis with low serum bicarbonate may develop

Drugs, disorders and other factors that may alter results
- Albumin is elevated in dehydration, and decreased in liver disease, nephrotic syndrome, rapid intravenous hydration, protein-losing enteropathies, severe burns, neoplasia, chronic inflammatory disease, pregnancy, oral contraceptives, prolonged immobilization, lymphomas, hypervitaminosis A, chronic glomerulonephritis
- Total serum protein is elevated in dehydration, multiple myeloma, macroglobulinemia, sarcoidosis, collagen-vascular disease, and decreased in malnutrition, low protein diet, overhydration, malabsorption, pregnancy, severe burns, chronic disease, cirrhosis, nephrosis

▒ Total cholesterol may be elevated in primary hypercholesterolemia, biliary obstruction, nephrotic syndrome, primary biliary cirrhosis, third trimester pregnancy, and decreased in starvation, malabsorption, hepatic failure

COMPLETE BLOOD COUNT
Description
Venous blood sample.

Advantages/Disadvantages
Disadvantage: nonspecific test.

Normal
▒ White blood cells: 3200–9800/mm^3 (3.2–9.8x10^9/L)
▒ Hemoglobin: men 13.6–17.7g/dL (8.4–11.0mmol/L); women 12–15g/dL (7.4–9.3mmol/L)
▒ Hematocrit: men 39–49% (0.39–0.49); women 33–43% (0.33–0.44)
▒ Platelets: 130–400x10^3/mm^3 (130–400x10^9/L)

Abnormal
▒ Values outside normal range
▒ Elevated platelet count may occur in nephrotic syndrome

Imaging
CHEST X-RAY
Description
▒ Plain posteroanterior film
▒ Nonspecific investigation for underlying diagnosis or complications in nephrotic syndrome

Abnormal
In nephrotic syndrome with massive edema, pleural effusion may be seen.

Cause of abnormal result
Generalized edema due to hypoalbuminemia.

Drugs, disorders and other factors that may alter results
Infection, congestive cardiac failure, other edematous states.

RENAL ULTRASOUND EXAMINATION
Description
Examines kidneys for size, shape, presence of hydronephrosis, and to rule out postvoiding vesicoureteral reflux.

Advantages/Disadvantages
Advantage: noninvasive and nontoxic.

Normal
Normal renal size and absence of obstruction and reflux.

Abnormal
Hydronephrosis.

Cause of abnormal result
Stones, malignancy; congenital vesicoureteral reflux causing FSGS.

TREATMENT

CONSIDER CONSULT
- All patients should preferably be referred to a nephrologist for supervision of treatment
- Patients with refractory edema may need admission for possible intravenous diuretic/intravenous albumin therapy and other special measures as recommended by renal consultants
- Patients who are steroid resistant may need cytotoxic therapy and hospital admission

IMMEDIATE ACTION
- Patients with acute renal failure with rapidly deteriorating renal function need urgent assessment in the hospital
- Patient's with complicating severe infections (e.g. peritonitis complicating ascites, septicemia) require urgent hospitalization and critical care

PATIENT AND CAREGIVER ISSUES
Impact on career, dependants, family, friends
- A large percentage of patients with nephrotic syndrome are children
- It is often a chronic relapsing remitting disease requiring long-term treatment
- Depending on etiology and response to therapy, may result in end-stage renal disease requiring dialysis or transplant

Patient or caregiver request
Many patients are concerned about use of long-term steroids.

MANAGEMENT ISSUES
Goals
- Treatment of symptoms (proteinuria, edema, hyperlipidemia) and, if necessary, complications of nephrotic syndrome
- To provide specific treatment as indicated depending on underlying or associated disease
- To preserve or improve renal function, especially with assiduous blood pressure control to minimize rate of progression of renal failure
- To reduce complications of the nephrotic syndrome, e.g. antithrombotic/antibiotic prophylaxis

Management in special circumstances
SPECIAL PATIENT GROUPS
Children:
- Corticosteroids are the mainstay of treatment
- Use of alkylating agents in children with steroid-responsive disease is controversial. Probably required if steroid dose is likely to interfere with growth (>0.5mg/kg on alternate days)
- Cyclophosphamide (2–2.5mg/kg/day) for 8 weeks is effective at reducing longer-lasting remissions
- Chlorambucil (0.2mg/kg/day) for 2 months seems to have a similar effect to cyclophosphamide
- Cyclosporin (up to 150mg/m^2/day) is usually effective in nephrotic children who relapse frequently. Relapse is almost invariable within 3 months of stopping treatment and there is risk of cyclosporin nephrotoxicity

SUMMARY OF THERAPEUTIC OPTIONS
Choices
Treatment can be considered as symptomatic, supportive, or specific to the underlying condition. Specific therapy is for the nephrologist to recommend.

- The specific therapeutic regimen depends on findings from renal biopsy and associated conditions and etiologies
- Corticosteroids are the mainstay of treatment for minimal change disease in children and adults

- In membranous glomerulopathy and focal segmental glomerulosclerosis, corticosteroids are also commonly used initially, but with less consistent results and longer periods of administration are required
- In cases of steroid failure or dependence, immunosuppressive therapy with cytotoxic drugs (cyclophosphamide or cyclosporin) has been used with varying results. Such therapy should not be attempted without prior consultation with an experienced nephrologist

General considerations:
- Edema may be controlled with diuretics but hypovolemia may precipitate renal failure. Intravenous treatments such as albumin, dopamine, or loop diuretic infusion may also be of use in a hospital setting under supervision by a nephrologist
- Angiotensin-converting enzyme (ACE) inhibitors may reduce proteinuria and are especially useful as antihypertensives. Blood pressure should be vigorously treated as effective control may slow rate of progression of renal failure irrespective of underlying cause
- Antithrombotic and antibiotic prophylaxis should be considered for severe nephrotics
- Hypercholesterolemia may need to be controlled with statins especially if the underlying condition is not curable
- A low salt, normal protein diet may be appropriate for nephrotics

Clinical pearls
- Minimal change glomerulopathy in adults is quite sensitive to steroid therapy and results are similar to those in children
- Morbidity from prolonged steroid therapy is serious and frequently life-threatening. To avoid serious complications, it is important to monitor the patient for them (especially growth retardation in children, osteoporosis, peptic ulcer disease, and serious infections such as tuberculosis) and to use the minimum dose required to initiate and maintain a remission. Also, when it is clear that the patient represents a treatment failure, steroids should be reduced or eliminated, and consideration given to possible use of steroid-sparing drugs
- Steroid therapy has no beneficial effects on the nephrotic syndrome caused by diabetic nephropathy, amyloidosis, reflux nephropathy, membranoproliferative glomerulonephritis, HIV nephropathy, chronic glomerulonephritis, and is contraindicated in these conditions
- Extreme caution must be exercised in the use of diuretics for fluid retention in nephrotics as they are quite susceptible to acute hypovolemia, and acute renal failure can be precipitated. Diuretics are really only indicated to treat symptoms that interfere with essential functions such as nutrition and ambulation. It is probably unwise to treat mild edema with intensive diuretic therapy

Never
Never initiate treatment of adult nephrotic syndrome with steroids or cytotoxic therapy without a renal consultation and a diagnostic renal biopsy.

FOLLOW UP
- Long-term follow up is required while the patient remains proteinuric
- Specific associated diseases may also require long-term follow up

DRUGS AND OTHER THERAPIES: DETAILS
Drugs
CORTICOSTEROIDS
- Mainstay of treatment for minimal change disease
- Patients with focal segmental glomerulosclerosis (FSGS) do not usually respond to the steroid regimens used for minimal change disease
- Steroids alone may hasten remission in membranous nephropathy
- Membranoproliferative glomerulonephritis is unlikely to respond to steroids
- Prednisone may be used.

Dose

Prednisone

Minimal change disease:

- Children: 2mg/kg/day (maximum 60mg) for 2–8 weeks until a complete remission occurs, followed by a slowly tapering dose for 4–8 weeks if remission is maintained. Subsequent therapy is quite variable and should only be undertaken under supervision by an experienced nephrologist
- Adults respond more slowly and should be treated with 1mg/kg/day for 8–12 weeks followed by 0.5mg/kg/day for a further 6–8 weeks, and then by a tapering dose over 8 weeks

FSGS:

- Some patients experience remission if treated with prolonged high-dose steroids, e.g. 60mg/day for 6 months

Efficacy

- In children with minimal change disease, remission of proteinuria and diuresis is usually seen in the first few weeks. Complete remission in about 90% of children occurs within 8 weeks of starting treatment
- Low-dose and abbreviated regimens carry a higher risk of early relapse
- 80–90% of adults with minimal change disease respond within 3–4 months
- Approx. 40% of patients with FSGS respond to prolonged steroid therapy with complete remission

Risks/Benefits

Risks:

- Slow acting
- False-negative skin allergy tests. Overwhelming septicemia if patient has an infection
- Loss of control of blood glucose in those with diabetes
- Use caution in elderly due to risk of diabetes and osteoporosis
- Use caution in patients with psychosis, seizure disorder, or myasthenia gravis
- Use caution in congestive heart failure, hypertension
- Use caution in ulcerative colitis, peptic ulcer, or esophagitis
- May mask the signs of an acute abdomen or intussusception

Side-effects and adverse reactions

- Side-effects are minimized by short duration of therapy
- Cardiovascular system: hypertension, thromboembolism
- Central nervous system: insomnia, euphoria, depression, psychosis
- Endocrine: adrenal suppression, impaired glucose tolerance, growth suppression in children, Cushing's syndrome
- Eyes, ears, nose, and throat: cataract, glaucoma, blurred vision
- Gastrointestinal: dyspepsia, peptic ulceration, esophagitis, oral candidiasis, nausea, diarrhea
- Musculoskeletal: proximal myopathy, osteoporosis
- Skin: delayed healing, acne, striae

Interactions (other drugs)

- Adrenergic neurone-blockers, alpha-blockers, beta-blockers, beta-2 agonists
- Aminoglutethimide ▪ Anticonvulsants (carbamazepine, phenytoin, barbiturates)
- Antidiabetics ▪ Antidysrhythmics (calcium channel blockers, cardiac glycosides)
- Antifungals (amphotericin, ketoconazole) ▪ Antihypertensives (ACE inhibitors, diuretics: loop and thiazide, acetazolamide; angiotensin II receptor antagonists, clonidine, diazoxide, hydralazine, methyldopa, minoxidil) ▪ Cyclosporine ▪ Erythromycin ▪ Methotrexate ▪ Nitrates ▪ Nitroprusside ▪ Nonsteroidal anti-inflammatory drugs (NSAIDs) ▪ Oral contraceptives ▪ Rifampin ▪ Ritonavir ▪ Somatropin▪ Vaccines

Contraindications
- Systemic infection ▪ Avoid live virus vaccines in those receiving immunosuppressive doses

Acceptability to patient
Most patients tolerate the long- and short-term side-effects of steroids in this situation.

Follow up plan
- Overall follow-up plan requires primary involvement of the consultant nephrologist
- Some adults develop transient non-nephrotic relapses and further treatment should be delayed until nephrotic syndrome develops

ANGIOTENSIN-CONVERTING ENZYME (ACE) INHIBITORS
- Blood pressure should be vigorously treated as effective control may slow rate of progression of renal failure irrespective of underlying cause
- ACE inhibitors are especially useful as antihypertensives and may reduce proteinuria and help to control edema independent of the cause

Dose
Dosages need to be individually titrated for the individual patient.

Efficacy
- Slow deterioration in renal function; greatest benefit has been shown in patients with nephrotic-range proteinuria
- Most efficacious agents available to reduce proteinuria and are increasingly used in normotensive nondiabetic nephrotic patients to prevent progression of underlying nephropathy

Risks/Benefits
Risks:
- Use caution in renal impairment
- Use caution in hypotension and aortic stenosis
- Use caution in hyperkalemia, neutropenia

Side-effects and adverse reactions
- Cardiovascular system: orthostatic hypotension and syncope, angina, palpitations, sinus tachycardia
- Central nervous system: headache, dizziness, fatigue
- Eyes, ears, nose, and throat: cough
- Gastrointestinal: nausea, vomiting, diarrhea, constipation, abdominal pain
- Genitourinary: renal damage, impotence
- Hematologic: neutropenia, agranulocytosis, aplastic and hemolytic anemia, pancytopenia, thrombocytopenia
- Metabolic: hyperkalemia, hyponatremia
- Skin: angioedema, maculopapular rash

Interactions (other drugs)
- Allopurinol ▪ Antihypertensives (loop and potassium-sparing diuretics, prazosin, terazosin, doxazosin) ▪ Azathioprine ▪ Heparin ▪ Insulin ▪ Iron ▪ Lithium ▪ NSAIDs ▪ Potassium ▪ Sodium ▪ Trimethoprim

Contraindications
- Pregnancy ▪ Angioedema ▪ Hypotension ▪ Children

Acceptability to patient
Generally acceptable.

Follow up plan
Regular follow up with monitoring of blood pressure, proteinuria, and renal function.

DIURETICS

- Edema may be treated with loop diuretics (e.g. furosemide), taking care to avoid hypovolemia which may worsen renal function or precipitate acute renal failure
- In children with evidence of hypovolemia, 20% albumin solution is recommended but can precipitate acute pulmonary edema if over used

Dose
- As advised by nephrologist
- May need to be reduced in renal disease

Efficacy
Effective at treating edema but worsen hypovolemia.

Risks/Benefits
Risks:
- Use caution with diabetes mellitus, systemic lupus erythematosus
- Use caution with renal and liver disease
- Use caution with pregnancy and nursing mothers
- Use caution with hypertension and gout
- Use caution with porphyria
- Reduces fluid congestion

Benefit: reduced symptoms of edema

Side effects and adverse reactions
- Cardiovascular system: chest pain, circulatory collapse, orthostatic hypotension
- Central nervous system: dizziness, headache, paresthesia, fever
- Eyes, ears, nose, and throat: visual disturbances, ototoxicity, tinnitus, hearing impairment, thirst
- Gastrointestinal: ischemic hepatitis, vomiting, pancreatitis, nausea, diarrhea, anorexia
- Genitourinary: glycosuria, hyperuricemia, bladder spasm, polyuria
- Hematologic: blood disorders
- Metabolic: hyperglycemia, hyponatremia, hypokalemia, hypomagnesemia, hypovolemia, hypochloremia, hypercholesterolemia, hypertriglyceridemia
- Skin: erythema multiforme, exfoliative dermatitis, urticaria

Interactions (other drugs)
- ACE inhibitors ▪ Alpha-adrenergic antagonists ▪ Amphotericin ▪ Antibiotics (aminoglycosides, polymixins, vancomycin, cephalosporins) ▪ Antidiabetics ▪ Antidysrhythmics (amiodarone, cardiac glycosides, disopyramide, flecainide, mexelitine, quinidine, sotalol) ▪ Beta-2 agonists ▪ Carbenoxolone ▪ Cholestyramine, colestipol ▪ Cisplatin ▪ Clofibrate ▪ Corticosteroids ▪ Diuretics (thiazides, metolazone, acetazolamide) ▪ Lignocaine ▪ Lithium ▪ NSAIDs ▪ Phenobarbital ▪ Phenytoin ▪ Pimozide ▪ Reboxetine ▪ Selective serotonin reuptake inhibitors ▪ Terbutaline ▪ Tubocurarine

Contraindications
- Renal failure with anuria ▪ Hepatic coma

Acceptability to patient
Generally acceptable.

Follow up plan
- Regular follow up with monitoring of renal function
- Patients must be closely monitored for volume depletion
- Hospital admission may be necessary for patients with gross edema

STATINS
- Hypercholesterolemia may need to be controlled, especially if underlying condition is not curable; statins are the most effective therapy
- Association between hyperlipidemia of nephrotic syndrome and accelerated atherosclerosis has not been proven conclusively
- Dietary manipulations are ineffective in nephrotic syndrome due to severity of hyperlipidemia
- Simvastatin is licensed as a hyperlipidemic agent

Dose
As advised by a nephrologist or cardiologist. Caution is required in patients with metabolic and electrolyte imbalances.

Efficacy
- Strong lipid-lowering effects
- Patients who respond to therapy with corticosteroids or cytotoxics without other cardiovascular risk factors are less likely to obtain benefit from treatment

Risks/Benefits
Risks:
- Marked response seen within 2 weeks of initiation, maximum therapeutic response occurring within 4–6 weeks. Response is maintained during chronic therapy
- Use caution with past liver disease, alcoholism
- Use caution with severe acute infections, trauma, hypotension
- Use caution with uncontrolled seizure disorders, severe metabolic and electrolyte disorders

Side-effects and adverse reactions
- Central nervous system: dizziness, peripheral neuropathy, headache, insomnia
- Gastrointestinal: nausea, vomiting, dyspepsia, pancreatitis, abdominal pain, liver dysfunction
- Genitourinary: erectile dysfunction
- Hematologic: blood cell disorders
- Musculoskeletal: muscle weakness and pain, rhabdomyolysis
- Skin: rash, Stevens-Johnson syndrome, abdominal pain

Interactions (other drugs)
- Azole antifungals ▪ Cholestyramine ▪ Colestipol ▪ Cyclosporine ▪ Danazol ▪ Fluoxetine ▪ Gemfibrozil ▪ Isradipine ▪ Macrolide antibiotics ▪ Nefazadone ▪ Niacin ▪ Warfarin

Contraindications
▪ Acute liver disease ▪ Pregnancy category X ▪ Nursing ▪ Safety and efficacy in pediatric patients have not been established

Acceptability to patient
Generally well tolerated. May cause muscle cramps and, occasionally, rhabdomyolysis.

Follow up plan
- Repeat cholesterol at 4–6 weeks (maximum response)
- Check liver function before therapy and at 12 weeks. If no change, no further monitoring necessary, if serum aspartate transaminase/alanine aminotransferase raised more than 3-fold above normal range, cease treatment
- Check creatine phosphokinase in patients with diffuse muscle pain or weakness

Patient and caregiver information
- Report symptoms of muscle aching or tenderness
- Take in the evening for increased effect

Chemotherapy
CYTOTOXIC DRUGS
- Cytotoxics/immunosuppressives may be useful for steroid-resistant cases or in conjunction with steroids as steroid-sparing drugs
- Should be used only upon specific recommendations of, and supervised by, a nephrologist experienced in their usage
- Drugs commonly used include: cyclophosphamide, cyclosporine, azathioprine, and chlorambucil (used rarely in adults); tacrolimus is a newer agent used in transplantation and may be useful in resistant cases
- Dose: as advised by a nephrologist

Efficacy
Minimal change disease:
- Cyclosporine is effective in maintaining remission and may be considered as a steroid-sparing agent in patients with frequent relapses. However, relapse commonly follows dose reduction or withdrawal
- Cyclophosphamide reduces risk of subsequent relapses but because of toxicity is only offered to those with frequent relapses

Membranous nephropathy:
- Combinations of steroids with chlorambucil induce remission and reduce loss of renal function but, as many of these patients are destined for spontaneous remission, this regimen is not widely used

FSGS:
- Prolonged courses of cyclophosphamide or azathioprine with steroids may induce lasting remission in at least some patients
- Cyclosporine is not thought to induce a lasting remission but may maintain remission as long as drug is used

Membranoproliferative glomerulonephritis:
- No evidence of benefit from cytotoxic agents
- Suggested that they stabilize renal function with antiplatelet agents or anticoagulants but have no effect on proteinuria

Risks/Benefits
Risks:
- Nephrotoxicity (patients with FSGS seem particularly susceptible) and hypertension with long-term use of cyclosporine
- Low risk of infertility in women and cystitis at moderate doses
- Secondary malignancy with cytotoxic treatments
- Use caution with radiation therapy

Benefit: in some cases may keep symptoms under control until spontaneous remission occurs

Side-effects and adverse reactions:
- Cardiovascular system: cardiotoxicity (at high doses)
- Central nervous system: dizziness, headache
- Gastrointestinal: nausea, vomiting, diarrhea
- Genitourinary: amenorrhea, azoospermia, ovarian fibrosis, sterility, hematuria, hemorrhagic cystitis, neoplasms
- Hematologic: leukopenia, myelosuppression, panycytopenia, thrombocytopenia
- Metabolic: bone marrow supression
- Respiratory: fibrosis
- Skin: alopecia, dermatitis

Interactions (other drugs):
- Allopurinol (increased cyclophosphamide toxicity) ■ Clozapine (may cause agranulocytosis) ■ Digoxin (decreased digoxin absorption from tablet form) ■ Pentostatin (increased toxicity with high-dose cyclophosphamide) ■ Phenytoin (reduced absorption of phenytoin) ■ Succinylcholine (prolonged neuromuscular blockade) ■ Suxemethonium (enhanced effect of suxemethonium) ■ Warfarin (inhibits hypoprothrombinemic response to warfarin)

Contraindications:
- Serious infections, including chicken pox and herpes zoster ■ Myelosuppression

Acceptability to patient
Generally acceptable.

Follow up plan
- Regular follow up with monitoring of hematologic indices and renal function
- Long-term surveillance for secondary malignancy

Other therapies
ANTITHROMBOTIC AND ANTIBIOTIC PROPHYLAXIS
- Prophylactic anticoagulants may be indicated for severe nephrotics as a hypercoaguable state exists, but long-term anticoagulation should not be necessary if underlying condition can be put into remission (e.g. minimal change disease). However, patients with nephrotic syndrome may be relatively resistant to effects of heparin as a result of antithrombin 111 losses in the urine
- Antibiotic prophylaxis may be considered in severe nephrotics
- Prophylactic penicillin may be considered in patients with ascites as they are at risk of spontaneous pneumococcal peritonitis

Risks/Benefits
Benefit: prevention of thromboembolic complications and infection which are both potentially life threatening.

Acceptability to patient
- Both treatments are generally acceptable
- Elderly patients are at greater risk of complications from anticoagulation

Follow up plan
Regular monitoring of heparin therapy.

399

LIFESTYLE

- Patients are at risk of malnutrition from persistent urinary protein losses, and gastrointestinal absorption may become suppressed due to edema of the bowel
- Adequate protein and calorie intake must be maintained
- Avoid high-protein diets as they exacerbate proteinuria. Dietary protein intake should not be lower than 1g/kg ideal bodyweight, and severe protein restriction has no demonstrable benefit
- Sodium restriction may help control edema and potentiates the antiproteinuric effect of ACE inhibitors. Limiting intake to 2g/day is usually sufficient to ameliorate fluid retention

RISKS/BENEFITS
Benefit: improvement in edema.

ACCEPTABILITY TO PATIENT
- Low-salt diets may initially be fairly tasteless to patients
- Many patients may dislike a reduced protein diet

FOLLOW UP PLAN
Ideally, patient should be advised by a renal dietitian.

EFFICACY OF THERAPIES

- Steroid therapy induces complete remission within 8 weeks of starting treatment in 90% of children with minimal change disease; 80–90% of adults with minimal change disease respond within 3–4 months
- In a significant proportion of patients with membranous glomerulopathy or focal segmental glomerulosclerosis (FSGS; 20–40%), longer-term administration of steroids may induce complete or partial remission
- For those who become steroid resistant there is no consensus as to what is the best treatment. Use of cytotoxic drugs is successful in some, depending on the underlying cause
- Chronic renal failure and end-stage renal disease will be the outcome for some patients despite therapy, depending on the underlying lesion in the kidney. More likely in nephrotic patients with morphologic glomerular abnormalities on renal biopsy (e.g. membranous glomerulopathy, FSGS, membranoproliferative glomerulonephritis)

PROGNOSIS

Depends on underlying cause of nephrotic syndrome and prognosis of any associated disorder.

Minimal change disease:
- Relapsing course
- In children, about 30% of steroid responders never have a relapse, and another 10–20% are cured after one to four episodes responsive to steroids. The remainder are frequent relapsers
- Adults tend to relapse less frequently than children
- Overall prognosis for eventual complete remission is excellent

FSGS:
- Traditionally thought to have poor prognosis
- 30–40% of patients respond to steroids with complete remission and in those that do respond renal survival at 5 years exceeds 95%
- Even in those who do not go into remission, renal survival at 5 years is 55%
- Remission of proteinuria in FSGS is associated with a greatly reduced risk of progressive renal disease

Membranous nephropathy:
- Clinical course is unpredictable
- Sustained remission may occur after years of nephrotic-range proteinuria; 20–30% have spontaneous remission and up to 40% have partial remission or remain stable
- Renal function may start to decline and then improve although, more commonly, there may be inexorable decline to end-stage renal disease once decline has started. Renal failure eventually develops in 15–20%
- Persistent nephrotic syndrome causes profound muscle wasting and malaise
- Prognosis is poorer for malignancy-associated patients than patients with the malignancy but no nephrotic syndrome
- Risk factors for poor prognosis are male gender, age >50, and heavy proteinuria
- Risk of recurrence of disease in renal transplant is around 10%

Membranoproliferative glomerulonephritis:
- End-stage renal disease occurs in 50% at 10 years and 90% at 20 years
- Spontaneous remission occurs in <20%

Therapeutic failure

- Cytotoxic drugs may be considered for patients not responding to steroids
- Patients who progress to end-stage renal disease require dialysis or renal transplantation for survival

Recurrence

- Relapses are treated similarly to initial presentation
- Children who are frequent relapsers may be managed by gradually tapering the steroid dose to the threshold at which relapse occurs and continuing this dose for 6–12 months. Safety depends on dose of steroid required

Deterioration

If renal function deteriorates progressively to end-stage renal disease, dialysis or transplant may be necessary.

COMPLICATIONS

- Renal vein thrombosis: important cause of renal impairment in patients with nephrotic syndrome, and often underdiagnosed. Frequently caused by membranous nephropathy, lupus nephritis, amyloidosis, and any form of glomerulonephritis causing nephrotic syndrome. May be completely asymptomatic or cause loin pain, hematuria, renal swelling, acute renal failure, or acute or chronic renal failure with oliguria. If it extends to the vena cava, may cause bilateral leg swelling or pulmonary emboli. Thrombosis of renal vein or its branches may be found in up to 50% of patients with membranous nephropathy and nephrotic syndrome but is symptomatic in only 5–15%
- Hypercholesterolemia: greatly raised serum cholesterol is nearly always seen in nephrotic patients and patients with a history of nephrotic syndrome have an increased risk of death from coronary heart disease. The mechanism is uncertain although increased hepatic synthesis appears to be switched on by decreased plasma oncotic pressure. Dietary treatment is usually disappointing and statins are effective and are the drugs of choice
- Infection: spontaneous bacterial peritonitis occurs particularly in nephrotic children and is frequently due to pneumococci. Cellulitis is a frequent problem in adults
- Acute renal failure with hypovolemia occasionally occurs, especially in adults after treatment with diuretics
- Chronic renal failure may develop and progress to end-stage renal disease
- Growth retardation is a potential complication in children treated with long-term steroids

CONSIDER CONSULT

- Any patient who relapses after discontinuation of therapy should be referred back to a nephrologist

PREVENTION

Very few preventive measures are applicable to this condition.

RISK FACTORS

Infections such as hepatitis B, hepatitis C, and HIV are associated with nephrotic syndrome. Patients who may be at increased risk of acquiring blood-borne infection, e.g. intravenous drug users, should be advised on risk reduction behaviors.

PREVENT RECURRENCE

Early detection of recurrence of minimal change glomerulopathy before the onset of severe proteinuria and edema can be achieved with careful monitoring with urine dipsticks and, if positive, reinstitution of treatment.

RESOURCES

ASSOCIATIONS

National Kidney Foundation
30 East 33rd St., Suite 1100
New York, NY 10016
Phone: (800) 622-9010 or (212) 889-2210
Fax: (212) 689-9261
E-mail: info@kidney.org
http://www.kidney.org

KEY REFERENCES

- Humes HD, Dupont HL, eds. In: Kelley's textbook of internal medicine. Philadelphia (PA): Lippincott Williams and Wilkins, 2000
- Siegel NJ. Minimal change disease. In: Greenberg A, ed. Primer on kidney diseases. New York: Academic Press, 2001: p143–7
- Hodson EM, Knight JF, Willis NS, Craig JC. Corticosteroid therapy for nephrotic syndrome in children (Cochrane Review). In: The Cochrane Library, 2001, 3. Oxford: Update Software
- Cameron JS. The nephrotic syndrome and its complications. Am J Kidney Dis 1987;10:157–71
- Schwarz A. New aspects of the treatment of nephrotic syndrome. J Am Soc Neph 2001;12(Suppl 17)
- Berns JS, Gaudio KM, Krassner LS, et al. Steroid-responsive nephrotic syndrome of childhood: a long term study of clinical course, histopathology, efficacy of cyclophosphamide therapy, and effects on growth. Am J Kidney Dis 1987;9:108–14
- Bergman JM. Management of minimal lesion glomerulonephritis: Evidence-based recommendations. Kidney Int 1999;55:S3–S16
- Korbet S. Primary focal segmental glomerulosclerosis. J Am Soc Nephrol 1998;9:1333–40

FAQS
Question 1
What is the role of diuretic therapy in nephrotic syndrome?

ANSWER 1
Diuretics may play a role, but they do not alter the natural history of the syndrome. Their use should be restricted to improving the patient's daily lifestyle to enable him/her to perform essential functions such as nutritional intake, appropriate ambulation, normal respiratory function. Minimal-to-moderate peripheral edema is not an urgent indication for diuretic usage. Remember nephrotic patients are vulnerable to episodes of acute hypovolemia with acute renal failure, and these are commonly precipitated by diuretics.

Question 2
Is nephrotic syndrome a manifestation of the nephropathy associated with systemic lupus erythematosus?

ANSWER 2
Yes, nephrotic syndrome is one type of lupus nephropathy (class V). A pure form of nephrotic syndrome in lupus is morphologically represented by the changes of membranous glomerulopathy on renal biopsy with subepithelial deposits in the basement membrane. This is uncommon compared to lupus glomerulonephritis which is typically manifested by a nephritic syndrome on urinalysis (proteinuria plus red blood cells and red blood cell casts). Also, lupus membranous nephropathy may spontaneously change, as manifested on biopsy and clinical manifestations, into a more common form of lupus glomerulonephritis.

Question 3
What is an effective way to treat nephrotic syndrome associated with systemic diseases and manifested on renal biopsy by focal segmental glomerulosclerosis (e.g. HIV nephropathy, heroin-associated nephropathy, reflux nephropathy)?

ANSWER 3
Unfortunately, these forms of nephrotic syndrome do not respond to conventional therapy used to treat idiopathic nephrotic syndrome such as corticosteroids or immunosuppressive therapy. The best approach is to provide supportive therapy including control of the major risk factors for progression to end stage, e.g. hypertension. Angiotensin-converting enzyme inhibitors or A11 receptor blockers may control the magnitude of the proteinuria as well as the hypertension.

CONTRIBUTOR
Fred F Ferri, MD, FACP

ORCHITIS

DESCRIPTION

- Most commonly viral (usually mumps) but may be bacterial
- Mumps is the commonest cause of viral orchitis
- Bacterial orchitis is treated with antibiotics
- Most patients recover fully, a few develop testicular infarction, atrophy or infertility
- Acute orchitis causes local testicular pain and tenderness, with scrotal swelling
- Primary orchitis is rare, most commonly associated with epididymitis

URGENT ACTION

Commence empirical antibiotic therapy if bacterial orchitis suspected.

ICD9 CODE
604.90 Orchitis (nonspecific septic)
604.91 Orchitis (in diseases classified elsewhere)
604.0 Orchitis (with abscess)
098.42 Orchitis (acute gonococcal)
098.13 Orchitis (chronic)
072.0 Orchitis (mumps)
604.99 Orchitis (suppurative)

SYNONYMS
If epldidymitis also involved, may be referred to as epididymo-orchitis.

CARDINAL FEATURES
- May be unilateral or bilateral
- May be due to either viral or bacterial infection, but isolated involvement of the testis without the epididymis, is more likely to be viral
- Mumps is the commonest cause of viral orchitis, is rare in prepubertal boys, but occurs in approximately 30% of postpubertal boys
- No specific treatment for mumps orchitis
- Bacterial orchitis treated with antibiotics, may be parenteral if infection severe
- Patients with bacterial orchitis may develop scrotal or testicular abscess, and require surgical drainage and occasionally orchidectomy
- Acute orchitis causes local testicular pain and tenderness, with scrotal swelling
- Most patients fully recover, but a small number develop testicular infarction, atrophy, or are rendered infertile

CAUSES
Common causes
May be due to viral or bacterial infection, if orchitis occurs without any involvement of the epididymis, cause is more likely to be viral.

Viral
- Mumps (most common)
- Coxsackie B virus

Bacterial (often associated with epididymitis)
- *Escherichia coli*
- *Klebsiella pneumoniae*
- *Pseudomonas aeruginosa*
- *Staphlococcus* species
- *Streptococcus* species
- *Chlamydia trachomatis*

Rare causes
Noninfectious orchitis (more commonly epididymoorchitis) usually secondary to chemical inflammation, secondary to sterile reflux of urine to the epididymis and testis via the vas deferens.

May occur in association with:
- Cytomegalovirus (CMV)
- Toxoplasmosis

- Cryptococcosis
- Histoplasmosis
- Candidiasis
- Blastomycosis
- Actinomycosis
- *Neisseria gonorrhoeae*
- Syphilitic gumma (may cause chronic orchitis)

Serious causes
Mycobacterium tuberculosis (tuberculosis): Usually associated with epididymitis

Contributory or predisposing factors
- Epididymitis
- Urinary tract infection
- Prostatitis
- Indwelling urethral catheter
- Recent urethral instrumentation or surgery
- Bladder outlet obstruction (e.g. urethral stricture, benign prostatic hyperplasia)
- Immunosuppression (e.g. infection with HIV)

EPIDEMIOLOGY
Incidence and prevalence
INCIDENCE
Incidence of orchitis is not known, but the incidence of mumps has decreased from 185,691 reported cases in 1968 to 906 reported cases in 1995.

FREQUENCY
Orchitis is common, although precise data are unavailable.

Demographics
AGE
- May occur at any age
- Mumps orchitis is rare in prepubertal boys, but occurs in about 30% of postpubertal males with mumps

RACE
- Racial differences in mumps incidence reflect immunization coverage
- Highest incidence of mumps in blacks
- Somewhat increased incidence of mumps in Hispanics
- Lowest incidence of mumps in whites

DIAGNOSIS

DIFFERENTIAL DIAGNOSIS

- The most important differential diagnoses are testicular torsion, testicular tumor, and Fournier's gangrene, all of which require urgent referral
- Other differential diagnoses include torsion of the testicular appendages, epididymitis, epididymal cyst, hydrocele, hematocele and testicular trauma

Testicular torsion
FEATURES
- Commonest at ages 12–18 years, but can occur at any age
- Usually present with testicular pain and swelling of sudden onset
- 10% have painless testicular swelling
- May have had previous episodes of testicular pain which settled spontaneously
- Refer immediately to urologist for scrotal exploration and detorsion
- If detorsion within 12 hours of onset, 80% chance of salvaging testis

Testicular tumor
FEATURES
- Commonest in young adults, but can occur at any age
- Higher incidence in patients with an undescended testicle (even if surgically corrected), previous contralateral testicular tumor and intersex disorders
- Painless swelling of the testis
- Usually no other symptoms, unless has metastasized
- May be found at time of evaluation for trauma or hydrocele

Fournier's gangrene
FEATURES
- Necrotizing fasciitis of the scrotum
- Variety of organisms may be responsible, most commonly E. coli
- Risk factors include recent scrotal trauma or surgery, or a history of diabetes mellitus
- Scrotal pain
- Foul smell
- Fever, tachycardia
- Dark discoloration of scrotal skin
- Crepitation may be felt if responsible organism is gas-producing
- Urgent surgical intervention required
- High mortality rate

Torsion of the testicular appendages
FEATURES
- Most common in prepubertal boys
- Severe testicular pain
- Scrotal swelling and induration
- May be clinically indistinguishable from testicular torsion
- Torted appendage may be visible through skin ('Blue dot sign')
- If sure of diagnosis, treat conservatively
- If any doubt, will require immediate urological consultation and may require scrotal exploration

Epididymitis
FEATURES
- Commonest in sexually active men, but can occur at any age
- Different causative organisms in each group

- In prepubertal boys, the commonest organisims are coliforms
- In sexually active young men, the commonest organisms are *Neisseria gonorrhoeae* and *Chlamydia trachomatis*
- In men over 35 years of age, the commonest organisms are Gram-negative bacteria
- Tender, erythematous scrotum
- Dysuria and/or urethral discharge
- May have fever and be systemically unwell
- May progress to involve testis, hence epididymo-orchitis
- Treat with antibiotics, choice depends on causative organism

Epididymal cyst
FEATURES

- Commonest in men over 40 years
- Palpable lump separate from testis
- No treatment required unless large or painful
- Treatment, if necessary, is by excision
- May need to do ultrasound to confirm if not distinguishable on physical exam or if there is a question of tumor

Hydrocele
FEATURES

- Occurs at any age
- Congenital or acquired
- Congenital hydrocele usually presents in childhood, and requires surgical repair of patent processus vaginalis if does not resolve by age 1
- Acquired hydrocele does not require treatment if asymptomatic, and underlying testis is normal

SIGNS & SYMPTOMS
Signs

- Pyrexia
- Tachycardia
- Swelling and erythema of the affected hemiscrotum
- Swollen, tender testis (and possibly epididymis)
- Reactive hydrocele
- Fluctuant area may be palpable, if abscess present
- Inguinal lymphadenopathy
- Urethral discharge

Symptoms

- Testicular pain
- Symptoms of urinary tract infection: frequency, dysuria
- Nausea and vomiting

CONSIDER CONSULT

- All young boys
- Patients in whom the diagnosis is in doubt
- Patients with systemic sepsis
- Patients suspected of having tuberculous orchitis
- Immunocompromized patients (e.g. those with HIV)
- Patients suspected of having gangrene, torsion, strangulated hernia or hydrocele
- If a scrotal abscess or gangrene is suspected
- If scrotal crepitus is present

INVESTIGATION OF THE PATIENT
Direct questions to patient
Q How old are you? In young men and boys testicular torsion and tumor must be excluded early.

Q Have you been passing urine more frequently than normal, and has it been painful?
A recent urinary tract infection may contribute to the development of orchitis.

Q Have you had any aching of the scrotum or pain on ejaculation? An episode of prostatitis may lead to the development of orchitis.

Q Have you recently had any surgery on the urinary tract? Instrumentation of the urinary tract may predispose to urinary tract infection.

Q Have you ever had any trauma to your urinary tract or genitalia? Trauma may predispose to the development of a urethral stricture.

Q Do you think that the strength of your flow when you urinate has changed at all? A slow flow may indicate the presence of a stricture.

Q Have you ever had any serious illness or infection? Patient may have a history of for example tuberculosis or HIV.

Q Does the patient have mumps? This is the most common cause of simple orchitis.

Contributory or predisposing factors
Q Any history of predisposing factors? For example, recent episode of epididymitis, prostatitis, urinary tract infection

Family history
Q Has anyone else in the family been unwell recently? Other members of the family may have had mumps.

Q Has anyone in the family had tuberculosis? If so, tuberculosis may need to be considered as a diagnosis, even if the patient is not known to have had it in the past.

Examination
- Check temperature: may be elevated
- Take pulse: may be tachycardic
- Measure blood pressure: if patient is hypotensive, with signs of systemic sepsis, suspect septic shock
- Examine the penis: crusting around the meatus suggests the patient may have a urethral discharge
- Examine the scrotum: affected hemiscrotum may be swollen and erythematous
- Examine the testis: the affected testis is hard, swollen, and may be surrounded by a reactive hydrocele; if the epididymis is involved (i.e. the patient has epididymo-orchitis), this will be tender and indurated

Summary of investigative tests
- Urinalysis (dipstick): should be performed in all patients, the presence of protein and/or leucocytes especially is suggestive of infection
- Urine culture: should be performed, as urinary tract infection may coexist
- Full blood count: if patient systemically unwell. Raised white cell count suggestive of significant infection, although a reduced white cell count may be seen in mumps
- Ultrasound scan of scrotal contents: to check for abscess, or any other pathology, particularly tumor
- Doppler ultrasound to assess blood flow
- Mumps viral titer: not performed routinely but may be useful in cases of diagnostic doubt
- Blood cultures: not performed routinely, but important in identifying bacterial pathogens

DIAGNOSTIC DECISION
Diagnosis based on clinical examination, supported by laboratory tests and ultrasound findings.

CLINICAL PEARLS

- The most common cause of simple orchitis is mumps
- Mumps orchitis can be severe enough to produce sufficient edema to result in bilateral atrophy and hypergonadotrophic hypogonadism with gynecomastia and infertility
- Aspiration of a tense inflammatory hydrocele (by a trained urologist) can result in symptomatic relief of pain and provide material for culture

THE TESTS
Body fluids
URINALYSIS (DIPSTICK)
Description
Midstream urine specimen.

Advantages/Disadvantages
Advantages:
- Quick and simple to perform at office level
- Provides information about a variety of urinary constituents very quickly

Disadvantages:
- Whether normal or abnormal, does not confirm or refute the diagnosis
- Is very nonspecific

Normal
No red or white blood cells, or protein identified.

Abnormal
- Red and/or white blood cells, and/or protein present
- Dipstick tests can be highly sensitive, a false positive result is possible

URINE CULTURE
Description
Midstream urine specimen.

Advantages/Disadvantages
- Confirms or refutes diagnosis of urinary tract infection
- Identifies bacteria responsible

Normal
No bacteria cultured.

Abnormal
Bacteria cultured.

Cause of abnormal result
- Presence of infection
- Contamination of specimen
- Improper handling of specimen

Drugs, disorders and other factors that may alter results
Urine sample may be contaminated, e.g. by skin or bowel commensal organisms.

FULL BLOOD COUNT
Description
Cuffed venous blood sample.

Advantages/Disadvantages
- Advantage: raised white cell count may indicate infection, although a decreased white cell count is often seen in mumps and other viral infections
- Disdvantage: nonspecific

Normal
WBC 4.0–11.0 x 10^9/l.

Abnormal
WBC:
- <4.0 x 10^9/l (may be seen in mumps)
- >11.0 x 10^9/l (especially if bacterial infection present)

Drugs, disorders and other factors that may alter results
- Many infections
- Immunocompromized state
- Some hematologic disorders
- Depending on the severity of the abnormality, may need investigation in its own right

VIRAL TITER (MUMPS)
Description
Isolation of the mumps virus from throat washings, urine, blood or spinal fluid using immunoflurescence assay for viral antigen.

Advantages/Disadvantages
- Advantage: confirmation of mumps infection
- Disdvantage: result not available immediately

Normal
Mumps virus not isolated.

Abnormal
- Mumps virus detected
- Keep in mind the possibility of a false positive result

Cause of abnormal result
Infection with mumps virus (a paramyxovirus).

BLOOD CULTURES
Description
Venous blood sample, usually taken while the patient is febrile.

Advantages/Disadvantages
Advantage: simple test

Disadvantages:
- Results not available immediately
- May be contaminated by skin organisms

Normal
No growth of organisms.

Abnormal
- Growth of organisms
- Keep in mind the possibility of a false positive result

Cause of abnormal result
Bacteremia.

Imaging
ULTRASOUND SCAN OF SCROTAL CONTENTS
Advantages/Disadvantages
Advantages:
- No exposure to ionizing radiation
- Identifies a variety of pathologies, e.g. abscess, tumor, torsion
- Done with Doppler ultrasound that can evaluate blood supply to testis
- Can be repeated as often as desired

Disadvantages:
- Often does not provide conclusive proof of a diagnosis
- If testicular torsion suspected, delay involved in organizing ultrasound will be unacceptable

Normal
Normal testes.

Abnormal
- Hypo- or hyperechoic area may be seen
- Considerable experience required to interpret scan
- Cystic area may represent abscess

Drugs, disorders and other factors that may alter results
Scarring or atrophy of testis due to previous trauma or infection.

DOPPLER ULTRASOUND
Advantages/Disadvantages
Advantages:
- No exposure to ionizing radiation
- Easy to perform
- Noninvasive, no patient discomfort
- Relatively inexpensive

Disadvantages:
- Nonspecific
- Operator-dependent
- Equivocal testing secondary to edema, hydrocele, and inflammation makes diagnosis the more difficult
- Adequate or increased blood flow may be present in early torsion
- Result is dependent on technique

Normal
Flow within normal guidelines.

Abnormal
- Increased flow-inflammation, e.g. epididymitis, early torsion
- Decreased flow-torsion

Drugs, disorders and other factors that may alter results
Trauma, scarring or torsion of testicular appendages.

TREATMENT

IMMEDIATE ACTION
Commence empirical therapy with a broad spectrum antibiotic, if bacterial orchitis suspected.

PATIENT AND CAREGIVER ISSUES
Patient or caregiver request
- Is the patient concerned that he may have testicular cancer?
- Is the patient concerned that he may be left infertile?
- Is the patient concerned that this may be sexually transmitted disorder?

Health-seeking behavior
Has the patient waited too long before presenting? If so, this might be due to fear or embarrassment.

MANAGEMENT ISSUES
Goals
- Treat infection
- Reduce pain and swelling
- Reduce chances of permanent sequalae
- Early recognition of need for specialist referral

Management in special circumstances
COEXISTING DISEASE
- Epididymitis: treat concurrently
- HIV: these patients often require complex care, and specialist advice should be sought

SPECIAL PATIENT GROUPS
Immunosuppressed patients: higher risk for unusual pathogens.

PATIENT SATISFACTION/LIFESTYLE PRIORITIES
- Small proportion of patients may be rendered infertile, this will have major implications if they wish children in the future
- Some patients require orchidectomy, which may lead to psychological distress

SUMMARY OF THERAPEUTIC OPTIONS
Choices
- There is no specific treatment for viral orchitis, and treatment is largely supportive
- Bacterial orchitis will require antibiotic therapy in most cases. If severe systemic sepsis is present, patient should be admitted to hospital for parenteral antibiotics. Often treatment needs to be commenced before the causative agent is identified
- Choice of antibiotic depends on suspected causative organism. No clear first choice, but suitable antibiotics include ciprofloxacin, levofloxacin, norfloxacin, amoxicillin-clavulanate and trimethoprim-sulfamethoxazole
- Analgesia is often required. Useful agents include NSAIDs (e.g. naproxen, ibuprofen), and acetaminophen
- Surgical therapy such as aspiration of hydrocele or scrotal exploration and/or orchiectomy may be required in some patients
- Scrotal supports may improve patient comfort

Clinical pearls
- There have been reports of systemic treatment with interferon-alpha 2B in the prevention of sterility after bilateral mumps orchitis

417

- A recent epidemic in Switzerland of mumps orchitis highlights the need for continued vaccination worldwide against the mumps virus
- Bacterial orchitis that fails to respond to oral agents require hospitalization and parenteral therapy

Never
Never commence a patient on antituberculous therapy without specialist referral.

FOLLOW UP
Plan for review
Review every 2–3 days, until patient obviously improving.

DRUGS AND OTHER THERAPIES: DETAILS
Drugs
CIPROFLOXACIN
Flouroquinolone antibiotic.

Dose
Adults:
- 250–500mg twice daily orally for 10–14 days

Children:
- Not recommended

Efficacy
- Effective against a wide range of Gram-positive and Gram-negative organisms
- Effective against most *Pseudomonas* spp.

Risks/Benefits
- Not suitable for children or growing adolescents
- Use caution in pregnancy, epilepsy, glucose-6-phosphate dehydrogenase deficiency
- Use caution in renal disease
- History of allergy

Side-effects and adverse reactions
- Gastrointestinal: abdominal pain, altered liver function, anorexia, diarrhea, heartburn, vomiting
- Central nervous system: anxiety, depression, dizziness, headache, seizures
- Eyes, ears, nose and throat: visual disturbances
- Skin: photosensitivity, pruritus, rash

Interactions (other drugs)
- Antacids - Beta-blockers - Caffeine - Cyclosporine - Diazepam - Didanosine - Mineral supplements (zinc, magnesium, calcium, aluminium, iron) - NSAIDs - Opiates - Oral anticoagulants - Phenytoin - Theophylline - Warfarin

Contraindications
Use is not recommended in children because arthropathy has developed in weight-bearing joints in young animals.

Acceptability to patient
High.

Follow up plan
Review every 2–3 days until clear evidence that infection is resolving.

Patient and caregiver information
- Take the tablets regularly
- Finish the course, even if you are feeling better
- Do not take antacids, or preparations containing iron or zinc for several hours before and after the time of taking your tablet
- Avoid sunbathing or using a sunbed whilst you are taking the treatment

LEVOFLOXACIN
Flouroquinolone antibiotic.

Dose
Adults:
- 250mg daily orally for 10–14 days

Children:
- Not recommended

Efficacy
- Effective against a wide range of Gram-positive and Gram-negative organisms
- Effective against most *Pseudomonas* spp.

Risks/Benefits
- History of allergy
- Use caution in adolescents
- Use caution in patients with a history of epilepsy and other seizure conditions, myasthenia gravis
- Use caution in renal disease
- Use caution in diabetes mellitus

Side-effects and adverse reactions
- Gastrointestinal: abdominal pain, altered liver function, anorexia, diarrhea, heartburn, pseudomembraneous colitis, vomiting
- Eyes, ears, nose and throat: visual disturbances
- Central nervous system: anxiety, depression, dizziness, headache, seizures
- Genitourinary: monoliasis, vaginitis
- Skin: photosensitivity, pruritus, rash

Interactions (other drugs)
- Antacids Anti-ulcer agents (cimetidine, famotidine, lansoprazole, nizatidine, omeprazole, ranitidine, sucralfate) Cyclosporine Didanosine Estrogens Iron, aluminium, magnesium, calcium, zinc NSAIDs Theophylline Typhoid vaccine Warfarin Zolmitriptan

Contraindications
- Pregnancy Nursing mothers

Acceptability to patient
High, once daily dose.

Follow up plan
Review every 2–3 days until clear evidence that infection is resolving.

Patient and caregiver information
- Drink plenty of fluids
- Take the tablets regularly
- Finish the course, even if you are feeling better
- Do not take antacids, or preparations containing iron or zinc for several hours before and after the time of taking your tablet
- Avoid sunbathing or using a sunbed whilst you are taking the treatment

NORFLOXACIN
Flouroquinolone antibiotic.

Dose
Adults:
- 400mg orally twice daily for 10–21 days

Children:
- Not recommended

Efficacy
- Effective against a wide range of Gram-positive and Gram-negative organisms
- Effective against most *Pseudomonas* spp

Risks/Benefits
- History of allergy
- Use caution in the elderly
- Use caution in renal disease and dehydration
- Use caution in seizure disorders

Side-effects and adverse reactions
- Gastrointestinal: nausea, vomiting, diarrhea, constipation, altered liver function tests, abdominal pain
- Hematologic: blood cell disorders
- Central nervous system: headache, dizziness, seizures, fatigue, anxiety
- Skin: rashes
- Ears, eyes, nose and throat: visual disturbances
- Genitourinary: crystalluria

Interactions (other drugs)
- Aluminium, calcium, magnesium, iron, zinc ■ Antacids ■ Antipyrine ■ Caffeine ■ Diazepam ■ Foscarnet ■ Metoprolol, propanolol ■ Pentoxyfilline ■ Phenytoin ■ Ropinirole ■ Sodium bicarbonate ■ Theobromine ■ Theophylline ■ Warfarin

Contraindications
- Children ■ Pregnancy ■ Nursing mothers

Acceptability to patient
High.

Follow up plan
Review every 2–3 days, until obviously improving.

Patient and caregiver information
- Drink plenty of fluids
- Take the tablets regularly
- Finish the course, even if you are feeling better

AMOXICILLIN-CLAVULANATE
Aminopenicillin antibiotic.

Dose
Adults
- 250–500mg (amoxicillin) every 8 hours for 10–14 days

Children:
- 20–40mg/kg per day (amoxicillin) in divided doses every 8 hours, for 10–14 days
- For children <40kg use chewable tablets for correct clavulanate dose

Efficacy
Effective against most Gram-positive and Gram-negative organisms.

Risks/Benefits
- Not effective against *Pseudomonas* spp.
- History of allergy
- Use caution if history of hypersensitivity to cephalosporins
- Use caution in renal failure
- Use caution in hepatic impairment
- Aviod use in mononucleosis
- Can be used in children

Side-effects and adverse reactions
- Gastrointestinal: diarrhea, abdominal pain, psuedomembranous colitis
- Eyes, ears, nose and throat: black tongue, oral thrush
- Central nervous system: headache, nausea
- Hematologic: bone marrow suppression
- Respiratory: anaphylaxis

Benefit: skin: allergic rashes, erythema multiforme

Interactions (other drugs)
- Atenolol ■ Chloramphenicol ■ Macrolide antibiotics ■ Methotrexate ■ Oral contraceptives
- Tetracyclines

Contraindications
Penicillin hypersensitivity.

Acceptability to patient
High.

Follow up plan
See every 2–3 days, until clear evidence that infection is resolving.

Patient and caregiver information
- Drink plenty of fluids
- Complete the course of tablets, even if you feel better

■ Take tablets with food
■ Oral suspension should be shaken before administering, refrigerated, any remaining solution should be discarded after 14 days

TRIMETHOPRIM-SULFAMETHOXAZOLE
Dose
Adults:
■ 160mg (trimethoprim)/800mg (sulfamethoxazole) twice daily for 10–14 days

Children (>2 months):
■ 8mg (trimethoprim)/kg per day in divided doses 12 hourly for 10–14 days

Efficacy
■ Effective against a wide range of Gram-positive and Gram-negative organisms
■ Not effective against *Pseudomonas* spp.

Risks/Benefits
■ History of allergy
■ Use caution in the elderly
■ Use caution in renal and hepatic impairment
■ Use caution in alcoholism, malnutrition, glucose-6-phosphate dehydrogenase deficiency

Benefit: can be used in children

Side-effects and adverse reactions
■ Gastrointestinal: nausea, vomiting, abdominal pain, hepatitis, pseudomembranous colititis
■ Central nervous system: headache, insomnia, anxiety, depression
■ Genitourinary: nephrosis, renal failure
■ Skin: Stevens-Johnson syndrome, rashes
■ Hematologic: blood cell disorders

Interactions (other drugs)
■ **Dapsone** ■ **Disulfiram** ■ **Methotrexate** ■ **Metronidazole** ■ **Warfarin** ■ **Phenytoin**
■ **Oral anticoagulants** ■ **Hypoglycemic agents**

Contraindications
■ **Pregnancy** ■ **Age less than 2 months** ■ **Folate deficiency**

Acceptability to patient
High.

Follow up plan
Review every 2–3 days, until clear evidence of improvement.

Patient and caregiver information
■ Drink plenty of fluids
■ Take the tablets regularly
■ Finish the course, even if you are feeling better

NAPROXEN
Nonsteroidal anti-inflammatory drug.

Dose
Adults
- Mild pain (OTC) 220mg 12 hourly orally
- Mild to moderate pain (PoM) 250mg 6–8 hourly orally

Efficacy
Good.

Risks/Benefits
- Use caution in hepatic, renal and cardiac disorders
- Propionic acids are effective and better tolerated than most other NSAIDs
- Use caution in elderly
- Use caution in bleeding disorders
- Use caution in porphyria

Benefit: effective pain relief

Side-effects and adverse reactions
- Gastrointestinal: diarrhea, vomiting, nausea, dyspepsia, peptic ulceration
- Central nervous system: headache, dizziness, drowsiness
- Hypersensitivity: rashes, bronchospasm, angioedema
- Thrombocytopenia
- Cardiovascular system: congestive heart failure, dysrhythmias, edema, palpitations
- Genitourinary: acute renal failure

Interactions (other drugs)
- Aminoglycosides ▪ Anticoagulants ▪ Antihypertensives ▪ Corticosteroids ▪ Cyclosporine ▪ Digoxin ▪ Diuretics ▪ Lithium ▪ Methotrexate ▪ Phenylpropanolamine ▪ Probenecid ▪ Triamterene

Contraindications
- Not recommended for children in this instance ▪ Hypersensitivity to NSAIDs or aspirin ▪ Previous gastrointestinal bleed or peptic ulceration ▪ Coagulation defects ▪ Do not use naproxen and naproxen sodium concomitantly

Acceptability to patient
Good, but significant incidence of gastrointestinal side-effects will make this unacceptable to some.

Patient and caregiver information
- Avoid aspirin, and aspirin-containing medications
- Avoid alcohol
- Take with food, milk or antacid to reduce the chance of indigestion or stomach upset
- If your stools turn black, see your doctor promptly

IBUPROFEN
Nonsteroidal anti-inflammatory drug.

Dose
Adults:
- 200–800mg orally four times daily (not to exceed 3200mg/day)

Children:
- 20–40mg/kg per day in three or four divided doses

Efficacy
Good.

Risks/Benefits
Risks:
- Use caution in elderly
- Use caution in hepatic, renal and cardiac failure
- Use caution in bleeding disorders

Benefits:
- May be used in children
- Inexpensive

Side-effects and adverse reactions
- Gastrointestinal: anorexia, nausea, dyspepsia, peptic ulceration, bleeding
- Central nervous system: headache, dizziness, tinnitus
- Hypersensitivity: rashes, bronchospasm, angioedema
- Cardiovascular system: hypertension, peripheral edema
- Genitourinary: nephrotoxicity
- Hematologic: blood cell disorders

Interactions (other drugs)
- **Aminoglycosides** ▪ **Anticoagulants** ▪ **Antihypertensives** ▪ **Baclofen** ▪ **Corticosteroids** ▪ **Cyclosporine, tacrolimus** ▪ **Digoxin** ▪ **Diuretics** ▪ **Lithium** ▪ **Methotrexate** ▪ **Phenylpropanolamine** ▪ **Warfarin**

Contraindications
- **Hypersensitivity to NSAIDs** ▪ **Renal disease** ▪ **Liver disease** ▪ **Coagulation defects**
- **Previous peptic ulcer or gastrointestinal bleed**

Acceptability to patient
Good, although incidence of gastrointestinal side-effects may make this unacceptable to some.

Patient and caregiver information
Take tablets either with food or an antacid.

ACETAMINOPHEN
Para-aminophenol derivative.

Dose
Adults and children >14 years:
- 325–650mg four hourly as required (not more than 4g/day), orally

Children <14 years:
- 10–15mg/kg four hourly as required (not more than 5 doses in 24 hours), orally

Efficacy
Good.

Risks/Benefits
Risks:
- Caution in hepatic and renal impairment
- Use caution in anemia

- Overdosage results in hepatic and renal damage unless treated promptly
- Overdose may lead to multiorgan failure and may be fatal
- Alcohol use should be restricted with acetaminophen use

Benefit: may be used in children

Side-effects and adverse reactions
- Acetaminophen rarely causes side-effects when used intermittently
- Rare: nausea, vomiting, rashes, blood disorders, acute pancreatitis, acute hepatic and renal failure

Interactions (other drugs)
- Alcohol ■ Anticoagulants ■ Anticonvulsants ■ Isoniazid ■ Cholestyramine ■ Colestipol
- Domperidone ■ Metoclopromide

Contraindications
Chronic alcoholism.

Acceptability to patient
High.

Patient and caregiver information
- Avoid alcohol
- Read labels of other over-the-counter drugs, many contain acetaminophen and may cause toxicity if taken concurrently

Surgical therapy

ASPIRATION OF HYDROCELE

Efficacy
- Good for relieving discomfort, but has no effect on the course of the infective process
- There is a high incidence of recurrence

Risks/Benefits
Risks:
- May introduce further infection
- Testis cannot be visually inspected

Benefits:
- Relieves discomfort
- Allows better examination of the testis by palpation

Acceptability to patient
High, as scrotal pain should be improved.

Follow up plan
Review daily until clear evidence of improvement.

Patient and caregiver information
If your scrotum becomes more swollen or painful, contact your doctor.

SCROTAL EXPLORATION
Efficacy
High.

Risks/Benefits
Risk: May need to proceed to orchiectomy

Benefits:
- Can drain infected material, or abscess if present
- If torsion or tumor present, will be identified, and treated appropriately

Acceptability to patient
Moderate, will require admission to hospital and a general anesthetic.

Follow up plan
Daily review until clear evidence that infection settling, then review weekly to fortnightly until wound healed.

Patient and caregiver information
- Wear a scrotal support after your operation until pain and swelling settled
- If your stitches are dissolveable do not spend a long time in the bath until the wound has healed, take a short bath or shower instead

ORCHIECTOMY
Efficacy
High.

Risks/Benefits
- Risk: patient left with a single testis, if develops orchitis in contralateral testis, could be left anorchic
- Benefit: infected organ removed, symptoms should now resolve

Acceptability to patient

Low, as most men would not wish removal of a testicle, even though in the presence of severe infection this may be inevitable.

Follow up plan
Daily review until clear evidence that infection settling, then review weekly to fortnightly until wound healed.

Patient and caregiver information
- The infected testis has been severely damaged, and probably has little or no normal function
- Normal sexual function and fertility are possible with a single testis
- A prosthetic testis can be inserted (later, when infection has resolved) to produce a more normal appearance
- If your stitches are dissolvable do not spend a long time in the bath until the wound has healed, take a short bath or shower instead

Other therapies
SCROTAL SUPPORT
Efficacy
- Highly effective for improving patient comfort, but does not influence course of infective process
- May be combined with ice packs for added relief of symptoms

Risks/Benefits
Increased patient comfort.

Acceptability to patient
High.

Patient and caregiver information
Wear the support all the time, except when washing, until scrotal swelling and pain has resolved.

EFFICACY OF THERAPIES
Evidence
PDxMD are unable to cite evidence which meets our criteria for evidence.

PROGNOSIS
Most patients make a full recovery, but a significant minority may develop testicular infarction, atrophy or be rendered infertile, especially if the orchitis was bilateral.

Clinical pearls
- Bacterial orchitis that is resistant to oral agents will require hospitalization, combination intravenous antibiotic therapy (quinolone plus aminoglycoside or aminoglycoside plus cephalosporin) and sequential imaging studies (color flow Doppler ultrasound both at the time of presentation and afterwards to document sequelae)
- All male patients in the reproductive age should probably have a FSH level drawn at 6 months post acute orchitis episode to assess the impact of the infectious process on the Sertoli cell compartment
- Warm tub soaks can help alleviate pain
- Pentoxifylline increases the oxygen carrying ability of red cells and so may further reduce the inflammation and provide more oxygen to the testis, this has also been recommended as a form of therapy to decrease the amount of inflammation and pain in men undergoing external beam radiation therapy for prostate cancer

Therapeutic failure
Refer patient urgently to a urologist.

Recurrence
- Any patient suffering from recurrent orchitis should be referred to a urologist
- Treatment initially will be an alternative antibiotic to that previously prescribed, and occasionally scrotal exploration or orchiectomy

Deterioration
If the patient's condition deteriorates, they should be referred urgently to a urologist, if this has not been done already.

COMPLICATIONS
Testicular infarction, atrophy and infertility may all occur following orchitis, even when it has been adequately treated. There is no specific treatment for any of these complications, although an atrophic testis may be replaced with a prosthesis to provide a better cosmetic appearance.

CONSIDER CONSULT
Patients who fail to respond to oral antibiotics.

Currently there is no specific preventative measures for orchitis, although the incidence of mumps orchitis may be reduced by childhood immunization against mumps.

RISK FACTORS

- Mumps: recent infection may lead to viral orchitis
- Urinary tract infection: may lead to bacterial orchitis
- Urinary tract surgery or urethral catheterization: resulting bacteremia/bactiuria may lead to bacterial orchitis
- Bladder outlet obstruction: treat etiology of obstruction

MODIFY RISK FACTORS
Lifestyle and wellness
IMMUNIZATION

Immunization against mumps will prevent mumps orchitis.

Cost/efficacy

- Measles, mumps, rubella (MMR) immunization, begun as a single dose in 1968 and increased to two doses in 1989, has reduced the incidence of mumps (the leading cause of orchitis) by over 99%
- However, the principal cost benefit of MMR immunization is the prevention of measles and rubella, diseases that have a much more important impact in prevention of morbidity and mortality than mumps

CHEMOPROPHYLAXIS

Patients undergoing catherization or surgery on the urinary tract should have prophylactic antibiotics.

Cost/efficacy

In most cases, a single preprocedure dose of an intravenous antibiotic will be sufficient to prevent a bacteremia and/or bactiuria leading to orchitis.

SCREENING
Screening is not appropriate for orchitis.

PREVENT RECURRENCE
In general, prevention of recurrence is not possible in this disorder.

RESOURCES

ASSOCIATIONS

American Urological Association
1120 N Charles St,
Baltimore,
MD 21201–559
Phone: 410-727-1100
Fax: 410-223-4373
http://www.amuro.org

KEY REFERENCES

Prostatitis, epididymitis and orchitis:
- Krieger JN. Prostatitis, epididymitis, orchitis. In: Mandell G, Bennett JE, Dolin R (eds). Mandell, Douglas and Bennett's Principles and Practice of Infectious Diseases, 5th edition. Churchill Livingstone, Philadelphia, 2000, pp 1244–1250

Orchitis:
- Mikolich DJ. Orchitis. In: Ferri F (ed). Ferri's Clinical Advisor, Instant Diagnosis and Treatment. Mosby, St Louis, 2001, p 483

Epididymitis:
- Nien PI. Epididymitis. In: Dambro MR (ed). Griffith's 5-Minute Clinical Consult. Lippincott Williams and Wilkins, Philadelphia, 2000, pp 370–371

Anaerobic and necrotizing infections:
- Furste W, Aguirre A. In: Dambro MR (ed). Griffith's 5-Minute Clinical Consult. Lippincott Williams and Wilkins, Philadelphia, 2000, pp 38–39

Urinary tract infections:
- Etheredge W. In: Rosen P (ed). Emergency Medicine Concepts and Clinical Practice, 4th edition. Mosby-Year Book, St Louis, 1998, pp2227–2258

Testes:
- Paulson DF. In Sabiston DC (ed). Textbook of Surgery. The Biological Basis of Modern Surgical Practice, 15th edition. WB Saunders, Philadelphia, 1997, pp1556–1560

Epididymitis:
- Holmes HK et al. Sexually Transmitted Diseases. Churchill Livingstone, Philadelphia, 1999, p855

Epididymitis:
- Ball TP. In: Seidmon JE, Hanno PM (eds). Current Urologic Therapy. WB Saunders, Philadelphia, 1994, p488

Acute epididymitis:
- Berger RE. Campbell's Urology WB Saunders, Philadelphia, 1997, pp672–673

Vaccination:
- Watson JC, Hadler SC, Dykewicz CA, Reef S, Phillips L. Measles, mumps, and rubella – vaccine use and strategies for elimination of measles, rubella, and congenital rubella syndrome and control of mumps: recommendations of the Advisory Committee on Immunization Practices (ACIP). MMWR Morb Mortal Wkly Rep 1998; 47RR-8: 1–57

FAQS
Question 1
What are the most common organisms in bacterial orchitis?

ANSWER 1
Neisseria gonorrhoeae, Treponema pallidum, Chlamydia spp; less common organisms include *Mycobacterium tuberculosis* and *Mycobacterium leprae.*

Question 2
What is orchitis?

ANSWER 2
It is a infection that is limited to the parenchyma of the testis.

Question 3
What are the radiologic findings of orchitis?

ANSWER 3
A radioisotope scrotal scan shows increased perfusion and scrotal ultrasonography will show focal or diffuse echo poor areas in the testicle.

Question 4
When is surgery indicated?

ANSWER 4
Surgery is indicated after referral to urologic specialist. The urologist will generally recommend surgery when there is the risk of gangrene, the presence of crepitus on examination, sepsis that fails to respond to parenteral antibiotics, and radiologic evidence to suggest that the testis is infracted.

Question 5
What is the connection between epididymitis and orchitis?

ANSWER 5
Orchitis usually occurs as a direct extension from epididymitis.

CONTRIBUTORS
Russell C Jones, MD, MPH
Philip J Aliotta, MD, MHA, FACS
Anuj K Chopra, MD

PEYRONIE'S DISEASE

SUMMARY INFORMATION

DESCRIPTION

- Fibrous plaques within the tunica albuginea of the corporal bodies of the penis
- Produces chordee (bending) of the penis with erection, sometimes with an hourglass constriction or rotational deformity
- Can produce pain at rest or especially with erection, during initial active phase of the disease
- Condition can evolve over 2 years
- The fibrous process often impairs erection
- Often results in penile shortening

KEY! DON'T MISS!

Syphilis and malignant metastases can lead to clinical features similar to Peyronie's disease.

ICD9 CODE
607.89 Peyronie's disease.

SYNONYMS
- 'Bent penis'
- Corporal fibrosis
- Chordee
- Plastic induration of the penis
- Penile fibromatosis
- 'Bent spike syndrome'

CARDINAL FEATURES
- Fibrous plaques within tunica albuginea of the penis
- Restricts or affects penile erection, with angulation, hourglass deformity, or corkscrew deformity
- Penile shortening does occur
- Onset is characteristically gradual over 3–6 months
- Condition can evolve over 2 years
- It can spontaneously resolve
- Pain is present during active phase only
- Commonly occurs in adult and older men

CAUSES
Common causes
- Idiopathic (microtrauma): the result of microtears in the albuginea dorsally occurring during intercourse. After such injuries, Peyronie's disease occurs due to excessive fibrosis. Resultant traction on that scar at subsequent activity leads to new trauma and scar extension
- Macrotrauma: fibrosis after penile fracture (rupture of the corpus cavernosum) or external contusion can be indistinguishable from Peyronie's disease, although the plaques in the former condition tend to be more localized at the base of the penis
- Intracavernous injection therapy for erectile dysfunction: papaverine has been reported to result in cavernosal scarring in 10–30% of patients; scarring with other mixtures (prostaglandin, phentolamine) is less common (<6%) and usually related to needle trauma
- Buckling injury with intercourse: trauma to the insertion of the septal fibers

Rare causes
- Low-flow priapism: can lead to scarring if treatment is delayed
- Penile surgery: most commonly when a penile prosthesis is removed due to infection or other reasons
- Autoimmune conditions: including scleroderma or systemic lupus, which cause atypically located scarring
- Malignant invasion of the corpora cavernosa: has been reported from carcinoma or sarcoma of the penis, prostate, bladder, rectum, kidney, and lung

Serious causes
- Postpriapism scarring should prompt a search to investigate a predisposing hematologic disorder, including sickle cell anemia, leukemia, or occult malignancy
- Corporal fibrosis due to intracavernous injection therapy should contraindicate this treatment

Contributory or predisposing factors

- An autoimmune basis has been suggested: patients with Dupuytren's contracture, Sjögren's syndrome, Behçet's syndrome, lederhosen disease, systemic sclerosis, and systemic lupus all have an increased rate of Peyronie's disease and, with Peyronie's patients, have an increased rate of DRw52 (human leukocyte antigen)
- Sickle cell anemia, leading to recurrent priapism
- Corporal invasion by malignancy should lead to a search for a primary tumor
- Intracavernous injection therapy, including papaverine
- Hypertension, diabetes mellitus, and gout are associated with Peyronie's disease

EPIDEMIOLOGY
Incidence and prevalence
INCIDENCE
10/1000.

PREVALENCE
32/1000.

FREQUENCY
Prevalence data vary depending on the investigation used. The best studies showed prevalence varied by age:
- 30–39 years: 15/1000
- 40–59 years: 30/1000
- 60–69 years: 40/1000
- >70 years: 65/1000

Demographics
AGE
Peyronie's disease is increasingly common from the third decade. However, the incidence of men reporting symptoms of Peyronie's disease peak at age 40–60, as interest in sexual performance, and elasticity of the tunica albuginea, may reduce thereafter.

GENDER
Exclusively a male disease.

RACE
No racial disposition to Peyronie's disease.

GENETICS
- A genetic link or defect has not been identified in Peyronie's disease
- Dupuytren's contracture is present in 15% of patients with Peyronie's disease and Peyronie's disease appears in 10–40% of descendants of those with Dupuytren's contracture

GEOGRAPHY
No geographical disposition to Peyronie's disease has been demonstrated.

DIFFERENTIAL DIAGNOSIS
Metastases to the penis
Malignancy metastases to the penis occur in both solid tumors (e.g. prostate) and in leukemia.

FEATURES
- Induration anywhere in the penis, not just tunica albuginea
- Pain and chordee less prominent in proportion to mass
- Primary tumor evident elsewhere, sometimes associated with hematuria

Syphilis
Syphilis is a sexually transmitted disease that can lead to penile lesions.

FEATURES
- Painless papules in the skin and mucous membranes, including the genitalia
- Generalized lymphadenopathy and malaise
- Cardiovascular manifestations include aortic inflammation, regurgitation, and aneurysm
- Neurosyphilis features include meninges involvement, tabes dorsalis, and paralysis
- Confirmable by serologic testing

Chordee with or without hypospadias
Usually present from birth.

FEATURES
- Curvature of penis without a palpable plaque, usually ventrally
- Usually present lifelong without progression

Ventral curvature secondary to urethral instrumentation
Trauma caused by instrumentation of the urethra.

FEATURES
- Fibroses can result from trauma of the urethra
- Palpable induration in corpus spongiosum and not the tunica albuginea

Dorsal vein thrombosis
Thrombosis of the dorsal vein can occur, which leads to pain and edema.

FEATURES
- Thrombosed dorsal vein is palpable superficial to tunica albuginea
- Sudden onset, short duration
- Penile edema and inflammation (not present in Peyronie's disease)

Acute penile fracture
Sudden onset of features.

FEATURES
- History of pain and loss of erection during intercourse
- Penile lesion may be tender
- Penile deformity and ecchymosis are present in the nonerect penis

Congenital curvature of the penis
Evident from childhood.

FEATURES

- Lifelong curvature of the penis with erection
- Pain is rarely a feature
- No history of trauma
- No evidence of plaque formation

SIGNS & SYMPTOMS
Signs

- Fibrous induration in tunica albuginea
- Angulation of penis with erection
- Hourglass deformity of penis shaft with erection
- Intromission may be prevented in severe disease

Symptoms

- Pain with erection (in initial and active phase)
- Shortening of penis
- Impairment of erections
- Physical difficulties with sexual intercourse

ASSOCIATED DISORDERS

- Dupuytren's contracture: the genetic link has not been identified
- Erectile dysfunction: a consequence of Peyronie's disease
- Secondary anxiety or depression leading to impaired libido is common in younger patients with disease presentation

KEY! DON'T MISS!
Syphilis and malignant metastases can lead to clinical features similar to Peyronie's disease.

CONSIDER CONSULT

- If the process is stable, i.e. past the acute phase when there is less pain, the plaque seems stable in size, there is more than 20 degrees of angulation, and the disease is interfering with successful intercourse. Remember that Peyronie's disease will regress spontaneously during the acute phase in 30–50% of cases
- If acute penile fracture is possible
- If the diagnosis of malignant invasion of the penis is made or needs to be ruled out

INVESTIGATION OF THE PATIENT
Direct questions to patient

Q When did you first notice the lump or penile deformity? Patients may delay their disease presentation until significant problems in attaining an erection develop.

Q Was there a traumatic event and did you notice any bruising to the shaft of the penis? Trauma to the penile shaft can cause fibroses leading to curvature of the penis.

Q Have you had penile surgery or infection? Both surgery and infection are predisposing factors to penile damage.

Q Was the onset sudden or gradual? Sudden onset of symptoms favor penile fracture over classic Peyronie's disease.

Q How has the deformity progressed until now? Slow progression is suggestive of Peyronie's disease.

Q Do you have pain with erections or difficulties maintaining an erection? This is often the cause of the patient presenting, although not diagnostic of Peyronie's disease.

Q Are there any mechanical problems with intercourse? The impairment of intercourse is a requisite for treatment, and the details of the impairment provide the benchmarks for progress in treatment.

Q With erections, how much (in degrees) and in what direction does the penis bend or have other deformities? At least 20 degrees of chordee are usually required before interference with intromission and penetration occurs. To follow the course of the disease, have the patient or partner take a Polaroid or digital photograph of his erection, and date it for the record.

Contributory or predisposing factors

Q Have you ever had a prolonged, unwanted, or painful erection? These would suggest postpriapism fibrosis, and prompt a work-up to exclude sickle cell disease.

Q Do you have Dupuytren's contracture or hand, wrist, or arm pain? These would suggest an association with Dupuytren's disease or an autoimmune disorder.

Q Do you have hypertension, diabetes, hypercholesterolemia? Risk factors for erectile dysfunction will need to be evaluated when making treatment decisions.

Q Do you smoke? Smoking is a contributory factor for erectile dysfunction.

Family history

Q Has another family member had Peyronie's disease or similar symptoms? Dupuytren's contracture, lupus, or systemic sclerosis are conditions showing an association with Peyronie's disease.

Examination

- Examination of the penis: this should include gently stretching the penis, measuring the stretch length, recording the number, size, location, and demarcation of each of the Peyronie's plaques. These are baseline measurements from which to follow progression and treatment
- Examination of the erect penis: only if the practitioner is trained in performing intracavernous injections. After the vasoactive injection, a drawing or photograph of the erect penis is made to document the degree of chordee or deformity
- Examination for any urethral, cutaneous infectious, or neoplastic lesions of the penis: this aids in the differential diagnosis for Peyronie's disease
- The prostate, scrotum, and abdomen should be examined: a full abdominal and genital examination, including per rectal to exclude evidence of urologic infection or malignancy, lymphadenopathy, vas beading, prostatic and testicular masses
- The hands and feet should be examined for the presence of Dupuytren's contractions: these are often associated with Peyronie's disease

Summary of investigative tests

Generally, most primary care physicians assess the plaque and then refer the patient to a urologist for further assessment if necessary and management. Investigative tests that may be helpful include:

- Penile ultrasound scan helps to define the penile structure and can identify calcification in the plaque and rule out tumor
- Intracavernous injection of vasoactive agents to produce erection for deformity measurement (normally performed by specialist)
- Magnetic resonance imaging scan of penis to visualize plaque and other penile structures (this test is rarely needed; when appropriate it would normally be ordered by specialist)
- Pharmacologic penile duplex Doppler to visualize penile vasculature if surgical therapy is contemplated (performed by a specialist)
- Dynamic infusion cavernosometry and cavernosography to investigate relation of plaque to cavernous body and to measure the extent of corporal-occlusive insufficiency (performed by a specialist)

DIAGNOSTIC DECISION

- Patients who do have fibrous plaques within the tunica albuginea and do not fulfill the criteria for any of the differential diagnoses have Peyronie's disease
- Diagnosis is usually provided by the history and examination, including careful palpation of the penis to determine if plaque or tumor is present, and a snapshot of the penis from above to show the degree of distortion. A penile ultrasound is usually performed to identify calcification in the plaque and to rule out tumor

THE TESTS
Imaging
PENILE ULTRASOUND SCAN
Description
B-mode ultrasound of the penis.

Advantages/Disadvantages
Advantages:
- Noninvasive examination
- No radiation risk
- Requires no preparation

Disadvantage: 40% of images are not able to demonstrate Peyronie's plaques clearly or completely

Normal
No plaques seen.

Abnormal
- The size, shape, and density of Peyronie's plaques may be demonstrated
- Impingement on other penile structures can be noted
- Fibrosis involving the corpus spongiosum
- Inflammatory or metastatic masses may be found
- Fibrosis of the whole corpus cavernosum may be demonstrated

Cause of abnormal result
- Peyronie's disease, urethral stricture or instrumentation, respectively
- Inflammatory masses suggest syphilis or leukemic infiltration
- Fibrosis of the whole corpus cavernosum is usually a consequence of priapism or an infected penile prosthesis

Drugs, disorders and other factors that may alter results
The patient who already had an indwelling penile prosthesis, or who has had paraffin injections into the penis, will give a striking picture on ultrasound!

CONSIDER CONSULT

- If there is pain in the penis with or without erection, patient dyspareunia, erectile dysfunction, inability to insert the penis into the vagina due to bend, spousal pain due to intromission, patient anxiety over the situation, palpable 'mass' in the penis

IMMEDIATE ACTION

Treatment: colchicine 1.2mg twice daily or 0.6mg three times daily after meals. Animal studies showed that, when given early, colchicines (not ibuprofen) could suppress the inflammatory response and prevent Peyronie's plaque formation.

PATIENT AND CAREGIVER ISSUES
Forensic and legal issues

Peyronie's disease can be debilitating and depressing. Very rarely such depression may present as parasuicidal.

Impact on career, dependants, family, friends

- Peyronie's disease which prevents intercourse can stress or contribute to the split of the marriage or significant-other relationship
- It is important to involve the patient and his sexual partner in the diagnosis and management of this disease

Patient or caregiver request

- Patients who have discovered Peyronie's plaques or chordee are often concerned that they have cancer or have an incurable condition
- Reassurance is helpful on both points

Health-seeking behavior

- Has the patient used any recreational drugs, or tried any home or herbal remedies?
- Does the patient smoke?

MANAGEMENT ISSUES
Goals

- Restore serviceable erections
- Reduce pain during active phase
- Reassure patient that he does not have cancer and that the condition is treatable

Management in special circumstances
COEXISTING DISEASE

Severe Peyronie's disease with significant organic erectile dysfunction is best treated with a penile prosthesis.

COEXISTING MEDICATION

- Patients on anticoagulants are not good candidates for intralesional injections
- Patients with decreased libido due to antiandrogen administration should expect limited improvements in erectile function as a result of treatment
- Patients with prostate cancer cannot use tamoxifen as oral therapy for Peyronie's disease

PATIENT SATISFACTION/LIFESTYLE PRIORITIES

- Once reassured about the benign nature of Peyronie's disease, most patients can be specific about their desired treatment goals
- A realistic picture of the natural history and prognosis should be given
- If oral treatments are not successful the patient may be put forward for surgery as other forms of treatment are not the mainstay of management

SUMMARY OF THERAPEUTIC OPTIONS
Choices

In most cases, management of Peyronie's disease will be carried out by a specialist urologist. Treatment approaches include:

- A conservative approach of reassurance and observation initially as the disease may be self-limiting
- Clinical evidence for the different treatment modalities is sparse
- If oral treatments are not successful the patient may be put forward for surgery as other forms of treatment are not the mainstay of management and not particularly successful
- Patients should be followed up for at least 2 years prior to considering invasive treatment and, if still present, patients should be counseled of the high likelihood of further progression before stabilization

If treatment is needed the following may be indicated.

Oral agents, including:
- Vitamin E
- Aminobenzoate potassium
- Tamoxifen
- Colchicine

Topical agents, including:
- Iontophoresis with verapamil, lidocaine, and dexamethasone
- Iontophoresis with orgotein, lidocaine, and verapamil
- Iontophoresis with dexamethasone and verapamil
- Extracorporeal shockwave (ESWL) treatment

Intralesional therapy (performed by a urologist):
- First choice: verapamil
- Second choice (expensive and toxic): interferon
- Third choice: orgotein (toxic) usually performed by a specialist
- Under FDA evaluation: collagenase
- Injections of steroids into the lesion will cause difficulties for future surgery

Surgical therapy:
- Penile plication
- Plaque excision or incision and grafting
- Penile prosthesis implantation with or without corporoplasty

Lifestyle issues:
- Assessment of sexual activity: types of sexual activity, intercourse positions
- Behaviors: smoking, use of intracavernosal injection therapy

Clinical pearls

- Evaluation of the erect penis after intracavernosal injection with or without high-resolution sonography is the method of choice for objectively assessing penile deformity
- Simple photography of the penis in the erect and 'affected' state helps further delineate the extent of the deformity

FOLLOW UP
Plan for review

- Patients under active treatment with oral medication should be seen at 3- to 6-month intervals to assess progress

- Once the condition is stable, annual follow-up should include penile examination and symptoms review
- Topical, intralesional, and surgical therapy are usually undertaken by the urologist

DRUGS AND OTHER THERAPIES: DETAILS
Drugs
VITAMIN E
- Oral medication for established Peyronie's disease
- No clear evidence for its efficacy
- Can reduce pain, curvature, and plaque lesions, particularly in the acute phase

Dose
Adult oral dose: 60–300 IU/day.

Efficacy
- Pain: 0–100%
- Curvature: 0–78%
- Plaque size reduction: 0–91%

Side-effects and adverse reactions
- Central nervous system: headache, tiredness
- Ears, eyes, nose, and throat: visual disturbances
- Gastrointestinal: nausea, diarrhea, vomiting, abdominal pain
- Metabolic: thyroid, pituitary, and adrenal hormone imbalances

Interactions (other drugs)
- Anticoagulants ■ Iron

Contraindications
No known contraindications.

Acceptability to patient
Side-effects and cost are low; therefore, vitamin E is usually well accepted.

Follow up plan
Re-evaluate every 3–6 months.

Patient and caregiver information
Reassure patient that spontaneous improvement rate is 50%.

AMINOBENZOATE POTASSIUM
- Indicated only for active phase of the disease
- Member of the vitamin B complex

Dose
Adult oral dose: 12g/day for 3 months.

Efficacy
Antifibrosis action may be due to increased oxygen uptake at the tissue level enhancing monoamine oxidase activity, which inhibits fibrosis.

Risks/Benefits
Risks:
- Should anorexia or nausea occur, therapy should be interrupted until the patient is eating normally again
- Use caution in renal disease
- If a hypersensitivity reaction occurs, treatment should be discontinued

Benefit: modest improvement in pain, curvature, and plaque size

Side-effects and adverse reactions
- Central nervous system: fever
- Gastrointestinal: anorexia, nausea, vomiting
- Skin: rash

Interactions (other drugs)
Sulfonamides.

Contraindications
- Drug should not be adminstered with sulfonamides ▪ Hypersensitivity to aminobenzoate potassium ▪ Renal disease

Acceptability to patient
- Patients have some difficulty with the number of pills required to ingest daily (24 pills at 500mg per pill; 12g/day)
- Patients have gastrointestinal problems with both the oral suspension and the pill forms

Follow up plan
Follow up is at 6-month intervals for 2 years.

TAMOXIFEN
In mild Peyronie's disease tamoxifen improves pain, penile angulation, and plaque size. This is an off-label indication.

Dose
Adult oral dose: 10–20mg twice daily.

Efficacy
Useful in mild disease to reduce penile angulation and plaque size.

Risks/Benefits
Risks:
- Use caution in menstrual irregularities or abnormal vaginal bleeding
- Use caution in leukopenia, neutropenia, or thrombocytopenia
- Use caution in cataracts or visual disturbances

Side-effects and adverse reactions
- Cardiovascular system: thromboembolic events (deep vein thrombosis, pulmonary embolism, or stroke)
- Central nervous system: headache, hot flashes
- Ears, eyes, nose and throat: visual impairments, retinopathy, cataracts
- Gastrointestinal: nausea, vomiting, elevated hepatic enzymes, hepatic necrosis, cholestasis, hepatitis
- Genitourinary: changes in libido

- Hematologic: anemia, thrombocytopenia, leukopenia, neutropenia
- Musculoskeletal: bone pain
- Metabolic: hypercalcemia, hyperlipidemia

Interactions (other drugs)
- Aminoglutethimide - Antivirals - Anticoagulants, nonsteroidal anti-inflammatory drugs (NSAIDs), platelet inhibitors, thrombolytic agents - Benzodiazepines - Bromocriptine - Cyclosporine - Diltiazem - Erythromycin - Nifedipine

Contraindications
Avoid intramuscular injections in patients with a platelet count <50,000/mm^3 (<50x10^9/L)

Acceptability to patient
Side-effects of gastrointestinal distress and alopecia are mild and patient compliance has been good.

Follow up plan
Evaluation at 3- to 6-month intervals until stable. Annual follow up thereafter.

COLCHICINE
Colchicine inhibits proliferation of anti-inflammatory cells and fibroblasts, increases collagenase activity, and reduces collagen synthesis.

Dose
Adult oral dose: 0.6–1.2mg/day for first week, then 1.8–2.4mg/day for 3 months.

Efficacy
May be beneficial in reducing plaque size and penile angulation.

Risks/Benefits
Risks:
- Use caution in the elderly and children
- Use caution in alcoholism, gastrointestinal disease, bone marrow suppression, and dental disease

Side-effects and adverse reactions
- Central nervous system: peripheral neuropathy, neuritis
- Gastrointestinal: nausea, vomiting, anorexia, abdominal pain, diarrhea, adynamic ileus
- Genitourinary: nephrotoxicity
- Hematologic: blood cell disorders
- Metabolic: hypothyroidism
- Musculoskeletal: myopathy
- Skin: injection site reaction, tissue necrosis, urticaria, angioedema, rashes, alopecia, purpura

Interactions (other drugs)
- Cyclosporine - Ethanol - Macrolide antibiotics - NSAIDs - Tacrolimus - Vitamin B12

Contraindications
- Severe cardiac, renal, or hepatic impairment - Blood dyscrasias - Intramuscular injections
- Intravenous administration of colchicine

Acceptability to patient
Gastrointestinal upset is common, but does not seem to dissuade motivated patients.

Follow up plan
- Patients on colchicine should be followed closely for gastrointestinal bleeding and/or anemia
- Upon completion of treatment, intervals of 3–6 months are appropriate for re-evaluation until stable
- Annual follow up is indicated

VERAPAMIL

Calcium channel blockers affect cytokine expression during early wound healing and inflammation, and increase the proteolytic activity of collagenase. This is an off-label indication.

Dose
Multiple injections totaling 10mg every 2–4 weeks for 12 weeks.

Efficacy
- Penile shaft narrowing improved in 100%
- Curvature improved in 42%
- Sexual performance improved in 58%
- 83% of patients reported that the disease had arrested or improved in the 8 months of follow up
- More useful in patients with small plaques

Risks/Benefits
Risks:
- The vasodilatory effects of verapamil may cause hemodynamic complications in patients with a substantial outflow gradient or markedly elevated pulmonary pressure
- Use caution with renal and hepatic disease
- Use caution with Duchenne muscular dystrophy
- Use caution with congestive heart failure, hypotension, acute phase of myocardial infarction, and concomitant beta-blocker therapy
- Use caution in children

Benefit: the 40–90% chance of improvement of Peyronie's symptoms are felt by some to outweigh the risks

Side-effects and adverse reactions
- Cardiovascular system: tachycardia, bradycardia, palpitations, congestive heart failure, atrioventricular block, hypotension, peripheral edema
- Central nervous system: dizziness, flushing, headache, fatigue
- Ears, eyes, nose, and throat: tinnitus
- Gastrointestinal: nausea, constipation, vomiting, abdominal pain
- Genitourinary: impotence, nocturia, polyuria, gynecomastia
- Skin: rash

Interactions (other drugs)
- Antidysrhythmics (amiodarone, digoxin, disopyramide, dofetilide, encainide, flecainide, procainamide, quinidine) ■ Antihypertensives (particularly alpha- and beta-blockers)
- Antivirals ■ Aspirin ■ Azole antifungals ■ Barbiturates ■ Benzodiazepines ■ Buspirone
- Calcium ■ Carbamazepine ■ Cardiac glycosides ■ Cimetidine ■ Cisapride
- Clarithromycin, erythromycin ■ Cyclosporine, tacrolimus ■ Dantrolene ■ Diclofenac
- Doxorubicin ■ Ethanol ■ Fentanyl ■ General and local anesthetics ■ Grapefruit juice
- Histamine H_2 antagonists ■ Imipramine ■ Lithium ■ Neuromuscular blockers ■ Phenytoin
- Rifampin ■ Statins ■ Selective serotonin reuptake inhibitors ■ Theophylline

Contraindications
- Cardiogenic shock ▪ Heart block ▪ Severe heart failure, history of heart failure ▪ Porphyria
- Hypotension ▪ Sick sinus syndrome ▪ Wolff-Parkinson-White syndrome

Acceptability to patient
- Less than 10% of patients decline intralesional injection therapy when offered; most patients continue the program once started
- No burdensome aspects of the treatment

Follow up plan
After completion of treatment, re-evaluate at interval of 3–6 months until condition is stable.

Patient and caregiver information
- Intercourse should be avoided for 24h after each injection
- Intralesional injection should only be performed with great caution if the patient is on anticoagulation

INTERFERON
In fibroblasts derived from Peyronie's plaques, interferon:
- Decreased the proliferation rate
- Decreased extracellular collagen
- Increased collagenase

Dose
Specialist will be required to formulate dosing regimen.

Efficacy
6/10 patients reported disappearance of pain on erection, but objective improvement in deformity was small (mean 20°).

Risks/Benefits
Risks:
- Use caution with children under 18 years
- Use caution with depression and mental disorders
- Use caution with seizure disorders and heart disease
- Use caution in photosensitivity and psoriasis
- All patients experienced brief influenza-like symptoms after interferon injection
- Long-term risk from interferon use is undefined

Benefit: the likelihood of objective improvement from interferon has not been established by published reports

Side-effects and adverse reactions
- Cardiovascular system: hypertension, palpitations, peripheral vascular disorders
- Central nervous system: dizziness
- Eyes, ears, nose, and throat: conjunctivitis
- Gastrointestinal: abdominal pain, constipation, diarrhea, vomiting
- Genitourinary: breast pain, cystitis, dysmenorrhea
- Hematologic: lymphadenopathy, leukopenia, lymphopenia
- Respiratory: dyspnea, sinusitis
- Skin: sweating, injection site reaction
- Other: flu-like syndrome, fever, myalgia, hepatic toxicity

Interactions (other drugs)
- Aminophylline ▪ Theophylline ▪ Zidovudine

Contraindications
Hypersensitivity to human albumin.

Acceptability to patient
The influenza-like symptoms after injection and the very high cost prevent interferon being used as a first-line treatment.

Follow up plan
After completion of treatment course, re-evaluate at 3- to 6-month intervals until stable.

Patient and caregiver information
Immunosuppressed patients should not have interferon.

COLLAGENASE
Purified clostridial collagenase alters the collagen content of penile plaque. This is an off-label indication.

Dose
Weekly to monthly intralesional injections have been used in trials.

Efficacy
In one reported trial, treatment out-performed placebo in improving plaque size and penile deformity ($p<0.007$), but primarily in patients with a lesser deformity, and with a small change in curvature.

Risks/Benefits
- Risk: the risks of pain or further scarring from collagenase use have been incompletely documented
- Benefit: the extent of improvement in plaque size and penile deformity are still under investigation

Acceptability to patient
- This modality is still investigational, relatively expensive, and painful
- Patient acceptability may be only moderate

Follow up plan
- Upon completion of treatment, will need a 3-month evaluation until stable
- Annual follow up thereafter

Patient and caregiver information
Intercourse should be avoided for 24h after intralesional injection.

STEROIDS
- Steroids are anti-inflammatory and decrease collagen synthesis
- Steroid injections into the lesion will make future surgery more difficult

Dose
Adult dose: dexamethasone 0.8–1.6mg or hydrocortisone sodium succinate 25–50mg, injected every 4–6 weeks for 6 months.

Efficacy
30–50% of patients, primarily younger patients with small discreet plaques in the distal penis, report improvement in chordee, pain, and plaque size. This same group of patients has the same incidence of spontaneous resolution.

Risks/Benefits
Risk:
- Local tissue atrophy and skin-thinning; subsequent surgery for Peyronie's disease becomes more complex due to difficulty in separating tissue planes

Risks – dexamethasone:
- Overwhelming septicemia if patient has an infection
- Loss of control of blood glucose in those with diabetes
- Use caution in renal disease, esophagitis, peptic ulcer, and ulcerative colitis
- Use caution in cerebral malaria, latent tuberculosis, and AIDS

Risks – hydrocortisone:
- False-negative skin allergy tests. Overwhelming septicemia if patient has an infection
- Loss of control of blood glucose in those with diabetes
- Use caution in the elderly due to risk of diabetes and osteoporosis
- Use caution in patients with psychosis, seizure disorders, or myasthenia gravis
- Use caution in congestive heart failure, hypertension
- Use caution in ulcerative colitis, peptic ulcer, or esophagitis

Benefit: 50% incidence of improvement in symptoms in mild cases

Side-effects and adverse reactions
- Side-effects are minimized by intralesional administration and short duration of therapy
- Cardiovascular system: hypertension, thromboembolism
- Central nervous system: insomnia, euphoria, depression, psychosis, seizures
- Eyes, ears, nose, and throat: cataract, glaucoma, blurred vision
- Endocrine: adrenal suppression, impaired glucose tolerance, growth suppression in children
- Gastrointestinal: dyspepsia, peptic ulceration, esophagitis, oral candidiasis, nausea, vomiting
- Musculoskeletal: proximal myopathy, osteoporosis
- Skin: delayed healing, acne, striae

Interactions (other drugs)
- Adrenergic neurone blockers, alpha-blockers, beta-blockers, beta-2 agonists
- Aminoglutethimide: increased elimination of hydrocortisone and reduced corticosteroid response
- Antidiabetic agents: increased blood glucose in patients with diabetes
- Antidysrhythmics (calcium channel blockers, cardiac glycosides)
- Antifungals (amphotericin, ketoconazole)
- Antihypertensives (angiotensin-converting enzyme (ACE) inhibitors, diuretics: loop and thiazide, acetazolamide; angiotensin II receptor antagonists, clonidine, diazoxide, hydralazine, methyldopa, minoxidil)
- Barbiturates: reduction in the serum concentrations of corticosteroids
- Cholestyramine: potential for reduced corticosteroid absorption
- Cyclosporine: increased level of hydrocortisone increases the risk of seizures
- Erythromycin
- Estrogens: increased corticosteroid effect
- Intrauterine contraceptive devices: contraceptive effect may be reduced by hydrocortisone
- Isoniazid: enhanced corticosteroid effect
- Methotrexate
- Nitrates
- Nitroprusside
- NSAIDs: increased risk of gastrointestinal ulceration
- Oral contraceptives
- Phenytoin: reduced efficacy of corticosteroids
- Ritonavir
- Rifampin: reduced efficacy of corticosteroids
- Salicylates: hydrocortisone increases the elimination of salicylates
- Somatropin

Contraindications
- Systemic infection
- Avoid live virus vaccines in those receiving immunosuppressive doses

Acceptability to patient
- Patients can be reassured that steroids used in Peyronie's disease have not resulted in side-effects seen with systemic steroids
- The medications used are not expensive

Follow up plan
- Patients completing steroids are re-evaluated at intervals of 3–6 months
- Follow up can then be annual

Patient and caregiver information
- Intercourse should be avoided for 24h after injection
- Patients should be aware that subsequent penile surgery would be more difficult

Physical therapy
IONTOPHORESIS
- Delivery of verapamil 10mg and/or dexamethasone 4mg with a local electric field
- Delivery of verapamil, lidocaine, and dexamethasone with a local electric field
- Delivery of orgotein, lidocaine, and verapamil with a local electric field

Efficacy
Beneficial effect in up to 60% of patients with Peyronie's disease undertaking this treatment regimen.

Risks/Benefits
Benefits:
- No untoward sequelae have been reported
- A 50% improvement rate has been claimed

Acceptability to patient
Treatment is painless, free of side-effects, and therefore well accepted.

Follow up plan
Evaluation of progress at 3- to 6-month intervals until the condition is stable or satisfactory to the patient.

EXTRACORPOREAL SHOCKWAVE (ESWL) TREATMENT
Delivery of shockwaves to the body in order to reduce the plaques.

Efficacy
- Small, uncontrolled studies report improvement in subjective symptoms in 90%
- Reduction in plaque occurred in 11/21 patients in a controlled study

Risks/Benefits
- Risk: because of short follow up in reported series, the risk of increased late progression of Peyronie's disease from ESWL is not established
- Benefit: the benefits remain to be established by long-term controlled studies

Acceptability to patient
- Side-effects were not reported
- In the US, the cost of ESWL may be prohibitive for many patients
- May be painful

Follow up plan
After completion of treatment, evaluation every 3–6 months until the condition is stable or satisfactory to the patient, and annually thereafter.

Patient and caregiver information
- Patients with cardiac pacemakers and defibrillators must have cardiology clearance and co-ordination before using ESWL
- Sexual intercourse should be avoided during the period of ESWL treatments

Surgical therapy
Indications for surgical treatment are that the patient has had Peyronie's disease for 2 years and one or more of the following are present:
- Severe curvature, narrowing, or indentation of more than one year's duration
- Sexual difficulty because of deformity
- Severe penile shortening

PENILE PLICATION
- Performed on the convex surface of the penis at the site opposite to the penile plaque
- Most appropriate for patients with good erections, adequate penile length, and without hourglass deformity

Efficacy
With appropriate patient selection, 80% report good results, with long-term satisfaction rates from 60–100%.

Risks/Benefits
Risks:
- Loss of penile length is certain
- Erectile dysfunction
- Penile hematoma
- Narrowing or indentation
- Urethral injury
- Suture granuloma
- Glans numbness
- Phimosis
- Very small risks from anesthesia, as in any surgery

Benefit: 80–98% correction of chordee

Acceptability to patient
Penile shortening always occurs with this technique, and for some patients is unacceptable.

Follow up plan
- Close follow up by the operating urologist for 1–3 months until healed
- Thereafter can be seen by primary care annually

Patient and caregiver information
- Loss of penile length will occur
- Erectile dysfunction can occur as a result of surgery
- Intercourse is avoided for 4 weeks after surgery, but thereafter is encouraged

PLAQUE EXCISION OR INCISION AND GRAFTING
- Lengthening of the tunica with graft is indicated with severe curvature resulting in shortened, narrowed, or hourglass penis
- Performed on the concave diseased side of the penis
- Very large, thick, or calcified plaques are often best excised; other plaques are incised in an 'H' fashion before graft placement

- Graft materials have evolved with improved results, from dermis, cadaveric pericardium to saphenous or dorsal penile vein, to small intestine submucosa

Efficacy
- Plaque excision and grafting resulted in a high incidence of erectile failure, graft contracture, late recurrence, and poor long-term results
- Plaque incision and grafting with vein have been reported to give successful straightening in 95% of patients, with only 13% complaining of decreased erections
- However, patients with large plaques or ventral grafts had loss of erections in over 85%

Risks/Benefits
Risk: erectile impairment, graft contracture, persistent curvature, and late failure or recurrence

Benefits:
- Penile straightening and repair of indentation
- Success of surgery is proportional to the urologist's experience with this condition

Acceptability to patient
This reconstructive surgery, with significant risk of complications or poor results, requires patient commitment and strong motivation.

Follow up plan
- The operating urologist will usually follow the patient for the first few months
- Thereafter, evaluation at 3- to 6-month intervals until stable
- Annual follow up by PCP from then onwards

Patient and caregiver information
After initial healing (3–6 weeks), patients may be required to use physical therapy devices (e.g. a vacuum erection device) to aid healing of the graft.

PENILE PROSTHESIS IMPLANTATION
- Patients with Peyronie's disease and erectile dysfunction that do not respond to medical therapy are treated with a penile prosthesis, with or without incision or excision of the plaque, and only rarely with grafting
- Penile straightening is usually done by placing the prosthesis, but can also be accomplished with penile modeling (manual fracture of the plaque over the implanted prosthesis)

Efficacy
- Provided the patient has realistic expectations, results are excellent
- A 95% rate of correction of chordee and restoration of erections can be expected

Risks/Benefits
Risks:
- Infection: 1.5%
- Mechanical revision or imperfect result: 2%

Benefits:
- Correction of chordee
- Restoration of erection

Acceptability to patient
Patient acceptance of penile prosthesis is high, as long as expectations are realistic.

Follow up plan
Once the prosthesis has healed, annual follow up is required.

Patient and caregiver information
- Patients with prostheses should use antibiotic prophylaxis when undergoing other surgery or dental extraction
- Erectile dysfunction can occur as a result of surgery and should be explained to the patient prior to surgery

LIFESTYLE
- Lifestyle changes that decrease risk of erectile dysfunction should be adopted if there is a component of erectile impairment in the clinical picture
- Smoking, alcohol, obesity, hyperlipidemia, and bicycling with a narrow seat should be avoided
- Regular exercise is beneficial
- Recreational drugs should be avoided, as they may increase the incidence of Peyronie's disease
- Diet favoring antioxidants may be protective, but the evidence in this regard is not conclusive

RISKS/BENEFITS
Benefit: all of the above have no risk, and may have benefit.

ACCEPTABILITY TO PATIENT
Lifestyle changes tend to be acceptable in proportion to motivation.

FOLLOW UP PLAN
At annual or other visits, these items should be queried.

PATIENT AND CAREGIVER INFORMATION
The natural history of Peyronie's disease should be made clear to the patient and his partner, to aid motivation.

OUTCOMES

EFFICACY OF THERAPIES

- Nonsurgical therapy tends to be of value, with an overall 50% improvement rate over a 6-month period, among those patients who have a significant incidence of spontaneous resolution
- Features associated with a lack of spontaneous resolution include duration >2 years at presentation, presence of Dupuytren's contractures, plaque calcification, and bending >45 degrees
- Surgical therapy is highly successful

Review period
Review annually.

PROGNOSIS

- The likelihood of a complete remission or cure of Peyronie's disease is poor. Of 97 University of California, Los Angeles (UCLA) patients with Peyronie's disease of 1–5 years' duration, 14% called their disorder resolving, 40% progressive, and 47% unchanging
- Only 40–60% have a response to oral or intralesional therapy
- A satisfactory long-term resolution of curvature or hourglass deformity is achieved with surgery in 60–90%
- Concomitant erectile dysfunction is an indication for early penile prosthesis implantation, and has a 95% cure rate

Clinical pearls

- Be sure to monitor blood pressure and heart rate after verapamil injection therapy
- Patients should maintain pressure over the plaque site post injection to prevent and/or reduce hematoma formation and secondary inflammation

Therapeutic failure
Patients should be advised that there are no guarantees with any of the interventions listed above. Failures generally progress along a continuum of therapeutic options and remedies.

Recurrence
Rare.

Deterioration

- Shrinkage of the penis
- Loss of sensation
- Penile pain

COMPLICATIONS
Peyronie's disease can be complicated by:

- Erectile dysfunction, which is an indication for penile prosthesis implantation
- Depression, which should be identified and treated

CONSIDER CONSULT

- If patient has failed oral therapy, or is unlikely to respond to oral therapy
- If the disease has been present more than 2 years

RISK FACTORS

- **Recreational drugs:** show a subsequent increased incidence of Peyronie's disease
- **Family history of Peyronie's disease:** a genetic link has not been identified but a familial association is present
- **Dupuytren's contracture:** decreased likelihood of spontaneous resolution
- **Recurrent priapism:** primarily due to sickle cell disease
- **Intracavernosal injection therapy:** risk of scarring increased with mixtures containing papaverine

For concomitant erectile dysfunction:
- Diabetes, hypertension, smoking, hyperlipidemia, alcoholism, lack of exercise

MODIFY RISK FACTORS

- Stop smoking
- Use antioxidants
- Lose weight
- Control diabetes
- Exercise
- Control gout
- Lower cholesterol
- Stop intracavernosal injection therapy

Lifestyle and wellness

TOBACCO
Smoking is a risk factor for erectile dysfunction, which can be a complication of Peyronie's disease.

ALCOHOL AND DRUGS
Men who take recreational drugs have an increased incidence of the development of Peyronie's disease.

DIET
Antioxidants are believed, but not proven, to decrease the development of Peyronie's disease in patients who have a predisposition to it.

PHYSICAL ACTIVITY
A sedentary lifestyle is a risk factor for erectile dysfunction, but not specifically for Peyronie's disease.

SEXUAL BEHAVIOR
Avoidance of unsafe sexual practices by using barrier contraception.

FAMILY HISTORY
A genetic link has not been identified, but a familial association is present.

DRUG HISTORY
Risk of scarring with intracavernosal injection therapy leading to Peyronie's disease is increased with mixtures containing papaverine.

SCREENING

Since treatment is not indicated unless there is interference with intercourse, screening for asymptomatic Peyronie's disease is not necessary; however, during annual physical examinations, men should be asked about their sexual function, and the penis should be examined for infection or malignancy.

ASSOCIATIONS

American Urological Association Inc.
1120 North Charles Street
Baltimore, MD 21201–5559
Tel: (410) 727-1100
Fax: (410) 223-4370
E-mail: aua@auanet.org
http://www.auanot.org

Sexual Medicine Society of North America
1111 N Plaza Drive, Suite 550
Schaumberg, IL 60173
Tel: (847) 517-7225
Fax: (847) 517-7225
E-mail: info@smsna.org
http://www.smsna.org

American Foundation for Urologic Disease
1128 North Charles Street
Baltimore, MD 21201
Tel: (800) 242-2383 or (410) 468-1800
E-mail: admin@afud.org
http://www.afud.org

National Organization for Rare Disorders
PO Box 8923
New Fairfield, CT 06812–8923
Tel: (800) 999-6673
E-mail: orphan@nord-rdb.com
http://www.rarediseases.org

National Kidney and Urologic Diseases Information Clearinghouse
3 Information Way
Bethesda MD 20892–3580
Tel: (800) 891-5390 or (301) 654-4415
E-mail: nkudic@info.niddk.nih.gov
http://www.niddk.nih.gov

KEY REFERENCES

- Gelbard MK, Dorey F, James K. The natural history of Peyronie's disease. J Urol 1990;144:1376–9
- Carson C. Potassium para-aminobenzoate for treatment of Peyronie's disease: is it effective? Tech Urol 1997;3:135–9
- Teloken C, Rhoden EL, Grazziotin TM, et al. Tamoxifen versus placebo in the treatment of Peyronie's disease. J Urol 1999;162:2003–5
- Riedl C, Plas E, Engelhardt P, et al. Iontophoresis for treatment of Peyronie's. J Urol 2000;163:95–9
- Hamm R, McLarty E, Ashdown J, et al. Peyronie's disease – the Plymouth experience of extracorporeal shockwave treatment. BJU Int 2001;87:849–52
- Levine LA. Treatment of Peyronie's disease with intralesional verapamil injection. J Urol 1997;158:1395–8
- Rehman J, Benet A, Melman A. Use of intralesional verapamil to dissolve Peyronie's disease plaque: a long-term single-blind study. Urology 1998;51:620–6

▨ Judge JS, Wisniewski ZS. Intralesional interferon in the treatment of Peyronie's disease: a pilot study. Br J Urol 1997;79:40–2

▨ Wegner HE, et al. Local interferon-alpha 2B is not an effective treatment in early-stage Peyronie's disease. Eur Urol 1997;32:190–3

▨ Gustafson H, Johansson B, Edsmyr F. Peyronie's disease: experience of local treatment with Orgotein. Eur Urol 1981;7:346–8

FAQS
Question 1
How long does it take for Peyronie's disease to stabilize?

ANSWER 1
One to two years.

Question 2
What is the difference between fracture of the penis and Peyronie's disease?

ANSWER 2
Patients who have penile fractures present with a different pattern of plaque formation and scarring than the type of Peyronie's disease. Fractures tend to occur laterally or ventrally in comparison to dorsal Peyronie's plaques.

Question 3
Why do patients have Peyronie's disease repeatedly?

ANSWER 3
Multiple occurrences of Peyronie's disease are due to repeated penile trauma with secondary inflammation and induration.

Question 4
What is the minimum amount of time someone should wait before more definitive treatment?

ANSWER 4
18–24 months from the initiation of the disease.

Question 5
Where does verapamil injection have the greatest utility?

ANSWER 5
In those patients with hourglass deformity and penile pain.

CONTRIBUTORS
Joseph E Scherger, MD, MPH
Philip J Aliotta, MD, MHA, FACS
Anuj K Chopra, MD

PHIMOSIS, PARAPHIMOSIS AND PRIAPISM

DESCRIPTION

Phimosis:

- Tightness of penile foreskin that prevents it from being drawn back from the glans
- Physiologic phimosis present at birth, resolves spontaneously during first 2–3 years of life. If the condition does not resolve spontaneously, it is defined as congenital phimosis
- Acquired phimosis is caused by recurrent foreskin tissue infection or irritation
- Circumcision may be required

Paraphimosis:

- Constriction of glans penis by proximally placed phimotic foreskin
- Occurs when the foreskin is not drawn back into place after being retracted (e.g. after cleaning, cystoscopy, or catheter insertion)
- Can result in such marked swelling of the glans penis that the foreskin can no longer be drawn forward
- If reduction of tissue cannot be performed manually, a dorsal slit procedure or circumcision is needed emergently
- If left untreated, can result in necrosis of the glans penis

Priapism:

- Painful and/or abnormally prolonged penile erection
- In idiopathic priapism, the erection is associated with prolonged sexual excitement and involves the corpus cavernosum only. Detumescence of tissue does not occur spontaneously
- In secondary priapism, the erection is not necessarily associated with sexual excitement, but all other signs and symptoms are the same as seen in idiopathic priapism
- Impotence is associated with the duration of priapism; 36h of erection considered the important prognostic threshold
- Two pathophysiologies can occur — low flow priapism (ischemic, associated with edema of the cavernosal trabeculae) and high-flow priapism (nonischemic, associated with cavernosal artery rupture)
- Treatment is generally a medical emergency

URGENT ACTION

Priapism:

- If surgical measures (blood aspiration from corpora cavernosa, followed by injection of medication) are needed to treat priapism, an emergency referral to a urologist may be indicated
- Remember, the length of time of erection impacts future impotence, therefore refer early in the course of the disease

ICD9 CODE

- 605 Redundant prepuce and phimosis
- 607.3 Priapism

CARDINAL FEATURES

Phimosis:

- Tightness of penile foreskin that prevents it from being drawn back from over the glans

Paraphimosis:

- When the foreskin is retracted and the glans penis is left behind, causing constriction of glans penis

Priapism:

- Painful and/or abnormally prolonged penile erection
- Erection involves only the corpora cavernosa, with the glans and corpora spongiosum remaining soft
- Detumescence does not occur spontaneously

CAUSES

Common causes

Phimosis:

- Physiologic phimosis is present at birth
- Acquired phimosis is caused by recurrent infection or irritation of the foreskin tissue

Paraphimosis:

- Occurs when the foreskin is not drawn back into place after being retracted (e.g. after cleaning, cystoscopy, or catheter insertion)

Priapism:

- Intracavernosal injections of vasoactive drugs used to treat erectile dysfunction
- Pelvic vascular thrombosis
- Prolonged sexual activity
- Sickle cell anemia
- Leukemia
- Total parenteral nutrition (especially after 20% lipid infusion)
- Medications (e.g. trazodone, phenothiazines, especially chlorpromazine, topical and systemic cocaine)
- Malignant penile infiltration
- Hyperosmolar intravenous contrast
- Spinal cord injury (usually self-limiting)
- Spinal or general anesthesia (usually self-limiting)

Rare causes

Priapism:

- Pelvic hematoma or neoplasm
- Bladder calculi
- Penile and perineal trauma or injury
- Urinary tract infection
- Intracavernous fat emulsion
- Black widow spider bite

Serious causes
Priapism:
- Leukemia and other blood dyscrasias
- Diabetes
- Cerebrospinal tumors
- Tertiary syphilis

Contributory or predisposing factors
Phimosis:
- Poor hygiene
- Diabetes
- Frequent diaper rash as infant

Paraphimosis:
- Presence of foreskin
- Inexperienced healthcare provider (leaving foreskin retracted after catheter placement)

Priapism:
- Dehydration
- Medication side effect (papaverine, phentolamine, sildenafil, prostaglandin E1, trazodone, hydralazine, prazosin, phenoxybenzamine, phenothiazines, butyrophenones, selective serotonin reuptake inhibitors, sedative-hypnotics, anticoagulants, cocaine, testosterone, and testosterone precursors)

EPIDEMIOLOGY
Incidence and prevalence
FREQUENCY
- Phimosis and paraphimosis: 1% of males over 16 years of age
- Priapism: unknown

Demographics
AGE
- Phimosis and paraphimosis: seen in infancy and adolescence
- Priapism: all ages, including children

GENDER
Phimosis, paraphimosis, and priapism: male only.

SOCIOECONOMIC STATUS
Phimosis and paraphimosis: less educated parents may not be aware of the required care of the infant penis and foreskin to prevent phimosis and paraphimosis.

DIFFERENTIAL DIAGNOSIS
Lymphedema
Chronic edema (due to insect bites, trauma, or allergic reactions) of the penis, which may be primary or secondary to lymphatic damage or obstruction; differential diagnosis for phimosis and paraphimosis.

FEATURES
- Painless
- Marked pitting edema (early stages)
- Tissue becomes indurated with nonpitting edema (chronic)

SIGNS & SYMPTOMS
Signs
Phimosis:
- Unretractable foreskin
- Superimposed balanitis

Paraphimosis:
- Drainage
- Ulceration
- Swelling

Priapism:
- Low-flow (ischemic) priapism presents with a flaccid glans penis
- High-flow (arterial) priapism presents with a rigid glans penis but can also be flaccid
- Erection involves the corpora cavernosa only

Symptoms
Phimosis:
- Usually not painful but may have pain on erection
- May produce urinary obstruction with ballooning of the foreskin and may lead to chronic inflammation and carcinoma

Paraphimosis:
- Penile pain

Priapism:
- Persistent, painful erection
- Difficulty in urination during erection
- Loss of sexual function (if treatment is not prompt and effective)

ASSOCIATED DISORDERS
Priapism: may be associated with sickle cell trait and disease, leukemia (especially chronic granulocytic leukemia), spinal cord injury.

CONSIDER CONSULT
- Priapism: penile Doppler testing may be needed to differentiate high-flow from low-flow priapism (i.e. ischemic vs arterial priapism), which requires referral to urologist

INVESTIGATION OF THE PATIENT
Direct questions to patient
Phimosis:

Q Are you (or is the child) diabetic? This could be a secondary cause for phimosis.

Q Does the infant have frequent episodes of diaper rash? Recurrent infection or irritation may contribute to acquired phimosis.

Q Has the child experienced recurrent bouts of balanitis (chemical or infectious)? This can lead to acquired phimosis.

Q Have you (or has the child) attempted to reduce the foreskin? Forced reduction of a foreskin can lead to chronic scarring and acquired phimosis.

Q Have you (or has the child) needed chronic use of a condom catheter? Recurrent infection and irritation from these devices could lead to phimosis.

Paraphimosis:

Q Have you (or has the child) needed chronic use of a condom catheter with home health aide assistance in its use? An inexperienced healthcare provider may leave foreskin retracted after catheter placement, leading to paraphimosis.

Q Have you (or has the child) been circumcised? An incomplete circumcision or lack of circumcision may contribute to this condition. Paraphimosis does not occur in a properly circumcised penis.

Priapism:

Q Are you (or is the child) diabetic? This could be a secondary cause for priapism.

Q Do you (or does the child) have sickle cell disease or leukemia? These conditions are both considered associated causes of priapism.

Q Do you have a prostate tumor or abdominal mass? Solid tumor penile infiltration may cause episodes of priapism.

Q Are you (or is the child) receiving total parental nutrition? Any nutritional plan that includes a fat emulsion may cause a fat embolus.

Q Have you (or has the child) recently received an injury to the penis or perineum? Blunt trauma to these tissues may cause swelling and alterations in blood flow through the penile vessels.

Q Are you using intracavernosal injections of vasoactive drugs for erectile dysfunction? This is the most common cause of priapism.

Contributory or predisposing factors
Phimosis:

Q How is your general physical condition? Poor hygiene is a contributing factor for possible acquired phimosis.

Q Are you (or is the child) diabetic? This could be a secondary cause for phimosis.

Q Does the infant patient have frequent episodes of diaper rash? Recurrent infection or irritation may contribute to acquired phimosis.

Paraphimosis:

Q Have you (or has the child) been circumcised? An incomplete circumcision or lack of circumcision may contribute to this condition.

Q Have you (or has the child) needed chronic use of a condom catheter with home health aide assistance in its use? An inexperienced healthcare provider may leave foreskin retracted after catheter placement, leading to paraphimosis. Pulling back a tight foreskin is by far the most common cause of paraphimosis.

Priapism:

Q **What medications are you (or the child) taking?** Several groups of medications have priapism as a known side-effect, including papaverine, phentolamine, sildenafil, prostaglandin E1, trazodone, hydralazine, prazosin, phenoxybenzamine, phenothiazines, butyrophenones, selective serotonin reuptake inhibitors, sedative-hypnotics, anticoagulants, cocaine, testosterone, and testosterone precursors.

Family history
Phimosis:

Q **Do you have a family member with diabetes?** The patient may be an undiagnosed diabetic.

Priapism:

Q **Do you have a family member with diabetes?** The patient may be an undiagnosed diabetic.
Q **Do you have a family member with sickle cell disease?** The patient may have undiagnosed sickle cell disease.

Examination
Phimosis:

- **Determine whether the patient has been circumcised.** An incomplete circumcision may contribute to this condition
- **Determine the patient's general physical condition.** Poor hygiene is a contributing factor for possible acquired phimosis
- **Determine whether attempted forced reduction of the foreskin has taken place.** Forced reduction of a foreskin can lead to chronic scarring and acquired phimosis

Paraphimosis:

- **Determine whether the patient has been circumcised.** An incomplete circumcision may contribute to this condition

Priapism:

- **Examine the patient for signs of dehydration.** This is considered a risk factor for priapism
- **Examine the patient for an arteriocavernosus fistula.** This fistula is indicative of arterial priapism
- **Examine the entire external genitalia.** Partial thrombosis of the corpora cavernosa will be seen, along with pelvic vascular thrombosis. In low-flow (ischemic) priapism, the corpus spongiosum and glans penis will be uninvolved. In high-flow (arterial) priapism, the glans penis will be rigid and the corpus spongiosum will be uninvolved

Summary of investigative tests
Phimosis and paraphimosis:

- No investigative tests applicable

Priapism:

- A complete blood count (CBC) or coagulation profile may be useful in determining whether leukemia or other blood dyscrasias may be the cause of this condition
- A sickle cell test and hemoglobin electrophoresis would be useful to determine whether sickle cell anemia is the cause of the condition
- Urinary tract infections could be identified as a possible cause by performing a routine urinalysis
- Penile Doppler ultrasound may be necessary to differentiate high-flow vs low-flow priapism (normally performed by a specialist; referral to a urologist)

DIAGNOSTIC DECISION

▨ Phimosis: diagnosis is based on physical findings – tight penile foreskin that cannot be drawn back from over the glans penis is the diagnostic key

▨ Paraphimosis: diagnosis is based on physical examination – constriction of the glans penis by proximally placed phimotic foreskin is the diagnostic key

▨ Priapism: diagnosis is based on physical examination – abnormally prolonged and/or painful erection with or without glans penis inflammation is the diagnostic key. Further details regarding ischemic or arterial priapism can also be obtained through physical examination

CLINICAL PEARLS

Distinctive features of priapism:

▨ Only the corpora cavernosa are erect

▨ The glans penis is small and flaccid

▨ The ventral surface of the erect penis is flat, since the bulge of the erect corpus spongiosum that surrounds the urethra in normal erection is absent

'Stuttering priapism' can occur:

▨ It consists of recurrent episodes of priapism

▨ Subside spontaneously after several hours or are successfully reversed by corporeal aspiration and phenylephrine injection

▨ These episodes can and do occur frequently

THE TESTS
Body fluids
COMPLETE BLOOD COUNT (CBC)
Description

A CBC consists of a white blood cell (WBC) count, red blood cell (RBC) count, hemoglobin, hematocrit, RBC indices, platelet count, and a WBC differential count. A random venous anticoagulated (EDTA) blood sample is collected, and the time of collection is noted.

Advantages/Disadvantages

▨ Advantage: rules out several conditions in differential diagnosis of priapism

▨ Disadvantage: does not confirm diagnosis of priapism

Normal
WBCs:

▨ Adults – 5000–10,000 cells/mm^3

▨ Children – 2 months to 6 years 5000–19,000 cells/mm^3; 6–17 years 4800–10,800 cells/mm^3

RBCs:

▨ Adults (male) – 4.2–5.4x10^6/mm^3

▨ Children – 6 months to one year 3.8–5.1x10^6/mm^3; 1–6 years 3.9–5.3x10^6/mm^3; 6–16 years 4.0–5.2x10^6/mm^3; 16–18 years 4.2–5.4x10^6/mm^3

Hemoglobin:

▨ Adults (male) – 14.0–17.4g/dL

▨ Children – 6 months to one year 9.9–14.5g/dL; 1–6 years 9.5–14.1g/dL; 6–16 years 10.3–14.9g/dL; 16–18 years 11.1–15.7g/dL

Hematocrit:

▨ Adults (male) – 42–52%

▨ Children – 6 months to one year 29–43%; 1–6 years 30–40%; 6–16 years 32–42%; 16–18 years 34–44%

Mean corpuscular volume (MCV):
- 82–98fL

Mean corpuscular hemoglobin concentration (MCHC):
- 31–37g/dL

Mean corpuscular hemoglobin (MCH):
- 26–34pg/cell

Platelet count:
- Adults – 140–400x10^3 cells/mm^3
- Children – 150–450x10^3 cells/mm^3

Abnormal
WBCs:
- Adults – <5000 or >10,000 cells/mm^3
- Children – 2 months to 6 years <5000 or >19,000 cells/mm^3; 6–17 years <4800 or >10,800 cells/mm^3

RBCs:
- Adults (male) – <4.2 or >5.4x10^6/mm^3
- Children – 6 months to one year <3.8 or >5.1x10^6/mm^3; 1–6 years <3.9 or >5.3x10^6/mm^3; 6–16 years <4.0 or >5.2x10^6/mm^3; 16–18 years <4.2 or >5.4x10^6/mm^3

Hemoglobin:
- Adults (male) – <14.0 or >17.4g/dL
- Children – 6 months to one year <9.9 or >14.5g/dL; 1–6 years <9.5 or >14.1g/dL; 6–16 years <10.3 or >14.9g/dL; 16–18 years <11.1 or >15.7g/dL

Hematocrit:
- Adults (male) – <42% or >52%
- Children – 6 months to one year <29% or >43%; 1–6 years <30% or >40%; 6–16 years <32% or >42%; 16–18 years <34% or >44%

MCV:
- <82 or >98fL

MCHC:
- <31 or >37g/dL

MCH:
- <26 or >34pg/cell

Platelet count:
- Adults – <140 or >400x10^3 cells/mm^3
- Children – <150 or >450x10^3 cells/mm^3

Keep in mind the possibility of a false-positive result.

Cause of abnormal result
Elevated WBCs:
- Leukemia
- Trauma or tissue injury
- Malignant neoplasms

- Toxins, uremia, coma, thyroid storm
- Drugs
- Acute hemolysis
- Acute hemorrhage
- Polycythemia vera
- Tissue necrosis

Decreased WBCs:
- Viral and bacterial infections
- Hypersplenism
- Bone marrow depression
- Leukemia
- Pernicious or aplastic anemia
- Myelodysplastic syndromes
- Congenital disorders
- Kostmann's syndrome
- Reticular agenesis
- Immune-associated neutropenia
- Marrow-occupying diseases (fungal infections, metastatic tumors)
- Iron-deficiency anemia

Elevated RBCs:
- Polycythemia vera
- Erythremic erythrocytosis
- Renal disease
- Extrarenal tumors
- Pulmonary disease
- Cardiovascular disease
- Alveolar hypoventilation
- Hemoglobinopathy
- Dehydration
- Gaisböck's disease

Decreased RBCs:
- Anemia
- Hodgkin's disease and other lymphomas
- Multiple myeloma
- Myeloproliferative disorders
- Leukemia
- Acute and chronic hemorrhage
- Lupus erythematosus
- Addison's disease
- Rheumatic fever
- Subacute carditis
- Chronic infection

Elevated hemoglobin:
- Polycythemia vera
- Congestive heart failure
- Chronic obstructive pulmonary disease

Decreased hemoglobin:
- Iron deficiency, thalassemia, pernicious anemia
- Liver disease

- Hypothyroidism
- Chronic or acute hemorrhage
- Hemolytic anemia

Elevated hematocrit:
- Erythrocytosis
- Polycythemia vera
- Shock

Decreased hematocrit:
- Anemia
- Leukemia
- Lymphoma
- Hodgkin's disease
- Myeloproliferative disorders
- Adrenal insufficiency
- Chronic disease
- Acute and chronic blood loss
- Hemolytic reactions

MCV:
- Elevated MCV – macrocytic anemia
- Decreased MCV – microcytic anemia

MCHC:
- Elevated MCHC – spherocytosis
- Decreased MCHC – iron deficiency, microcytic anemias, some thalassemias

MCH:
- Elevated MCH – macrocytic anemia
- Decreased MCH – microcytic anemia

Elevated platelet count:
- Essential thrombocythemia
- Chronic myelogenous and granulocytic leukemia, myeloproliferative disease
- Polycythemia vera and primary thrombocytosis
- Iron-deficiency anemia
- Hodgkin's disease, lymphomas, malignancies

Decreased platelet count:
- Idiopathic thrombocytopenic purpura
- Pernicious, aplastic, and hemolytic anemias
- Viral, bacterial, and rickettsial infection
- HIV infection
- Lesions involving the bone marrow

Drugs, disorders and other factors that may alter results
- RBCs: recumbent position for blood collection will decrease value by 5%; stress can elevate value
- Hemoglobin: excessive fluid intake decreases value; extreme physical exercise increases value
- Hematocrit: severe dehydration will cause falsely high values
- MCV: increased reticulocytes or marked leukocytosis increase values
- MCHC: falsely high in presence of lipemia, cold agglutinins, or rouleaux, and with high heparin concentrations
- MCH: falsely high in hyperlipidemia, elevated WBC counts, and high heparin concentrations
- Platelet count: increased after strenuous exercise, trauma, or excitement, and in winter

COAGULATION PROFILE

Description

A coagulation profile consists of a platelet count (as part of CBC), bleeding time, partial thromboplastin time (PTT), prothrombin time (PT), and fibrinogen level. A random venous anticoagulated (sodium citrate) blood sample is collected.

Advantages/Disadvantages
- Advantage: rules out several conditions in differential diagnosis of priapism
- Disadvantage: does not confirm diagnosis of priapism

Normal
- Bleeding time: 3–10min
- PTT: 21–35s
- PT: 11–13s
- Fibrinogen: 200–400mg/dL

Abnormal
- Bleeding time: <3 or >10min
- PTT: <21 or >35s
- PT: <11 or >13s
- Fibrinogen: <200 or >400mg/dL
- Keep in mind the possibility of a false positive result

Cause of abnormal result

Prolonged bleeding time:
- Thrombocytopenia
- Severe liver disease
- Advanced renal failure
- Leukemia, other myeloproliferative diseases
- Disseminated intravascular coagulation (DIC)

Prolonged PTT:
- Heparin therapy
- Vitamin K deficiency
- Liver disease
- DIC
- Congenital deficiencies of system coagulation factors

Shortened PTT:
- Extensive cancer
- Immediately after acute hemorrhage

Elevated PT:
- Vitamin K deficiency
- Liver disease
- Poor fat absorption
- DIC
- Zollinger-Ellison syndrome

Decreased PT:
- Regional enteritis or ileitis

Elevated fibrinogen:
- Inflammation
- Cancer, multiple myeloma, Hodgkin's disease

Decreased fibrinogen:
- Cancer
- DIC
- Primary fibrinolysis

Drugs, disorders and other factors that may alter results
- Bleeding time: excessive alcohol consumption, aspirin, fibrinolytic agents, extreme hot or cold conditions
- PTT: aspirin, antibiotics, antihistamines, heparin
- PT: alcoholism or excessive alcohol ingestion raises PT level, diarrhea and vomiting decrease PT level
- Fibrinogen: high levels of heparin interfere with results

SICKLE CELL TEST
Description
This blood measurement is routinely performed to screen for sickle cell anemia or trait and to confirm these diagnoses. A venous blood sample of 5mL with EDTA is obtained.

Advantages/Disadvantages
- Advantage: the test clearly indicates the presence of sickled RBCs
- Disadvantage: this test is not diagnostic for priapism. The distinction between sickle cell trait and sickle cell disease is made by electrophoresis

Normal
Normal erythrocyte shape.

Abnormal
- A positive test means that great numbers of erythrocytes have assumed the typical sickle cell (crescent) shape
- Keep in mind the possibility of a false-positive result

Cause of abnormal result
Both the presence of sickle cell trait and sickle cell anemia will produce a positive result.

Drugs, disorders and other factors that may alter results
False-negative:
- Will occur in infants
- Coexisting thalassemias or iron deficiency
- Pernicious anemia and polycythemia

False-positive:
- Can occur up to 4 months after transfusions with RBCs that have the sickling trait

HEMOGLOBIN ELECTROPHORESIS
Description
Normal and abnormal hemoglobin can be detected by electrophoresis. The most common forms of normal adult hemoglobin are Hb A1, Hb A2, and Hb F. Hb S is responsible for sickle cell anemia. A venous blood EDTA-anticoagulated sample is collected for analysis.

Advantages/Disadvantages
- Advantage: can clearly indicate presence of Hb S (sickle cell trait or anemia)
- Disadvantage: not diagnostic for priapism, only aids in differential diagnosis

Normal
- Hb A1: 96.5–98.5%
- Hb A2: 1.5–3.5%
- Hb F: 0–1%
- Hb S: 0%

Abnormal
- Hb A1: <96.5% or >98.5%
- Hb A2: <1.5% or >3.5%
- Hb F: >1%
- Hb S: >0%
- Keep in mind the possibility of a false-positive result

Cause of abnormal result
Elevated Hb A2:
- Beta-thalassemia major
- Sickle cell trait
- Sickle cell disease
- Megaloblastic anemia

Decreased Hb A2:
- Iron-deficiency anemia
- Sideroblastic anemia
- Erythroleukemia

Elevated Hb F:
- Thalassemias
- Sickle cell disease
- Anemia
- Acute or chronic leukemia
- Myeloproliferative disorders, multiple myeloma, lymphoma
- Metastatic carcinoma to the bone marrow

Presence of Hb S:
- Sickle cell trait
- Sickle cell anemia

Drugs, disorders and other factors that may alter results
- Hb F: increased during anticonvulsant therapy
- Hb S: coexisting thalassemias or iron deficiency can produce false-negative result
- False-positive results can occur up to 4 months after transfusion of RBCs with sickle cell trait

ROUTINE URINALYSIS
Description
Routine urinalysis testing involves the study of urine properties: color, appearance, specific gravity, pH, determination of the presence or absence of ketones, glucose, blood, protein, bilirubin, urobilinogen, nitrate, leukocyte esterase, and other abnormal constituents (via microscopic examination of urine sediment). A 10mL urine specimen (clean-catch) is usually sufficient for conducting these tests.

Advantages/Disadvantages
- Advantage: simple collection procedure, analysis often done in the primary care setting
- Disadvantage: not directly diagnostic for priapism, used to rule out other conditions

Normal
- Color: pale yellow to amber
- Appearance: clear to slightly hazy
- Specific gravity: 1.005–1.025
- pH: 4.5–8.0
- Glucose: negative
- Ketones: negative
- Blood: negative
- Protein: negative
- Bilirubin: negative
- Urobilinogen: 0.2–1.0 Ehrlich U/dL
- Nitrate: negative
- Leukocyte esterase: negative

Microscopic examination:
- Casts – negative, occasional hyaline cast
- RBCs – negative or rare
- Crystals – negative
- WBCs – negative or rare
- Epithelial cells – few; hyaline casts 0–1/low power field

Abnormal
- Color: anything other than pale yellow to amber
- Appearance: turbidity or cloudiness
- Specific gravity: <1.005 or >1.025
- pH: <4.5 or >8.0
- Glucose: positive
- Ketones: positive
- Blood: positive
- Protein: positive
- Bilirubin: positive
- Urobilinogen: <0.2 or >1.0 Ehrlich U/dL
- Nitrate: positive
- Leukocyte esterase: positive

Microscopic examination:
- Casts – >2/low power field
- RBCs – >3 cells/high power field
- Crystals – present
- WBCs – >4 cells/high power field
- Epithelial cells – >3 renal tubular epithelial cells/high power field

Cause of abnormal result
Color:
- Colorless urine – large fluid intake, untreated diabetes mellitus, diabetes insipidus, alcohol and caffeine ingestion, nervousness
- Orange urine – concentration (due to fever, sweating, reduced fluid intake), bilirubin, carrots or vitamin A ingestion, certain urinary tract medications
- Brownish-yellow or greenish-yellow urine – bilirubin in the urine oxidized to biliverdin
- Green urine – pseudomonal infection, indican
- Pink to red urine – RBCs, hemoglobin, methemoglobin, myoglobin, porphyrins
- Brown-black urine – RBCs oxidized to methemoglobin, methemoglobin, melanin or melanogen, phenol poisoning
- Smoky urine – RBCs
- Milky urine – fat, cystinuria, many WBCs, phosphates

Appearance:
- Turbidity may be caused by urinary tract infection
- Cloudiness may be due to presence of WBCs, RBCs, epithelial cells, or bacteria

Decreased specific gravity:
- Diabetes insipidus
- Glomerulonephritis and pyelonephritis
- Severe renal damage

Elevated specific gravity:
- Diabetes mellitus
- Nephrosis
- Dehydration, fever, vomiting, diarrhea
- Congestive heart failure

Low pH:
- Metabolic acidosis, diabetic ketosis, diarrhea, starvation, uremia
- Urinary tract infections caused by *Escherichia coli*
- Respiratory acidosis
- Potassium deficiency

Elevated pH:
- Urinary tract infections caused by proteus or pseudomonas
- Renal tubular acidosis, chronic renal failure
- Metabolic acidosis (vomiting)
- Respiratory alkalosis involving hyperventilation

Glucose:
- Diabetes mellitus
- Central nervous system disorders
- Impaired tubular reabsorption
- Thyroid disorders

Ketones:
- Diabetes mellitus
- Renal glycosuria
- Starvation, fasting, anorexia
- High-fat diet
- Prolonged vomiting
- Fever

Blood:
- Acute urinary tract infection
- Lupus nephritis
- Urinary tract or renal tumors
- Urinary calculi
- Glomerulonephritis
- Malignant hypertension
- Trauma to kidneys
- Leukemia
- Strenuous exercise
- Heavy smokers

Protein:
- Glomerular damage (diabetes mellitus, glomerulonephritis, malignant hypertension)
- Diminished tubular reabsorption (renal tubular nephrosis, pyelonephritis)
- Multiple myeloma, malignant lymphoma
- Acute infection
- Trauma
- Leukemia
- Sickle cell disease
- Tumors

Bilirubin:
- Hepatitis and liver disease
- Obstructive biliary tract disease

Elevated urobilinogen:
- Hemolytic anemia, pernicious anemia
- Malaria
- Hemorrhage into tissues
- Biliary disease, cirrhosis, acute hepatitis
- Cholangitis

Decreased urobilinogen:
- Cholelithiasis
- Biliary duct inflammation
- Cancer of the head of the pancreas
- Antibiotic therapy

Nitrate:
- Bacteriuria

Leukocyte esterase:
- Urinary tract infection

Microscopic examination
Casts:
- Glomerulonephritis
- Malignant hypertension
- Chronic renal disease
- Diabetic nephropathy
- Fever
- Emotional stress
- Strenuous exercise
- Heat exposure

RBCs:
- Pyelonephritis
- Renal stones
- Cystitis
- Prostatis
- Renal tuberculosis
- Genitourinary tract malignancies
- Trauma
- Tumors of the rectum, colon, pelvis

Crystals:
- Cystine crystals – cystinuria
- Leucine or tyrosine crystals – severe liver disease
- Calcium oxalate crystals: severe chronic renal disease
- Triple phosphate crystals – chronic infection
- Calcium phosphate crystals – chronic cystitis or prostatic hypertrophy

WBCs:
- Renal disease
- Urinary tract disease
- Viral infection
- Strenuous exercise
- Chronic pyelonephritis
- Bladder tumors
- Glomerulonephritis

Epithelial cells:
- Acute tubular necrosis
- Acute glomerulonephritis
- Pyelonephritis
- Salicylate poisoning
- Viral infections

Drugs, disorders and other factors that may alter results
- Color: beets turn urine red, rhubarb causes brown urine. Many drugs alter the color of urine
- Appearance: urates, carbonates, or phosphates from food may produce cloudiness. Fecal contamination or semen mixed with urine may cause turbidity
- Specific gravity: diuretics and antibiotics can cause high readings
- pH: ammonium chloride and mandelic acid produce acid urine, sodium bicarbonate, potassium citrate, and acetazolamide may produce alkaline urine
- Glucose: ascorbic acid, ketones, peroxide, stress, or excitement
- Ketones: levodopa, phenothiazines, insulin, aspirin, mettormin, captopril
- Blood: bacitracin, coumarin, aspirin, high doses of vitamin C, prostatic infection
- Protein: strenuous exercise, severe emotional stress, fever and dehydration, salicylate therapy
- Bilirubin: ascorbic acid, nitrate, drugs
- Urobilinogen: drugs that cause cholestasis
- Nitrate: azo dye metabolites, bilirubin, ascorbic acid
- Leukocyte esterase: trichomonas, parasites, histocytes, glucose, protein

Microscopic examination:
- RBCs- traumatic catheterization, after passing kidney stones

TREATMENT

CONSIDER CONSULT

Phimosis:

- If asymptomatic phimosis makes urethral catheterization difficult, the phimotic opening may need to be dilated, formally incised (dorsal slit procedure), and/or circumcised. If the patient is in urinary retention, this operative procedure should be performed following referral to the hospital's emergency department

Paraphimosis:

- If unable to reduce foreskin, refer immediately for dorsal slit or circumcision. This operative procedure should be performed following referral to the hospital's emergency department. It can be performed in the office by any physician familiar with the procedure, its complications, and their sequelae

Priapism:

- Important – no matter what the cause, urologic referral is an emergency!
- If surgical measures (blood aspiration from corpora cavernosa, followed by injection of medication) are needed to treat priapism, an emergency referral to a urologist is absolutely indicated
- If the etiology of the patient's priapism is found to be neurogenic, continuous caudal or spinal anesthesia may be needed, and the patient should be referred to a urologist. The urologist will treat and co-ordinate care and decide if the patient should be admitted to the hospital for further treatment
- In patients with sickle cell disease, oxygen, alkalinization of intravenous fluids while rehydrating, and transfusion may be required. The patient should be referred to a hospital where care will be co-ordinated from the emergency room or the patient will be admitted for treatment

IMMEDIATE ACTION

Phimosis:

- Immediate action not typically required. If patient's phimosis makes emergency urethral catheterization difficult, a dorsal slit procedure may be needed. Referral to a urologist is recommended

Paraphimosis:

- Immediate action should be taken to minimize edema and increase the chance of reduction without surgical intervention and decrease chance of necrosis of the glans. If patient's paraphimosis makes emergency urethral catheterization difficult, a dorsal slit procedure may be needed. Referral to a urologist is recommended

Priapism:

- If priapism is seen in patients with sickle cell disease, noninvasive standard antisickling measures, including exchange transfusion, may be needed. Oxygen and aggressive rehydration with alkalinized intravenous fluids should also be administered. Empiric terbutaline, given subcutaneously, is recommended for every patient presenting with priapism as soon as the diagnosis is made

PATIENT AND CAREGIVER ISSUES
Patient or caregiver request

Phimosis:

- We decided when my son was a baby not to have him circumcised; is this why he is having this problem now?/My son was circumcised as a baby; shouldn't that have prevented this condition? At birth, phimosis is physiologic; over time, the tissues loosen so that in over 90% of uncircumcised males, the prepuce becomes retractable by 3 years of age.

477

Circumcision may not have prevented this condition from occurring. Even after circumcision, phimosis can be caused by inflammation or forced retraction of the foreskin, leading to a scar that prevents foreskin retraction

- **My son had frequent diaper rashes as a baby; could it have caused this condition?** Frequent infection and scarring of the tip of the foreskin have been found to contribute to the occurrence of phimosis
- **I am diabetic and have a difficult time keeping my penis from being chronically irritated and infected; could this have caused this condition?** Following any injury or inflammatory event, the foreskin reacts by forming scar tissue, leading to difficulty in routine retraction of the tissue over the penis. Repeated infections and irritation may indeed lead to scarring sufficient to cause phimosis

Paraphimosis:

- **We decided when my son was a baby not to have him circumcised; is this why he is having this problem now?/My son was circumcised as a baby; shouldn't that have prevented this condition?** Paraphimosis occurs when the foreskin is retracted back and cannot be pulled back over the glans of the penis. Correct circumcision would have prevented this condition from occurring
- **I need to maintain a urinary catheter due to another medical condition; could it be contributing to this happening to my penis?** Leaving the penile foreskin retracted after catheter placement is, indeed, a risk factor in the development of paraphimosis

Priapism:

- **I have heard that the drugs I use to treat my erectile dysfunction could cause this to happen to my penis; is this true?** It is possible that this is a side-effect of the drugs used to treat your erectile dysfunction, especially if you use the injectable types of treatments
- **How can extended periods of sexual activity cause my penis to do this? I thought the opposite should happen.** This can occur due to failure of certain muscles in your penis to respond to your body's chemical signals to relax or contract in the process of removing blood from the engorged tissues
- **Will I become impotent because of this?** Even with early intervention, impotence following low flow priapism is up to 50%. The longer the duration of priapism, the higher the rate of impotence. High-flow priapism has a better prognosis, with a reported impotence rate of 20%

Health-seeking behavior

Phimosis and paraphimosis:

- **Have you (or the adult guardian) attempted to treat this condition in any way? What procedures have you performed? What was the outcome?** Unsuccessful physical manipulation of the penile foreskin may have worsened the patient's condition, requiring more extensive intervention by the physician. Use of lotions or ointments for foreskin lubrication may have contributed to infection of the tissues

Priapism:

- **Have you (or the adult guardian) attempted to treat this condition in any way? What procedures have you used? What was the outcome?** Unsuccessful physical manipulation of the penis may have worsened the patient's condition, requiring more extensive intervention by the physician. Use of cold or hot compresses may have damaged superficial tissues or worsened engorgement

MANAGEMENT ISSUES
Goals
Phimosis:

- Loosen penile foreskin to improve retraction
- Eliminate pain on erection
- Prevent recurrence

Paraphimosis:
- Return foreskin over glans
- Eliminate swelling and pain
- Prevent recurrence

Priapism:
- Achieve detumescence
- Preserve potency
- Prevent recurrence

Management in special circumstances
COEXISTING DISEASE
- Diabetic patients need to be counseled regarding prevention of possible penile infection and phimosis
- Patients with sickle cell disease (or trait) need to be aware of the possibility of priapism occurrence

COEXISTING MEDICATION
- Patients with erectile dysfunction and priapism need to have their erectile dysfunction medications titered to lower doses to aid in prevention of possible future priapism events
- Patients who are taking any of the medications where priapism is a possible side-effect should have their treatment regimens examined to determine whether the drugs can be changed to aid in preventing future priapism events
- All patients taking these medications must be aware of this as a possible side-effect and must notify their doctor if erection persists for >2h

SPECIAL PATIENT GROUPS
- Pediatric patients diagnosed with priapism need to be monitored for future priapismic events
- The elderly or other patients with chronic catheterization should be monitored for possible paraphimosis due to problems with catheterization procedures

PATIENT SATISFACTION/LIFESTYLE PRIORITIES
- Uncircumcised adult patients may feel uncomfortable having a circumcision performed. Physician should also be aware of any cultural or religious preferences regarding circumcision
- Patients experiencing priapism due to their medications used to treat erectile dysfunction may have problems with discontinuation of these medications. Physician should evaluate drug dose reduction before considering discontinuation

SUMMARY OF THERAPEUTIC OPTIONS
Choices
Phimosis:
- Elective circumcision is the definitive procedure of choice in the treatment of phimosis in the nonemergency situation
- Pediatric phimosis has been shown to be effectively treated with topical betamethasone – this is an off-label indication
- If phimosis prevents urethral catheterization, the phimotic opening may need to be dilated or crushed and formally incised (dorsal slit procedure). This procedure should be performed in the hospital emergency department

Paraphimosis:
- The first-line treatment for paraphimosis involves reduction of the foreskin, usually while the patient is sedated. It is performed by a healthcare provider trained in the procedure and with a knowledge of potential complications and their sequelae
- If mechanical reduction of the foreskin is not effective, referral to hospital may be needed for a dorsal slit procedure with subsequent circumcision

Priapism:

- Important – referral to a urologist is strongly recommended. This is an emergency condition! Primary care physicians and other healthcare providers are not encouraged to treat without urologic consultation!
- In patients with sickle cell disease, noninvasive standard antisickling measures, including exchange transfusion, should be pursued immediately if initial measures such as oxygen, intravenous hydration, alkalinization with bicarbonate in intravenous fluids, and analgesia are not successful
- Empiric terbutaline given subcutaneously is recommended for every patient presenting with priapism as soon as the diagnosis is made. This is an off-label indication, and should be adminstered under specialist supervision
- If detumescence does not occur with terbutaline, corporal aspiration alone, or corporal aspiration and irrigation with an alpha-agonist (epinephrine, ephedrine sulfate, or phenylephrine) are recommended. This is an off-label indication and should be administered under specialist supervision
- Should initial medical and corporal aspiration and irrigation fail, use of a shunt may be indicated

General:

- In addition to the treatment recommendations, certain lifestyle measures are appropriate

Never
Priapism:

- Conservative measures, such as sedation and algesia, oral estrogens, ice-water enemas, transurethral diathermy, spinal/epidural/general anesthesia, and local anesthetic injections have not been proven to be of value and should not be used in lieu of definitive intracavernosal therapy
- Early referral is key – time is the limiting factor in recovery of erectile function

FOLLOW UP

- Most cases of asymptomatic phimosis do not need treatment; however, repeated instances of infection or irritation should be monitored
- Patients should be reassured about the expected outcome of treatment for priapism, but physicians should not be overly optimistic regarding possible potency. Patients must be made aware of the high possibility of impotence

Plan for review
Phimosis and paraphimosis:

- Patient (or guardian) should be educated regarding appropriate hygiene and care of the foreskin
- If patient has undergone a procedure to treat his condition, the physician should schedule the patient for a follow-up visit one week after reduction of paraphimosis and 1–2 weeks after a circumcision

Priapism:

- Patient should receive information about long-term outlook, with possible referral for counseling regarding possible impotence
- Patient's vasoactive drug therapy should be evaluated, with possible reduction in dose or elimination if these drugs caused the priapic event
- If patient underwent surgery to treat the priapic event, close follow-up should be maintained, as detumescence may take several weeks

Information for patient or caregiver

Phimosis and paraphimosis:
- Patient (or guardian) should be educated regarding appropriate hygiene and care of the foreskin

Priapism:
- Patient should receive information about long-term outlook, possible referral for counseling regarding possible impotence
- If patient needs new medications or must change doses of existing medications for erectile dysfunction, he needs to receive instructions on these changes

DRUGS AND OTHER THERAPIES: DETAILS
Drugs
BETAMETHASONE

Topical betamethasone cream is indicated for use in reducing the phimotic ring.

Dose
0.05% betamethasone cream applied twice daily for one month.

Efficacy
This drug treatment is effective in reducing the inflammation associated with phimosis.

Risks/Benefits
Risks:
- Long-term use of potent topical corticosteroids can result in permanent thinning of sensitive skin, telangiectasias, or redness
- Caution needed in long-term use (10 days or more); may lead to secondary ocular infections, glaucoma, optic nerve damage, cataract
- May mask signs of pre-existing or secondary ocular infection
- Safe use in children has not been established
- Use caution in liver or renal disease
- Use caution in hypothyroidism, heart failure, hypertension, diabetes mellitus, myasthenia gravis, and pre-existing coagulopathy or thromboembolic disease
- Use caution in seizures or psychosis

Benefit:
- Simple, noninvasive treatment regimen

Side-effects and adverse reactions
Systemic absorption of topical betamethasone is minimal but theoretical:
- Endocrine – Cushing's syndrome; inhibition of the hypothalamic-pituitary-adrenal axis can occur if applied over large surface areas
- Metabolic – hyperglycemia, glucosuria, if used chronically (unlikely in these photodermatoses); growth retardation can occur in children
- Skin: rash, dermatitis, pruritus, atrophy, hypopigmentation, striae, xerosis, burning, stinging upon application, alopecia, conjunctivitis, cutaneous atrophy can occur after a few weeks

Interactions (other drugs)
No known interactions with topical betamethasone.

Contraindications
- Rosacea ■ Pruritus ■ Acne vulgaris ■ Use on face, axilla, or groin

Acceptability to patient
Highly acceptable to patient due to noninvasive aspect of treatment. If treating children, simple procedure for parent or caregiver.

Follow up plan
- Monitor potassium and blood sugar levels if long-term therapy is indicated
- Observe growth and development of infants and children on long-term therapy

Patient and caregiver information
- Medication should be used in the morning
- Discontinue medication if application area becomes infected or weepy

Surgical therapy
Depending on the severity of the phimosis/paraphimosis, two different procedures may be used: dorsal slit or circumcision. In priapism, corporal aspiration will often be performed, followed by a shunting procedure if significant detumescence does not occur following aspiration.

DORSAL SLIT PROCEDURE
- Dorsal slit of the foreskin is performed in any emergency situation to gain access to the urethral meatus for catheterization, or as a definitive treatment following simple foreskin reduction or phimotic ring incision and foreskin reduction in a patient with paraphimosis
- Local anesthesia (1% lidocaine) is infiltrated into the dorsal midline of the foreskin. Once local anesthesia is achieved, any preputial adhesions are separated. A hemostat is then placed on the plane between the glans penis and the superior overlying inner layer of foreskin. The hemostat is advanced to the level of the coronal sulcus and then closed. The closed hemostat is left in place for 3–5min, after which it is removed. The resulting serrated, crushed foreskin is cut longitudinally through the extent of the crushed tissue

Efficacy
After successful dorsal slit of the foreskin, the prepuce is easily retracted for cleansing of the glans penis or exposure of the urethral meatus.

Risks/Benefits
- Risk: possible injury to surrounding tissues or bleeding during procedure
- Benefit: surgical procedure resolves the anatomic difficulty

Acceptability to patient
Acceptable; however, some patients may complain about cosmetic appearance of the incised foreskin and relative inconvenience during urination.

Follow up plan
- Patient should return for visit 1–3 weeks after surgery
- If circumcision is needed following dorsal slit procedure, patient will need to be informed
- Patient (parental) education plan needed regarding tissue hygiene

Patient and caregiver information
- If circumcision is needed following dorsal slit procedure, inform patient regarding procedure and risks/benefits
- Patient (parental) education plan needed regarding tissue hygiene

CIRCUMCISION
- Elective circumcision is the definitive procedure of choice in the treatment of phimosis in the nonemergency situation

- Methods of circumcision in the pediatric population include the use of the Gomco clamp, the Plastibell device, or the Mogen clamp. Analgesia – local anesthetic, EMLA cream (lidocaine 2.5% and prilocaine 2.5%) dorsal penile nerve block, subcutaneous ring block – is recommended for all patients undergoing circumcision
- In adults, dorsal slit type and sleeve type of circumcision are performed under local anesthetic and other types, i.e. intravenous sedation, general anesthesia, spinal anesthesia

Efficacy
After successful circumcision, the prepuce is easily retracted for cleansing of the glans penis or exposure of the urethral meatus

Risks/Benefits
- Risks: bleeding, infection, other rare complications
- Benefits: possible reduced risk of urinary tract infection and penile cancer, possible reduced risk of acquiring a sexually transmitted disease

Acceptability to patient
Acceptable; however, adult patients may find the thought of undergoing the procedure distasteful.

Follow up plan
- Patient should return for visit 1–4 weeks after surgery
- Patient (parental) education plan needed regarding tissue hygiene and care of surgical site

Patient and caregiver information
- Patient (parental) education plan needed regarding tissue hygiene and care of surgical site
- Adult patient should be instructed to have no sexual activity until healing is complete

CORPORAL ASPIRATION
The mainstay of therapy for advanced priapism is aspiration of the corpora cavernosa combined with saline injection. This procedure is performed in the emergency room setting with a urology consult.

Efficacy
Simple aspiration in some cases can be successful if the priapism has been present for <24h. Because multiple anastomoses exist between the two corpora cavernosa, bilateral aspiration is not required.

Risks/Benefits
- Risk: hematoma and infection can occur following aspiration procedures. Impotence is a well-recognized complication following priapism, even with surgical intervention. Procedure is not beneficial after 48h and rarely beneficial in patients who have had major priapismic episodes
- Benefit: if detumescence is achieved after initial aspiration, no further treatment is required. Very effective in pain relief, minimal long-term complications

Acceptability to patient
Acceptable, as procedure is performed under local anesthesia and patient may expect rapid relief of symptoms, if successful; however, patients may have concerns regarding possible impotence.

Follow up plan
- Patient should return for visit 1–2 weeks after surgery
- Patient (parental) education plan needed regarding tissue hygiene and care of surgical site
- Patient may need referral for counseling regarding possible impotence

Patient and caregiver information
- Patient (parental) education plan needed regarding tissue hygiene and care of surgical site
- Adult patient should be instructed to have no sexual activity until healing is complete

SHUNT
Several types of shunting procedures are indicated in advanced priapism, depending on which tissues are most affected, including the glans-cavernosum shunt, the cavernosaphenous, dorsal vein corpora cavernosa shunt, and corporal saphenous vein bypass shunts.

Efficacy
To permit re-establishment of pelvic circulation, a shunt is recommended.

Risks/Benefits
- Risk: not successful if performed late in the priapismic attack
- Benefit: incision is small, procedure can be performed rapidly

Acceptability to patient
Acceptable, as procedure is performed under local anesthesia and patient may expect rapid relief of symptoms if procedure is successful; however, patients may have concerns regarding possible impotence.

Follow up plan
- Patient should return for visit 1–2 weeks after surgery
- Patient (parental) education plan needed regarding tissue hygiene and care of surgical site
- Patient may need referral for counseling regarding possible impotence

Patient and caregiver information
- Patient (parental) education plan needed regarding tissue hygiene and care of surgical site
- Adult patient should be instructed to have no sexual activity until healing is complete

Complementary therapy
Patients with sickle cell disease who experience priapic events may require additional therapy beyond that typically needed by nonsickle cell patients to treat priapism.

ANTISICKLING THERAPY
In the patient with sickle cell disease, intravenous hydration, alkalinization with bicarbonate in intravenous fluids, analgesia, and oxygen therapy should be initiated. If the above measures fail after 6–12h, then transfusion or exchange transfusion are indicated.

Efficacy
Transfusion in conjunction with corporal aspiration may allow for oxygenated blood to enter the cavernosa.

Risks/Benefits
- Risk: transfusion may not be useful if stasis in the cavernosa has occurred and venous return is obstructed
- Benefit: transfusion in conjunction with corporal aspiration may allow for oxygenated blood to enter the cavernosa

Acceptability to patient
Acceptable, but patient may be concerned regarding possible impotence.

Follow up plan
- If patient undergoes aspiration procedure as well as rehydration/transfusion, he should return for visit 1–2 weeks after surgery.
- Patient (parental) education plan needed regarding tissue hygiene and care of surgical site
- Patient may need referral for counseling regarding possible impotence

Patient and caregiver information
- Patient (parental) education plan needed regarding tissue hygiene and care of surgical site
- Adult patient should be instructed to have no sexual activity until healing is complete

Other therapies
FORESKIN REDUCTION
In cases of paraphimosis, manual reduction of the foreskin is the first procedure attempted to return the foreskin over the glans. The procedure involves gently pushing on the glans and pulling on the retracted foreskin, attempting reduction.

Efficacy
If reduction can be performed, foreskin should return to correct location.

Risks/Benefits
- Risk: if unsuccessful, a dorsal slit procedure may be indicated
- Benefit: does not require surgical intervention

Acceptability to patient
Acceptable, as patient will not require surgery and is sedated during the reduction procedure.

Follow up plan
Patient (parental) education plan needed regarding tissue hygiene.

Patient and caregiver information
Healthcare workers and patient (if paraphimosis due to catheterization procedure) need education plan regarding correct procedures.

LIFESTYLE
Modification of life practices will not change phimotic or paraphimotic penis. However, some changes in lifestyle may affect possible recurrence of priapism. Reduction of doses of vasoactive drug therapy, avoidance of dehydration, excess sexual stimulation, and causative drugs may all help in preventing recurrence.

RISKS/BENEFITS
Benefit: possible reduction in priapismic events.

ACCEPTABILITY TO PATIENT
Acceptable, but alterations in sexual lifestyle may be difficult for patient to accept.

FOLLOW UP PLAN
If patient needs support regarding lifestyle changes, counseling could be recommended.

PATIENT AND CAREGIVER INFORMATION
- Patient should be provided with information regarding changing doses or drugs used to treat erectile dysfunction
- Patient should be provided with counseling information regarding maintaining lifestyle changes

OUTCOMES

EFFICACY OF THERAPIES

- Phimosis and paraphimosis: complete resolution of condition should occur immediately after specific treatment is carried out effectively
- There should be some evidence of detumescence if any treatment that has been administered is to be considered effective. It may take several days to achieve complete resolution

Review period

- Phimosis and paraphimosis: if dorsal slit procedure or steroid cream (used for a month) is not effective in preventing foreskin constriction, a circumcision should be considered the next step in treating these patients
- Priapism: if the patient has a persistent erection for >2h, urologic intervention should be sought immediately

PROGNOSIS

- Phimosis and paraphimosis: complete resolution is expected if treatment is carried out effectively. If circumcision is required, outcome is excellent
- Priapism: even with excellent treatment, detumescence may take several weeks. Impotence is likely even if treatment is initiated early in event

COMPLICATIONS

- Phimosis and paraphimosis: unreduced paraphimosis can lead to gangrene of the glans. Inflammation of the prepuce can also occur
- Priapism: erectile dysfunction and impotence commonly occur

CONSIDER CONSULT

Phimosis and paraphimosis:

- If dorsal slit or circumcision procedures are complicated by injury to the urethral meatus or glans penis, referral to a reconstructive urologic surgeon or plastic surgeon for reconstructive procedures may be indicated

RISK FACTORS

Phimosis:

- **Poor hygiene** – infection or irritation may lead to acquired phimosis
- **Diabetes** – patients with diabetes are more prone to bacterial infection and irritation of penis

Paraphimosis:

- **Presence of foreskin** – constriction of the penis due to retracted foreskin
- **Inexperienced healthcare provider** – catheter placement and poor hygiene may lead in problems in returning foreskin to correct location

Priapism:

- **Drugs** – use of vasoactive drugs to treat erectile dysfunction
- **Medical history** – sickle cell anemia, leukemia, other blood dyscrasias, cerebrospinal tumors, tertiary syphilis, urinary tract infections
- **Excessive sexual stimulation** – tissue ischemia can result after several hours of continuous erection

MODIFY RISK FACTORS
SCREENING

- Screening for detection of phimosis or paraphimosis would not be useful, as many patients do not require medical or surgical treatment of these conditions
- Screening for priapism would not be useful, as this condition is manifested as an emergency condition

PREVENT RECURRENCE

- Recurrence of phimosis or parphimosis should not occur if the initial treatment is successful
- Recurrence of priapism may occur if patient has sickle cell disease or other contributing medical condition, or if he continues to take drugs for erectile dysfunction

Reassess coexisting disease

Several drugs used to treat erectile dysfunction have priapism as a side-effect. Reducing drug doses or modifying therapeutic regimen can reduce possibility of occurrence of priapism.

Phimosis, paraphimosis and priapism – RESOURCES

ASSOCIATIONS

National Kidney and Urologic Diseases Information Clearinghouse
3 Information Way
Bethesda, MD 20892–3580
Tel: (800) 891-5388 or (301) 654-4415
Fax: (301) 907-8906
E-mail: nkudic@info.niddk.nih.gov
http://www.niddk.nih.gov

The American Association of Sex Educators, Counselors, and Therapists (AASECT)
PO Box 5488
Richmond, VA 23220–0488
Tel: (319) 895-8407
E-mail: AASECT@aasect.org
Provides referrals for counselors and therapists in local area
http://www.aasect.org

American Foundation for Urologic Disease
1128 North Charles Street
Baltimore, MD 21201
Tel: (410) 468-1800
Fax: (410) 468-1808
E-mail: admin@afud.org
http://www.afud.org

American Academy of Pediatrics
141 Northwest Point Boulevard
Elk Grove Village, IL 60007–1098
Tel. (847) 434 4000
Fax: (847) 434-8000
E-mail: kidsdocs@aap.org
http://www.aap.org

American Urological Association
1120 North Charles Street
Baltimore, MD 21201
Tel:(410) 727 1100
Fax: (410) 223-4370
E-mail: aua@auanet.org
http://www.auanet.org

KEY REFERENCES

- Robert JR, Hedges JR. Clinical procedures in emergency medicine, 3rd edn. Philadelphia: WB Saunders, 1998, p947–949, 952–954
- Behrman RE, Kliegman RM, Jenson HB. Nelson textbook of pediatrics, 16th edn. Philadelphia: WB Saunders, 2000
- Circumcision policy statement. American Academy of Pediatrics. Task Force on Circumcision. Pediatrics 1999;103:686–93
- Chu CC, Chen KC, Diau GY. Topical steroid treatment of phimosis in boys. J Urol 1999;162:861–3
- Monsour MA, Rabinovitch HH, Dean GE. Medical management of phimosis in children: our experience with topical steroids. J Urol 1999;162:1162–4

FAQS

Question 1
What is priapism?

ANSWER 1
It is the persistence of erection that does not result from sexual desire.

Question 2
Are there different types of priapism?

ANSWER 2
Yes. Low-flow or veno-occlusive priapism – caused by decreased venous outflow resulting in increased intracavernosal pressure, resulting in erection; and high-flow priapism – caused by sustained increased arterial inflow without increased venous outflow resistance, resulting in high inflow and high outflow.

Question 3
What are some common causes of priapism?

ANSWER 3
- Low-flow priapism: sickle cell trait and disease, leukemia, total parenteral nutrition, medications, intracavernosal injections, malignant penile infiltration, hyperosmolar intravenous contrast, spinal cord injury, spinal or general anesthesia
- High-flow priapism: primarily from perineal or penile trauma causing injury to the cavernosal artery

Question 4
What is phimosis?

ANSWER 4
A condition in which the foreskin cannot be retracted behind the glans penis.

Question 5
What is paraphimosis?

ANSWER 5
A condition in which the foreskin has been retracted and left behind the glans, constricting the glans and causing painful vascular engorgement and edema.

CONTRIBUTORS
Joseph E Scherger, MD, MPH
Philip J Aliotta, MD, MHA, FACS
Stewart M Polsky, MD

POLYCYSTIC KIDNEY DISEASE

DESCRIPTION

- Autosomal-dominant polycystic kidney disease refers to a systemic hereditary disorder characterized by the formation of cysts in the cortex and medulla of both kidneys, as well as in other organs
- Affects about one in 1000 people and is the most common of the polycystic kidney diseases
- Expansion of cysts over time causes destruction of adjacent normal renal tissue
- Important cause of hypertension in younger patients and cause of progressive chronic renal failure, leading to end-stage renal failure in about 50% of affected patients
- Accounts for 10% of end-stage renal disease
- No specific therapy directed at the polycystic disease process is held to be of benefit. Complications such as hypertension and infection may be treated

URGENT ACTION

- Admission to hospital for treatment of sepsis, should manifestation of infection in one or more cysts develop
- Admission to hospital for suspicion of massive retroperitoneal hemorrhage associated with cyst rupture

ICD9 CODE
- 753.1 Polycystic kidney, unspecified type
- 7532.13 Polycystic kidney, autosomal dominant

SYNONYMS
- Autosomal-dominant polycystic kidney disease
- ADPKD
- Previously referred to as adult-onset polycystic kidney disease

CARDINAL FEATURES
- Multiple cysts develop in both kidneys. The disease process probably begins *in utero* in most patients although throughout its course probably <1% of the tubules become cystic. The kidneys increase in size and ultimately cause signs and symptoms in the fourth and fifth decades of life. Reported kidney weights vary from normal to over 4000g
- The cysts develop in the cortex and medulla, are lined by tubular-type cells, and may occur anywhere along the tubule. Most measure 2–5cm in diameter but may grow to >10cm, resulting in renal enlargement and palpable kidneys in 50% of patients. They contain uriniferous fluid, altered blood, or pyogenic secretions
- Normal renal tissue exists around the cysts but often shows nephrosclerosis and chronic interstitial nephropathy
- Progressive renal failure may occur as a result of matrix deposition and cellular infiltrate in the interstitium leading to loss of normal parenchyma rather than the cysts themselves. Recent studies report that there is no way to predict when or whether renal failure will develop in any given patient
- Cysts are also present in the liver in 30–50% of patients although there is no way to predict which patients will develop them. These develop after about the age of 30 years and increase in size and number, parallels renal progression. They are more common in women, probably owing to sex hormones. Although hepatocellular failure is rare and liver function is normally preserved, jaundice or portal hypertension can develop as a result of obstruction of major bile ducts or the portal venous system
- Cysts also occur in other organs such as the pancreas (10%), the spleen (<5%), and the ovary or testis (reported but rare)
- Disease may be detected during screening of family of affected patient
- Renal disease is often first detected on routine screening, e.g. hematuria or proteinuria on urinalysis, normochromic normocytic anemia, raised blood urea nitrogen and creatinine levels on biochemical screening
- Back or flank pain (60% of cases) and gross hematuria (30% of cases) are the major symptoms. Renal stones, cyst infections, and retroperitoneal hemorrhage also occur
- Hypertension develops in 60% of patients before the onset of measurable renal failure; it is found in 25% of children and 65% of adults

CAUSES
Common causes
- 90% of cases are inherited as autosomal-dominant trait
- Spontaneous mutation in 10% of cases
- Gene abnormality in the majority of cases (PKD1) is located on the short arm of chromosome 16. In the minority of cases (10%) the defect is on the long arm of chromosome 4 (PKD2)
- These genes are responsible for the large integral membrane proteins, polycystin 1 and 2 respectively, which interact in normal epithelial cell growth and proliferation

Contributory or predisposing factors

- Factors contributing to a worse prognosis include later age at diagnosis, male sex, hypertension, increased left ventricular mass, and larger renal volumes
- If diagnosed before age of one year, autosomal-dominant polycystic kidney disease may progress to renal failure in childhood; however, if it is detected in childhood it seems to follow same course as adult disease

EPIDEMIOLOGY

Incidence and prevalence

INCIDENCE

6000 new cases per year in the US.

PREVALENCE

- One in 200 to one in 1000 of the world population
- Approx. 500,000 people with autosomal-dominant polycystic kidney disease in the US

Demographics

AGE

Found in all ages.

GENDER

Affects males and females equally.

RACE

Appears to affect all races.

GENETICS

- Gene linkage is seen in 90–95% of affected families with abnormal gene on short arm of chromosome 16 (PKD1 families). A second genotype with abnormalities on the long arm of chromosome 4 also exists (PKD2 families). A third genotype is also proposed
- Inheritance shows autosomal dominance with nearly complete penetration but variable expression. It has been projected that 100% of gene carriers will show evidence of disease by age 80 but there is a possibility that environmental or epidemiologic factors strongly affect the expression of autosomal-dominant polycystic kidney disease
- A positive family history is obtained in the majority of cases (60%), although spontaneous mutation may occur

DIFFERENTIAL DIAGNOSIS
Simple cysts
FEATURES

- Cysts develop with aging and can be detected in one-third of people aged 60 and older
- Low incidence in those under 40, although they do occur rarely in infants and children
- Cysts may be single or multiple, and enlarge with time
- Most cysts are asymptomatic and are discovered incidentally
- Cysts may occasionally cause abdominal masses or abdominal or back pain from bleeding, sepsis from infection (uncommon), erythrocytosis, or hypertension
- Single cysts with smooth walls on ultrasound require no further evaluation. Renal cell carcinoma occurs only very rarely in the wall of a simple cyst (<0.1% of cases)

Autosomal recessive polycystic disease in children
FEATURES

- Rare disorder occurring one in 6000 to one in 55,000 live births
- Autosomal-recessive inheritance; may be seen in siblings but rarely in parents
- Considerable variability in expression
- Death occurs within hours or days of birth in 75% of cases. Those who survive the neonatal period have 50–80% chance of surviving to at least age 15 years
- Affects kidney and liver with innumerable small cysts

Tuberous sclerosis
Distinguishing features of tuberous sclerosis are as follows.

FEATURES

- Presents with hamartomas of skin, brain, eye, heart, and kidney
- 50% of patients are mentally handicapped and most have seizures
- Angiomyolipomas may occur in the kidney, as may renal cysts
- Autosomal-dominant inheritance with an incidence of one in 20,000 live births. Heterogeneous gene linkage with at least four identified loci, one on chromosome 16 next to the autosomal-dominant polycystic kidney disease gene

Von-Hippel Lindau syndrome
FEATURES

- Familial disorder with angiomatous or cystic lesions in the kidneys
- Also causes retinal angiomas, cerebellar and spinal hemangioblastomas, and adrenal pheochromocytomas
- May be confused with autosomal-dominant polycystic kidney disease
- Autosomal-dominant inheritance with gene defect on chromosome 3

Acquired renal cystic disease
FEATURES

- 40–90% of patients on chronic hemodialysis have multiple bilateral renal medullary and cortical cysts
- Less common (5%) in patients on continuous ambulatory peritoneal dialysis
- Usually asymptomatic, but may cause pain or palpable mass
- Renal carcinoma may develop in these cysts (in 7% of patients with these cysts) as well as serious hemorrhage

Medullary cystic disease
FEATURES
- Rare autosomal-dominant disorder of uncertain pathogenesis
- Small cysts in the medulla and corticomedullary areas of shrunken fibrotic kidneys
- Characterized by progressive renal insufficiency terminating in renal failure in childhood or adolescence

Renal carcinoma
Distinguishing features of renal carcinoma are as follows.

FEATURES
- Affects 30,600 people in the US annually; incidence is rising and 10,000 deaths occur each year
- Usually presents during fifth to seventh decades (median age 60), and is twice as common in men as in women
- Triad of hematuria, flank pain, and palpable mass seen in only 10% of patients, but presentation with one or two of these is common. 70% have hematuria (may be microscopic), 50% have abdominal or flank pain, and 40% have abdominal mass. 20–30% of cases are discovered incidentally
- 15% are complex cystic lesions

SIGNS & SYMPTOMS
Signs
- Hypertension occurs in 25% of children and young adults and in 65% of adults with autosomal-dominant polycystic kidney disease. Initially this may be a reflection of intrarenal ischemia and an activated renin-angiotensin system, but as chronic renal failure develops, salt and water retention play an increased part in the mechanism
- Hematuria occurs in over 50% of patients and may be microscopic or macroscopic. It is probably caused by the rupture of a cyst into the renal pelvis but it may also be caused by infection, stone, or neoplasm
- Abdominal mass may be found incidentally or noticed by the patient
- Chronic renal failure with elevated blood urea nitrogen and serum creatinine may be the first manifestation (usually after age 40), but this is variable. No specific physical signs of uremia present
- On urinalysis, proteinuria or hematuria may be present

Symptoms
- Autosomal-dominant polycystic kidney disease is not usually symptomatic until the third or fourth decade of life and is subsequently progressive. Onset of symptoms may be earlier if the disease is inherited from the mother. The rate of progression of chronic renal failure shows less variability within families than between families
- Pain is the most common symptom in autosomal-dominant polycystic kidney disease. It may be a unilateral or bilateral vague sense of heaviness or dull aching to knife-like and stabbing pain. It may be disabling when chronic and lead to analgesic abuse
- Loin or back pain may be severe and may be caused by cyst rupture, hemorrhage, infection within a cyst, or urolithiasis (20%)
- Urinary tract infection may not be more common than in the general population but it is often difficult to eradicate. Frequency, dysuria, fever, loin pain, smelly urine may alert to presence of infection
- Symptoms of chronic renal failure include anorexia, nausea and vomiting, itching, nocturia, restless legs, insomnia, and symptoms of anemia

ASSOCIATED DISORDERS

- Colonic diverticulosis is more common in patients with autosomal-dominant polycystic kidney disease than in the general population
- Heart valve abnormalities are more common than in the general population, occurring in about 30% of patients. The most common abnormality is mitral valve prolapses but aortic, tricuspid, and pulmonary valve incompetence are also seen
- Subarachnoid hemorrhage associated with berry aneurysms occurs in approx. 10% of patients and accounts for 7–13% of deaths in autosomal-dominant polycystic kidney disease
- Renal carcinoma is probably not more common than in the general population
- Ovarian cysts appear more common
- Inguinal hernias appear to develop more frequently

CONSIDER CONSULT

- Refer all patients with suspected autosomal-dominant polycystic kidney disease to a nephrologist for evaluation and development of a treatment plan as disease progresses
- Diagnostic imaging is needed; refer if necessary (ultrasound if feasible, computed tomography scanning if ultrasound result is equivocal)
- Referral for genetic counseling may be appropriate before screening family members

INVESTIGATION OF THE PATIENT
Direct questions to patient

Q **How old are you?** Autosomal-dominant polycystic kidney disease is not usually symptomatic until the third or fourth decade and is subsequently progressive, with about half of the patients having end-stage renal failure by age 70.

Q **Have you been advised to attend for screening?** Screening of family members is advised when a new case of autosomal-dominant polycystic kidney disease is identified and will initially include first-degree relatives, although many people with a 50% risk of autosomal-dominant polycystic kidney disease decide against screening.

Q **Have you undergone a periodic health examination recently?** Hypertension and proteinuria or hematuria on urinalysis may be the first clue to the presence of renal disease and instigate further investigation. A loin mass may be found incidentally.

Q **Do you feel well?** Symptoms of chronic renal failure are very nonspecific and may have been attributed elsewhere. They include malaise, tiredness, anorexia, nausea and vomiting, itching, thirst, polyuria and nocturia, restless legs, insomnia, and symptoms of anemia.

Q **Have you had any pain?** Loin pain may be severe and may be caused by cyst rupture, hemorrhage, infection within a cyst, or urolithiasis (20%). The size of the kidney alone may also cause pain.

Q **Have you had any symptoms to suggest urinary infection?** Urinary tract infection may not be more common than in the general population but it is often difficult to eradicate. Frequency, dysuria, fever, loin pain, and smelly urine may alert to the presence of infection but pyogenic cyst infection may occur in the absence of these symptoms.

Q **Have you had any previous history of kidney disease, urinary tract disease, or surgery?** Past episodes of infection, stones, pain, renal cysts may have been early manifestations of autosomal-dominant polycystic kidney disease, especially in younger patients with no family history.

Q **For women: have you had any fertility problems? Did you have any complications in any of your pregnancies?** Pregnancy-induced hypertension or pre-eclampsia may be retrospective clues to pre-existing renal disease. Women with moderate renal dysfunction are more likely to suffer pre-eclampsia and complications such as preterm labor. Women with severe renal dysfunction are less likely to conceive and more likely to suffer spontaneous abortion.

Q **Questions to evaluate presence or absence of associated disorders.** Questions should also be asked especially of patients with a known diagnosis of polycystic kidney disease: a survey of bowel symptoms to exclude diverticular disease, cardiovascular symptoms that may indicate mitral valve prolapse (present in approx. 25% of patients), presence of hernias, and ovarian or testicular cysts.

Contributory or predisposing factors
Family history

Q Is there a family history of kidney disease? This is of paramount importance in assessment. Familial diseases may not have been accurately diagnosed in the past.

Q Do you have a family history of autosomal-dominant polycystic kidney disease specifically? Which family member is affected? Family history is positive for autosomal-dominant polycystic kidney disease in about 60% of cases.

Q Has any family member suffered with brain hemorrhage? Subarachnoid hemorrhage associated with berry aneurysms occurs in approx. 10% of patients with autosomal-dominant polycystic kidney disease, and it may be worth screening patients with such a family history.

Examination

- **General examination** may reveal features of chronic renal failure, which are usually nonspecific (e.g. pallor, increased skin pigmentation). Wasting and weight loss may be evident. Glove-and-stocking neuropathy is a late feature. Anemia is less frequently seen than in other causes of chronic renal failure

- **Blood pressure** may be elevated. Hypertension is present in 65% of adults

- **Evaluate clinical evidence of hypertensive end organ damage**, including an examination of the fundi and the cardiovascular system

- **General abdominal examination** may reveal one or more masses or hepatomegaly. Bimanual palpation of the abdomen may detect bilaterally enlarged kidneys with an irregular surface in over 50% of cases of autosomal-dominant polycystic kidney disease

- **Urinalysis** should always be performed. Proteinuria or hematuria may be present in the later stages of the disease

Summary of investigative tests

- Urinalysis, microscopy, and culture should be performed, including a dipstick test for proteinuria and heme pigment; urine microscopy for hematuria, pyuria, casts; urine culture for infective organisms

- Complete blood count: erythrocyte count, hemoglobin, and hematocrit may be normal or elevated because of increased secretion of erythropoietin from functioning renal cysts. Anemia may also occur

- Renal function tests should be performed to evaluate the degree of chronic renal failure, including blood urea nitrogen, serum creatinine, and 24h creatinine clearance

- Ultrasound of the abdomen is extremely sensitive and specific in the diagnosis of autosomal-dominant polycystic kidney disease in patients over 30 years of age. Multiple cysts are seen in both kidneys and hepatic and pancreatic cysts may also be seen. Absence of cysts on ultrasound cannot completely exclude subsequent expression of autosomal-dominant polycystic kidney disease phenotype in patients under 30 years of age (and especially those under 10 years) (false-negative rate of 36%)

Investigations that would normally be performed by a specialist:

- Computed tomography scanning is more sensitive than ultrasound examination but the increased cost and radiation exposure militates against its initial use in asymptomatic people

- Intravenous urography is not indicated for diagnosis if either of ultrasound or computed tomography is available

- Cerebral arteriography is not routinely advised unless subarachnoid hemorrhage has occurred. Magnetic resonance angiography (MRA) is currently being evaluated in this role. It may be reasonable to perform MRA if there is a family history of ruptured cerebral aneurysm

- Gene linkage analysis is specific and available from commercial DNA-diagnostic laboratories. May be helpful in screening younger asymptomatic relatives when they seek advice about conception. Useful where cysts cannot be detected by imaging

DIAGNOSTIC DECISION

- Patient is considered to have polycystic kidney disease if three or more cysts are noted in both kidneys and there is a positive family history of autosomal-dominant polycystic kidney disease
- It is not difficult to diagnose in its fully developed form on history, family history, and examination of bilaterally enlarged kidneys. Ultrasound or computed tomography scan can confirm the diagnosis
- Diagnosis in the early stages is much harder. In children at risk even one cyst is considered suggestive and three or more cysts bilaterally distributed are diagnostic
- A cyst is considered to be present if it measures >2mm in diameter
- Up to 25% of patients may not have cysts before the age of 30

CLINICAL PEARLS

- The diagnosis of autosomal-dominant polycystic kidney disease is most specifically diagnosed by gene-linkage analysis, but this requires participation of more than one family member and is needed for diagnosis in only a minority of cases. The correct diagnosis can usually be made with the combination of historical information plus renal ultrasonography. If the latter is equivocal, then high-resolution computed tomography scanning is indicated
- To make a correct diagnosis in patients with a family history of autosomal-dominant polycystic kidney disease, specific age-dependent criteria have been developed, which have been validated by gene-linkage results: age 18–29 years, at least two renal cysts are required; age 30–59 years, at least two cysts in each kidney; age 60 years and over, at least four cysts in each kidney; for a child under 18 years, any renal cyst is highly specific for autosomal-dominant polycystic kidney disease

THE TESTS
Body fluids
URINALYSIS, MICROSCOPY AND CULTURE
Description

- Visual inspection of urine
- Dipstick urinalysis detects blood, albumin, pH, nitrite, leukocyte esterase
- Urine microscopy may detect pus cells, eosinophils, epithelial cells, red cells, casts, organisms. Culture may detect bacteria
- No salt wasting except in very late disease
- Massive proteinuria (>2g/24h) is rare and, if found, should prompt further investigation for another renal disorder
- In middle to late stages of disease (20–40 years) mild persistent qualitative proteinuria (>200mg/dL) may be found in 20–40% of cases

Advantages/Disadvantages
- Advantage: dipstick urinalysis is inexpensive and readily available
- Disadvantage: interpretation of microscopic examination of urine sediment requires an experienced observer

Normal
Inspection:
- Color – yellowish
- Clarity – crystal clear

Dipstick test:
- pH 4.6–8 (average 6)
- Protein – negative (<150mg/24h, protein is normally present in small quantities in urine)
- Blood – negative
- Nitrite – negative
- Leukocyte esterase – negative

Microscopy:
- Microscopy shows no pus cells or hyaline casts

Culture:
- No growth of organisms

Abnormal
- Color: may be red or reddish brown in presence of blood
- Clarity: cloudy urine may be due to infection with pyuria, crystalluria, or prolonged standing at room temperature
- Presence of protein (although normal concentrated urine may show 1+ of protein). Bacterial infection almost always causes mildly positive dipstick for protein. Strongly positive tests more often indicate renal disease
- Presence of blood
- Nitrite is usually positive in urine infection but not all organisms produce nitrite
- Leukocyte esterase present in significant urine infection (detects pyuria)
- Presence of bacteria on culture

Cause of abnormal result
- Color: hematuria from ruptured cyst in autosomal-dominant polycystic kidney disease
- Clarity: cloudy as a result of infection
- Protein present as a result of glomerular dysfunction
- Blood present as a result of cyst rupture, infection, stone
- Microscopic abnormalities: pus cells (usually as a result of infection); red blood cells (as a result of bleeding into cysts); white cell casts (in the presence of acute pyelonephritis); broad or waxy casts indicate chronic renal disease; infecting bacteria

Drugs, disorders and other factors that may alter results
- Protein elevated in renal disease, congestive heart failure, hypertension, neoplasms of renal pelvis and bladder, multiple myeloma
- Blood present with trauma to renal tract, renal disease, renal or ureteric calculi, carcinoma, prostatitis, menstrual contamination, hematopoietic disorders, anticoagulants, myoglobin cross-reacts on dipstick test
- Dipstick test is positive also for heme pigments (myoglobin, hemoglobin) whether inside or outside the cells

RENAL FUNCTION TESTS
Description
- Blood urea nitrogen, serum sample. Urea is a product of protein catabolism in the liver. Blood urea reflects balance between production and removal. Production is increased by steroids, catabolic stress, and gastrointestinal bleeding and decreased by liver disease. Removal is decreased by congestive cardiac failure, and hypovolemia
- Serum creatinine – produced at a constant rate from muscle and, except where there is acute muscle damage, endogenous creatinine production is directly related to muscle mass. Eliminated almost totally by glomerular filtration with very small amount of tubular secretion. Serum creatinine is inversely related to clearance rate. In patient of normal build, serum creatinine does not rise outside normal range until clearance is reduced to 50% of normal
- Creatinine clearance is a readily available way to assess glomerular filtration rate. Calculated by dividing 24-h creatinine excretion (measured by collecting urine for a 24-h period) by serum creatinine concentration. In the US, creatinine clearance is commonly expressed in units of mL/min

Advantages/Disadvantages
Advantage: serum creatinine is a good marker for significant renal impairment but not for early renal impairment

Disadvantages:

- Blood urea nitrogen is not alone a good indicator of renal excretory function because it is influenced by protein catabolism and urine flow
- Complete and accurate 24-h urinary collection is the main problem in determining creatinine clearance. In advanced renal disease, creatinine clearance may overestimate true renal function

Normal

- Blood urea nitrogen: 8–20mg/dL (3–6.5mmol/L)
- Serum creatinine: 0.7–1.4mg/dL (50–110mcmol/L); the normal range varies with age and sex because of variations in muscle mass
- Creatinine clearance: 75–124mL/min

Abnormal

Values outside the normal range.

Cause of abnormal result

- Deteriorating renal function in autosomal-dominant polycystic kidney disease
- Low protein intake or catabolic rate lowers blood urea nitrogen and hypercatabolism of protein raises it independently of any change in renal function

Drugs, disorders and other factors that may alter results

Blood urea nitrogen:

- May be elevated by renal insufficiency, drugs, dehydration, gastrointestinal bleeding, decreased renal blood flow, and urinary tract obstruction
- May be decreased in liver disease, malnutrition, third trimester of pregnancy, and overhydration

Serum creatinine:

- May be elevated in renal insufficiency, decreased renal perfusion, and rhabdomyolysis and by certain drugs (e.g. aminoglycosides, cephalosporins, diuretics, methyldopa)
- May be falsely elevated in ketosis and by some cephalosporins
- May be decreased in people with decreased muscle mass, in pregnancy, and in prolonged debilitation

Creatinine clearance:

- May be elevated in pregnancy
- May be decreased in renal insufficiency or by some drugs (e.g. cimetidine)

COMPLETE BLOOD COUNT

Description

- Serum sample
- Erythrocyte count, hemoglobin, and hematocrit may be increased above normal, possibly owing to abnormal erythropoietin production by cysts
- Patients with end-stage autosomal-dominant polycystic kidney disease do not have as profound an anemia as that seen in other end-stage renal disease
- Coagulation studies, leukocyte, and platelet counts are normal in the absence of complications

Normal

- Hemoglobin – male: 13.6–17.7g/dL; female: 12–15g/dL
- Hematocrit – male: 39–49%; female: 33–43%
- White cell count: 3200–9800/mm^3 (3.2–9.8x10^9/L)
- Red blood cells – male: 4.3–5.9x10^6/mm^3 (4.3–5.9x10^{12}/L); female: 3.5–5.0x10^6/mm (3.5–5.0x10^{12}/L)
- Mean corpuscular volume: 76–100 mcm^3 (76–100fL)
- Platelet count: 130,000–400,000/mm^3 (130–400x10^9/L)

Abnormal
- Results outside normal ranges
- Normochromic normocytic indices are characteristic in renal disease
- Iron deficiency may occur (hypochromic microcytic anemia)

Cause of abnormal result
- In autosomal-dominant polycystic kidney disease, the erythrocyte count and hematocrit may be increased above normal or may not be as low as in other renal diseases at comparable levels of renal insufficiency. This is due to increased erythropoietin production by cells that line the renal cysts
- Iron deficiency may result from poor dietary intake, low-grade gastrointestinal bleeding, menstrual loss, or frequent diagnostic tests

Drugs, disorders and other factors that may alter results
- Hematologic disease may coexist and contribute to anemia
- Occult infection in a nonfunctioning kidney is not uncommon and may contribute to anemia
- 'Uremic' marrow depression may occur as a result of the depressant effect on erythropoeisis of any of a number of poorly defined 'uremic toxins'

Imaging
ABDOMINAL ULTRASOUND
Description
- Very sensitive and specific in the diagnosis of autosomal-dominant polycystic kidney disease in patients over 30 years. Multiple cysts are seen in both kidneys and hepatic and pancreatic cysts may also be seen
- In younger patients there is increased incidence of false-negative examinations when compared with gene linkage analysis
- Absence of cysts on ultrasound cannot completely exclude subsequent expression of autosomal-dominant polycystic kidney disease phenotype in patients under 30 and especially those under 10 years (false-negative rate of 36%)

Advantages/Disadvantages
Advantages:
- Noninvasive, relatively inexpensive, widely available
- Useful for renal size, detection of hydronephrosis and cysts
- Can also examine other organs for cysts (e.g. liver)

Disadvantage: limited by its resolution and computed tomography scanning may be superior for detecting small cysts

Normal
No cysts present, although simple renal cysts may be present with advancing age and in patients with other chronic renal parenchymal diseases.

Abnormal
Ultrasound shows multiple echo-free areas in both kidneys.

Cause of abnormal result
Cysts in the kidneys.

Drugs, disorders and other factors that may alter results
- Simple cysts are usually single and smooth-walled
- 15% of renal cell carcinomas are cystic but usually have thick and irregular cyst walls and cyst fluid abnormalities
- Multiple simple cysts cannot be distinguished from the cysts of autosomal-dominant polycystic kidney disease by size or location

TREATMENT

CONSIDER CONSULT

- Refer to a nephrologist all patients with renal insufficiency, deteriorating renal function, difficult-to-control hypertension, recurrent infections, management of infected cysts, and renal stones
- Refer to a urologist patients with renal stones or recurrent episodes of gross hematuria, and patients in whom a nephrectomy is being considered before renal transplantation (e.g. nephrectomy for intractable renal infection or intractable pain)

IMMEDIATE ACTION

Hospitalize and consult nephrologist for evidence of sepsis or acute hemorrhage that is adversely affecting systemic hemodynamics.

PATIENT AND CAREGIVER ISSUES
Impact on career, dependants, family, friends

- Diagnosis may have a wide impact on the patient's family
- Other family members may be advised to be screened for the disease and will need to be counseled accordingly, taking into account benefits and disadvantages of knowledge of disease and likely outcomes, so that informed decisions can be made. Risks may include difficulty of insurability and employment, denial or loss of psychological defense, and lack of specific treatment or cure. Benefits may include freedom from worry if the person proves to be unaffected, as well as the opportunity for early management of treatable complications and family planning
- Patient and partner need to discuss issues relating to future pregnancies
- Treatment of condition may have an impact on the patient's career (e.g. time off work for dialysis)
- If a family member expresses a desire to donate a kidney, gene probing is more reliable than ultrasound to rule out the presence of cystic disease in the donor

Patient or caregiver request

The patient may be concerned that dialysis or renal transplant is the ultimate conclusion for all cases.

MANAGEMENT ISSUES
Goals

- Preservation of renal function as long as possible
- Optimum management of hypertension and renal tract infection
- Control of symptoms such as pain and hematuria
- Optimum management of chronic renal failure and timely intervention with dialysis or transplant when indicated
- Promotion of a healthy lifestyle with regard to smoking avoidance, exercise, weight control, and salt intake
- Education for the patient about the condition, including preparation for dialysis when indicated

Management in special circumstances
SPECIAL PATIENT GROUPS

- Pregnancy is generally well tolerated if renal function is near normal (serum creatinine <3.0mg/dL). Liver cysts may enlarge and gestational hypertension and pre-eclampsia are more common
- Women with mildly decreased and stable renal function generally do well in pregnancy, with the rate of live births exceeding 95%. Fetal growth is adequate in 75% of cases, and the underlying disorder is not usually exacerbated, nor is the long-term prognosis altered

- Women with moderate renal dysfunction have a more guarded prognosis, with one-third or more experiencing deterioration in renal function or significant hypertension/pre-eclampsia. Fetal growth restriction and preterm delivery occur in >50%
- Women with advanced or end-stage renal failure are generally infertile but occasionally conceive. Only about 50% of these pregnancies succeed and there is considerable maternal risk of cardiac failure, severe hypertension with cardiovascular accident, and maternal death
- Rarely, patients are symptomatic in childhood. Siblings of children presenting in the neonatal period have an increased risk of also presenting in childhood

PATIENT SATISFACTION/LIFESTYLE PRIORITIES
Patient occupation and lifestyle may need to be taken into account when considering management of end-stage renal disease (e.g. attending for hemodialysis or patient-controlled continuous ambulatory peritoneal dialysis, adherence to restrictive diets).

SUMMARY OF THERAPEUTIC OPTIONS
Choices
- There are no specific therapies aimed at the polycystic disease process itself
- Treatment is aimed at preserving renal function as far as possible by careful control of blood pressure, prompt treatment of bladder and kidney infection, and treatment of symptoms such as pain and hematuria
- A healthy lifestyle is advised
- Renal function is carefully monitored, with timely intervention with dialysis (hemodialysis or continuous ambulatory peritoneal dialysis) or renal transplant when appropriate

Blood pressure control:
- More than 80% of patients with autosomal-dominant polycystic kidney disease develop hypertension at some time during the course of the disease
- Hypertension typically antedates measurable change in renal function by several years
- Hypertension may accelerate renal destruction in some patients and is one of the most important risk factors for progression of renal insufficiency
- Angiotensin converting enzyme inhibitors (ACE-inhibitors) may be effective in treating hypertension in autosomal-dominant polycystic kidney disease, especially in the early stages, although they have (rarely) been associated with severe renal hemorrhage and sudden renal failure in patients with large kidneys. They are a rational choice of drug, provided that they do not compromise renal function, in light of the postulated role of activated renin-angiotensin system, although caution is advised
- Calcium channel blockers are also effective in treating hypertension in autosomal-dominant polycystic kidney disease
- Arterial blood pressure should be maintained throughout the course of the disease within a range of normal as defined by age and sex
- Referral to nephrologist is indicated for difficult-to-control hypertension

Eradication of intracystic infections:
- Suspected intracystic infection is an indication for urgent referral to nephrology and infectious disease
- Pyogenic bacterial infections are a major problem for patients with autosomal-dominant polycystic kidney disease, especially women
- Urinary tract infections may not respond well to conventional therapeutic regimens
- Water-soluble and cationic antibiotics (penicillins and aminoglycosides) penetrate cysts poorly. Quinolones may be more efficacious than aminoglycoside or beta-lactam antibiotics
- Drainage may rarely be necessary in resistant cases

Management of pain:

- Loin and/or back pain is the most common symptom in autosomal-dominant polycystic kidney disease and may become chronic and disabling complicated by analgesic abuse and addiction. Hematuria may be associated with intense discomfort but usually responds to bed rest and simple analgesia within a few days. Persistent pain should lead to consideration of infection, stone, or tumor especially if associated with other symptoms or hematuria
- Drugs that may cause further renal insult should be avoided (e.g. NSAIDs)

Specialist referral for the following may be helpful:

- Severe pain or massive renal enlargement that is compromising physical function may be treated by surgery such as surgical cyst deroofing, percutaneous cyst drainage, or ethanol sclerosis. Relief lasting years may be produced when performed in centers that treat large numbers of cases. Renal function does not appear to be either compromised or improved by these procedures

Treatment of hematuria:

- Hematuria caused by cyst rupture rarely requires specific treatment and it usually ceases with rest
- Occasionally, transcatheter arterial infarction may be used to control recurrent hemorrhage or surgical removal of clot and dome of cyst
- Hematuria resulting from infection, renal stone, or tumor requires treatment specific to the cause

Conservative management of chronic renal failure is generally supervised by a renal physician; therefore, early referral to nephrology to help develop a long-term treatment plan is essential:

- Control hypertension
- Search for and control hyperparathyroidism
- Erythropoieten for the treatment of severe anemia
- Correct acidosis to avert bone disease and muscle wasting
- Detect and treat hyperlipidemia
- Avoid further renal insults – NSAIDs, tetracyclines, aminoglycosides, and other nephrotoxic agents should be avoided
- Doses of drugs that are renally cleared require alteration; this is particularly important for hypoglycemic agents, digoxin, and antibiotics
- Preparation for end-stage renal failure – counseling on future need for dialysis or transplant. Creation of arteriovenous fistulae at least 3 months before use
- Patients are advised to keep their nondominant arm free from needle sticks and blood pressure checks
- Late referral for dialysis is associated with increased morbidity and mortality

Management of end-stage renal failure is supervised by a renal physician:

- Transplant if feasible
- Dialysis, generally either hemodialysis or continuous ambulatory peritoneal dialysis

Clinical pearls

- Hypertension is a major manifestation of autosomal-dominant polycystic kidney disease, occurring in 30% of children with the condition, 65% of adults over age 30 with the condition but normal renal function, and 80% of all adults over age 30 with the condition. Its treatment is important to prevent the cardiac complications of hypertension in these patients (especially left ventricular hypertrophy) and, theoretically, to slow progression to end-stage disease
- Nephrolithiasis occurs in 20–30% of patients, most commonly associated with low citrate excretion. Evaluation and treatment of patients with stones in autosomal-dominant polycystic kidney disease is similar to that in patients without the condition. Hypocitriuria is treated with oral potassium citrate in patients with normal renal function, but is contraindicated in patients with renal failure

- Acute loin or back pain in patients with autosomal-dominant polycystic kidney disease is usually self-limited and responds to rest and analgesics. Pain that is dull, chronic, and insidious in onset (more common in patients with large cysts) can be disabling and lead to narcotic addiction. Before this occurs, patients should be referred for a cyst decompression procedure, which does not adversely affect renal function

Never
Never use antikaliuretic drugs such as spironolactone, amiloride, or triamterene in patients with autosomal-dominant polycystic kidney disease and impaired renal function.

FOLLOW UP
- Further routine imaging is not required after the diagnosis has been established unless new symptoms require evaluation (e.g. diagnosis of an infected cyst using a computed tomography scan)
- Regular review for symptoms and biochemical evaluation of renal function is necessary

Plan for review
- Yearly review of symptoms, renal function, and urinalysis are advised for asymptomatic patients; in particular, since asymptomatic hypertension is the most common early manifestation of autosomal-dominant polycystic kidney disease, its discovery and treatment is essential to prevent cardiovascular complications and, possibly, to slow the rate of progression to end-stage renal disease
- More frequent review is required for those with established renal failure

DRUGS AND OTHER THERAPIES: DETAILS
Drugs
ANTIHYPERTENSIVE DRUGS
Angiotensin-converting enzyme (ACE) inhibitors and calcium channel blockers are the most commonly used antihypertensive drugs in autosomal-dominant polycystic kidney disease
- The large majority of patients with autosomal-dominant polycystic kidney disease experience hypertension at some time in the course of disease and this often antedates by several years any measurable change in renal function. Hypertension is probably one of the most important risk factors for progression of renal insufficiency
- Salt restriction, weight control, and appropriate exercise should be prescribed for patients with autosomal-dominant polycystic kidney disease
- Arterial blood pressure should be maintained throughout the course of the disease within a range of normal as defined by age and sex
- Angiotensin-converting enzyme inhibitors are a rational choice of drug in autosomal-dominant polycystic kidney disease since there is evidence that the renin-angiotensin system has an important role in the pathogenesis of hypertension in autosomal-dominant polycystic kidney disease. Enalapril and ramipril are suitable drugs
- Calcium blockers are also highly effective in autosomal-dominant polycystic kidney disease, e.g. amlodipine

Dose
ACE inhibitors
Ramipril:
- Dosage for hypertension: Initial starting dose should be 1.25 mg once daily, may be increased to 2.5mg orally daily
- Usual maintenance range: 2.5–20mg daily
- Dose reduced in chronic renal failure: 25–50% reduction for creatinine clearance 10–50mL/min and 50–75% reduction for <10mL/min

Enalapril:
- Dosage for hypertension: 2.5–5mg daily
- Usual range: 10–40mg daily in divided doses

Dose reduction in nephropathy and renal impairment: 5–20mg daily

Calcium channel blockers
Amlodipine:
- Dosage for hypertension: 2.5–10mg daily

Efficacy
- ACE inhibitors are highly effective in treating hypertension in autosomal-dominant polycystic kidney disease, especially in the early stages of the disease
- Calcium channel blockers are also highly effective in autosomal-dominant polycystic kidney disease but may not have the other beneficial effects of ACE inhibitors

Risks/Benefits
Risks
ACE inhibitors:
- Use caution in renal impairment, hypotension, aortic stenosis, hyperkalemia, neutropenia

Amlodipine:
- Use caution in congestive heart failure, hypotension, hepatic insufficiency, aortic stenosis
- Use caution in elderly

Benefit: good blood pressure control may delay or slow renal deterioration

Side-effects and adverse reactions
ACE inhibitors:
- Cardiovascular system: orthostatic hypotension and syncope, angina, palpitations, sinus tachycardia
- Central nervous system: headache, dizziness, fatigue
- Eyes, ears, nose, and throat: cough
- Gastrointestinal: nausea, vomiting, diarrhea, constipation, abdominal pain
- Genitourinary: renal damage, impotence
- Hematologic: neutropenia, agranulocytosis, aplastic and hemolytic anemia, pancytopenia, thrombocytopenia
- Metabolic: hyperkalemia, hyponatremia
- Skin: angioedema, maculopapular rash

Amlodipine:
- Cardiovascular system: bradycardia, arrhythmias (including ventricular tachycardia and atrial fibrillation), hypotension, palpitations, chest pain, peripheral edema, syncope, tachycardia, postural dizziness
- Central nervous system: anxiety, asthenia, depression, fatigue, headache, insomnia, malaise, tremor
- Gastrointestinal: constipation, dyspepsia, diarrhea, flatulence, pancreatitis, vomiting, gingival hyperplasia
- Genitourinary: nocturia, polyuria
- Musculoskeletal: arthralgia, arthrosis, muscle cramps, myalgia
- Skin: angiodema, erythema multiforme, pruritus, rash, rash erythematous, rash maculopapular

Interactions (other drugs)
ACE inhibitors:

■ Allopurinol ■ Antihypertensives (loop and potassium sparing diuretics, prazosin, terazosin, doxazosin) ■ Azathioprine ■ Heparin ■ Insulin ■ Iron ■ Lithium ■ Nonsteroidal anti-inflammatory drugs ■ Potassium ■ Trimethoprim ■ Sodium

Amlodipine:

■ Barbiturates ■ Diltiazem ■ Erythromycin ■ Fentanyl ■ H-2 blockers ■ Proton pump inhibitors ■ Quinidine ■ Rifampin ■ Vinoriotinc

Contraindications
ACE inhibitors:
■ Pregnancy ■ Angioedema ■ Hypotension ■ Children

Amlodipine:
■ Sensitivity to amlodipine ■ Pregnancy and breast-feeding ■ Significant aortic stenosis ■ Cardiogenic shock ■ Unstable angina

Acceptability to patient
■ ACE inhibitors are generally well tolerated although some patients may discontinue treatment because of irritating cough
■ Calcium blockers are generally well tolerated. Some patients may have problems with flushing or 'woody' peripheral edema, which may take a long time to settle once established

Follow up plan
■ Regular blood pressure checks and monitoring of renal function are required. Check blood urea nitrogen, creatinine, and potassium within 2 weeks of initiation
■ Potassium levels should be checked periodically while on ACE inhibitor therapy

Patient and caregiver information
■ If patient is taking ACE inhibitors: do not use salt substitutes containing potassium; dizziness, light headedness, or fainting may occur during first few days of therapy. Therefore, get up slowly to sitting and standing and take dose at night to minimize orthostatic problems
■ If patient is taking calcium blockers: notify clinician of irregular heart beat, shortness of breath, swelling of feet and hands, or pronounced dizziness

ANTIBIOTIC THERAPY FOR INTRACYSTIC CYST INFECTION
■ Appropriate specific therapy of intracystic infections requires consultation with infectious disease specialist and nephrologist
■ Coliform, staphylococcal and *Bacteroides* organisms have been isolated from cyst aspirates in occasional patients
■ Choice of appropriate antibiotic depends on results of culture and sensitivity and identification, if possible, of type of cyst. Since penicillins and sulfonamides are not likely to penetrate cyst walls, ciprofloxacin is often used as initial therapy until culture results are obtained
■ Infection may be impossible to eradicate until any intrapelvic urinary stones are removed
■ Occasionally renal infection is so serious and intractable that nephrectomy is necessary. Should be used only as a last resort where parenteral antibiotics have been unsuccessful. Oral antibiotics for an indefinite period may also be recommended by some physicians

Dose
Ciprofloxacin:
■ Complicated or severe urinary tract infection – 500mg orally twice daily for 14 days
■ Uncomplicated urinary tract infection – 100–250mg orally twice daily for 7 days

Efficacy
- Penetrate into infected cysts
- Active against enterococci, staphylococci, streptococci, *Escherichia coli*, *Hemophilus* spp., *Klebsiella* spp., and *Proteus* spp.
- Most strains of *Pseudomonas* and anaerobic bacteria including *Bacteroides* spp. and clostridia are resistant

Risks/Benefits
Risks:
- Not suitable for children or growing adolescents
- Caution in adolescents, pregnancy, epilepsy, G6PD deficiency
- Use caution in renal disease

Benefit: wide range of activity

Side-effects and adverse reactions
- Central nervous system: anxiety, depression, dizziness, headache, seizures
- Eyes, ears, nose, and throat: visual disturbances
- Gastrointestinal: abdominal pain, altered liver function, anorexia, diarrhea, vomiting
- Skin: photosensitivity, pruritus, rash

Interactions (other drugs)
- Antacids ■ Beta-blockers ■ Caffeine ■ Cyclosporine ■ Didanosine ■ Diazepam
- Mineral supplements (zinc, magnesium, calcium, aluminium, iron) ■ NSAIDs ■ Opiates
- Oral anticoagulants ■ Phenytoin ■ Theophylline

Contraindications
■ Use is not recommended in children because arthropathy has developed in weight-bearing joints in young animals ■ Pregnancy category B

Acceptability to patient
Generally well tolerated.

Follow up plan
- Clearance of uncomplicated urinary tract infection/bacteruria should be documented with negative midstream urine
- Patient with cyst infection should be carefully followed, as these may be very difficult to eradicate. Specialist consultation and management is required

Patient and caregiver information
Prevention of infection is as important as treatment: shower rather than bath, frequent voiding, good perineal hygiene, voiding immediately after sexual intercourse. Avoid urinary tract instrumentation unless absolutely necessary.

Surgical therapy
SURGICAL CYST DEROOFING, PERCUTANEOUS CYST DRAINAGE, OR ETHANOL SCLEROSIS
- Severe pain or massive renal enlargement that is compromising physical function may be treated by surgical cyst deroofing, percutaneous cyst drainage, or ethanol sclerosis
- Renal function does not appear to be either compromised or improved by these procedures

Efficacy
Good long-lasting effects of deroofing of cysts have been obtained in the management of pain in centers that perform large numbers of procedures.

Risks/Benefits
- Risk: usual risks of anesthesia
- Benefit: may provide long-lasting pain relief

Acceptability to patient
Patients will generally accept surgery and its risks.

Follow up plan
Routine postoperative follow-up should be provided by the surgical team.

RENAL TRANSPLANT
- In selected patients, nephrologist may recommend transplantation to treat end-stage autosomal-dominant polycystic kidney disease
- Contraindicated in the presence of malignancy, active infection, patient unfit for general anesthesia, extremes of age, and advanced cardiac or pulmonary disease
- Most patients with autosomal-dominant polycystic kidney disease receive allograft with native kidney in place, but bilateral nephrectomy may be indicated for severe pain, unrelenting infection, recurrent severe hemorrhage, neoplasm, extreme kidney size

Efficacy
Post-transplant survival rates for the patient and the kidney appear equal to those in patients with other renal disorders.

Risks/Benefits
Risks:
- Post-transplantation complications associated with autosomal-dominant polycystic kidney disease include ruptured cerebral berry aneurysm and peritonitis secondary to ruptured colonic diverticuli
- Acute rejection may occur
- Chronic renal allograft dysfunction may occur
- Opportunistic infections such as cytomegalovirus and *Pneumocystis* are more prevalent in immunocompromised patients
- There is an increased risk of lymphoproliferative disease and other malignancies
- Hypertension and hyperlipidemia are very common after transplantation, particularly with cyclosporine treatment, and many successful recipients die prematurely from cardiovascular disease

Acceptability to patient
- Releases patient from dialysis
- Requires life-long immunosuppression, often with potentially toxic drugs such as cyclosporine, corticosteroids, or azathioprine

Follow up plan
Regular follow-up by renal transplant team with assessment of renal function is required.

Patient and caregiver information
- Potential living related donors need to be carefully screened for subclinical renal disease
- Outcome depends on human leukocyte antigen matching, surgical complexity, and comorbid conditions. One-year graft survival is approx. 80–90% for first cadaveric grafts, >90% for living related grafts, and 75% for highly sensitized patients and those with comorbid conditions such as diabetes mellitus
- Despite major advances in prevention of acute rejection, 10-year graft survival is only about 50%

Other therapies
HEMODIALYSIS

- Hemodialysis is most widely and extensively used modality for treatment of end-stage renal failure. Practically any patient can be treated with hemodialysis provided access to the circulation is available
- Dialysis machines consist of blood pump, dialysate delivery system, and a range of safety features to monitor integrity of extracorporeal circuit, prevent air embolism, and maintain standard dialysate concentration
- Long-term access to the circulation is usually via an autologous arteriovenous fistula or a synthetic arteriovenous graft
- Anticoagulation is achieved with systemic unfractionated heparin
- Solute removal occurs by diffusion down a concentration gradient across a semipermeable membrane
- Used three times weekly for most patients, typically for a period of 4h per treatment

Efficacy
As renal replacement therapy it prevents death from uremia and its complications.

Risks/Benefits
Risks:

- Muscle cramps and hypotension during dialysis are frequent in some patients
- Dialysis-associated amyloidosis may occur in long-term hemodialysis patients with arthropathies (50% patients after 10 years). Carpal tunnel and scapulohumeral periarthritis are earliest clinical manifestations of dialysis-associated amyloidosis

Acceptability to patient

- Patients must comply with fluid, salt, and other dietary restrictions
- Patients may find that large amount of time spent in dialysis interferes greatly with other activities

Follow up plan

- Follow-up is likely to be provided by the patient's nephrologist
- End-stage renal failure survival reflects comorbid cardiovascular disease, although evidence of better survival with more efficient dialysis
- Principal cause of death is cardiovascular disease; sepsis also is common

CONTINUOUS AMBULATORY PERITONEAL DIALYSIS (CAPD)

- CAPD is provided under supervision of a nephrologist as an alternative to hemodialysis
- Indicated for treatment of end-stage renal failure in patient capable of self-care or who has a carer to assist with exchanges
- 1–3L sterile dialysate are infused into peritoneal cavity via a catheter, left to dwell for 1–8h and subsequently drained
- Solute removal achieved by diffusion from blood into dialysate
- Water removal achieved by establishing an osmotic gradient into the peritoneal cavity (usually by adding glucose to dialysate)
- Usually four exchanges of 2–2.5L daily are performed
- Presence of polycystic disease is not a contraindication

Efficacy
Low-efficiency system compared to hemodialysis, and repeated exchanges needed on a more or less continuous basis.

Risks/Benefits
Risks:
- Peritonitis is major problem with an infection rate of one per 20 patient months
- Exit site infections can be protracted and are more predictive of catheter loss than peritonitis rates. Elimination of nasal carriage of staphylococci is important in reducing those infections
- Weight gain is frequently seen, with absorption of glucose from dialysate being the main problem
- Abdominal wall hernias may develop or worsen due to raised intra-abdominal pressure

Acceptability to patient
Generally acceptable to patient, but requires a capable patient and willing assistant at home.

Follow up plan
Follow-up is likely to be provided by the patient's nephrologist.

Patient and caregiver information
Limited duration of use – few patients remain on CAPD for more than 10 years.

LIFESTYLE
Diet:
- Some studies suggest that reducing protein intake in patients with chronic renal failure before the end-stage is reached may reduce the occurrence of renal death by about 40% compared with higher or unrestricted protein intake
- Optimum level of protein intake cannot be confirmed from available studies, but nephrologists commonly recommend that protein intake not be <0.6g/kg body weight/day to avoid undernutrition

Exercise:
- Exercise levels need not be modified in the early stages of disease
- There is evidence that recurrent bouts of gross hematuria, usually related to direct trauma, are associated with an increased rate of decline in renal function, and it would seem sensible to avoid contact sports if this is a problem

ACCEPTABILITY TO PATIENT
Interventions are generally acceptable to patients.

FOLLOW UP PLAN
Supervision by dietician may improve compliance with low-protein and other special diets.

EFFICACY OF THERAPIES

- Control of hypertension within values appropriate for age and sex is thought to attenuate progression to end-stage renal failure
- Urinary tract infection, especially cyst infection, may be very difficult to eradicate
- Good results may be obtained from surgical procedures for intractable pain relief such as deroofing of cysts
- Reducing protein intake in patients with chronic renal failure may be beneficial in reducing progression to need for dialysis
- Patients with autosomal-dominant polycystic kidney disease appear to have less complications from hemodialysis than patients with end-stage renal disease from other causes
- Continuous ambulatory peritoneal dialysis has limited duration of use; few patients remain on it for >10 years. Peritonitis is a significant problem
- Post-transplant survival rates for the patient and the kidney in autosomal-dominant polycystic kidney disease appear equal to those in patients with other renal disorders

PROGNOSIS

- Prognosis is variable and difficult to predict. Renal function usually normal until after the age of 30 years. Some degree of renal failure develops in about 90% of patients
- For patients with autosomal-dominant polycystic kidney disease, the probability of being alive and not having end-stage renal failure is about 77% at age 50, 57% at age 58, and 52% at age 73 years

Clinical pearls

It should be emphasized that the pattern of progression to end-stage renal disease is highly variable, particularly from family to family and even within families. It is highly debatable whether screening young family members before they consider marriage or pregnancy is useful or desirable for the individual, the family, or the general population.

Deterioration

- If blood pressure is difficult to control, consultation with the nephrologist for consideration of other drug therapy is indicated
- If pain is increasingly severe, referral for consideration of surgical procedures is indicated
- Chronic renal failure may progress to end-stage renal failure, when treatments such as dialysis (hemodialysis, continuous ambulatory peritoneal dialysis) or transplant will be required to sustain life

COMPLICATIONS

- Chronic renal failure may be complicated by anemia, hypertension, left ventricular hypertrophy, increased cardiovascular mortality, hypertriglyceridemia, impaired drug elimination, bone disease, vascular and extra-articular calcification, pericarditis, neuropathy
- Hematuria occurs in over 50% of patients and may be microscopic or macroscopic. It is usually due to rupture of a cyst into the pelvis. It may also be due to renal stone, infection in a cyst, malignant tumor
- Urinary tract infection: parenchymal pyogenic bacterial infection is a major problem for patients with autosomal-dominant polycystic kidney disease, especially women. Coliform, staphylococcal, and *Bacteroides* organisms have all been implicated. Cysts may become infected and behave like a deep-seated abscess. This may be accompanied by bacteria and/or bacteremia. Diagnosis may prove difficult without computed tomography scanning
- Loin or back pain may be due to cyst rupture, hemorrhage, or infection within a cyst or to urolithiasis (10% of patients pass renal stones). Intractable pain may be caused by enlarging cysts
- Nephrolithiasis develops with a frequency of about 20%. Computed tomography is the most sensitive technique for the detection of renal stones and differentiating them from nephrocalcinosis. Treatment is no different to that of patient without polycystic kidney disease
- Liver cysts may cause enlargement of the liver, but symptoms and complications from hepatic cysts are rare
- Subarachnoid hemorrhage occurs in <10% patients with autosomal-dominant polycystic kidney disease

CONSIDER CONSULT

- If blood pressure is difficult to control, consultation with the nephrologist for consideration of other drug therapy is indicated
- If pain is increasingly severe, referral for consideration of surgical procedures is indicated
- Refer early for dialysis. Late referral to a nephrologist for dialysis is associated with increased morbidity and mortality

PREVENTION

- Currently there are no techniques for the prevention of this hereditary disorder
- Genetic counseling may potentially reduce the number of people affected with autosomal-dominant polycystic kidney disease, but since the majority of affected people are asymptomatic until much later in reproductive life and autosomal-dominant polycystic kidney disease is not an inevitably lethal condition, counseling at a young age is generally not recommended
- Prenatal diagnosis by linkage analysis is not indicated in this disease

RISK FACTORS

Risk factors that may influence the rate of progression toward end-stage renal disease:
- Hypertension
- Infection, particularly within cysts
- High-protein diet
- Cardiac disease

MODIFY RISK FACTORS
Lifestyle and wellness
TOBACCO
Renal patients are at increased risk of cardiovascular disease and it is appropriate to advise against smoking.

ALCOHOL AND DRUGS
Drugs that may further damage renal function should be avoided, e.g. over-the-counter NSAIDs.

DIET
- Low-protein diet may prolong the useful life of the kidneys if renal failure is present
- Salt restriction will aid the management of hypertension
- Renal patients are at increased risk of cardiovascular disease and it is appropriate to advise about weight loss

PHYSICAL ACTIVITY
Renal patients are at increased risk of cardiovascular disease, and it is appropriate to advise exercise programs. Patients with large kidneys should avoid contact sport to avoid repeated trauma to large cysts.

SEXUAL BEHAVIOR
Void immediately after sexual intercourse and maintain good perineal hygiene to help to prevent urinary tract infection.

SCREENING

- Population screening is not warranted
- Targeted screening of relatives of affected patients allows detection of more cases, both asymptomatic and those with complications. At the time of diagnosis, 30–40% of affected relatives will already have unsuspected complications. Such screening must, however, be carried out with informed consent of the person being screened
- The appropriate time to screen adult relatives has not been determined and screening may create major problems, such as loss of health insurance. It is probably appropriate for asymptomatic adults over the age of 18 years who plan marriage or pregnancy. Typical screening tests would include physical examination, renal ultrasound, urinalysis, and determination of serum creatinine and blood urea nitrogen
- Screening of patients with autosomal-dominant polycystic kidney disease for cerebral aneurysm is not recommended unless there is a positive family history of cerebral aneurysms or a family member with subarachnoid hemorrhage

ASSOCIATIONS

National Kidney Foundation
30 East 33rd Street, Suite 1100
New York, NY 10016
Tel: (800) 622-9010 or (212) 889-2210
Fax: (212) 689-9261
E-mail: info@kidney.org
http://www.kidney.org

KEY REFERENCES

- Fick GM, Gabow PA. Hereditary and acquired cystic disease of the kidney (review). Kidney Int 1994;46:951–964
- Watson ML. Complications of polycystic kidney disease (review). Kidney Int 1997;51:353–365
- Ecder T, Chapman A, Godela M, Brosnahan M. Effect of antihypertensive therapy on renal function and urinary albumin excretion in hypertensive patients with ADPKD. Am J Kid Dis 2000;35:427–432
- Fouque D, Wang P, Laville M, Boissel JP. Low protein diets for chronic renal failure in non-diabetic adults (Cochrane review). In The Cochrane Library , 3, 2001. Oxford: Update Software
- Steinman T. Pain management in polycystic kidney disease. Am J Kidney Dis 2000;35:770–772

FAQS

Question 1

At what point is dialysis indicated?

ANSWER 1

Dialysis is indicated when reasonable medical therapy can no longer reverse, prevent, or control the clinical manifestations of uremia. The level of serum creatinine when this occurs is variable, but usually this point occurs when creatinine exceeds 7–8mg/dL (or creatinine clearance <15mL/min). The clinical manifestations of uremia include severe anorexia, vomiting, severe anemia, asterixis, and weight loss. Intractable fluid overload with congestive heart failure may require initiation of dialysis at lower levels of serum creatinine.

Question 2

What antibiotic should be used to treat lower urinary tract infection in, e.g., a middle-aged woman with symptoms suggesting urinary tract infection, *Escherichia coli* in midstream urine, and a known history of autosomal-dominant polycystic kidney disease but normal renal function?

ANSWER 2

Lower urinary tract infection (i.e. cystitis) should be treated similarly to how it is treated in patients without polycystic kidney disease, as determined by culture and sensitivities. Trimethaprim-sulfamethoxazole and cephalosporins are still useful drugs in this condition. In contrast, intracystic infections are more serious and require other antibiotics that are likely to penetrate cyst walls, such as ciprofloxacin.

Question 3

Is antibiotic prophylaxis ever indicated and, if so, what drug would be appropriate?

ANSWER 3

Antibiotic prophylaxis is not useful or indicated in the prevention of serious intracystic infections. On the other hand, prophylaxis with drugs such as trimethaprim-sulfamethoxazole might be useful in uncomplicated recurrent lower urinary tract infections (similar to this use in the general population).

CONTRIBUTORS

Dennis F Saver, MD
Martin Goldberg, MD, FACP
Ganesh G Shenoy, MD

PROSTATIC CANCER

SUMMARY INFORMATION

DESCRIPTION

- Neoplasm involving the prostate
- Over 99% are adenocarcinomas
- Most are silent until an advanced stage, then present with features of local or distal spread
- Digital rectal examination may be abnormal
- Benign prostatic hyperplasia often coexists

URGENT ACTION

Admit to hospital immediately if suspected:

- Spinal cord compression – actual or imminent
- Hypercalcemia
- Renal failure

KEY! DON'T MISS!

- Spinal cord compression
- Hypercalcemia

ICD9 CODE
185 Malignant neoplasm of prostate

CARDINAL FEATURES
- Usually silent disease until reaches advanced stage
- The most common symptoms are of urinary outflow obstruction – hesitancy, poor stream, chronic retention of urine, acute retention of urine
- Lower urinary tract symptoms may also occur – frequency, nocturia
- Bone pain and pathologic fractures may be presenting features
- Rarer presentations are with reduced ejaculate volume (caused by obstruction of the ejaculatory ducts), hematospermia (caused by involvement of the seminal vesicle) or impotence (caused by invasion of the neurovascular bundle)
- May present with unexplained deep vein thrombosis or recurrent thrombophlebitis
- Digital rectal examination may reveal an area of increased firmness, loss of the median sulcus, or an irregularly enlarged prostate
- Benign prostatic enlargement does not exclude prostatic cancer; 10–30% of men with benign prostatic hyperplasia have occult prostatic cancer
- Disease progression is by local extension via lymphatics or by hematologic spread to distant sites, particularly bone. Local extension tends to be into and through the prostatic capsule, the bladder base, and the seminal vesicles. Extension to the urethra or rectum is uncommon
- Unusually, anemia, marrow suppression, retroperitoneal fibrosis, or disseminated intravascular coagulation may occur
- Rarely, paraneoplastic syndrome from ectopic hormone production may occur
- In advanced stage, prostate may be enlarged, hard, and fixed, with extension to seminal vesicles
- In advanced stage, patient may present with acute renal failure due to bilateral ureteric involvement
- In advanced stage, the patient may present with lower body edema

CAUSES
Contributory or predisposing factors
- Risk factors may include high dietary monosaturated fat intake (especially alpha-linoleic acid, found in red meat and butter); this factor is crudely estimated to account for 10–15% of geographical differences in incidence). In contrast, genistein, an isoflavonoid found in soy, is believed to be protective (it inhibits 5-alpha reductase)
- Increased age
- Family history
- African race
- Vasectomy has been proposed as a risk factor but the issue has been revisited in a large analysis and no relationship was found. The American Urological Association states that there is no risk of prostate cancer from vasectomy

EPIDEMIOLOGY
Incidence and prevalence
- The most common nondermatologic malignancy worldwide
- One-third to one-half of all men have prostatic carcinoma identifiable at necropsy by the end of their lives
- Accounts for 70% of all male cancers
- Only lung cancer has a higher mortality

INCIDENCE

- 100,000 new cases diagnosed per year in the US
- Nearly 30,000 deaths per year
- For a 50-year-old man with a life expectancy of 25 years, the lifetime risk of microscopic prostate cancer is about 42%, the risk of clinically evident prostatic cancer is 10–15%, and that of fatal prostatic cancer is 3%. Risk increases with age
- The chance of developing invasive prostate cancer is 1/100,000 from age 0–39 years, 1/103 from age 40–59 years, and 1/8 from age 60–79 years

PREVALENCE

- Estimates are that 50–70% of men over 80 years of age have histologic evidence of carcinoma in their prostate, but the majority will never develop symptoms since many tumors are very slow growing and other comorbidities may intervene. Moreover, it is estimated that one in 10 histologic tumors will never progress
- Men in their 30s and 40s have a high incidence of small foci of prostatic intraepithelial neoplasia, whereas older men have larger lesions
- Most men die with their prostate cancer rather than from it

Demographics

AGE

- Incidence increases with age
- Uncommon in those <50 years of age
- 80% of new cases are in patients >65 years of age
- Average age at diagnosis is 72 years

RACE

- African-Americans have the highest incidence of prostate cancer in the world – one in every nine males. They also present later with higher-grade tumors and have poorer survival (66% at 5 years vs 81% for Caucasian Americans)
- Incidence is low in Asians
- Asian men have a lower level of 5-alpha reductase whereas African men have high serum testosterone levels, which has been postulated as the link

GENETICS

- Approximately 9% of all cases and 40% of early-onset cancers are familial
- Inheritance is believed to be Mendelian. Frequency of the predisposing allele is believed to be 0.36% but the men who inherit it have a 90% chance of developing the disease by age 85 years. The genes are currently being sought
- If a first-degree relative is affected, chances of developing disease is increased 2- to 3-fold
- If two first-degree relatives are affected, the risk is increased 4-fold
- New evidence has emerged linking the breast cancer gene mutations BRCA I and BRCA II to an increased risk of prostate cancer; therefore, consider screening men with high familial incidence of breast cancer

GEOGRAPHY

Clinical incidence varies around the world – high in the US, UK, Scandinavia; low in Hong Kong, Japan, Singapore.

DIFFERENTIAL DIAGNOSIS
Benign prostatic hyperplasia
Benign prostatic hyperplasia (BPH) occurs progressively with age and is not always symptomatic. Incidence of acute urinary retention increases with age. Symptoms correlate poorly with increased prostatic size – but prostate size greater than 30mL is associated with 3-fold increased risk of acute retention. 10–30% of men with BPH have occult prostatic cancer.

FEATURES
Lower urinary tract symptoms:
- Frequency
- Urgency
- Nocturia

Bladder outflow obstruction:
- Hesitancy
- Poor urinary stream
- Terminal dribbling
- Acute retention of urine
- Chronic retention of urine
- Digital rectal examination reveals a smoothly enlarged prostate
- Prostate-specific antigen (PSA) levels may be raised

Prostatitis
Asymptomatic inflammatory prostatitis – includes acute or chronic infection of the prostate (bacterial or granulomatous) and nonbacterial or chronic pelvic pain syndromes of the prostate (types IIIa and IIIb).

FEATURES
- Perineal pain
- Systemic disturbance/malaise
- Pain on ejaculation
- Hematospermia
- Prostate usually very tender on digital rectal examination – may be indurated
- Requires antibiotics for 4–6 weeks
- Can cause marked rise in prostate-specific antigen (PSA) levels

Prostatic stones
Stones forming in the prostate (e.g. secondary to infection).

FEATURES
- Perineal pain
- Pain on ejaculation
- Prostatitis
- Abnormality on digital rectal examination possible
- Hematospermia

SIGNS & SYMPTOMS
Signs
- Often none
- May be nonuniformly enlarged prostate on digital rectal examination – area of increased firmness, hard or irregular prostate with abnormal feel, loss of median sulcus

- Benign prostatic hyperplasia and carcinoma commonly coexist, so smoothly enlarged prostate does not exclude the diagnosis of prostatic carcinoma
- Urinary tract infection and prostatic carcinoma may also coexist
- In advanced disease, prostate may be enlarged, hard, and fixed with extension to seminal vesicles
- Bone pain is typically an aching pain that is worse on movement
- Neuropathic pain is common. The pelvis and vertebrae are often involved
- Hypercalcemia may be a feature of metastatic disease
- Acute spinal cord compression is a risk if there is vertebral involvement

Symptoms
- Usually silent disease until advanced stage
- May cause symptoms of urinary outflow obstruction – hesitancy, poor stream, chronic retention of urine, acute retention of urine
- May cause lower urinary tract symptoms – frequency, nocturia, urinary tract infection
- Bone pain and pathologic fractures may be presenting features
- May present with features of spinal cord compression – these are, progressively, lumbar vertebral tenderness; central back pain; radicular pain exacerbated by neck tension, coughing, and straining and more marked in recumbent position; sphincter disturbance; weakness; and sensory loss
- May present with features of hypercalcemia – bone pain, calculus formation, anorexia, constipation, dehydration, confusion
- May present with features of renal failure – malaise, reduced urine volume, edema, anuria

ASSOCIATED DISORDERS
- Benign prostatic hyperplasia
- Urinary tract infection (UTI) – all male patients with a UTI who have induration on digital rectal examination must be examined 6 weeks after antibiotic therapy to make sure that the induration has resolved

KEY! DON'T MISS!
- Spinal cord compression
- Hypercalcemia

CONSIDER CONSULT
Almost all patients should be referred for investigation if prostatic cancer is suspected. There is very occasionally an option of nonreferral in a small number of patients who:
- Are very frail with a short life expectancy
- Have contraindications to transurethral biopsy (e.g. poor health plus anticoagulants)
- Opt for nonreferral after a full, informed discussion (nonreferral is a big decision in primary care and risks litigation unless the patient is very clear on the facts and has made an informed decision; a primary care physician should choose this option only after specialist advice because watchful waiting may prove highly detrimental to the patient)
- However, prognosis in prostate carcinoma is very much based on tumor classification; without biopsy this information is not available and it is difficult to make a truly informed decision

INVESTIGATION OF THE PATIENT
Direct questions to patient
Q Is there a history of some weeks or months of bladder irritability (frequency, nocturia)? Exclude urinary tract infection if the history is short, or if dysuria is a major feature. Remember that acute urinary tract infection may be the first sign of prostate cancer.
Q Is there a history of difficulty stopping or starting micturition, and is the strength of the stream deteriorating? These are cardinal symptoms of prostatic enlargement and may not necessarily indicate prostate cancer.

Q **Is there any pain in the perineum?** Nonspecific perineal pain, perhaps worse on micturition or ejaculation, may be the presenting feature.

Q **Is there any pain in the bones?** Prostate cancer often spreads to the bones early, and bone pain may be the first symptom. The pain is usually localized, constant, and severe, and it may be worse on moving.

Q **Is there any pain on ejaculation or blood in the ejaculate?** These symptoms do not necessarily indicate any disease, and they may indicate prostatitis as well as prostate cancer.

Q **Is the patient feeling generally unwell, tired, or 'low', or has there been any weight loss, anorexia, thirst, memory disturbance, or confusion – perhaps noted by family or friends?** These nonspecific features indicate possible systemic disease from cancer dissemination, renal failure, or hypercalcemia.

Q **Is there any lower limb numbness or weakness, difficulty walking, or problems with emptying the bowels or bladder?** These features all suggest possible spinal cord problems and warrant rapid, complete investigations.

Family history

Q **Has anyone in your family ever had any prostate trouble?** Be particularly interested in first-degree relatives.

Q **Has anyone had a prostate operation?** Determine if this was for cancer or for benign prostatic hyperplasia.

Q **Does anyone in your family have regular injections for his prostate?** Likely to be goserelin.

Examination

- **Digital rectal examination.** Remember, however, that about 10% of patients with carcinoma have a normal digital rectal examination
- **Examination of painful areas as dictated by history.** Is this pain acute or chronic in onset?
- **If back pain is present, essential to check for vertebral tenderness and sensory loss.** If in doubt, refer. Remember that about 10% of cases of cord compression do not have associated tenderness over the vertebrae, so this finding is not essential for diagnosis. Be highly suspicious in anyone who suddenly ceased to be able to walk or stand as well as before

Summary of investigative tests

- Prostate-specific antigen (PSA): in all cases of suspected carcinoma of the prostate, including patients with bone pain alone. May prove that disease is present; however, 20% of cases have a normal PSA level, and slightly raised PSA may occur in benign prostatic disease and prostatitis. This test is likely to be initially ordered in primary care
- Prostatic acid phosphatase: now out of favor as a diagnostic test for prostatic carcinoma
- Free PSA percentage: in patients with a normal digital rectal examination and a PSA in the range 4–10ng/mL. This test may be ordered in primary care in the future, although if suspicion exists it is likely that the primary care physician will already have made a referral
- PSA density: this test is under evaluation but is likely to be ordered by specialist. To calculate the PSA density, divide serum PSA level by the prostatic volume as determined by transurethral ultrasound. Based on the result, serial digital rectal examinations and PSA would be advised for men with a PSA density <0.15, and biopsy would be advised for men with a PSA density >0.15
- Renal function tests: blood urea nitrogen and creatinine should be performed to rule out impending renal failure caused by ureteric involvement
- Midstream urine for microscopy, culture and sensitivity should be performed to exclude active urinary infection
- Transrectal ultrasound-guided biopsy of the prostate may be performed by a urologic specialist, although primary care physicians should be aware of the procedure and its risks in order to understand the problems inherent in any screening program involving PSA
- Fine-needle aspiration of the prostate (no longer commonly performed) would be performed by a urologic specialist

- Transrectal ultrasound may be used alone in some patients to assess extent of disease or presence of disease in cases in which digital rectal examination is normal (normally performed by a urologic specialist)
- Computed tomography scanning may be useful in assessing spread of disease (performed by a specialist)
- Bone scan is used to evaluate presence and degree of bony metastasis (normally performed by specialist)

DIAGNOSTIC DECISION

Biopsy of the prostate gives definite diagnosis; indications for prostate biopsy are one of:
- An abnormality on digital rectal examination
- An elevation in the serum prostate-specific antigen (PSA) level
- An elevated PSA velocity (an increase in PSA level of >0.75mg/mL in 12 months is considered an elevated PSA velocity)
- A high PSA density
- Prostatic intraepithelial neoplasia on an earlier biopsy

Guidelines

The following guidelines are available at the National Guidelines Clearinghouse:
- Prostate specific antigen [1]
- The American Cancer Society. Recommendations from the American Cancer Society Workshop on Early Prostate Cancer Detection [2]

The American Academy of Family Physicians have produced the guidelines on:
- Diagnosis and treatment of prostate cancer [3]

CLINICAL PEARLS

- One of the most important points is to recognize that at least 25% of the men with normal prostate-specific antigen (PSA) levels will have biopsy proven prostate cancer. The PSA blood test is one of many diagnostic tools at our disposal. However, elevations in PSA level precede detection by digital rectal examination or by symptoms by about 10 years
- Do not use the standard PSA value guide of 0.0–4.0ng/mL as an absolute; PSA levels increase with age

THE TESTS
Body fluids
PROSTATE SPECIFIC ANTIGEN (PSA)
Description
- Blood test useful in early diagnosis and monitoring. This is a protease secreted by prostate epithelial cells
- Has been proposed as screening tool
- Use of PSA for diagnostic testing was approved in the US by the FDA in 1994
- Test may be the trigger for more invasive investigations with their associated morbidity and mortality (e.g. transrectal prostatic biopsy)
- In one study, 75% of PSA-detected cancers and 56% of digital rectal examination-detected prostate cancers were confined to the prostate

Advantages/Disadvantages
Disadvantages:
- False negative rate. Over 20% of patients with prostatic cancer have normal PSA levels
- False positive rate. 30–50% of patients with benign prostatic hyperplasia (BPH) have elevated PSA; levels depend on prostate volumes, and each 1g of BPH increases the PSA level by 0.2ng/mL

- PSA is not a highly discriminatory test, particularly in the case of localized and curable cancers
- PSA is highly elevated for about 18 days by transrectal biopsy, rigid cystoscopy, catheterization, and transurethral resection of the prostate; it is recommended that PSA is not checked for at least 6 weeks after these procedures

Normal
- <4ng/mL – but around 20% of patients with prostatic cancer have results in this range, and these include some of the patients with small, potentially curable disease
- In men on finasteride, normal is <2ng/mL since finasteride halves the PSA levels
- PSA levels increase with age

Abnormal
- >4ng/mL (but for men on finasteride, values >2ng/mL is abnormal; and values increase with age)
- Where the result is in the range 4–10ng/mL there is still a high false-positive rate. In these cases the risk of cancer is 25% – measuring 'free' PSA may be helpful
- >10ng/mL is highly suggestive of prostatic carcinoma – few false-positive results occur in this range
- With cut-off of 4ng/mL, overall sensitivity is 46%, specificity 91%, positive predictive value 32% (compared with 21% for digital rectal examination)

Cause of abnormal result
- Prostatic carcinoma
- Benign prostatic hyperplasia
- Prostatic inflammation – prostatitis, stones

Drugs, disorders and other factors that may alter results
- PSA is elevated by prostatitis
- Finasteride lowers PSA
- PSA is slightly elevated by digital rectal examination, but the elevation (0.4ng/mL on average) is not clinically significant
- Flexible cystoscopy does not significantly elevate PSA
- PSA is highly elevated by transrectal biopsy and transurethral resection of the prostate for about 18 days – it is recommended that PSA is not checked for at least 6 weeks after these procedures
- PSA levels in aging prostates may also be influenced by prostatic schema or infarction and subclinical prostatitis

PROSTATIC ACID PHOSPHATASE
Description
Enzyme blood test that was widely used before the discovery of prostate-specific antigen for diagnosis, staging, and monitoring. It was initially used as a marker for metastatic disease.

Advantages/Disadvantages
Disadvantages:
- Use is limited, owing to cross-reactivity with serum acid phosphatases from other tissues, diurnal variations, and elevations after digital rectal examination
- Not recommended

Cause of abnormal result
- Cross-reaction with serum acid phosphatases from other tissues
- Diurnal variations
- Elevated levels after digital rectal examination

'FREE' PROSTATE SPECIFIC ANTIGEN (PSA) PERCENTAGE

Description
Venous blood test.

Advantages/Disadvantages
Advantages:

- Useful in patients with PSA levels of 4–10ng/mL (risk of carcinoma of prostate is 25% if digital rectal examination normal) to attempt to assess probability of prostate cancer
- Useful only when not investigating the patient further is an option that the patient or his caregiver can understand and contemplate
- Also useful as evaluator of aggressiveness of known tumor: low free PSA percentage suggests high-grade, faster growing cancer whilst higher free PSA suggests slower growing tumor
- May be helpful in making decisions with those patients whose life expectancy is not long and in whom invasive investigation might therefore be less appropriate

Disadvantage: does not provide certainty

Normal
Free PSA percentage >25% (lowers risk of prostatic cancer from 25% to 8% and indicates that a prostatic tumor, if present, is likely to be of the low-grade, slow-growing variety).

Abnormal
Free PSA <10% (increases risk of prostatic carcinoma to 56% and indicates that a prostatic tumor, if present, is likely to be for the higher-grade, more aggressive type).

Cause of abnormal result

- Prostatic carcinoma
- Benign prostatic hyperplasia

RENAL FUNCTION TESTS – BLOOD UREA NITROGEN AND CREATININE

Description
Blood test.

Advantages/Disadvantages
Advantages:

- Easy, inexpensive, and readily available
- Can rule out impending renal failure caused by ureteric involvement

Normal
Normal range for local laboratory usually given on form, but approximately:

- Blood urea nitrogen: 7–18mg/dL (1.16–3.0mmol/L)
- Creatinine (adult male): 0.7–1.3mg/dL (62–115mcmol/L)

Abnormal
Raised urea and creatinine.

Cause of abnormal result
Renal failure.

Drugs, disorders and other factors that may alter results
- Renal failure from another cause
- Dehydration
- Metabolic disturbance
- Various drugs
- Hypertension
- Renal artery stenosis
- Infection or inflammation
- Gastrointestinal bleeding

URINE MICROSCOPY
Description
Midstream urine specimen.

Advantages/Disadvantages
- Advantage: useful for identifying a urinary tract infection
- Disadvantage: presence of a urinary tract infection does not exclude carcinoma of prostate

Normal
Clear urine, no white cells or organisms.

Cause of abnormal result
Urinary tract infection.

Biopsy
TRANSRECTAL ULTRASOUND-GUIDED BIOPSY OF THE PROSTATE
Description
- Ultrasound-guided biopsy or fine needle aspiration
- Performed by specialist but included here because primary care physicians need to be fully aware of the procedure and its risks in order to understand the problems inherent in any screening program involving PSA
- Six cores are advised – three from the left and three from the right plus ultrasound-guided sampling of abnormal foci

Advantages/Disadvantages
Disadvantages:
- Painful
- Invasive
- Mortality 0.8%
- Only 25–50% of men with an abnormal rectal examination will be found to have cancer
- May cause retrograde ejaculation

TREATMENT

CONSIDER CONSULT

Always refer for therapy unless the patient declines diagnosis and treatment, and then only with full documentation in the patient record with patient's witnessed signature – the primary care physician should only choose this option after obtaining the specialist's advice. Otherwise always refer to a urologist for treatment; the urologist will make the decision over which treatment to use. 'Watchful waiting' is especially likely to be an indefensible treatment choice in:

- Young patients (those with a life expectancy >10 years)
- Symptomatic patients
- Patients with high prostate-specific antigen levels (>10ng/mL)

IMMEDIATE ACTION

- Consider treating spinal cord compression with high-dose oral corticosteroids (dexamethasone 16mg stat) while waiting for the patient to be transferred to hospital
- Consider commencing fluid hydration/resuscitation if patient is dehydrated, when hypercalcemia is suspected, or if the patient's transfer to hospital might be prolonged

PATIENT AND CAREGIVER ISSUES
Patient or caregiver request

- Patients often request a prostate-specific antigen (PSA) test – they may have read about it or heard about it from friends, or they may have experience of friends or family whose prostate cancer has been diagnosed and treated following an abnormal PSA reading
- In the US this does not present the primary care physician with a problem since there is a clear screening program with criteria for entry
- It is important that an asymptomatic patient who is to have a PSA test should understand that there is a significant risk of an inconclusive result, which is likely to result in invasive testing that may have long-term consequences and that carries a significant mortality. On the other hand, in advanced disease (which may still be asymptomatic), deferred treatment carries a significantly worse prognosis in terms of complications and death. Truthful presentation of the exact morbidity and mortality rates is essential. Physicians should not discriminate on the basis of age
- Older patients can be told that most patients die with rather than from their prostate cancer and that with advancing age the presence of some abnormal cells in the prostate is extremely common

Health-seeking behavior

- What has the patient read? You need to know if the patient has been advised on the basis of what he has read to have a test, and if the material he has read has given him an accurate picture of the problems inherent in prostate-specific antigen (PSA) screening
- What experience has the patient had of prostate cancer (e.g. from friends or relatives)? The patient may not understand that many men die with their cancer and many cancers do not progress in the patient's lifetime
- What experience has the patient had of other cancers? Prostate cancer is unusual in its sometimes long latent phase compared with other cancers, and many patients are unaware that this is often not an aggressive disease. It is always important to talk through these ideas and concerns to alleviate anxiety and misconception as far as possible
- Patients with experience of other cancer particularly need to be reassured that surgery is an aggressive procedure and that medical therapy can be equally successful

MANAGEMENT ISSUES
Goals

- Prevent further progression of disease, preventing premature death and disability
- Control symptoms and maximize quality of life

- Minimize adverse effects of treatment
- Select those patients in whom careful observation is appropriate
- Make sure that patients understand clearly what their options are
- Select those patients in whom disease is more aggressive for more radical treatment

Management in special circumstances

Treatment may not be appropriate in unwell patients with a low life expectancy (due to great age or poor general medical condition), and so investigation is also unlikely to be appropriate.

SPECIAL PATIENT GROUPS

Sexually active patients need to be aware of the risk of retrograde ejaculation and of erectile dysfunction following biopsy and, more importantly, following prostatectomy. They may need psychologic help or counseling.

PATIENT SATISFACTION/LIFESTYLE PRIORITIES

- Never assume that patients are too old to care about their sexual function
- Where there is a choice in treatment (e.g. radical surgery and radiotherapy vs hormonal treatment), patients should be enabled to be partners in making that choice

SUMMARY OF THERAPEUTIC OPTIONS
Choices

Choice of therapy depends on:
- Patient's age and life expectancy
- His health and fitness for surgery
- The staging of the tumor and the presence of metastatic disease (i.e. disease prognosis)
- Patient choice

Choices are:
- Watchful waiting alone: this choice is only applicable when the patient is fully informed and agrees to it. However, it is difficult for the patient to be fully informed without information from biopsy. Caution is advised in counseling a patient with confirmed cancer to follow watchful waiting
- Hormonal therapy (androgen deprivation): gonadotropin releasing hormone (GnRH) analogs such as leuprolide or goserelin are the mainstays of treatment in nonlocalized disease. They may also be used in some centers as adjunct therapy to prostatectomy, external beam radiotherapy, and brachytherapy for localized disease
- Chemotherapy treatments such as paclitaxel, docetaxel, estramustine, cyclophosphamide with doxorubicin, and cyclophosphamide with ketoconazole decrease pain and prolong palliation and may be seen increasingly in the future
- Immune therapy is a possible new development (in the trial stages), which may be seen in the future; it uses targeted chemotherapy to deliver chemotherapeutic agents directly to tumor cells. Several groups are studying retroviruses that have been altered to carry cytokine genes such as interleukins-2, -4, -6, and -7, interferon-gamma, tumor necrosis factor-alpha and granulocyte-macrophage colony stimulating factor
- Orchiectomy is the 'gold standard' of androgen deprivation in that it provides the most total androgen deprivation possible. As such it may be the treatment of first choice for many specialists for patients with disease spread and for patients who do not wish radical prostatectomy, and frequently as an addition to radical prostatectomy. Patients may not wish to opt for this choice for psychologic reasons
- Radical prostatectomy is usually the treatment of choice in young patients with localized disease. It probably offers greater psychologic relief in the younger patient, but it is radical surgery and may result in erectile and urinary problems in some patients
- Cryotherapy is a newer treatment modality. It has recently been approved as a first line of treatment modality as well as for salvage therapy from failed first line therapies

- External beam radiation therapy is another established first choice in therapy
- Brachytherapy (radioactive seed treatment – i.e. targeted radiotherapy): 10-year survival rates with the implantation of radiotherapeutic sources rivals survival rates with radical prostatectomy and external beam radiation; it is a definite first-line therapy in the US

Other drug therapy:
- Adrenal enzyme synthesis inhibitors (e.g. ketoconazole): not a first-line therapy but available for specialist use if side-effects of other therapies not tolerated; there is no FDA approval for the use of ketoconazole at the high doses required
- Nonsteroidal androgen receptor blockers (e.g. flutamide, bicalutamide): first-line choice to cover an androgen flare when GnRH analogs are started. It is widely accepted practice to add these to androgen deprivation when hormonal escape occurs (e.g. if prostate-specific antigen (PSA) starts to rise during treatment with GnRH analogs)
- Steroidal androgen receptor blockers (e.g. cyproterone, medroxyprogesterone): second-line choice after androgen blockers as adjunct treatment when tumor escapes GnRH control
- Diethylstilbestrol fulfills the same role as androgen receptor blockade; the choice is essentially a matter of specialist preference
- 5-alpha reductase inhibitors (e.g. finasteride) are of unproven benefit at present and are not recommended for therapy in the US

Combination therapy:
- Therapy depends on the staging of the tumor
- Adjuvant therapy (chemotherapy, hormonal therapy, or radiotherapy) to surgical or medical castration confers little benefit in nonmetastatic prostate cancer
- For patients with metastatic disease, combination of leuprolide and flutamide provides best results. Alternatives include adrenalectomy, hypophysectomy, estrogen administration or medical adrenalectomy with aminoglutethimide

Tumor staging
The Gleason scale can be used: histologic patterns are assigned numbers 1 to 5 (best differentiated to least differentiated). These numbers are added to give a total tumor score of 2 to 10:
- Score 2–4: good prognosis
- Score 5–7: intermediate prognosis
- Score 8–10: anaplastic lesions with poor prognosis

Alternatively the following staging system can be used:
- Stage A: no palpable tumor
- Stage B: tumor confined to the prostate gland
- Stage C: extracapsular extension
- Stage D: metastatic prostatic cancer
- Stage D1: pelvic lymph node metastases
- Stage D2: distant metastases

Stages A-B:
- No clear evidence of superiority of any single treatment

Stage C:
- Early androgen deprivation (surgical or chemical) improves survival and reduces complication risks
- Androgen deprivation with radiation therapy improves survival compared with radiation alone

Stage D:

- Androgen deprivation (surgical or chemical) improves symptoms and objective signs of disease in most patients
- Deferring androgen deprivation results in reduced survival and increased complication rates
- Chemotherapy decreases pain and prolongs palliation in some men with symptomatic androgen independent prostate cancer

Guidelines

The American Academy of Family Physicians have produced the guidelines on:
Diagnosis and treatment of prostate cancer [3]

Clinical pearls

- Watchful waiting is a valid treatment for some patients and the decision should be made by the patient, the physician, and the patient's family. A statement, consenting with this process, signed by the patient and the family can prevent future legal and emotional complications
- Patients older than 70 years are in many places treated with radiation (brachytherapy with or without external beam radiation) instead of radical prostatectomy
- Intermittent androgen ablation therapy is not a recognized standard of care for prostate cancer. There are no set guidelines for this form of therapy and it should be offered only with great caution until a standard delivery regimen is researched, outcomes are obtained, and survival predictability is available
- Presently, it appears likely that brachytherapy as a solitary therapy or in combination with external beam radiotherapy will be demonstrated to be as effective (or as ineffective) as surgery
- For localized disease regardless of grade, many urologists still offer all forms of treatment and aim at helping their patients to select treatment based on their age, comorbid factors, and their life expectations

FOLLOW UP

- Follow-up is usually by the specialist
- Primary care physician might be asked to arrange regular prostate-specific antigen (PSA) checks before review appointments
- PSA and digital rectal examination is usually offered by the specialist every 3 months for anywhere from 1–2 years, then at 6-month intervals for 3 years, and annually from the 5-year anniversary
- Patient will be instructed to see the primary care physician if new symptoms develop between review appointments; if this occurs, consider appropriate investigations and ask for early specialist review

Plan for review

Review with urologist and see patient at 3–6 monthly intervals to check:

- Clinical examination
- Digital rectal examination
- Prostate-specific antigen (PSA) level: if symptoms suggestive of metastasis develop or if PSA level starts to rise, a bone scan and chest X-ray are indicated

Information for patient or caregiver

- Explain expected side-effects of treatment
- Advise to seek early review if new symptoms – urinary or general – develop
- Discuss natural history of carcinoma of the prostate, its frequency, and the chance of progression

DRUGS AND OTHER THERAPIES: DETAILS
Drugs
ANDROGEN DEPRIVATION: GONADOTROPIN RELEASING HORMONE (GNRH) ANALOGS

- Androgen deprivation is the mainstay of treatment for advanced prostate cancer
- GnRH analogs include leuprolide and goserelin

Dose

- Leuprolide acetate: 1mg (subcutaneously); 7.5mg monthly (intramuscularly), 22.5mg 3-monthly (intramuscularly), or 30mg 4-monthly (intramuscularly)
- Goserelin: at a dosage of 3.6mg, this should be administered subcutaneously every 28 days into the upper abdominal wall using an aseptic technique under the supervision of a physician; at a dosage of 10.8mg, this should be administered subcutaneously every 12 weeks into the upper abdominal wall using an aseptic technique under the supervision of a physician
- Initiation of treatment is covered with an antiandrogen, either steroidal or nonsteroidal, to reduce flare phenomenon

Efficacy

- Increasingly the first-line therapy for both nonmetastatic and metastatic prostate cancer, either alone or in combination
- Usually preferred by patients and specialists to orchiectomy
- Initial rise in luteinizing hormone (LH) and follicle-stimulating hormone may cause worsening of pain and other symptoms if not covered by an antiandrogen

In nonmetastatic disease:

- Antiandrogen therapy from diagnosis reduces complications and may improve survival. It also improves survival over and above radiotherapy
- Immediate antiandrogen therapy after radical prostatectomy and pelvic lymphadenectomy improves survival and reduces risk of recurrence
- In clinically localized disease, no direct evidence has been found that early androgen treatment improves length or quality of life in asymptomatic men

In locally advanced disease:

- Androgen deprivation improves survival in men with locally advanced disease treated with radiotherapy
- Immediate antiandrogen treatment after radical prostatectomy and pelvic lymphadenectomy improves survival and reduces the risk of recurrence in men with node-positive prostate cancer

In metastatic disease:

- Androgen deprivation may reduce mortality in metastatic prostatic cancer
- Immediate androgen deprivation generally offers no survival benefit over deferring treatment until progression occurs; it may improve survival in men with locally advanced disease but no bony metastases
- Maximal androgen blockade plus orchiectomy offers a modest benefit but with increased adverse events compared with orchiectomy or androgen deprivation alone
- Delaying treatment only to when symptoms progress leads to increased mortality and complication rates
- Controversy remains as to whether combining androgen deprivation with androgen blockade is better than androgen deprivation alone

Risks/Benefits

Risks:

- Risks include the flare phenomenon, defined as an initial stimulation of LH and testosterone secretion during the first 2–3 weeks

(Goserelin)
- Use caution in patients with depression
- Use caution in patients with hypertension

(Leuprolide)
- Use caution in hepatic disease or cardiac disorders (edema, cerebrovascular accident, myocardial infarction, hypertension)
- Use caution in seizures, diabetes mellitus, or thromboembolic disease

Benefit: an appropriate form of treatment for nonsurgical candidates

Side-effects and adverse reactions
Goserelin:
- Gastrointestinal: diarrhea, constipation, nausea, vomiting
- Genitourinary: decreased libido
- Skin: sweating, rash
- Miscellaneous: gynecomastia
- Central nervous system: depression, anxiety, headaches, spinal cord compression
- Cardiovascular system: cerebrovascular accident, dysrhythmias, hot flashes, myocardial infarction

Leuprolide:
- Cardiovascular system: edema
- Central nervous system: pain, headache, dizziness, paresthesias
- Gastrointestinal: nausea, vomiting, diarrhea, constipation
- Genitourinary: hot flashes, sweating, urinary frequency and urgency disorders
- Musculoskeletal: joint pain, myalgia, neuromuscular disorders
- Skin: rashes

Interactions (other drugs)
None listed.

Contraindications
None listed.

Evidence
- A RCT compared immediate (at time of diagnosis) vs delayed (at time of disease progression) androgen deprivation in men with node-positive disease following radical prostatectomy. GnRH agonists or orchiectomy were used. There was significant improvement in overall survival in the immediate treatment group [4] *Level P*
- Another RCT compared immediate vs delayed androgen deprivation in men with stage C or D prostate cancer. GnRH agonists or orchiectomy were used. Disease-related mortality was reduced in patients with stage C disease receiving immediate treatment [5] *Level P*
- A nonsystematic review of RCTs compared different types of androgen deprivation (diethylstilbestrol, orchiectomy and GnRH agonists) in men with metastatic prostate cancer. Disease-related symptoms, laboratory results and radiographic findings improved in most men. There were no significant differences in response rates, time to progression, or survival. Duration of response was 12–18 months for all treatments [6] *Level M*

Acceptability to patient
- Side-effects are difficult – counseling is essential
- Poor tolerance by asymptomatic men

Follow up plan
Review 3-monthly then 6-monthly with digital rectal examination and prostate-specific antigen.

Patient and caregiver information
Patients should be made aware of the side-effects and of the availability of treatments for impotence.

DIETHYLSTILBESTROL
Nonsteroidal synthetic estrogen derivative that suppresses testosterone production.

Dose
- Oral: initiate with 50mg tablet three times daily and increase this dose level to 4 or more tablets three times daily, depending on the tolerance of the patient. Maximum daily dose not to exceed 1g
- Intravenous injection (ampules, 0.25g): 0.5g (2 ampules) dissolved in approximately 250mL of normal saline for injection or 5% dextrose for injection to be given by slow intravenous infusion the first day, and each day thereafter 1g (4 ampules) to be similarly administered in approximately 250–500mL of normal saline for injection or 5% dextrose for injection

Efficacy
Effectively suppresses testosterone production.

Risks/Benefits
Risks:
- Use caution in hypertension, congestive heart failure and hypertriglyceridemia
- Use caution in diabetes mellitus

Benefit: an option for patients not considering surgery

Side-effects and adverse reactions
- Gastrointestinal: nausea, pancreatitis, vomiting
- Genitourinary: testicular atrophy, breast changes
- Central nervous system: headache
- Cardiovascular system: myocardial infarction, pulmonary embolism, stroke

Interactions (other drugs)
- Anticonvulsants ▪ Corticosteroids ▪ Rifampin ▪ Warfarin

Contraindications
- Thromboembolic disorders ▪ Estrogen-dependent cancers ▪ Abnormal bleeding
- Pregnancy ▪ Breast cancer

Evidence
A nonsystematic review of RCTs compared different types of androgen deprivation (diethylstilbestrol, orchiectomy and GnRH agonists) in men with metastatic prostate cancer. Disease-related symptoms, laboratory results and radiographic findings improved in most men. There were no significant differences in response rates, time to progression, or survival. Duration of response was 12–18 months for all treatments [6] *Level M*

Acceptability to patient
May have lower incidence of sexual dysfunction than goserelin.

Follow up plan
Review every 3–6 months.

Patient and caregiver information
Patients should be advised about side-effects.

ADRENAL ENZYME SYNTHESIS INHIBITORS
- Usually second line therapy
- Ketoconazole (an imidazole derivative) at high doses is used – there is no FDA approval for ketoconazole at these high doses (this is an off label indication)

Dose
- Ketoconazole 1200mg daily (six times the antifungal dose) results in chemical castration in less than 24h
- There is no FDA approval for ketoconazole at these high doses
- Often given with citrus juices to improve absorption

Efficacy
- Effects are not durable – testosterone levels return to baseline shortly after the drug has been discontinued
- Can be useful for the atypical patients with cord compression and coagulopathy

Risks/Benefits
Risks:
- Risk of fatal hepatic toxicity
- Use caution in renal and hepatic disease
- Use caution in patients with sulfite sensitivity

Benefits:
- Decreases androgen metabolism
- Significant impact on liver metabolism, with elevation of serum triglycerides and abnormal levels of liver enzymes; hepatotoxicity limits long-term use

Side-effects and adverse reactions
- Central nervous system: headache, dizziness
- Gastrointestinal: nausea, vomiting, diarrhea, abdominal pain
- Hematologic: blood cell disorders
- Skin: rashes, urticaria, irritation, stinging

Interactions (other drugs)
- Alfentanil - Antacids - Antimuscarinics - Antiulcer agents (cimetidine, famotidine, omeprazole, nizatidine) - Antivirals (amprenavir, didanosine, indinavir, ritonavir, nelfinavir, saquinavir) - Anxiolytics (buspirone, chlordiazepoxide) - Astemizole - Benzodiazepines - Calcium channel blockers (dihydropyridines) - Cisapride - Corticosteroids - Cyclosporine - Estrogens - Ethanol - Isoniazid - Methadone - Oral anticoagulants - Phenytoin - Quinidine - Rifampin - Sildenafil - Statins - Sucralfate - Tacrolimus - Terfenadine - Tolteridine - Warfarin

Contraindications
- Hypersensitivity to ketoconazole - Fungal meningitis

Follow up plan
Monitor liver function and hematologic indices before starting and every 3 months while the patient continues on this treatment.

ANDROGEN BLOCKADE – NONSTEROIDAL ANTIANDROGENS

- Inhibits androgen binding by competitive block
- Decreases testosterone and dihydrotestosterone
- Increases luteinizing hormone so that potency can be maintained

Dose
Flutamide: two 125mg capsules three times daily at 8h intervals for a total daily dose of 750mg.

Efficacy
- Effective at blocking flare phenomenon in patients taking gonadotropin releasing hormone (GnRH) analogs
- Antiandrogens as monotherapy are considered inferior to conventional castration with respect to antitumor effects, but some patients may be willing to accept this risk in order not to be impotent

Risks/Benefits
Risks:
- Avoid exposure to sunlight due to photosensitivity
- Use caution in renal, cardiac or hepatic impairment
- Evidence for combined long-term androgen deprivation and androgen blockade remains controversial

Side-effects and adverse reactions
- Cardiovascular system: edema
- Central nervous system: fatigue, insomnia, dizziness
- Eyes, ears, nose, and throat: blurred vision, thirst
- Gastrointestinal: nausea, vomiting, diarrhea, anorexia, hepatotoxicity, altered hepatic enzymes, cholestatic jaundice, increased appetite, abdominal pain
- Genitourinary: decreased libido, inhibition of spermatogenesis, gynecomastia, mastalgia
- Hematologic: anemia, leukopenia
- Skin: photosensitivity, rashes

Interactions (other drugs)
Warfarin (increased hypoprothrombinemic effect).

Contraindications
- Pregnancy category D
- Severe hepatic disease

Evidence
Inconclusive evidence from systematic reviews suggests that combined androgen blockade (with orchiectomy or GnRH agonists) plus nonsteroidal antiandrogens improves survival in patients with metastatic prostate cancer, compared with androgen deprivation alone [7] *Level M*

ANDROGEN BLOCKADE – STEROIDAL ANTIANDROGENS

- Used on initiation of gonadotropin releasing hormone (GnRH) analogs to block initial surge
- Medroxyprogesterone acetate is sometimes used, which has progestagen and glucocorticoid activity

Dose
Medroxyprogesterone acetate: 400–1000mg/week.

Efficacy
Effective at blocking flare phenomenon in patients taking GnRH analogs.

Risks/Benefits
Risks:

- The drug should be discontinued immediately if any of the following should occur or be suspected: thrombophlebitis, cerebrovascular disorders, pulmonary embolism, and retinal thrombosis
- Medication should be discontinued pending examination if there is a sudden partial or complete loss of vision, or if there is a sudden onset of proptosis, diplopia or migraine. If examination reveals papilledema or retinal vascular lesions, medication should be withdrawn
- Anaphylaxis and anaphylactoid reactions have been reported

Side-effects and adverse reactions

- Central nervous system: headache, insomnia, dizziness, depression, asthenia, nervousness, hot flashes
- Gastrointestinal: nausea, vomiting, diarrhea, weight gain, abdominal pain or discomfort
- Genitourinary: hot flushes, decreased libido
- Skin: rashes, urticaria, pruritus, alopecia

Interactions (other drugs)
Aminoglutethimide (may significantly depress the serum concentrations of medroxyprogesterone acetate).

Contraindications

- Active thrombophlebitis, or current or past history of thromboembolic disorders, or cerebral vascular disease ▪ Liver dysfunction or disease

Follow up plan
Monitor liver function and hematologic indices before starting treatment and every 6–12 weeks while the patient remains on it.

Surgical therapy
RADICAL PROSTATECTOMY

- Surgical removal of the prostate with its capsule, the seminal vesicles, the ducts deferens, some pelvic fasciae, and sometimes pelvic lymph nodes
- Performed via the retropubic or perineal route

Efficacy

- Logic certainly suggests that in selected patients with small localized tumors of aggressive potential, radical prostatectomy can prevent progression. Evidence for this is not yet clear
- Should be reserved for those who will live long enough to benefit from this control

Risks/Benefits
Risks:

- Mortality 1.5–5% (increases with increasing age); fatal complications have been reported in 0.5–1% of men treated with radical prostatectomy and may exceed 2% in men aged 75 years and older
- Retrograde ejaculation (100%)
- Impotence: potency (i.e. ability to achieve and sustain an erection sufficient for intercourse) is lost immediately but when operation is successful it is regained over one year in up to two-thirds of patients. Chance of preserving potency is greater in younger men (90% of those under 50 years of age)
- Urinary retention
- Postoperative pain
- Urinary incontinence: reported rates of pad requirement vary from 6% to >50%

- Nearly 8% of men older than 65 years suffer major cardiopulmonary complications within 30 days of operation
- Urethral stricture in 18% of patients
- Fecal incontinence in 5% of patients
- Total urinary incontinence in 3% of patients
- Bowel injury requiring surgical repair in 1% of patients
- Deep vein thrombosis in 1% of patients
- Rectal injury in 0.6% of patients
- Colostomy in <0.1% of patients

Evidence
- A small RCT compared radical prostatectomy with watchful waiting in men with clinically localized prostate cancer. A nonsignificant increase in survival was found for patients treated with prostatectomy after median follow-up of 23 years [8] *Level P*
- A RCT compared radical prostatectomy with external beam radiation in men with clinically localized prostate cancer. There was a higher rate of metastatic disease in patients treated with radiotherapy [9] *Level P*

Acceptability to patient
- Depends on patient counselling
- Essential to warn thoroughly of risks
- Younger patients are possibly more likely to want radical surgery
- Evidence shows that younger patients are more likely to get radical surgery

Follow up plan
- Postoperative review
- Review with new symptoms
- 3 to 6 monthly review for regular measurements of prostate-specific antigen

Patient and caregiver information
Risks of surgery, including sexual and urinary dysfunction, should be discussed with the patient.

ORCHIECTOMY
The 'gold standard' of androgen deprivation (i.e. the longest-standing and most effective treatment against which others can be compared but which cannot so far be bettered in terms of degree of androgen deprivation).

Efficacy
- The gold standard in advanced disease – provides the most total androgen deprivation possible
- Also included in radical approach to early disease that is confined to prostate
- Patients with metastatic disease who present with pain often show significant palliation within 48h

Risks/Benefits
Risks:
- Risks of major surgery
- Voice changes
- Anxiety
- Depression
- Hot flushes
- Loss of libido
- Impotence
- Dysrhythmia
- Osteoporosis

- Alopecia
- Dry skin
- Rash
- Sweating
- Gynecomastia

Evidence
- A RCT compared immediate (at time of diagnosis) vs delayed (at time of disease progression) androgen deprivation in men with node positive disease following radical prostatectomy. GnRH agonists or orchiectomy were used. There was significant improvement in overall survival in the immediate treatment group [4] *Level P*
- Another RCT compared immediate vs delayed androgen deprivation in men with stage C or D prostate cancer. GnRH agonists or orchiectomy were used. Disease-related mortality was reduced in patients with stage C disease receiving immediate treatment [5] *Level P*
- A RCT compared orchiectomy, radiotherapy, and both treatments in combination for the treatment of locally advanced prostate cancer. There was no significant difference between the groups for overall survival or need for further treatment of local disease progression [10] *Level P*
- A nonsystematic review of RCTs compared different types of androgen deprivation (diethylstilbestrol, orchiectomy and GnRH agonsits) in men with metastatic prostate cancer. Disease-related symptoms, laboratory results and radiographic findings improved in most men. There were no significant differences in response rates, time to progression, or survival. Duration of response was 12–18 months for all treatments [6] *Level M*

Acceptability to patient
- Often unacceptable
- Testicular prostheses may be inserted for cosmetic effect

Follow up plan
Review 6-monthly with prostate-specific antigen levels and digital rectal examination.

Radiation therapy
EXTERNAL BEAM RADIATION (EBR)
Three types of external beam radiotherapy are used:
- External beam radiotherapy alone: delivered by radiation oncologists at dosage levels between 7400cGy and 8400cGy. It can be given as full-pelvis therapy or conformal therapy (in which the dose delivery is limited to the conforms of the prostate shape and the immediate periprostatic area). Historically, survival rates are comparable to radical prostatectomy
- External beam radiotherapy plus brachytherapy: a dose of 4500cGy is delivered to the prostate and the periprostatic region followed by brachytherapy. This is generally reserved for patients with a prostate specific antigen (PSA) level >10ng/mL, a Gleason score of 7 or more, and palpable disease
- Salvage external beam radiotherapy: for failed primary therapies. It is usually given if there is evidence of biochemical failure (rising PSA level) after radical prostatectomy surgery

Efficacy
- Uncertain
- Up to 30% of men with clinically localized prostate cancer treated with radiotherapy still have positive biopsies 2–3 years after treatment
- One retrospective, nonrandomized, multicenter pooled analysis found 5-year estimates of overall survival, disease-specific survival, and freedom from biochemical failure (as defined by raised prostate-specific antigen (PSA)) to be 85%, 95%, and 66%, respectively
- Estimated 5-year rates of no biochemical recurrence according to PSA concentrations before treatment and Gleason histologic scores ranged from 81% for pretreatment PSA <10ng/mL to 29% for PSA of 20ng/mL or more, and a Gleason score from 7 to 10

Risks/Benefits

Risks:

- Urethral and bladder symptoms occur predominantly in those patients who had transurethral resection of the prostate before radiation therapy
- Risk of complications is greater for doses >7000cGy

Complications include:

- Damage to skin
- Scarring of pelvic structures
- 60% develop rectal and bladder symptoms during the third week of treatment; this usually resolves on completion of treatment
- Diarrhea in 10% of patients
- Rectal bleeding in 4% of patients (and may persist)
- Sexual function is preserved in 73–82% of patients in the first year, but erectile potency diminishes with time, and 30–60% of patients maintain potency at 5 years plus

Persistent symptoms and late complications are less common:

- Chronic cystitis in 12% of patients
- Diarrhea persists in 0.4–3.0% of patients
- Proctitis in 8% of patients
- Urethral stricture in 3% – one in three need dilatation
- Hematuria in 3%

Evidence

- A RCT compared radical prostatectomy with external beam radiation therapy in men with clinically localized prostate cancer. There was a higher rate of metastatic disease in patients treated with radiotherapy [9] *Level P*
- Conformal and conventional radiotherapy were compared in a RCT of patients with non-metastatic prostate cancer. At median 3.6 years follow-up, there was no significant difference in tumor control (by PSA level) between the groups. Significantly fewer men treated with conformal radiation suffered from radiation proctitis [11] *Level P*
- A RCT compared external beam radiation therapy with strontium-89 in patients with metastatic prostate cancer. Strontium-89 was associated with significantly fewer new sites of pain, and a reduced need for further radiotherapy [12] *Level P*
- A RCT compared orchiectomy, radiotherapy, and both treatments in combination for the treatment of locally advanced prostate cancer. There was no significant difference between the groups for overall survival, or need for further treatment of local disease progression [10] *Level P*

Acceptability to patient

Radiation dose may worry some patients.

BRACHYTHERAPY

Radioactive seed treatment (i.e. targeted radiotherapy). Works on the principle that deposition of radiation energy decreases as a square function of the distance from the radiation source. Two forms are recognized:

- Permanent seed implant, which utilizes iodine-125 or palladium-103
- Temporary high-dose interstitial seed therapy with iridium

Efficacy

Uncertain, but initial results are encouraging.

Risks/Benefits

Risks:

- Urinary bladder toxicity is substantial – nearly half of all patients require medication for symptoms, and 14% have severe symptoms 2 years after implantation
- Complications reported in case series include urinary retention (6–8%), incontinence (13–18%), cystitis/urethritis (4–7%), proctitis (6–14%), and impotence (6–50%)
- Long-term outcomes from a representative national sampling of men have not been reported

Benefit: >80% retain potency at 3 years, which is the major advantage of this treatment

PATIENT AND CAREGIVER INFORMATION
Chemotherapy
CHEMOTHERAPY WITH CONVENTIONAL AGENTS
Efficacy

- May have an increasing role in prostate cancer therapy
- No single agent or combination has been shown to improve survival in a randomized trial. However, preliminary results from laboratory studies suggest that prostate cancer is not as resistant to treatment as has been supposed
- Newer agents that have been tried include estramustine (a combination of estrogen and a mustine agent) and paclitaxel (a taxane)
- Many standard agents are now being evaluated again; they include cyclophosphamide with granulocyte-macrophage colony stimulating factor (GM-CSF), cyclophosphamide with doxorubicin plus GM-CSF, and cyclophosphamide with ketoconazole

Risks/Benefits

Risks:

- Toxicities are significant

Side-effects:

(Paclitaxel)

- Hypersensitivity reactions (can be severe); premedication with dexamethasone for 3 days may mitigate these
- Myelosuppression
- Persistent fluid retention
- Peripheral neuropathy
- Cardiac conduction defects and arrhythmias
- Alopecia, myalgia, fatigue, vomiting, nausea

(Estramustine)

- Decreased gametogenesis
- Myelosuppression
- Nausea, vomiting, malaise
- Gynecomastia
- Deranged liver function
- Cardiovascular damage including angina and myocardial infarction

Interactions:

(Paclitaxel)

- Antibacterials ■ Antifungals ■ Cyclosporin

There are no recorded interactions for estramustine.

Evidence
Patients with symptomatic metastatic prostate cancer (androgen independent) may benefit from chemotherapy. RCTs have shown that some men have reduced pain and prolonged palliation with chemotherapy, but there is no evidence of improved survival [7] *Level P*

Other therapies
WATCHFUL WAITING
- Reasonable in patients with early-stage disease and a life expectancy <10 years, or in patients with focal, moderately differentiated disease
- It is not an option in patients with advanced, metastatic, or symptomatic disease
- Patients must struggle with the trade-off between avoiding the complications of treatment against the potential increase in life expectancy
- The decision should be made by the patient, the physician, and the patient's family. A statement, consenting with this process, signed by the patient and the family can prevent future legal and emotional complications

Efficacy
- Possibly as good as other options in localized disease
- Recent studies show 5- and 10-year survival rates of 67% and 41%, respectively, for all mortality, but 94% and 87% for cancer specific mortality, suggesting that most deaths were not cancer-related
- 5-year survival depended on histologic grade – 98% for well differentiated tumors, 92% for moderately differentiated tumors, 29% for poorly differentiated tumors
- Overall progression-free survival was 53% at 10 years

Risks/Benefits
Risk: the psychologic stress of being aware that a cancer is present but untreated must be considered

Benefits:
- Benefit of no treatment – but may be at expense of patient anxiety
- Overall it is an approach that can be considered for patients with life expectancy <10 years and a favorable histology

Evidence
- Two large prospective clinical cohort studies found that watchful waiting had a 15-year disease specific survival rate of 80% in men with clinically localized disease. This ranged from 95% for well differentiated tumors to 30% for poorly differentiated tumors [13,14] *Level P*
- A small RCT compared radical prostatectomy with watchful waiting in men with clinically localized prostate cancer. A nonsignificant increase in survival was found for patients treated with prostatectomy after median follow-up of 23 years [8] *Level P*

Acceptability to patient
Acceptable if patients agrees.

Follow up plan
- Review with any new symptoms
- Consider review for rechecking PSA every 6–12 months

EFFICACY OF THERAPIES

- Choice of therapy depends on tumor grade and degree of spread
- In early aggressive disease, it appears that aggressive treatment improves survival. Radical therapy in early disease involves radical prostatectomy with lymphadenectomy, orchiectomy and combined androgen deprivation, and androgen blockade (either steroidal or nonsteroidal)
- Side-effects and complications of this approach are high, particularly in older patients, and expected survival arising from other medical disease is likely to continue to influence treatment choice, even when evidence becomes clearer in the future
- Hormonal treatment, either chemical androgen deprivation or by orchiectomy, remains the usual choice in patients in whom disease has spread beyond the prostate, although radical prostatectomy with gland clearance may be a possibility if spread is very localized
- Watchful waiting is reserved for those with less aggressive tumors and a life expectancy <10 years
- New treatments such as targeted immune therapy and chemotherapy are under evaluation
- Some specialists currently agree that combined radical prostatectomy with radiotherapy and sometimes also orchiectomy or other androgen deprivation offers the best chance of cure in localized disease
- It is accepted practice to add androgen blockade to androgen deprivation either from the outset or when PSA rises on androgen blockade – there is evidence that this prolongs survival
- With the advent of chemotherapy and immune therapy further combinations will become possible

Evidence

- A small RCT compared radical prostatectomy with watchful waiting in men with clinically localized prostate cancer. A nonsignificant increase in survival was found for patients treated with prostatectomy after median follow-up of 23 years [8] *Level P*
- A higher rate of metastatic disease was found in patients treated with external beam radiation compared with radical prostatectomy in men with clinically localized prostate cancer [9] *Level P*
- Two large prospective clinical cohort studies found that watchful waiting had a 15-year disease-specific survival rate of 80% in men with clinically localized disease. This ranged from 95% for well differentiated tumors to 30% for poorly differentiated tumors [13,14] *Level P*
- RCTs found limited evidence of a survival benefit for patients with locally advanced disease treated with immediate androgen suppression therapy at the time of diagnosis [15] *Level P*
- Immediate androgen deprivation in men with node positive disease following radical prostatectomy has been shown to significantly improve overall survival compared with delayed androgen deprivation [4] *Level P*
- Early androgen suppression improved overall 5-year survival compared with deferred treatment in patients with locally advanced prostate cancer who were receiving external beam radiation [16] *Level M*
- A RCT found no significant difference between orchiectomy, radiotherapy, and both treatments in combination for overall survival or need for further treatment of local disease progression in patients with locally advanced prostate cancer [10] *Level P*
- A systematic review found limited evidence suggesting that early androgen suppression in patients with advanced prostate cancer reduces disease progression and complications due to progression. Early androgen suppression may provide a small but statistically significant improvement in overall 10-year survival [17] *Level M*
- No significant differences in response rates, time to progression, or survival has been found between different types of androgen deprivation (diethylstilbestrol, orchiectomy and GnRH agonists) in men with metastatic prostate cancer. Duration of response was 12–18 months for all treatments [6] *Level M*

- Inconclusive evidence from systematic reviews suggests that combined androgen blockade (with orchiectomy or GnRH agonists) plus nonsteroidal antiandrogens improves survival in patients with metastatic prostate cancer [7] *Level M*
- Patients with symptomatic metastatic prostate cancer (androgen independent) may benefit from chemotherapy. RCTs have shown that some men have reduced pain and prolonged palliation with chemotherapy, but there is no evidence of improved survival [7] *Level P*

Review period

- 3–6 months
- 6-monthly digital rectal examination and prostate-specific antigen (PSA) levels thereafter
- More intensive follow-up will be necessary if metastatic symptoms develop, and referral to a palliative care specialist for joint care is appropriate

PROGNOSIS

- Prognosis varies with tumor stage and spread
- The risk that a patient with well differentiated or moderately differentiated, clinically palpable, localized prostate cancer will remain free of symptomatic progression is 70% at 5 years and 40% at 10 years
- The risk of progression is higher in men with poorly differentiated prostate cancer
- The median actuarial time from the increase in prostate-specific antigen (PSA) concentration to the development of metastatic disease was 8 years in a retrospective analysis of large surgical series; once metastatic disease developed, median actuarial time to death was 5 years

Tumor staging:
- Stage A: confined to the prostate, no nodule palpable
- Stage B: palpable nodule confined to the gland
- Stage C: local extension
- Stage D: regional lymph nodes (D1 pelvic) or distant metastasis (D2)

Gleason classification:
- Histologic patterns are assigned numbers 1 to 5 (best differentiated to least differentiated). These numbers are added to give a total tumor score of 2 to 10
- Score 2–4: good prognosis
- Score 5–7: intermediate prognosis
- Score 8–10: anaplastic lesions with poor prognosis

The TNM (tumor, nodes, metastasis) method is also used for staging:
- T0: clinically unsuspected
- T1: clinically unapparent
- T2: confined within prostate
- T3: outside capsule or extension into vesicle
- T4: fixed to other tissue
- N0: no evidence of nodal involvement
- N1: regional node involvement
- M0: no evidence of distant metastases
- M1: evidence of distant metastases

Grade 1 tumors 10-year survival:
- After prostatectomy: 94%
- After radiotherapy: 90%
- With conservative management: 93%

Grade 2 or 3 localized tumors:

- Survival rate is better with surgery than with radiotherapy or conservative management. Data are incomplete, however.

Deterioration

- If prostate-specific antigen (PSA) rises, start hormone therapy or progress through therapeutic choices
- Repeat transurethral resection of prostate if obstructive symptoms occur
- Targeted radiotherapy is a useful treatment for bone pain caused by metastatic disease

Terminal illness

- Continue hormone therapy
- Use radiotherapy for bone pain; nonsteroidal anti-inflammatory drugs can also be helpful
- Use brachytherapy for salvage
- Give appropriate analgesia for pain, bearing in mind that morphine and diamorphine are renally excreted, and so if renal function is deteriorating, build-up of toxic metabolites and hence side-effects is likely. Fentanyl is metabolized by the liver and may be a better choice
- Nausea and vomiting are common in prostatic carcinoma – antiemetics that work on the chemoreceptor trigger zone (e.g. haloperidol) are likely to be the most effective
- Pathologic fractures are common; pain may be eased by pinning
- Cachexia and anorexia may respond to small doses of corticosteroids (e.g. dexamethasone 2mg once daily)
- Hypercalcemia is treated by intravenous rehydration plus intravenous pamedronate on a sliding scale. Clinical improvement takes 3–5 days
- Laxatives are always necessary when opiate analgesia is being used regularly

COMPLICATIONS

Hypercalcemia presents with:

- Bone pain
- Calculus formation
- Constipation
- Anorexia
- Dehydration
- Confusion
- Treatment improves clinical condition and well-being. Poor prognostic sign

Bony complications present with:

- Bone pain, typically pain described as aching or gnawing, worse on movement, may be tender spot
- Pathologic fractures: fracture on minimal or no impact
- Spinal cord compression: presents with lumbar vertebral tenderness, central back pain, radicular pain exacerbated by neck tension, coughing and straining (more marked in the recumbent position), sphincter disturbance, weakness, and sensory loss

Local complications:

- Renal failure: malaise, reduced urine volume, edema, anuria, raised urea and creatinine
- Acute retention of urine

PREVENTION

Studies are ongoing to look at finasteride, a 5-alpha reductase inhibitor, to prevent the development of prostate cancer in older men.

RISK FACTORS
Some evidence of dietary risk factors.

MODIFY RISK FACTORS
Some evidence for dietary modification.

Lifestyle and wellness
DIET

Risk factors may include high dietary intake of monosaturated fat (especially alpha-linoleic acid, found in red meat and butter). In contrast genistein, an isoflavonoid found in soy, is believed to be protective (it inhibits 5-alpha reductase).

SCREENING
In the US, there has been widespread prostate-specific antigen (PSA) testing since 1992, with increased rates of radical prostatectomy and radiotherapy but a decline in the death rate by only 1/100,000 men. Regions in the US with the greatest decreases actually have the lowest rates of testing. Moreover, countries with low rates of testing do not have higher age-adjusted rates of death.

The US National Cancer Institute PLCO cancer screening trial is looking at 74,000 men to determine whether screening followed by appropriate treatment will save lives.

The American Cancer Society, the American Urological Association, and the American College of Radiology currently recommend that all men aged over 50 years who have an anticipated survival of 10 years or more (based on medical comorbidities) should undergo (for the purpose of early detection of prostatic cancer).
- Annual digital rectal examination
- Annual serum PSA measurement

It is further recommended that screening begins at age 40 years in:
- African-American men
- Patients with a known history of prostatic cancer

However, many groups are concerned about the suboptimal sensitivity, specificity, and positive predictive values of digital rectal examination, PSA levels, and transrectal ultrasound. The psychologic and economic cost is significant. For example, the United States Preventive Services Task Force and the Canadian Task Force on Periodic Health Examination do not recommend screening.

PROSTATE SPECIFIC ANTIGEN FOLLOWED BY BIOPSY WHEN RESULT ABNORMAL
Cost/efficacy

It is unclear whether PSA screening would do more harm than good. Present evidence suggests this may be so. Nevertheless this method is widely used in the US.

In prostatic carcinoma, screening criteria are not met at present. PSA screening in asymptomatic men at specified ages at specified intervals, followed by transrectal biopsy where PSA is raised, does not meet the criteria because:

- There is no clear evidence that early intervention in prostatic cancer alters the outcome. Logic suggests that there are some small early tumors that are entirely within the prostate where prostatectomy is more likely to be curative – but these are likely to be the tumors with the lower and possibly normal PSA values
- At-risk group would be all men. The screening interval would need to be small and the age range covered very large, so this would be an expensive program
- The PSA level is not highly specific in the range 4–10ng/mL (25% chance of prostatic carcinoma)
- The PSA level is not highly selective – around 20% of patents with carcinoma of the prostate have a normal PSA value (<4ng/mL)
- Transrectal biopsy is highly specific and selective, but it is invasive and not entirely safe.

Screening of symptomatic patients also fails to fulfill the criteria because:

- Symptoms are very likely to be due to benign prostatic hyperplasia (not a predictor of risk)
- Patients with early but aggressive disease, the most important to pick up, are less likely to be symptomatic

Recommendations:

- Consider screening any man with symptoms of benign prostatic hyperplasia who has a raised PSA level
- Screen any man with possible bone pain
- Screen any man with suspected malignancy and an unknown primary (e.g. a man with an unexplained deep vein thrombosis)
- Screen any man with an abnormal digital rectal examination
- Review men with proven urinary tract infection to make sure symptoms settle – if not, consider screening

PREVENT RECURRENCE

If prostate-specific antigen (PSA) rises, start hormone therapy or progress through the therapeutic choices.

RESOURCES

ASSOCIATIONS
American Urological Association
1120 North Charles Street
Baltimore, MD 21201
Tel: 410-727-1100
Fax: 410-223-4370
E-mail: aua@auanet.org
www.auanet.org

KEY REFERENCES
- Anonymous. Screening for prostate cancer. Ann Intern Med 1997;126:480–484
- Beduschi MC, Oesterling JE. Prostate specific antigen. Urol Clin North Am 1997;24(2):323–32
- Bennett CL, Tosteson TD, Schmitt B, et al. Maximum androgen-blockade with medical or surgical castration in advanced prostate cancer: a meta-analysis of published randomized controlled trials and 4128 patients using flutamide. Prostate Cancer Prostatic Dis 1999;24–8
- Bertelsen S. Transrectal needle biopsy of the prostate. Acta Chir Scand 1966; 357:226–231
- Bishoff JT, Motley G, Optenberg SA, et al. Incidence of fecal and urinary incontinence following radical perineal and retropubic prostatectomy in a national population. J Urol 1998;160:454–458
- Byar DP, Corle DK. Hormone therapy for prostate cancer: results of the Veterans Administration cooperative urologic research group studies. Nat Cancer Inst Monogr 1988;7:165–170
- Catalona WJ, Partin AW, Slawin KM, et al. Use of the percentage of free PSA to enhance differentiation of prostate cancer from benign prostatic disease: a prospective multicentre cliical trial, JAMA 1998;279:1542–7
- Caubet JF, Tosteson TD, Dong EW, et al. Maximum androgen blockade in advanced prostate cancer: a meta-analysis of published randomized controlled trials using nonsteroidal antiandrogens. Urology 1997;49:71–78
- Crook J, Perry G, Robertson S, Esche B. Routine prostate biopsies: results for 225 patients. Urology 1995;45:624–632
- D'Amico AV, Whittington R, Malkowicz SB, et al. Biochemical outcome after radical prostatectomy, external beam radiation therapy, or interotitial radiation therapy for clinically localized prostate cancer, JAMA 1998;280:969–974

Key references and guidelines
1. Prostate specific antigen (PSA): best practice policy. Baltimore (MD): American Urological Association, Inc; 1999. Oncology (Huntingt) 2000;14:267–86 available at the National Guidelines Clearinghouse
2. The American Cancer Society. Recommendations from the American Cancer Society Workshop on Early Prostate Cancer Detection, May 4–6, 2000 and ACS guideline on testing for early prostate cancer detection: update 2001. In: American Cancer Society guidelines for the early detection of cancer. CA Cancer J Clin 2001;51:39–44 available at the National Guidelines Clearinghouse
3. The American Academy of Family Physicians. Naitoh J, Zeiner RL, Dekernion JB. Diagnosis and treatment of prostate cancer. Am Fam Physician 1998;57:1531–9,1541–2,1545–7
4. Messing EM, Manola J, Sarodsy M, et al. Immediate hormonal therapy compared with observation after radical prostatectomy and pelvic lymphadenectomy in men with node-positive prostate cancer. N Engl J Med 1999;341:1781–1789. Reviewed in: Clinical Evidence 2001;6:674–681
5. Medical Research Council Prostate Cancer Working Party Investigators Group. Immediate versus deferred treatment for advanced prostatic cancer: initial results of the Medical Research Council trial. Br J Urol 1997;79:235–246. Reviewed in: Clinical Evidence 2001;6:674–681
6. Robson M, Dawson N. How is androgen-dependent metastatic prostate cancer best treated? Hematol Oncol Clin North Am 1996;10:727–747. Reviewed in: Clinical Evidence 2001;6:674–681
7. Michaelson D, Talcott J, Smith M. Prostate cancer: metastatic. In: Clinical Evidence 2001;6:674–681. London: BMJ Publishing Group
8. Iverson P, Madsen PO, Corle DK. Radical prostatectomy versus expectant treatment for early carcinoma of the prostate: 23 year follow-up of a prospective randomized study. Scan J Urol Nephrol Suppl 1995;172(suppl.):65–72. Reviewed in: Clinical Evidence 2001;6:682–692

9 Paulson DF, Lin GH, Hinshaw W, Stephani S, and the uro-oncology research group. Radical surgery versus radiotherapy for adenocarcinoma of the prostate. J Urol 1982;128:502–504. Reviewed in: Clinical Evidence 2001;6:682–692

10 Fellows GJ, Clark PB, Beynon LL, et al. Treatment of advanced localised prostatic cancer by orchiectomy, radiotherapy, or combined treatment. Br J Urol 1992;70:304–309. Reviewed in: Clinical Evidence 2001;6:682–692

11 Dearnaley DP, Khoo VS, Norman AR, et al. Comparison of radiation side-effects of conformal and conventional radiotherapy in prostate cancer: a randomized trial. Lancet 1999;353:267–272. Reviewed in: Clinical Evidence 2001;6:682–692

12 Quilty PM, Kirk D, Bolger JJ, et al. A comparison of the palliative effects of strontium-89 and external beam radiotherapy in metastatic prostate cancer. Radiother Oncol 1994;31;33–40. Reviewed in: Clinical Evidence 2001;6:674–681

13 Albertsen PC, Hanley JA, Gleason DF, Barry MJ. Competing risk analysis of men aged 55 to 74 years at diagnosis managed conservatively for clinically localized prostate cancer. JAMA 1998;280:975–980. Reviewed in: Clinical Evidence 2001;6:682–692

14 Lu-Yao GL, Yao S. Population-based study of long-term survival in patients with clinically localised prostate cacner. Lancet 1997;349–906–910. Reviewed in: Clinical Evidence 2001;6:682–692

15 Wilt T. Prostate cancer: non-metastatic. In: Clinical Evidence 2001;6:682–692. London BMJ Publishing Group

16 Agency for Health Care Policy and Research. Relative effectiveness and cost-effectiveness of methods of androgen suppression in the treatment of advanced prostatic cancer: Summary. Rockville, MD: Agency for HealthCare Policy and Research, 1999. Reviewed in: Clinical Evidence 2001;6:682–692

17 Nair B, Wilt T, MacDonald R, Rutks I. Early versus deferred androgen suppression in the treatment of advanced prostatic cancer (Cochrane Review). In: The Cochrane Library, 1, 2002. Oxford: Update Software

FAQS
Question 1
What are the types of prostate cancer?

ANSWER 1
Multiple types of prostate malignancy exist: adenocarcinoma (>90% of cases), transitional cell carcinoma, sarcoma, and metastatic disease.

Question 2
In which portion of the prostate does cancer usually occur?

ANSWER 2
Approximately 75% of the cancers occur in the peripheral zone of the prostate, 20% in the transition zone of the prostate, and between 5 and 10% in the central zone.

Question 3
What is the Gleason's score?

ANSWER 3
Gleason's score is based on the histopathologic pattern of cancer cell distribution in the tumor. Two areas of the cancer are examined, and each area is graded between 1 and 5 on the basis of the degree of anaplasia. The sum of the assigned Gleason score for the two areas is the Gleason's score – it can range from 2 (1+1) to 10 (5+5). The histologic patterns are identified as: well differentiated pattern (scored 2, 3, or 4); moderately differentiated pattern (scored 5, 6, or 7); and poorly differentiated pattern (scored 8, 9, or 10). The higher the Gleason's score, the poorer the prognosis.

Question 4

When should referral be made to a urologist?

ANSWER 4

Referral to a urologist should be made when there is:

- A palpable nodule on digital rectal examination
- Any irregularity to the prostate is identifiable on digital rectal examination
- Elevated prostate-specific antigen (PSA) (i.e. >4.0)
- Elevated PSA velocity (i.e. PSA increases by >0.75 in one year)

Question 5

What is the evaluation of a patient with an elevated prostate-specific antigen (i.e. >4.0) and a benign-feeling prostate?

ANSWER 5

Such a patient should have a urologic consult, a transrectal ultrasound of the prostate, and sextant biopsies (one or two cores of tissue from each sextant).

CONTRIBUTORS

Randolph L Pearson, MD
Philip J Aliotta, MD, MHA, FACS
Julian N Anthony, MD

PROSTATITIS

SUMMARY INFORMATION

DESCRIPTION

- Disorder of the prostate, usually painful
- May or may not be due to bacterial infection
- Voiding difficulties are often present
- Can be divided into four types: acute bacterial prostatitis; chronic bacterial prostatitis; chronic non-bacterial prostatitis, or chronic pelvic pain syndrome, which may either be inflammatory or non-inflammatory; and asymptomatic inflammatory prostatitis
- Bacterial forms are treated with antibiotics

URGENT ACTION

Patients with acute bacterial prostatitis should be started immediately on a broad-spectrum antibiotic, after collecting samples for urine and blood culture.

KEY! DON'T MISS!

- A fluctuant prostate on palpation in a patient with acute bacterial prostatitis suggests an abscess, which must be treated by drainage and antibiotic therapy
- Prostatic massage is contraindicated in patients with acute bacterial prostatitis, because of the risk of precipitating bacteremia

ICD9 CODE

601.0 acute prostatitis
601.1 chronic prostatitis
601.9 prostatitis, unspecified

SYNONYMS

- Inflammatory chronic pelvic pain syndrome (for non-bacterial prostatitis)
- Non-inflammatory chronic pelvic pain syndrome (for non-inflammatory non-bacterial prostatitis)
- Pelviperineal pain syndrome (for non inflammatory non-bacterial prostatitis)
- Prostatodynia (for non-inflammatory non-bacterial prostatitis)

CARDINAL FEATURES

- Disorder of the prostate, usually painful
- Urogenital pain is the primary symptom; voiding difficulties or sexual dysfunction may also be present
- Voiding difficulties can be obstructive or irritative
- Acute bacterial prostatitis is readily treatable with antibiotics; chronic forms of prostatitis are more difficult to treat

CAUSES

Common causes

Acute bacterial prostatitis:

- *Escherichia coli* is the most common cause

Less common causes are:

- *Klebsiella* species
- *Pseudomonas* species
- *Proteus* species
- *Enterococcus* species
- *Serratia* species
- *Enterobacter* species
- Gram-positive bacteria such as *Enterococci*

Chronic Prostatitis:

The pathogenesis of chronic prostatitis may or may not be associated with bacteria and leukocytosis with prostatic inflammation.

Non bacterial prostatitis:

- Etiology is unknown
- Possibly due to infection with organisms that are difficult to culture, e.g. *Chlamydia trachomatis,* or may represent a noninfectious disease

Rare causes

- Gram-positive bacteria other than *Enterococci*
- *Neisseria gonorrhoeae*
- Mycobacterium tuberculosis – sequela of miliary TB
- Parasitic prostatitis – common in certain parts of the world
- Fungi-associated with systemic mycosis, ie: blastomycosis, coccidioidomycosis, cryptococcosis, histoplasmosis, paracoccidioidomycosis, and candida

Other Causes:

- Autoimmune
- Neuromuscular: nonbacterial prostatitis is a form of reflex sympathetic dystrophy
- Dysfunctional high pressure voiding which may occur through presumed obstruction to urine flow in the lower urinary tract from anatomic and/or physiologic abnormalities such as bladder neck contraction, detrusor-sphincter dyssynergia, urethral stricture
- Prostatic duct reflux that occurs as a result of dysfunctional high pressure voiding

EPIDEMIOLOGY
Incidence and prevalence
INCIDENCE
50–80 per 1000.

PREVALENCE
50–80 per 1000.

FREQUENCY
In the early 1990s, the diagnosis of prostatitis resulted in more than 2 million office visits per year. Prostatitis accounts for 8% of urology office visits and 1% of primary care visits.

Demographics
AGE
- Rarely affects prepubertal boys
- Can affect adult males of any age

DIFFERENTIAL DIAGNOSIS
Benign prostatic hyperplasia
FEATURES
- Not usually painful
- Micturition symptoms are similar to those of prostatitis, but dysuria is less common
- Rare in men under the age of 50
- Prostate feels smooth on examination

Prostatic cancer
FEATURES
- Symptoms of lower urinary tract obstruction
- Prostate feels hard and irregular on palpation
- Prostate specific antigen is elevated (although high levels are also sometimes seen in prostatitis)

Interstitial cystitis
FEATURES
- Dysuria
- Urinary frequency
- Suprapubic pain
- Sterile urine culture
- Prostate normal on palpation

Urinary tract infection
FEATURES
- Dysuria
- Difficulty voiding
- Bacteria in urine, but not increased after prostatic massage. Prostate normal on palpation

Prostatic abscess
FEATURES
- Fever
- Dysuria
- Urinary frequency
- Perineal pain
- Hematuria
- Urethral discharge
- Pain in the lower back
- Acute urinary retention

Seminal vesiculitis
FEATURES
- Fever
- Perineal pain
- Urinary frequency
- Hemospermia
- Hematuria
- Urinary tract infection

SIGNS & SYMPTOMS
Signs
Acute bacterial prostatitis:
- Prostate tender, warm, swollen, irregular on palpation
- Bacteria in urine

Chronic prostatitis:
- Variable prostatic tenderness on palpation
- Anal sphincter spasm (sometimes)

Symptoms
Type I: Acute bacterial prostatitis:
- Malaise
- Fever
- Chills
- Low back, abdominal, pelvic, or perineal pain
- Myalgia
- Pain on voiding
- Difficulty voiding, i.e., dysuria, frequency, urgency, nocturia

Type II: Chronic prostatitis (bacterial and non-bacterial forms cannot be distinguished on the basis of symptoms):
- Pain or discomfort in perineum, low back, scrotum, or penis
- Voiding symptoms: dysuria, urgency, frequency, nocturia, hesitancy, slow stream, and poor bladder emptying
- Sexual dysfunction
- Pain or discomfort on ejaculation
- Psychological stress
- Traditionally, symptoms are present for at least 3 months for a diagnosis of chronic prostatitis. The patient may present with recurrent urinary tract infections caused by the same pathogen. The organism may persist unaltered in prostatic fluid during therapy with most antimicrobial agents because it accumulates poorly in prostatic secretions

Types IIIA and IIIB: (non-bacterial prostatitis)
- Pelvic pain
- Ejaculatory pain
- Frequency/urgency
- Psychological stress
- Myalgias
- Dysuria

Type IV: Asymptomatic inflammatory prostatitis (AIP):
- Asymptomatic
- Diagnosis established by testing and/or biopsy

ASSOCIATED DISORDERS
Other urinary tract infections frequently coexist with prostatitis.

KEY! DON'T MISS!
- A fluctuant prostate on palpation in a patient with acute bacterial prostatitis suggests an abscess, which must be treated by drainage and antibiotic therapy
- Prostatic massage is contraindicated in patients with acute bacterial prostatitis, because of the risk of precipitating bacteremia

CONSIDER CONSULT

- Hematuria and hemospermia are indications for further investigation by a urologist
- Male factor infertility in a patient with prostatitis is an indication for urologic consultation
- Consider referring patients with severe psychological stress to a psychiatrist or clinical psychologist

INVESTIGATION OF THE PATIENT
Direct questions to patient

Q Have you felt feverish or generally unwell? Fever and malaise are symptoms of acute bacterial prostatitis.

Q What symptoms do you have when urinating? Pain on urination is more common in prostatitis than in benign prostatic hyperplasia.

Q Do you feel pain in the pelvic or genital area when not urinating? Pain is a symptom of prostatitis but not of benign prostatic hyperplasia or of urinary tract infection.

Q How long have your symptoms lasted? Symptoms must have persisted for at least 3 months for a diagnosis of chronic prostatitis.

Examination
Perform a digital rectal examination, checking prostate for:

- Tenderness (usually tender in acute bacterial prostatitis, may or may not be tender in chronic prostatitis)
- Consistency (a hard, irregular prostate could suggest prostatic cancer, and a fluctuant prostate in a patient with acute bacterial prostatitis could suggest an abscess)

Summary of investigative tests

- Because bacteriuria usually accompanies acute bacterial prostatitis, the pathogen is generally identified by culture of the voided urine
- Acute bacterial prostatitis can normally be diagnosed on clinical grounds alone, but a sample should be collected for urine culture to identify the responsible pathogen
- A blood sample should also be taken from patients with acute bacterial prostatitis for blood culture and complete blood count
- The traditional gold standard test for diagnosing chronic prostatitis is the Meares-Stamey four-glass test, which provides information about prostatic infection and inflammation. However, pre- and post- massage urine testing is now more widely used as a simpler alternative to the Meares-Stamey test
- Transrectal ultrasound (normally performed by a specialist) is not generally useful as a diagnostic test for prostatitis but can confirm the presence of a suspected prostate abscess
- Tests of serum prostate specific antigen (PSA) (normally performed by a specialist) are not generally useful in ruling out malignant disease, as PSA is often also elevated in prostatitis
- Prostate biopsy is useful when suspecting malignant disease
- As a general rule, identifying inflammatory cells in prostatic fluid (10 leukocytes/high power field and 1 or 2 lipid-laden macrophages/high power field) indicate prostatic inflammation (normally performed by a specialist)

DIAGNOSTIC DECISION
Guidelines for the diagnosis and management of prostatitis have been published:

- National Institute of Health consensus definition and classification of prostatitis [1]
- Research guidelines for chronic prostatitis [2]

Type I: Acute bacterial prostatitis
Can be diagnosed on clinical grounds alone, based on symptoms of:

- Difficult and painful urination
- Systemic symptoms (fever and malaise)
- Tender, swollen prostate on examination

Type II: Chronic bacterial prostatitis

- Appropriate symptoms last for at least 3 months
- Positive bacteria culture from post-massage urine
- Positive prostate localization tests, i.e., semen analysis, expressed prostatic secretions (EPS), and voided bladder sample-3 (VB-3)

Type IIIA: Inflammatory chronic pelvic pain syndrome

- Appropriate symptoms last for at least 3 months
- Negative bacteria culture
- Elevated leukocytes from post-massage urine
- Variable voiding
- Sexual symptoms

Type IIIB: Non-inflammatory chronic pelvic pain syndrome

Diagnosis of exclusion, based on:

- Appropriate symptoms last for at least 3 months
- Negative bacteria culture and negative leukocytes from post-massage urine
- Variable voiding
- Sexual symptoms

Type IV. Asymptomatic inflammatory prostatitis

- Prostate inflammation discovered incidentally during other investigations: biopsy, semen, elevated PSA, EPS, VB-3
- Absence of prostate-specific symptoms

CLINICAL PEARLS

- Prostatitis is the most common urologic diagnosis in men younger than 50
- Prostatitis is the third most common urologic diagnosis in men older than 50
- Prostatitis is present in half of all concordant prostate glands
- Drainage of the prostate abscess can be most effectively done with transrectal ultrasound and CT scan directed drainage procedures

THE TESTS
Body fluids
URINE CULTURE

Description

Culture of midstream urine.

Advantages/Disadvantages

Advantages:

- Ease of collection of sample
- Routine laboratory test

Disadvantages:

- Can provide useful information only in acute bacterial prostatitis
- A patient with chronic prostatitis may present with recurrent UTI

Normal

No bacteria can be cultured.

Abnormal

- Uropathogenic bacteria are cultured in urine
- Culture of bacteria does not rule out other types of urinary tract infection
- Keep in mind the possibility of a false-positive result

Cause of abnormal result
Urinary tract infection, which may or may not be localized to the prostate.

Drugs, disorders and other factors that may alter results
Other urinary tract infections.

BLOOD CULTURE
Description
Culture of venous blood.

Advantages/Disadvantages
Advantages:
- Ease of collection of sample
- Routine laboratory test

Disadvantage: can provide useful information only in acute bacterial prostatitis

Normal
No bacteria can be cultured.

Abnormal
- Bacteria are cultured from the blood sample
- Keep in mind the possibility of a false-positive result; culture of bacteria does not prove that infection originated in the prostate

Cause of abnormal result
Acute bacterial prostatitis which is causing systemic infection.

Drugs, disorders and other factors that may alter results
Other forms of systemic infection.

COMPLETE BLOOD COUNT
Description
Venous blood sample.

Advantages/Disadvantages
Advantages:
- Ease of collection of sample
- Routine laboratory test

Disadvantage: nonspecific

Normal
- Red blood cells: 4.33–5.67 1012/liter
- White blood cells: 3.83–11.0 109/liter
- Neutrophils: 1.94–7.78 109/liter
- Lymphocytes: 1.08–3.10 109/liter
- Monocytes: 0.240–0.870 109/liter
- Eosinophils: 0.028–0.531 109/liter
- Basophils: 0.011–0.106 109/liter
- Platelets: 156–352 109/liter

Abnormal
- Elevated white cell counts
- Keep in mind the possibility of a false-positive result

Cause of abnormal result
Systemic infection, which may or may not originate in the prostate.

Drugs, disorders and other factors that may alter results
Other infections.

MEARES-STAMEY FOUR-GLASS TEST
Description
Four samples are taken: a first voided urine specimen and subsequent midstream urine are first collected. Prostatic massage is then done, and any expressed prostatic secretions are collected. Finally, a first voided urine specimen after the prostatic massage is collected.

NB: prostatic massage is contraindicated in acute bacterial prostatitis.

Advantages/Disadvantages
Advantage: gold standard for localization of urinary tract infections

Disadvantages:
- Complicated sample collection process
- Prostatic massage is uncomfortable for the patient
- Many false-negative and false-positive results

Normal
No bacteria can be cultured from any of the samples, and all samples give negative leukocyte counts.

Abnormal
- Bacteria are cultured from any or all of the samples
- Any or all of the samples have elevated leukocyte counts
- Keep in mind the possibility of a false-positive result

Cause of abnormal result
- Positive bacterial culture in first voided urine specimen (pre-massage) suggests urethritis
- Positive bacterial culture in midstream urine specimen (pre-massage) suggests cystitis
- Positive bacterial culture in expressed prostatic secretions or post-massage urine, in the absence of positive bacterial culture in pre-massage specimens, or bacterial culture at least 10 times higher in post-massage samples than in pre-massage samples suggests bacterial prostatitis
- Elevated leukocyte counts in expressed prostatic secretions or post-massage urine in the absence of positive bacterial culture suggests inflammatory non-bacterial prostatitis

Drugs, disorders and other factors that may alter results
Other urinary tract infections.

PRE AND POST MASSAGE URINE TEST

Description
Two urine samples are collected, a midstream urine specimen before prostatic massage, and a first voided urine specimen immediately after prostatic massage.

NB: prostatic massage is contraindicated in acute bacterial prostatitis

Advantages/Disadvantages
Advantage: simpler than Meares-Stamey test, but provides almost as much information

Disadvantages
- Prostatic massage is uncomfortable for the patient
- Slightly higher false-positive rate than Meares-Stamey test

Normal
No bacteria can be cultured from either sample, and both samples give negative leukocyte counts.

Abnormal
- Bacteria are cultured from either or both of the samples
- Either or both of the samples have elevated leukocyte counts
- Keep in mind the possibility of a false-positive result

Cause of abnormal result
- Positive bacterial culture in pre-massage urine suggests cystitis
- Positive bacterial culture in post-massage urine, in the absence of positive culture in pre-massage urine, or bacterial culture at least 10 times higher in the post-massage sample than in the pre-massage sample suggests bacterial prostatitis
- Elevated leukocyte counts in the post-massage urine in the absence of positive bacterial culture suggests inflammatory non-bacterial prostatitis

Drugs, disorders and other factors that may alter results
Other urinary tract infections.

TREATMENT

CONSIDER CONSULT

- Patients with severe acute bacterial prostatitis and septicemia should be referred for urgent inpatient treatment with parenteral antibiotics. Inpatient treatment may also be necessary if patient has acute bacterial prostatitis and is in urinary retention
- Patients with suspected prostate abscess should be referred for urgent surgical treatment
- Patients whose symptoms do not respond to initial treatment should be assessed by a urologist
- Patients with obstructive voiding symptoms

IMMEDIATE ACTION

Patients with acute bacterial prostatitis should be started immediately on a broad-spectrum antibiotic, after collecting samples for urine and blood culture.

PATIENT AND CAREGIVER ISSUES
Patient or caregiver request

Patients with sexual dysfunction may request treatment with sildenafil. Evidence is limited. Ensure that the patient has been appropriately worked up for erectile dysfunction and has no contraindications to sildenafil.

Health-seeking behavior

- Patients with acute bacterial prostatitis are unlikely to have waited long before seeking medical attention because of the dramatic nature of symptoms, but those who have waited too long may have progressed to septicemia or prostatic abscess
- Symptoms of chronic prostatitis are less dramatic, so patients may not present until symptoms have persisted for several months

MANAGEMENT ISSUES
Goals

- Treatment of acute bacterial prostatitis should aim to eradicate infection and lead to complete resolution of symptoms
- Treatment of chronic bacterial prostatitis should ideally be curative, although results are often disappointing; if curative treatment is unsuccessful, treatment should aim to reduce symptoms and improve quality of life
- Treatment of chronic pelvic pain symptom is unlikely to be curative and should aim to reduce symptoms and improve quality of life

Management in special circumstances

If left untreated, acute bacterial prostatitis can progress to life-threatening septicemia.

PATIENT SATISFACTION/LIFESTYLE PRIORITIES

- Patients with mild symptoms of chronic prostatitis may prefer to live with their symptoms rather than undergo extensive tests and treatment that may ultimately be unsuccessful
- Surgical treatment of prostatitis, particularly radical prostatectomy, carries a high risk of impotence, which must be discussed with the patient; it must not be assumed that elderly patients are not sexually active
- Sexual dysfunction as a symptom of prostatitis should not be assumed to be unimportant on the basis of age alone

SUMMARY OF THERAPEUTIC OPTIONS
Choices

Guidelines for the management of prostatitis have been published [3]

Type I: Acute Bacterial Prostatitis:

Broad spectrum antibiotics (trimethoprim/co-trimoxazole or fluoroquinolones – norfloxacin, ciprofloxacin, or ofloxacin), which should continue for 4 weeks, are the treatment of choice for acute bacterial prostatitis.

Type II: Chronic Bacterial Prostatitis:

Antibiotics (mainly fluoroquinolones – norfloxacin, ciprofloxacin, or ofloxacin) are also the treatment of choice for chronic bacterial prostatitis; treatment should continue for 4–6 weeks for asymptomatic patients between episodes of recurrent urinary tract infections and for 12 weeks for symptomatic patients.

Type IIIA: Inflammatory Chronic Pelvic Pain Syndrome:

- Antibiotics can also be tried in patients with inflammatory prostatitis without demonstrable infection, as patients may be infected with bacteria that are hard to culture
- Repetitive prostate massage may be helpful in relieving symptoms of chronic prostatitis
- Alpha-blockers may help to relieve obstructive voiding symptoms
- Analgesics can be useful
- Finasteride may improve symptoms in chronic prostatitis
- Cernilton (a pollen extract) may improve symptoms in some patients, but evidence is limited
- Immune modulators: experimental
- Pentosan polysulfite (Elmiron, Alza): experimental
- Supportive therapy, such as relaxation exercises, may be helpful if symptoms cannot be otherwise controlled
- Surgery is occasionally indicated, although in general the risks outweigh the benefits
- Sildenafil may be requested by the patient. Ensure that the patient has been appropriately worked up for erectile dysfunction and has no contraindications to sildenafil
- Anti-inflammatory agents (ibuprofen) and stool softener should be considered as palliative measures
- Dietary restrictions are unnecessary unless spicy foods or alcoholic beverages seem to cause or aggravate symptoms
- Hot sitz baths may soothe painful symptomatic episodes
- Patients who respond poorly to medical management or with significant emotional problems should be referred to a psychologist or psychiatrist for stress management

Type IIIB: Noninflammatory Chronic Pelvic Pain Syndrome

- Does not respond to antibiotics
- Recommend high dose alpha blockers, consider analgesics and amitriptyline and a short course of muscle relaxant (Valium or baclofen)
- Consider pelvic/perineal trigger point massage
- Prostatic massage not likely to be helpful
- Symptomatic relief can take place with heating pads, sitz baths, air ring or cushion, and the use of anatomically correct bicycle seats
- Biofeedback is especially helpful when detrusor-sphincter-dyssynergia occurs.

Type IV: Asymptomatic Inflammatory Prostatitis:

No treatment in asymptomatic individuals unless the patient is infertile, has an elevated PSA, or pre-op prophylaxis.

Clinical pearls

- In Type I, acute bacterial prostatitis, failure to respond to antimicrobial therapy requires transrectal ultrasound of the prostate or CT scan assessment to rule out prostate abscess
- In Type II, chronic bacterial prostatitis, if the organism persists after antimicrobial therapy, repetitive prostatic massage plus antibiotic therapy may help

- In Type IIIA refractory cases, transurethral microwave thermotherapy appears in limited reports to benefit some patients [4]
- A fluoroquinolone and tetracycline sequentially or concurrently will determine whether the patient has a clinical response. TMP/SMX can be substituted for the fluoroquinolone

Never

Prostate massage is contraindicated during acute bacterial prostatitis because of the risk of precipitating bacteremia.

Patients with acute prostatitis that are in acute urinary retention should have no urethral instrumentation – a urologist should be called immediately (patient most likely will require suprapubic tube placement).

FOLLOW UP
Plan for review

- Symptoms of acute bacterial prostatitis should begin to resolve within days after starting antibiotic treatment; if they do not by the completion of therapy, this could suggest a prostatic abscess or resistant organisms
- Patients with a suspected prostatic abscess should be referred for urgent surgical treatment
- Treatment of patients with resistant organisms should be based on antibiotic sensitivity from cultures taken at initial presentation
- Parenteral antibiotic treatment may be necessary if patients have deteriorated on oral antibiotics
- Patients with chronic prostatitis who do not respond to 8–12 weeks of antibiotic therapy should be referred to a urologist

Information for patient or caregiver

- Patients with acute bacterial prostatitis should return for urgent treatment if their symptoms worsen despite antibiotic treatment
- Patients with acute bacterial prostatitis must complete 4 weeks of antibiotic treatment to reduce the risk of developing chronic bacterial prostatitis

DRUGS AND OTHER THERAPIES: DETAILS
Drugs
NORFLOXACIN
Dose
400mg twice daily.

Efficacy
Symptoms of acute bacterial prostatitis generally subside within a few days; efficacy in chronic bacterial prostatitis is variable, and treatment may take weeks to have an effect.

Risks/Benefits
- Generally few risks, although benefits are likely only in bacterial prostatitis
- Use caution in children and the elderly
- Use caution in renal disease and dehydration
- Use caution in seizure disorders

Side-effects and adverse reactions
- Gastrointestinal: nausea, vomiting, diarrhea, constipation, altered liver function tests, abdominal pain
- Hematological: blood cell disorders
- Central nervous system: headache, dizziness, seizures, fatigue, anxiety

- Skin: rashes
- Ears, eyes, nose and throat: visual disturbances
- Genitourinary: crystalluria

Interactions (other drugs)
- Aluminium, calcium, magnesium, iron, zinc ▪ Antacids ▪ Antipyrine ▪ Caffeine
- Diazepam ▪ Foscarnet ▪ Metoprolol, propanolol ▪ Pentoxyfilline ▪ Phenytoin
- Ropinirole ▪ Sodium bicarbonate ▪ Theobromine ▪ Theophylline ▪ Warfarin

Contraindications
No known contraindications.

Evidence
Norfloxacin has been shown to be superior to co-trimoxazole in a controlled clinical study and has also been shown to be effective in patients refractory to co-trimoxazole treatment [5,6]

Acceptability to patient
High, however medication is expensive.

Follow up plan
- Patients with acute bacterial prostatitis who fail to respond to treatment within a few days should be urgently reassessed
- Patients with chronic bacterial prostatitis who fail to respond to treatment should be referred to a urologist

Patient and caregiver information
Treatment of acute bacterial prostatitis should continue for 4 weeks to reduce the risk of developing chronic bacterial prostatitis.

CIPROFLOXACIN

Dose
500mg twice daily.

Efficacy
Symptoms of acute bacterial prostatitis generally subside within a few days; efficacy in chronic bacterial prostatitis is variable, and treatment may take weeks to have an effect.

Risks/Benefits
- Generally few risks, although benefits are likely only in bacterial prostatitis
- Not suitable for children or growing adolescents
- Caution in adolescents, pregnancy, epilepsy, G6PD deficiency

Side-effects and adverse reactions
- Gastrointestinal: abdominal pain, altered liver function, anorexia, diarrhea, heartburn, vomiting
- Central nervous system: anxiety, depression, dizziness, headache, seizures
- Eyes, ears, nose and throat: visual disturbances
- Skin: photosensitivity, pruritus, rash

Interactions (other drugs)
- Theophylline ▪ Cyclosporine ▪ Oral anticoagulants ▪ NSAIDs ▪ Opiates ▪ Didanosine
- Beta-blockers ▪ Phenytoin ▪ Antacids ▪ Diazepam ▪ Caffeine ▪ Mineral supplements (zinc, magnesium, calcium, aluminum, iron)

Contraindication

Use is not recommended in children because arthropathy has developed in weight-bearing joints in young animals.

Evidence

Ciprofloxacin has been studied in several clinical trials, generally with favorable results [7,8,9,10].

Acceptability to patient

High, however medication is expensive.

Follow up plan

- Patients with acute bacterial prostatitis who fail to respond to treatment within a few days should be urgently reassessed
- Patients with chronic bacterial prostatitis who fail to respond to treatment should be referred to a urologist

Patient and caregiver information

Treatment of acute bacterial prostatitis should continue for 4 weeks to reduce the risk of developing chronic bacterial prostatitis.

OFLOXACIN

Dose

300mg orally twice daily for 6 weeks.

Efficacy

Symptoms of acute bacterial prostatitis generally subside within a few days; efficacy in chronic bacterial prostatitis is variable, and treatment may take weeks to have an effect.

Risks/Benefits

- Generally few risks, although benefits are likely only in bacterial prostatitis
- Use caution with the elderly and children
- Use caution in renal disease and seizure disorders

Side-effects and adverse reactions

- Gastrointestinal: vomiting, altered liver function, anorexia, diarrhea, heartburn, abdominal pain, pseudomembraneous colitis
- Central nervous system: dizziness, headache, anxiety, depression, seizures
- Eyes, ears, nose and throat: visual disturbances
- Skin: rash, photosensitivity, pruritus

Interactions (other drugs)

- Aluminum, magnesium, iron, zinc, calcium ▪ Antacids ▪ Didanosine ▪ Procainamide ▪ Sodium bicarbonate ▪ Sulcrafate ▪ Warfarin

Contraindications

No known contraindications.

Evidence

Ofloxacin has shown promising results in a number of clinical trials, although many were uncontrolled [11].

Acceptability to patient

High, however medication is expensive.

Follow up plan
- Patients with acute bacterial prostatitis who fail to respond to treatment within a few days should be urgently reassessed
- Patients with chronic bacterial prostatitis who fail to respond to treatment should be referred to a urologist

Patient and caregiver information
Treatment of acute bacterial prostatitis should continue for 4 weeks to reduce the risk of developing chronic bacterial prostatitis.

TRIMETHOPRIM
Dose
100mg twice daily.

Efficacy
Symptoms of acute bacterial prostatitis generally subside within a few days; efficacy in chronic bacterial prostatitis is variable, and treatment may take weeks to have an effect. Efficacy is generally less good than that of fluoroquinolones.

Risks/Benefits
- Generally few risks, although benefits are likely only in bacterial prostatitis
- Use caution in renal impairment
- Inexpensive
- Suitable antibiotic for patient on warfarin

Side-effects and adverse reactions
- Gastrointestinal: nausea, vomiting, hepatic disease
- Hematologic: leukopenia, megaloblastic anemia, neutropenia, thrombocytopenia
- Skin: rashes, Stevens-Johnson syndrome

Interactions (other drugs)
- **Dapsone** ▪ **Phenytoin** ▪ **Procainamide**

Contraindications
- **Severe renal impairment** ▪ **Folate deficiency** ▪ **Blood dyscrasias**

Acceptability to patient
High.

Follow up plan
- Patients with acute bacterial prostatitis who fail to respond to treatment within a few days should be urgently reassessed
- Patients with chronic bacterial prostatitis who fail to respond to treatment should be referred to a urologist

Patient and caregiver information
Treatment of acute bacterial prostatitis should continue for 4 weeks to reduce the risk of developing chronic bacterial prostatitis.

CO-TRIMOXAZOLE
A combination of trimethoprim and sulfamethoxazole.

Dose
960mg (160mg trimethoprim, 800mg sulfamethoxazole) twice daily.

Efficacy

Symptoms of acute bacterial prostatitis generally subside within a few days; efficacy in chronic bacterial prostatitis is variable, and treatment may take weeks to have an effect. Efficacy is generally less good than that of fluoroquinolones.

Risks/Benefits

- Generally few risks, although benefits are likely only in bacterial prostatitis
- Use caution in the elderly
- Use caution in renal and hepatic impairment
- Use caution in alcoholism, malnutrition, G6PD deficiency

Side-effects and adverse reactions

- Gastrointestinal: nausea, vomiting, abdominal pain, hepatitis, pseudomembranous colitis
- Central nervous system: headache, insomnia, anxiety, depression
- Genitourinary: nephrosis, renal failure
- Skin: Stevens-Johnson syndrome, rashes
- Hematological: blood cell disorders

Interactions (other drugs)

- Dapsone ▪ Disulfiram ▪ Methotrexate ▪ Metronidazole ▪ Warfarin ▪ Phenytoin
- Oral anticoagulants ▪ Hypoglycemic agents

Contraindications

- Hepatic or renal failure ▪ Folate deficiency

Evidence

Evidence for efficacy of co-trimoxazole has come from a number of studies, although many were uncontrolled [12,13,14]

Acceptability to patient

High.

Follow up plan

- Patients with acute bacterial prostatitis who fail to respond to treatment within a few days should be urgently reassessed
- Patients with chronic bacterial prostatitis who fail to respond to treatment should be referred to a urologist

Patient and caregiver information

Treatment of acute bacterial prostatitis should continue for 4 weeks to reduce the risk of developing chronic bacterial prostatitis.

ANALGESICS

Dose

Anti-inflammatory: ibuprofen 600mg orally every 6 hours.

Efficacy

May help some patients when pain is an important symptom, but little evidence of long-term efficacy.

Risks/Benefits

- Risk of gastrointestinal side-effects with NSAIDs
- Risk of dependence or abuse with opioids

- Benefits in pain relief variable
- Anti-inflammatory effect of NSAIDs may be helpful in inflammatory prostatitis
- All currently available NSAIDS have unwanted effects especially in the elderly
- Substantial individual variation in clinical response to NSAIDs
- Have a range of actions: anti-inflammatory, analgesic, anti-pyretic
- Use caution in renal, cardiac and hepatic impairment

Side-effects and adverse reactions
- Gastrointestinal: diarrhea, dyspepsia, nausea, vomiting, gastric bleeding and perforation
- Skin: rashes, urticaria, photosensitivity
- Genitourinary: reversible renal insufficiency, renal disease (high doses over long periods)
- Respiratory: worsening of asthma
- Ears, eyes, nose and throat: tinnitus, decreased hearing
- Central nervous system: headache, dizziness

Interactions (other drugs)
- Aspirin ■ Baclofen ■ Cyclosporine ■ Corticosteroids ■ Heparins ■ Ketorolac ■ Lithium ■ Methotrexate ■ Moclobemide ■ Other NSAIDs ■ Nitrates ■ Pentoxifylline (oxpentifylline) ■ Phenindione ■ Phenytoin ■ Quinolones ■ Ritonavir ■ Sulphonylureas ■ Tacrolimus ■ Antihypertensives (ACE inhibitors, adrenergic neurone blockers, alpha-blockers, angiotensin-II receptor antagonists, beta-blockers, clonidine, diazoxide, diuretics, hydralazine, methyldopa, minoxidil, nitroprusside) ■ Antiplatelet agents (clopidogrel, ticlopidine) ■ Zidovudine ■ Antidysrhythmics (calcium channel blockers, cardiac glycosides)

Contraindication
NSAIDs are contraindicated in patients with peptic ulceration and coagulation defects.

ALPHA-BLOCKERS
Dose
Alpha blockers:
- Doxazosin 1,2,4,8mg at bedtime
- Terazosin 1,2,5,10mg orally at bedtime
- Tamsulosin 0.4–0.8mg orally every day 30 minutes after same meal (dinner)

Efficacy
May help improve urinary flow and possibly other symptoms if prostatitis is due to dysfunctional voiding.

Risks/Benefits
- Generally few risks, variable benefits
- Orthostatic hypotension – particularly in patients taking other antihypertensive, diuretic, vasodilator medications
- Improved bladder control
- Use caution in hepatic disease
- Use caution in nursing mothers

Side-effects and adverse reactions
- Cardiovascular system: chest pain, palpitations, hypotension
- Eyes, ears, nose and throat: visual disturbances, tinnitus
- Gastrointestinal: abdominal cramps, constipation, diarrhea, dry mouth, vomiting
- Central nervous system: dizziness, headache, fever, paresthesia
- Genitourinary: incontinence, polyuria
- Respiratory: dyspnea
- Skin: pruritus, rash

Interactions (other drugs)
- ACE inhibitors ■ Indomethacin ■ Calcium channel blockers ■ Beta-blockers

Contraindications
No absolute contraindications recorded.

Evidence
Alpha-blockers have been studied in a number of clinical trials, alone and in combination with antibiotics. Results have generally been favorable [15,16,17,18].

FINASTERIDE
Dose
5mg once daily.

Efficacy
May relieve symptoms of prostatitis, but evidence is not yet clear.

Risks/Benefits
- Balance of risks and benefits for this disorder requires further research
- Use caution in hepatic disease
- Use caution in obstructive uropathy
- Condoms should be used if partner is pregnant or likely to become pregnant (finasteride is excreted in semen)
- Women of child bearing age should avoid handling crushed or broken tablets

Side-effects and adverse reactions
- Genitourinary: decreased libido, impotence, ejaculation disorders, breast tenderness and enlargement
- Hypersensitivity reactions

Interactions (other drugs)
No known interactions.

Contraindications
- Children ■ Women

Evidence
Finasteride has shown promising preliminary results in a small placebo-controlled study [19].

Acceptability to patient
Impotence and decreased libido as well as gynecomastia may occur as side-effects.

Follow up plan
Prostate specific antigen will be decreased by 50%. This must be kept in mind when following patient for possible prostate cancer.

Complementary therapy
CERNILTON
A pollen extract.

Efficacy
May improve symptoms in some patients, but takes several months to have an effect.

Risks/Benefits
Very little known risk, but benefit uncertain.

Evidence
Evidence of efficacy is from small, uncontrolled trials [20,21]

Acceptability to patient
High, particularly in patients favorably disposed to complementary therapies.

Patient and caregiver information
Treatment should continue for several months to be effective.

Other therapies
REPETITIVE PROSTATE MASSAGE
NB: Contraindicated in acute bacterial prostatitis.

Efficacy
May be beneficial, particularly in combination with antibiotics, as a result of draining occluded prostatic ducts and improving antibiotic penetration.

Risks/Benefits
Little risk involved (although the technique is unpleasant), benefit variable.

Evidence
Although the technique has been used for a long time, evidence is mostly anecdotal or from small, uncontrolled studies [22]

Acceptability to patient
- Always uncomfortable for patient
- May be painful

Follow up plan
The follow-up plan should be based upon the clinical picture of the patient.

LIFESTYLE
- Dietary restrictions are unnecessary unless spicy foods or alcoholic beverages seem to cause or aggravate symptoms
- Avoidance of bicycle riding

RISKS/BENEFITS
- If bicycle riding is an important form of exercise for the patient, avoiding it may harm general physical fitness
- May improve symptoms

ACCEPTABILITY TO PATIENT
Will depend on the importance of bicycle riding to the patient and the improvement in symptoms brought about by discontinuing it.

PATIENT AND CAREGIVER INFORMATION
If bicycle riding was an important form of exercise for the patient, he should be encouraged to replace it with another exercise to maintain general physical fitness.

EFFICACY OF THERAPIES

■ Acute bacterial prostatitis is normally responsive to antibiotic treatment; failure to respond quickly could suggest a prostatic abscess or resistant organisms

■ Fluoroquinolone treatment of chronic bacterial prostatitis should cure over half of patients, although many will require specialist referral

■ Treatment of chronic pelvic pain syndrome has variable efficacy in improving symptoms but is rarely curative

Evidence

■ Evidence for treatment of prostatitis is generally poor

■ Clinical trials have shown the benefits of antibiotic therapy, particularly fluoroquinolones, for bacterial prostatitis [23]

■ There is also specific evidence for norfloxacin, ciprofloxacin, and ofloxacin

■ A number of clinical trials have shown benefit of alpha-blockers, alone or in combination with antibiotics

■ Evidence for other treatments is generally anecdotal or from small and poorly controlled clinical trials

Review period

Patients are seen according to type of prostatitis:

■ Type I: 6–8 weeks
■ Type II: 8–12 weeks
■ Type III: 8–12 weeks
■ Type IV: 6 months-1 year

PROGNOSIS

■ Acute bacterial prostatitis is generally cured by prompt antibiotic treatment, although patients may subsequently develop chronic bacterial prostatitis, particularly if antibiotic treatment is insufficient

■ Chronic bacterial prostatitis may be cured by antibiotic treatment, although therapeutic failures and recurrences are common

■ Recurrent bacterial prostatitis can be treated with prophylactic antibiotic therapy

■ Prognosis of chronic pelvic pain syndrome is poor, and relief of symptoms should be the goal of treatment

Clinical pearls

Refer all clinical failures to a urologic specialist.

Therapeutic failure

- Patients with acute bacterial prostatitis who fail to respond to treatment should be treated aggressively. Parenteral antibiotic treatment may be necessary if patients have deteriorated on oral antibiotics
- Patients with chronic prostatitis who fail to respond to initial antibiotic therapy should generally be referred to a urologist
- Patients with a suspected prostatic abscess should be referred for urgent surgical treatment

Recurrence

Consider long-term prophylactic antibiotic treatment for patients with recurrent bacterial prostatitis; trimethoprim, co-trimoxazole, and nitrofurantoin are appropriate treatments for long-term antibacterial prophylaxis.

Deterioration

Deterioration in patients with acute bacterial prostatitis may be due to antibiotic resistance or complications and should be treated aggressively.

COMPLICATIONS

- Acute bacterial prostatitis may progress to pyelonephritis or septicemia, which require aggressive parenteral antibiotic treatment
- Acute bacterial prostatitis may also progress to prostatic abscess, which requires urgent referral for surgical drainage in addition to antibiotic treatment

CONSIDER CONSULT

If acute bacterial prostatitis progresses to prostatic abscess, refer for surgical drainage in addition to antibiotic treatment.

PREVENTION

PREVENT RECURRENCE

Patients with recurrent bacterial prostatitis should be considered for long-term low-dose prophylactic antibiotic therapy.

ASSOCIATIONS

The Prostatitis Foundation
1063 30th Street Box 8
Smithshire, Illinois 61478
Tel: 1-888-891-4200
Fax: 309-325-7184

American Urological Association
1120 North Charles Street
Baltimore, MD 21201
Tel: 410-727-1100
Fax: 410-223-4370
Email: aua@auanet.org

KEY REFERENCES

- Nickel JC. Prostatitis: evolving management strategies. Urol Clin North Am 1999;26:737–751.
- Nickel JC. Effective office management of chronic prostatitis. Urol Clin North Am 1998;25:677–684.
- Schaeffer AJ. Prostatitis: US perspective. Int J Antimicrob Agents 1999;11:205–211.
- Pewitt EB, Schaeffer AJ. Urinary tract infections in urology, including acute and chronic prostatitis. Infect Dis Clin North Am 1997;11:623–646.
- Stevermer JJ, Easley SK. Treatment of prostatitis. Am Fam Physician 2000;61:3015–3026.

Evidence references and guidelines

1 Krieger JN, Nyberg L Jr, Nickel JC. National Institute of Health consensus definition and classification of prostatitis. JAMA 1999;282(3):236–237.
2 Nickel JC, Nyberg LM, Hennenfent M. Research guidelines for chronic prostatitis: consensus report from the first National Institutes of Health International Prostatitis Collaborative Network. Urology 1999;54:229–233.
3 National guideline for the management of prostatitis. Clinical Effectiveness Group (Association of Genitourinary Medicine and the Medical Society for the Study of Venereal Diseases). Sex Transm Infect 1999;75 Suppl 1:S46–S50.
4 Nickel JC, Sorenson R. Transurethral microwave thermotherapy for nonbacterial prostatitis. J Urol 1996;155(6):1950–1954.
5 Sabbaj J, Hoagland VL, Cook T. Norfloxacin versus co-trimoxazole in the treatment of recurring urinary tract infections in men. Scand J Infect Dis Suppl 1986;48:48–53.
6 Schaeffer AJ, Darras FS. The efficacy of norfloxacin in the treatment of chronic bacterial prostatitis refractory to trimethoprin-sulfamethoxazole and/or carbenicillin. J Urol 1990;144:690–693.
7 Weidner W, Schiefer HG. Chronic bacterial prostatitis: therapeutic experience with ciprofloxacin. Infection 1991;19 Suppl 3:S165-S166
8 Naber KG, Busch W, Focht J. Ciprofloxacin in the treatment of chronic bacterial prostatitis: a prospective, non-comparative multicenter clinical trial with long-term follow-up. The German Prostatitis Study Group. Int J Antimicrob Agents 2000;14:143-149
9 Weidner W, Ludwig M, Brähler E, Schiefer HG. Outcome of antibiotic therapy with ciprofloxacin in chronic bacterial prostatitis. Drugs 1999;58 Suppl 2:103-106
10 Weidner W, Schiefer HG, Brähler E. Refractory chronic bacterial prostatitis: a re-evaluation of ciprofloxacin treatment after a median follow-up of 30 months. J Urol 1991;146:350-352
11 Aagaard J, Madsen PO. Diagnostic and therapeutic problems in prostatitis. Therapeutic position of ofloxacin. Drugs Aging 1992;2:196-207
12 Meares EM. Long-term therapy of chronic bacterial prostatitis with trimethoprim-sulfamethoxazole. Can Med Assoc J 1975;112:22-25
13 Foltzer MA, Reese RE. Trimethoprim-sulfamethoxazole and other sulfonamides. Med Clin North Am 1987;71:1177-1194
14 Ronald AR. Urinary tract infections: the efficacy of trimethoprim/sulfamethoxazole. Clin Ther 1980;3:176-189
15 Barbalias GA, Nikiforidis G, Liatsikos EN. Alpha-blockers for the treatment of chronic prostatitis in combination with antibiotics. J Urol 1998;159:883-887

16 Neal DE, Moon TD. Use of terazosin in prostatodynia and validation of a symptom score questionnaire. Urology 1994;43:460-465

17 Lacquaniti S, Destito A, Servello C, et al. Terazosine and tamsulosin in non bacterial prostatitis: a randomized placebo-controlled study. Arch Ital Urol Androl 1999;71:283-285

18 de la Rosette JJ, Karthaus HF, van Kerrebroeck PE, de Boo T, Debruyne FM. Research in 'prostatitis syndromes': the use of alfuzosin (a new alpha 1-receptor-blocking agent) in patients mainly presenting with micturition complaints of an irritative nature and confirmed urodynamic abnormalities. Eur Urol 1992;22:222-227

19 Leskinen M, Lukkarinen O, Marttila T. Effects of finasteride in patients with inflammatory chronic pelvic pain syndrome: a double-blind, placebo-controlled, pilot study. Urology 1999;53:502-505

20 Buck AC, Rees RW, Ebeling L. Treatment of chronic prostatitis and prostatodynia with pollen extract. Br J Urol 1989;64:496-199

21 Rugendorff EW, Weidner W, Ebeling L, Buck AC. Results of treatment with pollen extract (Cernilton N) in chronic prostatitis and prostatodynia. Br J Urol 1993;71:433-438

22 Nickel JC, Alexander R, Anderson R, et al. Prostatitis unplugged? Prostatic massage revisited. Tech Urol 1999;5:1-7

FAQS
Question 1
How does bacterial prostatitis occur?

ANSWER 1
Bacterial prostatitis probably evolves from ascending urethral infection or reflux of infected urine into prostatic ducts that empty into the posterior urethra. Other possibilities include invasion by rectal bacteria (by direct extension or lymphogenous spread) and hematogenous infection.

Question 2
What are the types of prostatitis?

ANSWER 2
Traditionally, acute and chronic bacterial prostatitis, nonbacterial prostatitis, and prostatodynia. The NIH has recategorized the types of prostatitis into four types: acute, chronic, chronic pelvic pain, and asymptomatic.

Question 3
What percentage of prostatitis is bacterial prostatitis?

ANSWER 3
Approximately 5%.

Question 4
What are the causative organisms in bacterial prostatitis?

ANSWER 4
The causative organisms in bacterial prostatitis are similar in type and incidence to those responsible for UTI: common strains of Escherichia coli clearly predominate. Infections are less frequently caused by species of Proteus, Klebsiella, Enterobacter, Pseudomonas, Serratia, and other less common Gram-negative organisms.

Question 5
What are the symptoms/signs of acute bacterial prostatitis?

ANSWER 5
Sudden onset of moderate to high fever, chills, low back and perineal pain, urinary frequency and urgency, nocturia, dysuria, generalized malaise with accompanying arthralgia and myalgia, and varying degrees of bladder outlet obstruction.

Rectal palpation usually discloses an exquisitely tender, swollen prostate gland that is partially or totally firm, irregular, and warm to the touch.

CONTRIBUTORS
Fred F Ferri, MD, FACP
Philip J Aliotta, MD, MHA, FACS
Stewart M Polsky, MD

PYELONEPHRITIS

SUMMARY INFORMATION

DESCRIPTION

- Acute infection of the renal pelvis or parenchyma
- Acute pyelonephritis is usually due to ascending infection; in uncomplicated cases the offending organism is usually *Escherichia coli* (75%)
- Rare severe variants of pyelonephritis are seen where complicating factors or stasis, stones, impaired immunity, or diabetes exists

URGENT ACTION

- Patients with pyelonephritis and severe concomitant illness have serious tissue infection and are at risk of bacteremia; they merit admission for consultation and intensive parenteral antimicrobial therapy
- Patients with uncomplicated pyelonephritis can be treated as outpatients with a 14-day course of oral antibiotics that should be instituted immediately. Trimethoprim/sulfamethoxazole or ciprofloxacin is recommended for adults, and cefixime for children
- Patients with complicated pyelonephritis need inpatient treatment – coexisting diabetes, stones, previous pyelonephritis, known renal damage, known renal anatomic abnormalities, and pregnancy are indications for admission

KEY! DON'T MISS!

Exclude underlying serious causes of renal tract obstruction.

ICD9 CODE
- 590.1 Acute pyelonephritis
- 590.8 Nonspecific pyelonephritis
- 590.10 Acute pyelonephritis without lesion of medullary necrosis

SYNONYMS
- Acute pyelonephritis
- Pyonephrosis
- Renal carbuncle
- Lobar nephronia
- Acute bacterial nephritis
- Upper urinary tract infection (UTI)

CARDINAL FEATURES
- Acute infection of renal pelvis or parenchyma
- Abscess formation but sparing of glomerulus
- May be asymptomatic
- Classical presentation is with rigors, fever, nausea, vomiting, and unilateral or bilateral loin pain radiating to iliac fossae and suprapubic area
- Fever and loin pain are frequently also present in uncomplicated lower UTI, and may be absent in pyelonephritis
- Lumbar tenderness and guarding are usual
- Dysuria, frequency, and urgency due to associated cystitis occur in 30%
- Septicemia, shock, and hypotension may supervene in severe cases
- Urine microscopy reveals: red and white blood cells; white blood cell casts if renal parenchyma is involved; organisms; and epithelial cells
- Children may present with fever alone or with vomiting, apathy, convulsion, abdominal distension, irritability, poor perfusion, poor color, flank mass, enuresis, diarrhea, or vulval pruritus
- In the absence of urinary tract abnormalities, pyelonephritis rarely leads to serious chronic renal disease above the age of 5 years
- May rarely result in acute papillary necrosis or, in the presence of obstruction, may progress to chronic pyelonephritis

CAUSES
Common causes
- Ascending UTI: 75% of cases of pyelonephritis are due to *E. coli*; 10–15% are caused by other Gram-negative rods, *Klebsiella*, *Proteus*, *Enterobacter*; others include *Pseudomonas*, *Serratia*, and *Citrobacter*. Gram-positive agents include *E. faecalis* and less commonly *Staphylococcus aureus*, anaerobes
- Fungal agents in immunocompromised patients and diabetics, especially *Candida* spp.

Rare causes
- Other infecting organisms may include *Salmonella*, *Leptospira*, *Mycoplasma*, *Chlamydia*
- In travelers the possibility of tropical infection and echinococcus can be borne in mind

Contributory or predisposing factors
- Diseases or conditions that cause stasis of urine in the urinary tract promote multiplication of organisms in the urinary tract and ascension of infection
- Diseases that impair immunity promote multiplication of organisms in the urinary tract and ascension of infection
- Presence of a device in the urinary tract

Obstructions to urine flow:

- Vesicoureteric reflux (VUR) is the most important predisposing factor in children <6 years of age
- Obstruction of outflow of bladder – benign prostatic hypertrophy, prostatic carcinoma, bladder tumors
- Carcinoma arising from renal tract, e.g. renal cell carcinoma, bladder cancer, ureteric tumors; carcinoma arising outside renal tract and impinging on it, e.g. bowel, cervix, prostate
- Radiotherapy or surgical damage to ureters
- Pregnancy – encourages reflux by dilatation of the ureters and probably reduces immunity of renal parenchyma
- Calculi – cause obstruction and stasis, and act as foci for infection
- Neurologic abnormality, e.g. spina bifida, multiple sclerosis
- Polycystic kidney disease – affects 0.8 per 1000 of the population and is inherited as an autosomal dominant trait
- Renal parenchymal damage due to tuberculosis
- Neurogenic bladder following trauma or secondary to neurologic disorders such as diabetic neuropathy

Impaired immunity:

- HIV
- Myeloproliferative disorders
- Diabetes
- Organ transplantation
- Chemotherapy

Stasis and impaired immunity may coexist in patients with:

- Malignancy, especially after chemotherapy
- Diabetes

Devices in the urinary tract:

- Indwelling bladder catheters (Foley catheters)
- Ureteral stents

EPIDEMIOLOGY
Incidence and prevalence

- 20–50% of children <6 years of age with pyelonephritis have vesicoureteric reflux, but only 4% of adults
- About 12% of patients in Europe requiring dialysis are said to have renal scarring secondary to recurrent pyelonephritis in early childhood

INCIDENCE

- Community-acquired acute pyelonephritis: 15.7 per 100,000 per year
- Hospital-acquired acute pyelonephritis: 7.3 per 10,000 hospital persons
- About 3% of girls and 1% of boys develop a prepubertal UTI; of these 17% develop infection-related scarring, and of these 10–20% develop hypertension. Rarely, progressive renal dysfunction with eventual failure results

Demographics

AGE

- Acute pyelonephritis occurs more commonly in sexually active women
- Acute pyelonephritis occurs more commonly in men over 50 years of age

GENDER

Women are more commonly affected than men.

GENETICS

- Vesicoureteric reflux is familial, with 10% of first degree relatives affected
- Polycystic renal disease has an autosomal dominant inheritance

SOCIOECONOMIC STATUS

Increased rates of asymptomatic bacteriuria in pregnancy have been noted in patients of lower socioeconomic class and higher multiparity.

DIAGNOSIS

DIFFERENTIAL DIAGNOSIS
Acute appendicitis
In appendicitis, pain from a retroperitoneal appendix may mimic pyelonephritis particularly well.

FEATURES
- Patient may give history of pain, which began around umbilicus before moving to right iliac fossa
- Pain may be aggravated by movement of the hip
- Guarding
- Rebound tenderness
- Pyrexia

Diverticulitis
Diverticulitis is caused by infection of large bowel diverticula with abscess formation, and perforation is a risk.

FEATURES
- Pyrexia
- Patient toxic and unwell
- Abdominal pain may be localized or diffuse
- History of diverticular disease or constipation, 'lazy bowels'
- More common in older patients

Cholecystitis
Cholecystitis is acute inflammation of the gallbladder. There may be abscess formation and bile flow obstruction with cholangitis and hepatitis resulting. Gallstones usually underlie the problem.

FEATURES
- Pyrexia
- Right upper quadrant pain – constant or colicky
- Jaundice may be present
- Rigors may be present and suggest ascending cholangitis
- More common in overweight women over 40 years of age

Salpingitis
Salpingitis is caused by an ascending female genital tract infection with abscess formation.

FEATURES
- Fever – may be low-grade
- Abdominal pain
- Cervical motion tenderness
- Dyspareunia
- Discharge is not invariable
- Fluid in pouch of Douglas may cause pain of filling bladder

Perinephric abscess
Usually due to *Staph. aureus* infection and may occur by hematogenous spread.

FEATURES
- Acute loin pain and tenderness
- Loin may bulge on affected side

- Patient usually extremely ill
- Fever
- Leukocytosis
- Positive blood culture
- Urinary symptoms are absent
- Urine may contain no pus cells or organisms

Hemorrhage into renal cyst

Single or multiple renal cysts are common – polycystic renal disease is found in 0.8 per 1000 of the adult population and may be asymptomatic. Hemorrhage into a cyst is an uncommon presentation.

FEATURES

- Acute loin pain of sudden onset
- Renal colic of sudden onset
- Other symptoms of polycystic renal syndrome may be present: hypertension, hematuria, renal failure
- Positive family history

Lower urinary tract infection

Lower urinary tract infections include urethritis, cystitis, and prostatitis.

FEATURES

- Frequency of micturition
- Dysuria
- Not usually febrile

Acute muscle injury

History of injury is not always clear.

FEATURES

- Pain and tenderness may overlie loin
- Patient is otherwise well, afebrile, and not toxic
- Urine microscopy is clear
- Pain is aggravated by movement of affected muscles

Ectopic pregancy

Intrauterine device or history of tubal ligation should increase suspicion of ectopic pregnancy.

FEATURES

- Amenorrhea of varying length
- Vaginal bleeding
- Abdominal pain which may localize to right or left iliac fossa
- Guarding and rebound tenderness
- Increasing pain as bladder fills
- Adnexal mass on bimanual examination
- If ruptured ectopic pregnancy, hypotension and collapse may result

SIGNS & SYMPTOMS
Signs

- Costovertebral angle tenderness and abdominal guarding
- Pyrexia, often paroxysmal; peaks as high as 103.5–104°F are not uncommon
- Kidney may be palpable and tender

Symptoms
- Can be asymptomatic

Localized symptoms:
- Unilateral or bilateral loin pain radiating to iliac fossae and suprapubic area
- Fever and loin pain are frequently present in uncomplicated lower UTI, but may be absent in upper UTI
- Dysuria, frequency, or urgency due to associated cystitis occurs in 30%

Generalized symptoms:
- Rigors, fever
- Nausea, anorexia, vomiting, and diarrhea
- Hypotension and shock with septicemia, particularly in complicated cases with obstruction

In children:
- Fever alone
- Apathy, irritability, convulsion, septicemia
- Abdominal distension, flank mass, diarrhea
- Poor perfusion, poor color
- Enurosis, vulval pruritus
- In febrile infants, occult UTIs are as common as suspected UTIs; 3.5% of infants with another infection source, e.g. otitis media, also have a UTI

KEY! DON'T MISS!
Exclude underlying serious causes of renal tract obstruction.

CONSIDER CONSULT
- Generally children under 2 years of age with first or second proven UTIs are always referred for investigation with renal ultrasound, voiding cystourethrography, and radionuclide scanning; under some guidelines all children under 5 years are investigated in this way
- Older children are usually offered ultrasound scan and abdominal plain film, and if there are no abnormalities referral is not usually necessary in this group for first or second uncomplicated UTI. However, clinical judgment and local guidelines may apply
- Children with complicated UTI (including suspected pyelonephritis) should all be referred for investigation, even if treated as outpatients
- Men: since uncomplicated acute pyelonephritis is most unusual, all adult males with first episode of acute pyelonephritis should be referred to urology for evaluation for possible obstruction or other complicating condition
- Women: recurrent acute pyelonephritis should trigger referral to a urologist to rule out complicating conditions; women with first UTIs do not merit further investigation

INVESTIGATION OF THE PATIENT
Direct questions to patient
History of complaint to identify likelihood of diagnosis:
Q What is the nature and site of the pain? Look for loin pain or features suggesting other diagnoses.
Q For how long has it been present? A very prolonged history in a well patient may make muscular pain more likely and renal pain less so.
Q Does anything make it worse or better? Muscular pains and stones cause pain, which is worse on movement.
Q Have you had any urinary symptoms such as pain on passing urine, frequency of micturition, or urgency? Urinary symptoms are unusual in men without underlying renal tract abnormality such as prostatic hypertrophy.
Q Do you have any loin pain and have you had previous episodes? This may suggest underlying renal disease.

Ask about complicating factors:

Q Do you have urinary hesitancy, frequency, urgency, poor stream, nocturia?

Q Have you ever had these symptoms before? Recurrent problems suggest malformation, stones, chronic disease.

Q Does anyone in your family have any kidney problems? Both reflux and polycystic kidney disease run in families.

Q Are you diabetic? Diabetes can cause urinary tract obstruction, impaired immunity, and consequently severe pyelonephritis. It is advised to admit the diabetic patient with pyelonephritis.

Q Have you traveled abroad recently? Consider infection by unusual organisms or HIV.

Contributory or predisposing factors

Q Have you ever suffered from gout? This may suggest uric acid stones.

Q Have you ever thought you passed a kidney stone or had renal colic? Patients who form one stone are likely to form others.

Family history

Q Does anyone in your family have any kidney abnormalities? This is suggestive of inherited renal abnormalities, either of structure (e.g. polycystic disease, vesicoureteric reflux) or function (e.g. cystinuria and other disorders of tubular function).

Q Does anyone in your family suffer from blood pressure problems? Early onset or severe hypertension in the family may indicate familial renal disease such as polycystic kidney disease.

Examination

- **Vital signs examination** for fever, hypotension, and orthostasis
- **General examination** for dehydration, fever, and blood pressure (hypotension in an unwell patient suggests sepsis and mandates hospitalization)
- **Abdominal examination** with attention to palpable kidneys, abdominal masses, tenderness, guarding, suprapubic tenderness
- **Rectal examination** to determine presence of enlarged prostate gland in men
- **Consider pelvic examination** if gynecologic differential diagnoses have not been excluded

Summary of investigative tests

- Urine dipstick examination for blood, protein, glucose, nitrites
- Urine microscopy to look for white cells, red cells, casts
- Midstream urine for culture and sensitivity to look for organisms
- White blood count and differential for polymorphonuclear leukocytosis
- Blood urea nitrogen (BUN) and creatinine to look for acute or chronic renal failure
- Blood culture to look for sepsis
- Abdominal plain film of abdomen may show calculi and renal outline
- Renal ultrasonography to identify obstruction, abscess, cysts, renal pelvis dilatation
- Voiding cystourethrography to look for vesicoureteric reflux in children and in patients thought to have disturbance of bladder emptying. Normally ordered after resolution of acute infection to avoid false-positive result
- Intravenous urography including film of bladder postvoiding (looks for stones and obstruction, outlines renal pelvis – parenchyma less well; clubbing of adjacent calyces suggests chronic pyelonephritis). Now infrequently ordered due to availability of ultrasonography
- Renal radioisotope scan is useful in showing early cortical scarring in children
- CT scan for suspected abscess or renal mass and in patients refractory to treatment

DIAGNOSTIC DECISION

Indications for radiologic and/or urologic examination of the urinary tract:

- Patients requiring hospital admission for acute pyelonephritis should have a renal ultrasound, especially if infection is slow to respond to antimicrobials; patients with urinary infection and septic shock should have an emergency renal ultrasound

- Children with first or second UTIs, particularly those under 2 years, require excretory urography and voiding cystourethrography to detect obstruction, vesicoureteric reflux, and renal scarring. DMSA scanning is a sensitive technique for detecting scars but does not reveal pyelocalyceal or ureteric anomalies. These studies are undertaken after resolution of the acute infection
- Most adult men with UTI have anatomic abnormality of the urinary tract, most commonly prostatic enlargement; renal ultrasound is required, including postvoiding views to look for residual urine
- First UTIs in women do not require radiologic or urologic study
- Recurrent UTIs in women are more controversial and cost-effectiveness has not been properly evaluated. The few women who might benefit from investigation include those refractory to appropriate antimicrobial therapy or with rapid relapse, continuing hematuria, night sweats, and symptoms of possible obstruction including back or pelvic pain

CLINICAL PEARLS

- Use urine culture and sensitivity to guide modification of antibiotic choice. Switch drugs if indicated by antibiotic-sensitivity testing
- Pyelonephritis can be initial presentation of previously undiagnosed diabetes. Have a high degree of suspicion if blood sugar is elevated and follow-up with further diabetes testing

THE TESTS
Body fluids
URINE DIPSTICK EXAMINATION
Description
- Dipstick testing for markers of infection or renal disease
- Dipstick examination may reveal presence of hemoglobin, protein, nitrites, and leukocyte esterase

Advantages/Disadvantages
Advantages.
- Easy to perform and inexpensive
- Although positive dipstick examination does not distinguish lower UTI from pyelonephritis, it may be helpful to locate focus of infection to renal tract if symptoms are vague

Normal
Negative for all test squares.

Abnormal
Positive result.

Cause of abnormal result
- Nitrites – highly suggestive of organisms (90% sensitivity)
- Hemoglobin – suggests bleeding from bladder, ureter, or renal pelvis or parenchyma, which may be due to infection, tumor, bleeding cyst, chronic pyelonephritis, analgesic nephropathy or glomerulonephritis
- Leukocyte esterase – suggests infection or inflammation in renal tract (not all dipsticks show white cells)
- Protein – infection, acute renal failure

Drugs, disorders and other factors that may alter results
- Diabetes may cause glycosuria and eventually proteinuria
- Lower UTI or tumor will also give positive results
- Contaminant, e.g. menstrual blood or cross-reaction with myoglobin (rhabdomyolysis)

URINE MICROSCOPY
Description
- Laboratory test that can usually be ordered urgently from hospital laboratory, but formed elements such as casts are more readily recognized by trained nephrologists
- Examination of urine under microscope to look for white cells, red cells, organisms, casts, debris, papillary fragments
- Gram staining to look for organisms

Advantages/Disadvantages
Advantages:
- Easy and quick
- If presence of organisms can be confirmed, then it is highly helpful in diagnosis and management

Disadvantage: gram staining only shows organisms present at very high concentration

Normal
No organisms or cells.

Abnormal
10 or more white blood cells per high-power field (HPF).

Cause of abnormal result
- >10 white blood cells per HPF is compatible with, but not diagnostic of, UTI and does not confirm whether the upper urinary tract is involved
- Presence of white cells and casts may also indicate recent inflammation or glomerular disease
- Presence of red cells requires further investigation unless there is active infection, in which case repeat examination once infection has been treated

Drugs, disorders and other factors that may alter results
- False-negative may be due to patient maintaining a high volume and voiding frequently – sample may appear normal but culture should demonstrate bacteria
- False-negative may be due to antibiotics – oral trimethoprim is active in the bladder within 15min of ingestion

MIDSTREAM URINE FOR CULTURE AND SENSITIVITY
Description
Midstream specimen for laboratory analysis.

Advantages/Disadvantages
- Advantage: easy, noninvasive test
- Disadvantage: results not available for 48h

Normal
No growth at 48h.

Abnormal
- UTI is usually considered proven if there are $>10^5$ colony-forming units/mL urine
- Occasionally, mixed bacterial growths of 10^5 colony-forming units/mL ($10,000/cm^3$) of various organisms may be considered significant where there are other risk factors (e.g. indwelling catheter, obstruction) but in these cases judgment depends on organisms grown and clinical situation

- Usually less than a significant (10^5 colony-forming units/mL) pure growth is assumed to be contaminant, but 20% of patients with acute pyelonephritis have urine cultures with <100,000 colony-forming units/mL

Cause of abnormal result
- Infection anywhere in urinary tract
- Contamination from genital infection, skin, handling
- Keep in mind the possibility of a false-positive result, although where a clear 100,000/cm^3 pure growth of organisms is required for a positive result this is less likely

WHITE BLOOD COUNT AND DIFFERENTIAL
Description
Venous blood sample.

Advantages/Disadvantages
Advantages:
- Simple, inexpensive test
- Quick and relatively noninvasive

Disadvantages:
- Requires laboratory analysis of blood constituents
- Information is nonspecific for renal disease

Normal
White cell count: 3200–9800/mm^3 (3.2–9.8x10^8/L).

Abnormal
Results outside the normal range

Cause of abnormal result
- Low white blood cell count may result from myelosuppression due to marrow invasion, marrow disease, HIV
- In babies, low neutrophil count can be indicative of sepsis
- Raised white blood cell count is usually due to infection

Drugs, disorders and other factors that may alter results
Many drugs may cause impairment of white cell production, particularly chemotherapeutic agents and cytotoxic drugs.

BLOOD UREA NITROGEN (BUN) AND CREATININE
Description
Blood test assessing various markers of renal function.

Advantages/Disadvantages
Advantages:
- Simple, inexpensive test
- Quick and relatively noninvasive

Disadvantages:
- Requires laboratory analysis of blood constituents
- Information is nonspecific for renal disease

Normal
- BUN: 8–18mg/dL (3–6.5mmol/L)
- Creatinine: 0.6–1.2mg/dL (50–110mmol/L)

Abnormal
Outside the reference values.

Cause of abnormal result
Renal failure due to any cause with glomerular insufficiency elevates BUN and creatinine.

Drugs, disorders and other factors that may alter results
Urea:
- Raised by factors increasing protein catabolism (e.g. blood in gut, steroids, sepsis) and slow rate of urine flow (e.g. acute urinary tract obstruction). May also be raised by drugs (aminoglycosides, lithium, steroids), dehydration, bleeding, congestive heart failure, reduced glomerular filtration rate due to renal disease
- Decreased by liver disease, malnutrition, pregnancy (third trimester), celiac disease, acromegaly

Creatinine:
- Raised by high-meat diet
- Decreased in decreased muscle mass, pregnancy, prolonged debility

BLOOD CULTURES
Description
- Blood samples sent off in culture media to obtain information about organisms that may be responsible for sepsis
- 15–20% of patients hospitalized for pyelonephritis will show bacteremia on blood culture

Advantages/Disadvantages
Disadvantages:
- Contamination is common, leading to false-positive results
- Result not available for 48h

Normal
No organisms identified.

Abnormal
- Organisms identified in peripheral blood
- Keep in mind the possibility of a false-positive result

Cause of abnormal result
- Septicemia
- Bacteremia

Imaging
RENAL ULTRASOUND
Description
- All patients requiring hospital admission for acute pyelonephritis should have a renal ultrasound, especially if infection is slow to respond to antimicrobials
- Patients with urinary infection and septic shock should have an emergency renal ultrasound

Advantages/Disadvantages
Advantages:

- Noninvasive, easy test that does not expose patient to radiation
- Shows renal size and position, dilatation of collecting ducts, tumors, cysts, and other abdominal and pelvic pathology
- Can also image bladder and assess residual urine
- Particularly suitable for pediatric patients as it is noninvasive and does not involve gonadal radiation

Disadvantages:

- Poorer image in obese patients
- Cannot show the ureters
- Operator-dependent
- Printed images show less than the real-time operation

Abnormal
Abnormal renal tract images.

Cause of abnormal result
Renal pelvic and duct dilatation, cysts, tumors, and stones.

INTRAVENOUS UROGRAM
Description
Most commonly used to evaluate renal size and to rule out hydronephrosis.

Advantages/Disadvantages
Advantage:

- Provides excellent definition of collecting system and is better than ultrasound for evaluating renal papillae, stones, and uroepithelial malignancy

Disadvantages:

- Need for injection, time requirement, dependence on adequate renal function, risk of exposure to contrast medium (allergy, nephrotoxicity); latter is most likely when diabetes or underlying renal insufficiency is present
- Not the investigation of choice in children due to high level of radiation involved in serial X-rays and limited likelihood of finding obstruction by stones
- Contraindications include severe reactions to contrast media, and moderate or severe renal failure

Abnormal

- Renal scarring or distortion
- Reduction of renal size
- Clubbing of calyces
- Obstruction of renal outflow, most commonly by stones at the pelviureteric junction
- When obstruction is present, the nephrogram and pyelogram are both delayed, and dilatation of the outflow system is seen

Cause of abnormal result
Acute pyelonephritis:

- Kidney may be grossly or focally enlarged (20%)
- Lesion may resemble neoplasm or abscess

Drugs, disorders and other factors that may alter results
Congenitally abnormal kidneys and single kidneys may also be seen for the first time.

VOIDING CYSTOURETHROGRAM
Description
- Used to look for vesicoureteric reflux in children and in patients suspected of having disturbance of bladder emptying
- Bladder is filled with contrast medium through a urinary catheter, and films are taken while the patient voids

Advantages/Disadvantages
Advantages:
- Used to diagnose vesicoureteric reflux and assess its severity
- Used in combination with urodynamic studies in the assessment of bladder and urethral abnormalities, recurrent renal infections, renal scars, or renal failure of unknown cause

Abnormal
- Grade I and II reflux: reflux up the ureters but not reaching the renal pelvis; may drop back into bladder as bladder relaxes resulting in residual urine
- Grade III–V reflux: urine goes all the way up the ureters and into the renal pelvis and parenchyma during voiding

Cause of abnormal result
Reflux.

RENAL RADIOISOTOPE SCAN
Description
- DPTA is injected, taken up by the kidney, and excreted by the glomeruli. This is monitored by an external gamma camera
- DMSA is filtered by glomeruli and partially bound to proximal tubular cells

Advantages/Disadvantages
Advantages:
- DPTA scans assess arterial perfusion of each kidney
- DMSA scans of the renal cortex show shape, size, and function of each kidney and can demonstrate early cortical scarring, which is of particular value in children

Abnormal
Scarring, abnormal renal outline, and reduced excretion.

Cause of abnormal result
- Reflux nephropathy
- Anatomic abnormality
- Glomerular disease
- Renal vascular disease

PLAIN ABDOMINAL X-RAY
Advantages/Disadvantages
Advantages:
- May show renal outlines
- Opaque calculi and calcification within the renal tract may also be shown

Disadvantages:
- Urate stones are radiolucent
- Bowel gas and perinephric fat may occlude imaging of renal tract rendering this test particularly useless

Abnormal
Opaque calculi and calcification.

Cause of abnormal result
Calculi.

CT SCAN
Advantages/Disadvantages
Advantages:
- Can define extent of collections of pus
- Useful for characterizing mass lesion within kidney or cystic masses identified with renal ultrasound
- Gives clearer definition of retroperitoneal tissues
- Excellent images even in obese patients

Abnormal
Abnormal renal image.

Cause of abnormal result
- Abscess of renal parenchyma and perinephric space
- Renal malignancy
- Renal cysts
- Renal calculi

TREATMENT

CONSIDER CONSULT

- Admit clinical cases of acute pyelonephritis for inpatient treatment (parenteral antimicrobials) if there are systemic features or nausea and vomiting, which prevent treatment with oral antibiotics
- Admit patients with complicated pyelonephritis for inpatient treatment. Coexisting diabetes, stones, previous pyelonephritis, known renal damage, known renal anatomic abnormalities (at risk for intrarenal abscess formation), and pregnancy are indications for admission

IMMEDIATE ACTION

If transit time to hospital is prolonged and patient is severely unwell with suspected sepsis, initiate antimicrobial therapy, preferably parenterally, with ampicillin and gentamicin.

PATIENT AND CAREGIVER ISSUES
Health-seeking behavior

- **How long did you wait before seeking treatment?** Patients may delay seeking treatment
- **(In the case of a child) Has there been a previous episode(s) for which treatment was never sought?** Failure to thrive could be evidence of repeated episodes indicating vesicoureteric reflux
- **Have you been taking any over-the-counter medication, including herbal medicines?** No over-the-counter or herbal medications are efficacious in urinary tract infection (UTI)
- **Do you have an abnormality of the renal tract?** Patients with known urinary tract abnormalities may not realize that UTI symptoms require urgent treatment to prevent serious complications

MANAGEMENT ISSUES
Goals

- To treat pyelonephritis swiftly and effectively, to relieve symptoms without causing toxicity to patient, and to prevent complications
- To give comprehensive antibiotic therapy that covers all likely pathogens to prevent or relieve systemic sepsis
- To assess for presence of risk factors which might predispose patient to renal scarring
- In pregnancy, to prevent fetal complications of acute pyelonephritis, including low birth-weight and prematurity

Management in special circumstances
COEXISTING DISEASE

- Pre-existing renal failure: makes further impairment of renal function more critical, and decreases immune response and resistance to infection. Further, adjustment of doses of drugs that are excreted by kidneys is required
- Immunosuppression makes pyelonephritis and sepsis more likely, so treatment should be aggressive
- Diabetes: particular vigilence is need as diabetics are at risk for asymptomatic bacteriuria; control of blood sugar is particularly important in treating diabetics with pyelonephritis

SPECIAL PATIENT GROUPS
Pregnant women:
- At risk for asymptomatic bacteriuria
- Treat aggressively to prevent reflux and scarring as asymptomatic bacteriuria and pyelonephritis are associated with preterm delivery
- Avoid drugs contraindicated in pregnancy, including gentamicin, sulfa drugs in the third trimester, quinolones
- Although antibiotic treatment is effective, there are insufficient data to recommend any specific oral regimen during pregnancy

Children:
- Initiate investigations appropriate to age, looking for scarring and reflux and aiming to prevent further damage

PATIENT SATISFACTION/LIFESTYLE PRIORITIES
Patients with recurrent problems are likely to prefer a long-term solution, particularly if stones or renal tract abnormalities are causing chronic reinfection.

SUMMARY OF THERAPEUTIC OPTIONS
Choices
- Choice of antibiotic should take account of setting, medical history of patient, urine Gram stain, previous infecting organism, and local antibiotic sensitivities (there is widespread resistance to *Escherichia coli*, the most common infecting organisms – 75% – and it is necessary to refer to local guidelines for antimicrobial therapy)
- Patients with mild-to-moderate uncomplicated pyelonephritis, who are able to take oral medication, can be treated as outpatients with a 14-day course of oral antibiotics that should be instituted immediately; early review is necessary to ascertain clinical improvement
- Patients with severe concomitant illness, complicated UTI, obstruction, severe illness, pregnancy, or nausea and vomiting are not suitable for outpatient treatment
- Intravenous antibiotics are used if patient is systemically unwell and vomiting: ampicillin, gentamicin, ciprofloxacin, cefoxitin/ceftriaxone, and vancomycin
- Oral antibiotics are used if patient is systemically unwell and not vomiting: amoxicillin, cefixime, trimethoprim/sulfamethoxazole, and ciprofloxacin or other fluoroquinolones
- Sulfonamides and quinolones are the antibiotics of choice due to their good activity against Gram-negative rods and good oral bioavailability
- Complicated infection in the immunosuppressed patient requires the use of empirical therapy until laboratory sensitivities become available. Other organisms including candidiasis may be involved
- High fluid intake may be effective

Clinical pearls
- Antibiotics alone will not adequately treat the obstructed patient; drainage of infected urine is paramount
- Frequent changes of antibiotic therapy can lead to resistance and should be avoided
- Control of blood sugar is very important in treating the diabetic with pyelonephritis
- Single-daily dosing of gentamicin is simple and has not been associated with adverse outcomes

FOLLOW UP
- If offering oral treatment, arrange to review patient if symptoms worsen over the next 24h or are not improved markedly after 24–48h
- If treating orally with good response, no need to recheck urine culture
- All other patients with acute pyelonephritis will have been admitted to hospital
- Pregnancy: screening for bacteriuria should be continued through pregnancy with regular midstream urine specimen

Plan for review
- All patients treated as outpatients should be instructed to return if symptoms worsen or are not markedly relieved at 48h
- Patients should be reassessed at 48h
- Urine culture and microscopy need not be repeated unless there is a failure of therapy

Information for patient or caregiver

- Patients should be instructed to drink large volumes, and to void without waiting or hanging on
- Patients need to be informed that UTI can lead to renal damage, and about potential seriousness of UTI in young children
- Use of cranberry juice or capsules is controversial but without evident harm unless patient is diabetic. It has been proposed that cranberries, in addition to acidifying the urine, prevent *Proteus* and *E. coli* spp. from adhering to bladder walls

DRUGS AND OTHER THERAPIES: DETAILS
Drugs
AMPICILLIN

- Broad spectrum of action
- First-line parenteral treatment (with gentamicin) in complicated UTI

Dose
Adult intravenous dose: 1.5–3.0g every 6h.

Efficacy
Effective against both Gram-positive and -negative bacteria: Gram-positive organisms include *Staphylococcus*, *Enterococcus*, *Streptococcus*; Gram-negative organisms include *Hemophilus*, *Escherichia coli*, *Klebsiella*, *Proteus*, *Providencia*.

Risks/Benefits
Risks:

- Risk of fatal anaphylactoid reactions
- Use caution in renal disease and mononucleosis
- Use caution in neonates or the elderly
- Do not administer for prolonged or repeated treatment
- Contraindicated in penicillin hypersensitivity
- Use as a single agent for treatment of pyelonephritis is inadvisable due to resistance of *Escherichia coli* and other urinary pathogens being nearly 30%

Benefits:

- Low incidence of side-effects
- Inexpensive and good tolerability

Side-effects and adverse reactions

- Central nervous system: seizures, hallucinations, coma, anxiety
- Gastrointestinal: nausea, diarrhea, vomiting, altered liver function tests, pseudomembranous colitis
- Genitourinary: urinary problems, renal damage, moniliasis, vaginitis
- Hematologic: bleeding disorders, bone marrow depression
- Hypersensitivity reactions

Interactions (other drugs)

- Allopurinol (may increase incidence of rash) ■ Atenolol ■ Chloramphenicol (inhibit effect of ampicillin) ■ Macrolide and tetracycline antibiotics (inhibit effect of ampicillin) ■ Methotrexate ■ Oral contraceptives ■ Probenecid (decreases renal tubular secretion of ampicillin) ■ Phenindione ■ Warfarin

Contraindications
Hypersensitivity to penicillins.

Acceptability to patient
Dependent on any side-effects or pain at injection site.

Follow up plan
- Daily review of clinical condition
- Observe intravenous site at injection

GENTAMICIN
- One of the two drugs (with ampicillin) of first-line empirical choice; reserved for hospital usage
- Used particularly for its broad coverage against Gram-negative organisms
- Its nephrotoxicity means careful monitoring of blood levels and renal function are necessary

Dose
Adults with normal renal function:
- 3–5mg/kg intravenously daily, titrated against peak and trough levels
- Dilute in 50–100mL of normal saline or 5% dextrose in water and infuse over 30–60min in divided doses 8-hourly; alternatively give as single dose once daily

Children with normal renal function:
- Under 5 years: 2.5mg/kg/dose intravenously 8-hourly
- Over 5 years: 1.5–2.5mg/kg/dose intravenously 8-hourly

Efficacy
- Broad spectrum of action – used where serious Gram-negative infection is suspected
- Gram-positive organisms include *Staphylococcus* (including penicillin and methicillin-resistant strains) and *Streptococcus faecalis*; Gram-negative organisms include *Escherichia coli*, *Proteus* spp., *Pseudomonas aeruginosa*, *Enterobacter*, *Serratia*, *Citrobacter*, *Providencia*, *Salmonella*, *Shigella*, *Yersinia*

Risks/Benefits
Risks:
- Use caution in prolonged use (may lead to overgrowth of resistant organisms)
- Use caution in pregnancy and lactation, neonates, and the elderly
- Use caution in Parkinson's disease, renal disease, and hypokalemia
- Use caution in hearing deficit
- Potentially toxic
- Blood levels need monitoring for safety

Benefit:
- Drug of choice in severe infection

Side-effects and adverse reactions
- Cardiovascular system: changes in blood pressure, palpitations
- Central nervous system: neurotoxicity dizziness, confusion, convulsions
- Eyes, ears, nose, and throat: irritation, tinnitus, deafness, ototoxicity, visual disturbances
- Gastrointestinal: altered liver function tests, anorexia, nausea, vomiting
- Genitourinary: nephrotoxicity
- Hematologic: blood cell disorders
- Respiratory: respiratory depression
- Skin: rash

Interactions (other drugs)
▪ Amphotericin B ▪ Antibiotics (penicillins, cephalosporins, polymyxins, vancomycin) ▪ Anticholinesterases (neostigmine, pyridostigmine) ▪ Cyclosporine ▪ Loop diuretics ▪ Neuromuscular blocking agents (atracurium, vecuronium) ▪ Nonsteroidal anti-inflammatory drugs (NSAIDs) ▪ Platinum compounds (carboplatin, cisplatin) ▪ Succinylcholine

Contraindications
▪ Myasthenia gravis ▪ Pre-existing deafness ▪ Renal impairment ▪ Hypersensitivity to gentamicin or other aminoglycosides

Acceptability to patient
Patient may be concerned by risks and a full explanation of monitoring and follow up is required.

Follow up plan
- Monitor urine output and perform urinalysis for protein, casts, cells
- Serum peak drawn 30–60min postdose
- Serum trough drawn just before next dose
- Serum creatinine and creatinine clearance
- Calcium, magnesium, sodium
- Audiometric testing – assess hearing before, during, and after treatment, especially in babies and children
- Observe intravenous site at injection

Patient and caregiver information
- Inform patient concerning risks of treatment and follow up required
- Patient should be informed to report headache, dizziness, tinnitus, or feeling of fullness in head

CIPROFLOXACIN
Good spectrum of activity, especially against Gram-negative organisms.

Dose
Adult intravenous and oral dose: 500mg twice daily for 14 days.

Efficacy
- Effective especially against Gram-negative bacteria: *Escherichia coli, Proteus, Klebsiella, Serratia, Citrobacter, Enterobacter,* and certain *Pseudomonas*
- Gram-positive organisms: *Enterococcus, Staphylococcus,* and *Streptococcus*

Risks/Benefits
Risks:
- Not suitable for children or growing adolescents
- Use caution in pregnancy, epilepsy, G6PD deficiency, renal disease
- Serious and fatal reactions have been reported with concurrent use of ciprofloxacin and theophylline
- Serious anaphylactic reactions have been reported
- Severe hypersensitivity reactions have been reported with concurrent use of ciprofloxacin and other drugs
- Risk of pseudomembranous colitis
- Risk of crystalluria – keep patients well hydrated
- Advise caution with driving or operating machinery

Benefits:

- Good spectrum of activity
- Good safety profile and tolerability
- Intravenous and oral regimen interchangeable

Side-effects and adverse reactions

- Cardiovascular system: rare serious cardiovascular events
- Central nervous system: anxiety, depression, dizziness, headache, seizures, confusion, tremors, hallucinations, suicidal ideation, increased intracranial pressure, toxic psychosis
- Eyes, ears, nose, and throat: visual disturbances, tinnitus, hearing loss, bad taste
- Gastrointestinal: abdominal pain, altered liver function, anorexia, diarrhea, vomiting, gastrointestinal bleeding, intestinal perforation, cholestatic jaundice
- Genitourinary: nephrotoxicity
- Musculoskeletal: rare arthralgia and other joint conditions
- Respiratory system: rare, sometimes serious, events
- Skin: photosensitivity, pruritus, rash, angioedema, edema, cutaneous candidiasis, hyperpigmentation, erythema nodosum, rare serious reactions

Interactions (other drugs)

- Antacids
- Beta-blockers
- Caffeine
- Cyclosporine
- Diazepam
- Didanosine
- Mineral supplements (zinc, magnesium, calcium, aluminum, iron)
- NSAIDs
- Opiates
- Oral anticoagulants
- Phenytoin
- Theophylline
- Warfarin

Contraindications

- Use is not recommended in children because arthropathy has developed in weight-bearing joints in young animals
- Pregnancy category C
- Nursing
- Safety and efficacy in patients under 18 years of age have not been established

Acceptability to patient
Usually well tolerated.

Follow up plan

- Observe intravenous site at injection
- Observe patient's clinical condition to check for drug effectiveness

CEFOXITIN/CEFTRIAXONE

- Good spectrum of activity
- Has the advantage of being a once-daily dose
- Intravenous therapy is required for pyelonephritis

Dose

- Adult intravenous dose for ceftriaxone: 1–2g/day
- Adult intravenous dose for cefoxitin: 1–2g, 6- to 8-hourly

Efficacy

- Effective against sensitive organisms with broad spectrum
- Gram-positive organisms include: *Streptococcus, Staphylococcus*; Gram-negative organisms include *Escherichia coli, Proteus, Serratia, Providencia, Klebsiella, Citrobacter, Salmonella,* certain *Pseudomonas*; anaerobes include certain *Bacteroides*

Risks/Benefits

Risks

Cefoxitin:

- Use caution in hypersensitivity to penicillins, history of gastrointestinal disease
- Use caution in pregnancy and breast-feeding
- Use caution in renal disease, pre-existing coagulopathy
- Use caution with intramuscular injections
- Use caution in the elderly

Ceftriaxone:

- Use caution in patients with penicillin hypersensitivity, renal disease
- Risk of serious acute hypersensitivity reactions
- Risk of pseudomembranous colitis, and of reversible gall bladder disease
- Use caution with pregnancy and breast-feeding

Benefits:

- Effective against sensitive organisms with broad spectrum
- Low incidence of side-effects

Side-effects and adverse reactions

Cefoxitin:

- Cardiovascular system: hypotension
- Central nervous system: malaise, headache, dizziness, fever
- Gastrointestinal: nausea, vomiting, diarrhea, pseudomembranous colitis, abdominal pain, liver enzyme disturbances, transient hepatitis, and cholestatic jaundice
- Genitourinary: nephrotoxicity, interstitial nephritis
- Hematologic: blood cell dyscrasias
- Muscularskeletal: exacerbation of myasthenia gravis
- Skin: maculopapular rash, urticaria, injection site reaction, rashes, pruritus

Ceftriaxone:

- Central nervous system: headache, sleep disturbance, confusion, dizziness
- Gastrointestinal: anorexia, nausea, diarrhea, abdominal pain, bleeding, raised liver enzymes, reversible gall bladder disease
- Genitourinary: nephrotoxicity
- Hematologic: bone marrow suppression, leukocytosis, lymphocytosis, monocytosis, basophilia, decrease in prothrombin time
- Skin: rash

Interactions (other drugs)

Cefoxitin:

- Aminoglycosides Chloramphenicol Estrogens Loop diuretics Oral anticoagulants Polymyxin B Probenecid Typhoid vaccine Vancomycin

Ceftriaxone:

- Aminoglycosides Chloramphenicol Oral anticoagulants Polymyxin B Probenecid Vancomycin

Contraindications
Cefoxitin:

- Hypersensitivity to cephalosporins ■ Porphyria ■ Safety and efficacy in pediatric patients less than 3 months of age have not yet been established

Ceftriaxone:

- Patients less than one month of age ■ Pregnancy category B ■ Hypersensitivity to ceftriaxone

Acceptability to patient
Low incidence of side-effects and high effectivity make these drugs acceptable.

Follow up plan

- Observe patient's clinical condition for drug effectiveness
- Observe intravenous site at injection

VANCOMYCIN

- Alternative to ampicillin in accordance with local guidelines where there is known resistance to ampicillin
- Effective against Gram-positive bacteria resistant to penicillins

Dose
Should only be administered by or under supervision of an experienced clinician who will recommend the appropriate intravenous dose.

Efficacy
Bactericidal against Gram-positive organisms except enterococci where it is bacteriostatic.

Risks/Benefits
Risks

- Use caution in renal disease, inflammatory bowel disease
- Use caution in neonates and the elderly

Side-effects and adverse reactions

- Cardiovascular system: cardiac arrest, cardiovascular collapse, phlebitis
- Ears, eyes, nose, and throat: hearing disturbances, ototoxicity
- Gastrointestinal: nausea
- Genitourinary: renal damage
- Hematologic: neutropenia, eosinophilia, leukopenia
- Skin: rashes, chills, fever, 'red man's syndrome'

Interactions (other drugs)

- Aminoglycosides ■ Amphotericin B ■ Capreomycin ■ Cholestyramine, colestipol (oral vancomycin) ■ Cidofovir ■ Cisplatin ■ Cyclosporine ■ Ethacrynic acid ■ Indomethacin ■ Methotrexate ■ Neuromuscular blockers ■ Paramomycin ■ Pentamidine ■ Polymyxin B ■ Salicylates ■ Streptozocin ■ Surfactants

Contraindications

- Hearing deficit ■ Cidofovir (vancomycin should be discontinued 7 days before cidofovir treatment) ■ Intramuscular administration

Acceptability to patient
Medication has serious side-effects but may be necessary for severe Gram-positive infections not treatable by other antibiotics.

Follow up plan
Due to side-effects the following monitoring is necessary during treatment: audiograms, blood urea nitrogen (BUN) and serum creatinine, and serum vancomycin concentrations.

AMOXICILLIN
- Useful drug for uncomplicated pyelonephritis
- Good activity against Gram-negative rods
- Useful in both adults and children

Dose
- Adult oral dose: 500mg every 8h
- Child oral dose: 125mg every 8h

Efficacy
Effective against Gram-negative organisms.

Risks/Benefits
Risks:
- Erythematous rashes common in mononucleosis, chronic lymphocytic leukemia, HIV
- Caution in renal impairment

Benefits:
- Inexpensive and well tolerated
- Good oral absorption

Side-effects and adverse reactions
- Central nervous system: fever, headache
- Gastrointestinal: diarrhea, nausea
- Hematologic: bone marrow suppression
- Respiratory: anaphylaxis
- Skin: erythema multiforme, rash, urticaria

Interactions (other drugs)
- Atenolol ▪ Chloramphenicol ▪ Macrolide antibiotics ▪ Methotrexate ▪ Oral contraceptives
- Tetracyclines

Contraindications
- Penicillin hypersensitivity ▪ Mononucleosis

Acceptability to patient
Usually very acceptable as good tolerability and effective against pathogens causing pyelonephritis.

Follow up plan
- Encourage patient to make contact at once if symptoms become more severe
- Review at 48h for clinical improvement – if not, consider admission

Patient and caregiver information
Patient must return if illness becomes more severe, and must agree to review in 48h to assess for clinical improvement.

CEFIXIME
Oral cefixime is especially beneficial in children, with good effectiveness and tolerability for pyelonephritis.

Dose
- Adult oral dose: 400mg/day or 200mg twice daily for 14 days
- Children under 12 years or <50kg: 8mg/kg/day as a single dose or 4mg/kg/day as a twice-daily dose

Efficacy
Especially beneficial in children.

Risks/Benefits
Risks:
- Use caution in renal imapirment, hypersensitivity to penicillins
- Risk of pseudomembranous colitis

Benefits:
- Effective medication
- Good tolerability

Side-effects and adverse reactions
- Central nervous system: headache, sleep disturbance, confusion, dizziness
- Gastrointestinal: anorexia, nausea, diarrhea, abdominal pain, bleeding, raised liver enzymes, pseudomembranous colitis
- Genitourinary: nephrotoxicity
- Hematologic: bone marrow suppression
- Skin: rash

Interactions (other drugs)
- Aminoglycosides ▪ Chloramphenicol ▪ Oral anticoagulants ▪ Polymyxin B ▪ Probenecid ▪ Vancomycin

Contraindications
- Hypersensitivity to cefixime ▪ Age less than 6 months

Acceptability to patient
Usually very acceptable as effective and well tolerated.

Follow up plan
- Encourage patient to make contact at once if symptoms become more severe
- Review at 48h for clinical improvement – if not, consider admission

Patient and caregiver information
Patient must return if illness becomes more severe, and must agree to review in 48h to assess for clinical improvement.

TRIMETHOPRIM/SULFAMETHOXAZOLE
Main choice for pyelonephritis.

Dose
Adult oral dose: 160mg trimethoprim/800mg sulfamethoxazole twice daily for 14 days.

Efficacy
Effective for pyelonephritis in adults.

Risks/Benefits
Risks:

- Use caution in renal and hepatic function impairment, and G6PD deficiency
- Use caution in elderly patients receiving diuretics
- Risk of streptococcal pharyngitis

Benefits:

- Effective for uncomplicated pyelonephritis in adults
- Inexpensive

Side-effects and adverse reactions

- Central nervous system: seizures, anxiety, aseptic meningitis, ataxia, chills, depression, fatigue, headache, insomnia, vertigo
- Hematologic: agranulocytosis, aplastic anemia, thrombocytopenia, leukopenia, neutropenia, hemolytic anemia, megaloblastic anemia, hypoprothrombinemia, methemoglobinemia, eosinophilia
- Gastrointestinal: hepatitis (including cholestatic jaundice and hepatic necrosis), elevation of serum transaminase and bilirubin, pseudomembranous enterocolitis, pancreatitis, stomatitis, glossitis, nausea, emesis, abdominal pain, diarrhea, anorexia
- Genitourinary: renal failure, interstitial nephritis, BUN and serum creatinine elevation, toxic nephrosis with oliguria and anuria, and crystalluria
- Musculoskeletal: arthralgia, myalgia
- Respiratory: pulmonary infiltrates
- Skin: Stevens-Johnson syndrome, erythema multiforme, exfoliative dermatitis, generalized skin eruptions, photosensitivity, pruritus, urticaria, rash

Interactions (other drugs)

- Dapsone (may cause increased serum concentrations of both dapsone and trimethoprim-sulfamethoxazole) ■ Disulfiram, metronidazole ■ Methotrexate (increases methotrexate level) ■ Oral anticoagulants (increases hypoprothrombinemic response) ■ Oral hypoglycemics (may cause hypoglycemia) ■ Phenytoin (may increase phenytoin concentration to toxic levels) ■ Procainamide (increases procainamide level)

Contraindications

- Megaloblastic anemia secondary to folate deficiency ■ Neonates under 2 months of age ■ Renal disease manifested by serum creatinine <15mL/min ■ Should not be used in breast-feeding woman or in pregnant women near term

Acceptability to patient
Usually acceptable, although risk of potentially serious side-effects and hypersensitivity.

Follow up plan

- Encourage patient to make contact at once if symptoms become more severe
- Review at 48h for clinical improvement – if not, consider admission

Patient and caregiver information
Patient must return if illness becomes more severe, and must agree to review in 48h to assess for clinical improvement.

LIFESTYLE
High fluid intake.

ACCEPTABILITY TO PATIENT
Variable.

FOLLOW UP PLAN
Patients at high risk of renal failure should be kept under regular (3- to 6-monthly at least) review of blood pressure and renal function.

PATIENT AND CAREGIVER INFORMATION
Patients need to understand reasons for dietary adjustments and want to co-operate.

EFFICACY OF THERAPIES

- Acute uncomplicated pyelonephritis shows a 95% response to treatment within 48h, although fever may take longer to resolve
- 10–30% of acute pyelonephritis relapse after a 14-day course of therapy
- Patients who relapse are usually cured by a second 14-day course of therapy, but occasionally a 6-week course is necessary

Review period

6 months.

PROGNOSIS

- In the absence of urinary tract abnormalities, pyelonephritis rarely leads to serious renal disease above the age of 5 years
- Of children who develop a urinary tract infection (UTI) prepubertally, about 17% will develop infection-related scarring. Of those who scar, 10–20% become hypertensive, and rarely progressive renal dysfunction with eventual failure may result

Clinical pearls

- Women with recurrent upper or lower UTIs should be asked explicitly about relation of infection to sexual intercourse, and antibiotic prophylaxis should be attempted if there is an association
- Patients with recurrent pyelonephritis almost certainly have a urologic abnormality and should be referred for urologic evaluation

Therapeutic failure

- If failure after 48h in a patient being treated with the right antibiotic in the community, refer to hospital
- If failure of intravenous therapy occurs or sepsis supervenes, radiologic investigation is indicated under supervision of a specialist

Recurrence

- Recurrence/relapse is common
- If recurrence post 14-day oral antibiotics, a second 14-day course is appropriate as long as the indications for outpatient treatment still remain
- If there is further recurrence after this, a 6-week course may be initiated but referral for investigation at this time is appropriate
- In men, the threshold for further investigation should be very much lower

Deterioration

- Outpatients should be admitted acutely if deterioration occurs on therapy
- Repeat midstream urine analysis is appropriate in case organism has been missed/error on sensitivities
- Deterioration in clinical condition despite treatment, or failure to improve within 48h of correct treatment, is an indication for referral for further investigation

COMPLICATIONS

- Kidney scarring in children and hence abnormal kidney growth and development. Vesicoureteric reflux in children. Infants with grade III–V reflux should be treated initially with continuous antibiotic prophylaxis. There is no consensus on ongoing management of children with grades I and II reflux. Surgical repair is the preferred option for more severe and bilateral disease (grades III–V), particularly if disease persists or there is scarring at diagnosis. Disease persisting beyond age 6 is likely to require surgical repair even if there is no scarring
- Rarely, acute papillary necrosis, when fragments of renal papillae are excreted in the urine
- Gram-negative septicemia may occur and produce hyper- or hypodynamic septic shock in adults or children and requires urgent inpatient treatment with antibiotics, inotropes, and intravenous fluid management
- Acute renal failure with sepsis may occur and is particularly likely in patients with diabetes mellitus or chronic urinary obstruction
- Renal abscess can occur due to ascending infection combined with urinary tract obstruction. Diagnosis of a renal abscess is usually on CT and treatment may be surgical drainage with antimicrobial cover
- Perinephric abscess may arise from ascending UTI (or from hematogenous seeding) with the history and examination being nonspecific, although fever and malaise are usual. Perinephric abscess may burst into the pararenal space resulting in paranephric abscess. 30% of perinephric abscesses are due to *E. coli* and 40% *Proteus*, and mortality is 50%
- Pyelonephritis in pregnancy increases rate of preterm delivery, premature rupture of membranes, and requirement for special care

CONSIDER CONSULT

- Women who are refractory to antibiotic therapy, who relapse rapidly and repeatedly, and who continue to have bacteriuria should be referred for further investigation to rule out possible obstruction

PREVENTION

RISK FACTORS
- Dehydration
- Intercourse-related urinary tract infections (UTIs)
- Previous episode of pyelonephritis
- In men, prostatic hypertrophy
- Pregnancy

MODIFY RISK FACTORS
General measures for all patients to prevent UTI:
- Avoid dehydration – adequate hydration; drink more fluids in a hot climate or work environment
- Women prone to UTI should have a high fluid intake, void before and after intercourse, and use the double micturition technique
- Treat stones and obstructive lesions appropriately
- Aim for optimal control of underlying conditions such as diabetes

Other measures:
- Pregnant women – screening at 12–16 weeks for bacteriuria and treat positive findings appropriately
- Men – treat symptoms of prostatic hypertrophy

Lifestyle and wellness
ALCOHOL AND DRUGS
Alcohol is dehydrating and high intake may be associated with increased risk of pyelonephritis.

DIET
Adequate hydration.

SEXUAL BEHAVIOR
Women prone to UTI should void before and after intercourse.

DRUG HISTORY
Prolonged abuse of combinations of over-the-counter analgesics risks analgesic nephropathy and papillary necrosis, which then predispose to renal infection by stasis and obstruction.

CHEMOPROPHYLAXIS
Selected groups who are at high risk of further scarring are given prophylactic low-dose antibiotics under the supervision of an experienced specialist.

Cost/efficacy
Cost of these low-dose antibiotics is low financially, although pathogen resistance can develop.

SCREENING

- Screening of asymptomatic patients for bacteriuria: there is insufficient evidence to recommend screening even in diabetic and older patients
- Screening of asymptomatic children for bacteriuria: there is fair evidence to exclude dipstick analysis to detect bacteriuria and renal abnormalities from the urine of healthy infants and children

SCREENING PREGNANT WOMEN FOR ASYMPTOMATIC BACTERIURIA

- Screening pregnant women for asymptomatic bacteriuria is recommended at 12–16 weeks with urine culture. Prevalence has been found to be 2.5–8.7% and, although no different from nonpregnant women, up to 30% of those with asymptomatic bacteriuria develop pyelonephritis, which is associated with preterm delivery, prematurity, and need for special care
- Antibiotic treatment is effective in reducing risk of pyelonephritis in pregnancy and seems to reduce preterm delivery
- Women with a higher frequency of prepregnancy symptomatic UTI have a higher incidence of asymptomatic bacteriuria in pregnancy
- Women with known renal scars have a 3.3-fold increased incidence of hypertension, a 7.6-fold increased risk of pre-eclampsia, and a higher rate of obstetric interventions

PREVENT RECURRENCE

- Avoid dehydration by maintaining adequate hydration in hot climate or working environment, and limiting alcohol consumption
- If intercourse-related UTIs, consider voiding before and after intercourse, and double micturition
- If previous episode of pyelonephritis, educate patient about symptoms and encourage early attendance if these develop
- In men, treat symptoms of prostatic hypertrophy

ASSOCIATIONS
National Kidney and Urologic Diseases Information Clearinghouse
3 Information Way
Bethesda, MD 20892–3580
http://www.niddk.nih.gov/health/kidney/kidney.htm

American Urological Association
1120 North Charles Street
Baltimore, MD 21201
Tel: (410) 727-1100
Fax: (410) 223-4370
E-mail: aua@auanet.org
http://www.auanet.org

KEY REFERENCES
- Nicolle LE. Urinary tract infection. In: Greenberg A, ed. Primer on kidney diseases. New York: Academic Press, 2001: p354–60
- Stamm WE, Hooton TM. Management of UTI in adults. N Engl J Med 1993;329:1328–34
- Brenner and Rector's the kidney, 6th edn. Philadelphia: WB Saunders, 2000
- Arant BS Jr. Chapter on: Vesicoureteral reflux and reflux nephropathy. In: Greenberg A, ed. Primer on kidney disease. New York: Academic Press, 2001, p345–54
- Collins TR, Devries CR. Recurrent urinary tract infection in children: A logical approach to diagnosis, treatment and long term management. Comprehensive Ther 1997;23:44–8

FAQS
Question 1
How does pyelonephritis occur?

ANSWER 1
Most commonly caused when bacteria in the bladder ascend the ureters and invade the renal parenchyma.

Question 2
What are the common clinical features of pyelonephritis?

ANSWER 2
Dysuria, fever, flank pain, nausea and vomiting.

Question 3
What are the common pathogens causing pyelonephritis?

ANSWER 3
Escherichia coli is the most common pathogen (75% of cases). Other causal pathogens include *Klebsiella, Proteus, Enterobacter, Pseudomonas, Serratia, Citrobacter, E. faecalis,* and less commonly *Staph. aureus.*

Question 4
How do I know if the patient with pyelonephritis is also obstructed?

ANSWER 4
Check a postvoid residual for incomplete bladder emptying and do a renal ultrasound to evaluate for hydronephrosis.

Question 5
Should patients with neurogenic bladders or chronically indwelling Foley catheters receive suppressive antibiotics to prevent urinary tract infections (UTIs)?

ANSWER 5
Generally, no. Suppressive antibiotics tend to breed resistant organisms and make it very difficult to treat subsequent UTIs.

CONTRIBUTORS
Dennis F Saver, MD
Martin Goldberg, MD, FACP
Jennifer F Weil, MD
Rakesh Gulati, MD

RENAL ARTERY STENOSIS

SUMMARY INFORMATION

DESCRIPTION

- Narrowing or complete occlusion of one or both renal arteries
- Cause of hypertension in up to 5% of all hypertensive patients
- Different etiology in different age groups
- Bilateral renal-artery stenosis may give rise to acute or chronic progressive renal failure

URGENT ACTION

Urgent evaluation is necessary when there is suspicion of renal artery stenosis, as well as evidence of renal insufficiency, manifested by elevation of the BUN (blood urea nitrogen) and creatinine.

ICD9 CODE
440.1 Renal artery stenosis

SYNONYMS
- Renal artery obstruction
- Renovascular hypertension
- Ischemic nephropathy

CARDINAL FEATURES
- Complete or partial occlusion of one or both renal arteries
- One of the most frequent causes of curable hypertension
- One of the few causes of hypertension that can be treated surgically
- Can cause hypertension in individuals aged <30 years
- Bilateral renal-artery stenosis is now recognized as an important cause of ischemic nephropathy with chronic renal failure in the elderly

CAUSES
Common causes
Chronic
- Atherosclerosis in patients aged >50 years
- Fibromuscular dysplasia in patients aged <30 years

Rare causes
Chronic
- Extrinsic compression of renal artery (e.g. by a tumor)

Acute
- Trauma – resulting from surgery or angiography (with or without underlying atherosclerotic disease or fibromuscular dysplasia)
- Embolism (associated with atrial arrhythmias, prior myocardial infarction, etc.)
- Dissection or rupture of renal artery aneurysm
- Inadvertent ligation during surgery in the region
- Fat/cholesterol or tumor emboli

Contributory or predisposing factors
Chronic
- Generalized atherosclerosis
- Fibromuscular dysplasia

EPIDEMIOLOGY
Incidence and prevalence
PREVALENCE
- Renal artery stenosis will be found in 0.2–5% of all patients with hypertension
- Atherosclerosis accounts for 90% of cases of renal artery stenosis

Demographics
AGE
- Chronic renal artery stenosis due to atherosclerosis is more common at age >50 years
- Chronic renal artery stenosis due to fibromuscular dysplasia is more common at age <30 years
- Renal artery stenosis occurring in children is most commonly due to intimal fibroplasia

GENDER

- Renal artery stenosis secondary to atherosclerosis is more common in men
- Fibromuscular dysplasia is more common in young women

RACE

- Can occur in all races, but less frequently found as a cause of severe hypertension in African-Americans in comparison to Caucasians
- Both atherosclerotic and fibromuscular causes of renal artery stenosis are more common in Caucasians

SOCIOECONOMIC STATUS

Lipid status, diet, and tobacco abuse, as well as type II diabetes mellitus may be related to socioeconomic status and contribute to the development of atherosclerosis.

DIFFERENTIAL DIAGNOSIS
Essential hypertension
FEATURES
- Accounts for 90% of all causes of hypertension
- Defined as a systolic blood pressure of 140mmHg or more, and/or diastolic blood pressure of 90mmHg or more
- Essential hypertension is a diagnosis of exclusion

Acute renal failure
FEATURES
- Nausea, vomiting, weakness are features of acute renal failure
- Hypertension, edema, oliguria may be present
- Symptomatology will be determined by the cause of the acute renal failure

Chronic renal failure
FEATURES
- Weakness, lethargy, anemia, shortness of breath are features of chronic renal failure
- Hypertension, edema may be present
- Symptomatology will be determined by the cause of the chronic renal failure

SIGNS & SYMPTOMS
Signs
Hypertension: The physician should suspect renal artery stenosis in the following circumstances
- Caucasian female aged <30 years, with hypertension not attributed to any other cause
- Caucasian male aged >50 years, with or without hypertension and known atheromatous disease
- Diabetic male or female >50 years, with or without hypertension
- Poor response to medical treatment for hypertension at any age
- Patients aged <20 years with hypertension

Abdominal bruit

Embolic infarction: In cases of cholesterol emboli, there may be vasculitic-type multisystem manifestations, e.g. fever, retinal ischemia, neurologic deficits, toe gangrene

Symptoms
Renal artery stenosis is usually asymptomatic, unless bilateral renal-artery stenosis with renal failure is present, in which case the clinical picture is that of renal failure or uremia.

ASSOCIATED DISORDERS
Other manifestations of atherosclerotic disease may be present (e.g. peripheral vascular disease, coronary atherosclerotic disease, or cerebrovascular disease)

CONSIDER CONSULT
All cases of suspected renal artery stenosis should be referred to a nephrologist for diagnosis and therapy. Urgent evaluation is necessary when there is suspicion of renal artery stenosis, as well as evidence of renal insufficiency manifested by elevation of the BUN (blood urea nitrogen) and creatinine. Also:
- If the patient is aged <30 years with hypertension that cannot be attributed to any other cause and which seems difficult to control

- If the patient is aged >50 years and has other evidence of atherosclerotic disease with hypertension that is poorly responsive to medical treatment
- If a hypertensive patient develops impaired renal function after administration of ACE (angiotensin-converting enzyme) inhibitors

INVESTIGATION OF THE PATIENT
Direct questions to patient

Q How old were you when you were first noted to have high blood pressure? Early onset of hypertension, age <30 years, might suggest renal artery stenosis.

Q Do you have any problems with your circulation in addition to your high blood pressure? Coexisting peripheral vascular disease may suggest atherosclerotic renal arterial disease.

Q Do you have coronary or cerebrovascular disease? Atherosclerotic disease is a common cause of renal artery stenosis.

Contributory or predisposing factors

Q Do you have high blood pressure? Secondary causes of hypertension must be considered.

Q Do you smoke? Smoking is associated with an increased risk of atherosclerotic disease.

Q Are you known to have a high cholesterol level? High cholesterol may be significant in the development of atherosclerosis.

Q Do you have diabetes? Type I or type II diabetes is a significant risk factor for the development of atherosclerosis.

Q Do you have peripheral, coronary, or cerebrovascular disease? The presence of claudication, angina, history of myocardial infarction, transient ischemic attacks, or stroke suggest the presence of diffuse atherosclerotic disease.

Q Have you ever had problems with your kidneys? Renal artery stenosis in one kidney only will not affect renal function; however, it suggests that renal artery stenosis may develop in the remaining kidney, leading to a significant decline in renal function.

Family history

Q Do you have a family history of hypertension, diabetes, hypercholesterolemia, peripheral vascular disease, coronary atherosclerotic disease, or cerebrovascular disease?

Examination

- Measure blood pressure. Be sure to use the correct size blood pressure cuff for an accurate reading. Hypertension alone does not suggest renal artery stenosis but warrants consideration of secondary causes of hypertension
- Listen for carotid and femoral bruits. Always auscultate before palpating. The presence of atherosclerotic disease in another part of the body increases the chance that hypertension may be caused by renal artery stenosis
- Palpate peripheral pulses to ascertain if there is widespread atherosclerosis. Carotid, brachial, radial, femoral, popliteal, dorsalis pedis, and posterior tibial pulses should be checked
- Listen for abdominal bruits: These are only audible in about 50% of patients with renal artery stenosis and are best heard at the costovertebral angles
- Examine fundi for hypertensive retinopathy

Summary of investigative tests

Investigations that would normally be performed by a primary care physician

- Renal function tests: particularly creatinine levels; these are indicated in the investigation of both acute and chronic renal artery stenosis
- Urinalysis: gross or microscopic hematuria may occur in acute renal-artery occlusion. In chronic disease, proteinuria may indicate renal pathology
- Renal ultrasound: asymmetry of kidney size is suggestive of renovascular disease

Investigations that would normally be performed by a specialist

- Renal-vein renin levels: more accurate than measuring peripheral plasma renin levels but more invasive
- Captopril nuclear renogram: this is the first procedure in the investigation of renovascular hypertension. It demonstrates the presence of renal ischemia but cannot actually show the location or quality of a stenosis in the renal artery
- Digital subtraction angiography: requires catheterization of the aorta and all of its concomitant risks including renal embolization. May be performed with renal-vein renin levels
- Magnetic resonance angiography: not yet widely used as an investigative procedure in renal artery stenosis but has significant advantages over several others, totally noninvasive, no contrast medium required

DIAGNOSTIC DECISION

- The diagnosis may be suspected in patients who develop hypertension before the age of 30 years, after 50 years, or in those with previously diagnosed hypertension that is accelerating or unresponsive to therapy
- The presence of a bruit in the epigastric region is indicative of renal artery stenosis
- Definitive diagnosis can be made with renal arteriography

CLINICAL PEARLS

- Bilateral renal-artery stenosis is now recognized increasingly as an important cause of progressive renal failure, with or without hypertension, in patients with generalized atherosclerosis, particularly diabetics
- An important clue to possible bilateral renal-artery stenosis is acute deterioration in renal function following administration of angiotensin-converting enzyme inhibitors

THE TESTS
Body fluids
DIPSTICK URINALYSIS
Description
A midstream specimen of urine is required.

Advantages/Disadvantages
Advantages:

- Quick
- Simple
- Noninvasive

Disadvantages:

- Accuracy of urinalysis is dependent on skill of observer and on type of dipstick used
- May also be affected by dilution/concentration of urine or dietary factors

Normal
There should be no protein, blood, or glucose detected.

Abnormal

- Proteinuria greater than a trace
- Microscopic nonhemolysed blood
- Keep in mind the possibility of a false-positive result

Cause of abnormal result
Renal or urinary tract disease.

Drugs, disorders and other factors that may alter results
Proteinuria is not specific for renal disease and can occur in other disorders such as congestive cardiac failure, multiple myeloma, and essential hypertension.

RENAL-VEIN RENIN LEVELS
Description

- Venous blood samples taken directly from renal vein
- This test is rarely done but can be performed simultaneously with renal arteriography

Advantages/Disadvantages
Advantages:

- More accurate way to determine if only one kidney is involved in overproduction of renin, contributing to hypertension
- May predict the potential success or otherwise of revascularization

Disadvantages:

- Highly invasive procedure as it involves placing a catheter into the renal veins via the femoral vein, external iliac vein, and inferior vena cava
- Results not foolproof

Normal
1.6 (+/- 1.5 SE)

Abnormal
A level of 1.5 times greater on the 'affected' or 'more affected' side than on the 'unaffected' or 'lesser affected' side may indicate that one kidney is responsible for the hypertension.

Cause of abnormal result

- Renal artery stenosis
- Keep in mind the possibility of a false positive or false negative result

Drugs, disorders and other factors that may alter results
May be affected by antihypertensive medication.

Tests of function
RENAL FUNCTION
Description
Venous blood sample

Advantages/Disadvantages

- Advantage: Simple and straightforward.
- Disadvantage: Not specific for renal artery stenosis or renovascular hypertension

Normal
Serum creatinine: normal adult range 0.6–1.2mg/dL.

Abnormal
Serum creatinine: >1.2mg/dL.

Cause of abnormal result
Most commonly due to acute or chronic renal impairment secondary to renal disease, renal hypoperfusion, or urinary tract obstruction.

Imaging
RENAL ULTRASOUND
Description
Ultrasound imaging of the renal tract with or without color Doppler.

Advantages/Disadvantages
- Advantage: Noninvasive
- Disadvantage: Color Doppler required to demonstrate reduced renal-artery flow volume

Normal
- Normal size kidney
- Normal calyces and ureters
- Color Doppler: normal blood flow to kidneys

Abnormal
- Small, atrophic kidney
- Color Doppler: reduced renal-artery blood flow

Cause of abnormal result
Atrophic kidneys, which may be:
- Congenital
- Secondary to pyelonephritis
- Secondary to renal infarction

Drugs, disorders and other factors that may alter results
Obesity may obscure ultrasonic visualization of the renal tract.

CAPTOPRIL NUCLEAR RENOGRAM
Advantages/Disadvantages
Advantages:
- Noninvasive
- Captopril enhances abnormalities that may not be so easily visualized in a conventional nuclear renogram

Normal
Uptake of the tracer and accumulation time are the same for both kidneys.

Abnormal
On affected side (renal artery stenosis present) in comparison to nonaffected side there is slower uptake of tracer, prolonged accumulation time, and a delay in peak time.

Cause of abnormal result
- Renal artery stenosis
- Keep in mind the possibility of a false-positive or false-negative result

Drugs, disorders and other factors that may alter results
Patients must be withdrawn from any ACE (angiotensin-converting enzyme) inhibitor prior to the test being done.

DIGITAL SUBTRACTION ANGIOGRAPHY
Advantages/Disadvantages
Advantages:
- Provides very clear detail of renal arterial system
- Defines size and location of lesion

Disadvantages:

- Highly invasive, requiring intra-aortic catheterization, which can lead to trauma of the aorta and renal artery, with complications of dissection, rupture, thrombosis, or embolization
- Iodinated contrast media may be nephrotoxic
- If patient is at high risk for contrast nephrotoxicity, carbon dioxide angiogram may be performed

Normal
Normal flow of contrast through renal arterial system with no narrowing or stenoses.

Abnormal

- > 70% stenosis of the renal arterial system anywhere from the ostium (the beginning of the renal artery at the aorta) to the kidney
- Appearances will differ depending on etiology of narrowing, e.g. the stenoses of fibromuscular dysplasia have a different appearance from those of atherosclerosis

Cause of abnormal result
Renal artery stenosis.

MAGNETIC RESONANCE ANGIOGRAPHY

Advantages/Disadvantages
Advantages:

- Totally noninvasive
- Does not involve exposure to radioactivity

Disadvantages:

- It may not be possible to visualize smaller vessels in as much detail as conventional angiography
- The MRI machine may provoke claustrophobia in susceptible patients

Normal
No renal artery stenosis.

Abnormal
Narrowing of affected renal artery.

PATIENT AND CAREGIVER ISSUES
Patient or caregiver request

- How successful is angioplasty for treating this problem? Percutaneous transluminal angioplasty (PCTA) is 80–90% successful in patients with fibromuscular dysplasia. Atherosclerotic lesions have a 50% risk of recurrence within 2 years. The use of a stent may reduce the risk of recurrence. Patients may have persistent hypertension despite dilation of the affected renal artery
- Will I still need drug treatment even if I have angioplasty? This depends on how successful the angioplasty is – most patients will still need antihypertensive medication, even after PCTA
- What will happen to my kidneys? In disease affecting only one side, even if the stenosis cannot be corrected, renal function should not be impaired, as the kidney on the nonaffected side will continue to work normally. In cases where disease affects both renal arteries, or if the disease occurs where there is already only one kidney, and treatment is ineffective, then renal failure may occur

MANAGEMENT ISSUES
Goals
Chronic

- Correctly identify those patients who require referral for more detailed investigation to confirm the diagnosis and therapy
- In patients receiving antihypertensive medication, maintain an acceptable target blood pressure
- Monitor renal function and identify patients with deteriorating function

Acute

- This always occurs in the hospital as an adverse result of a procedure. The course of action will be dictated by what occurred

Management in special circumstances
In cases of acute renal-artery occlusion, the rapid confirmation of the diagnosis is essential if thrombolytic or anticoagulant therapy is to be of benefit.

COEXISTING DISEASE

- If there is coexisting acute or chronic renal failure, care must be taken when prescribing antihypertensive medication such as ACE (angiotensin-converting enzyme) inhibitors
- Referral to a specialist is certainly indicated

COEXISTING MEDICATION
The usual recommendations regarding interactions between different antihypertensives and other medications will apply.

SPECIAL PATIENT GROUPS
Pregnancy

- In pregnancy the choices of antihypertensives are more limited due to teratogenic effects
- Percutaneous transluminal angioplasty could be carried out during pregnancy but may be more hazardous
- Control of renovascular hypertension during pregnancy may be more difficult if there is concomitant pre-eclampsia

Children and teenagers

- Children or teenagers presenting with renovascular hypertension should be referred to a pediatric nephrologist

PATIENT SATISFACTION/LIFESTYLE PRIORITIES

■ Life-long drug therapy for hypertension secondary to chronic renal-artery stenosis may seem unacceptable to some patients

■ The choice of antihypertensive may need to be influenced by the patient's lifestyle, e.g. beta-blockers can be a problem for those who engage in very active exercise or who work outdoors in cold climates

SUMMARY OF THERAPEUTIC OPTIONS
Choices

■ Percutaneous transluminal angioplasty (PCTA): (with or without stenting): this is the first-choice treatment for patients with renal artery stenosis secondary to fibromuscular dysplasia. It is often the first choice for older patients with atherosclerosis but is not as effective since the failure rate is high and the restenosis rate is also high. Newer techniques using stents are improving the long-term outcome of PCTA

■ Surgical revascularization: generally reserved for cases where PCTA is unlikely to be effective and where drug treatment alone is insufficient. Hazardous for patients with concomitant atherosclerotic disease because of the elevated risk of perioperative myocardial infarction and stroke

■ Drug therapy: antihypertensive medication, particularly angiotensin-converting enzyme inhibitors (combined with beta-blockers, diuretics, calcium channel antagonists, and alpha-adrenergic antagonists in these very refractory patients), is the treatment of choice for older patients with unilateral atherosclerotic disease and unimpaired renal function. In cases of suspected bilateral renal-artery stenosis, particularly if there is impaired renal function and angioplasty, or surgery is not feasible, angiotensin-converting enzyme (ACE) inhibitors are contraindicated and other drugs must be used. A large number of effective antihypertensive agents are available, any of which may be used in the treatment of hypertension secondary to renal artery stenosis.

Guidelines

■ Guidelines for percutaneous transluminal angioplasty [1]

Clinical pearls

■ For patients with hypertension and atherosclerotic renal-artery stenosis, ACE inhibitors and angiotensin-receptor blockers are effective in controlling hypertension in 86–92% patients, but loss of renal mass is not ameliorated

■ Hypertension is more likely to be cured with a revascularization procedure in patients with fibromuscular dysplasia than in patients with atheromatous renal-artery stenosis

■ In addition to any revascularization procedure, successful therapy requires the use of cholesterol-lowering drugs, aspirin, and smoking cessation

Never

Never use ACE inhibitors to treat renovascular hypertension in the presence of known bilateral renal-artery disease, if there is only one functioning kidney, or if there is impaired renal function.

FOLLOW UP

Regardless of the cause of the renal artery stenosis all patients with this diagnosis will require regular follow-up to ensure that hypertension is well controlled and that renal function is monitored.

Plan for review

■ Regardless of the mode of treatment, e.g. surgical, medical, or both, these patients will need regular life-long follow-up under the auspices of a specialist to monitor and treat their hypertension and to monitor renal function

- Frequency of follow-up will depend on the severity of their disease and their response to treatment but should be at no less than 6-monthly intervals with checking of blood pressure and monitoring of renal function
- Repeat of imaging tests should be carried out if there is a deterioration in the patient's condition, with reduced renal function or a sudden rise in blood pressure not responding to drug treatment

Information for patient or caregiver

- If drug therapy is recommended it is essential that this is followed carefully to ensure optimum blood pressure control
- Drug treatment will not cure the problem and there will be a life-long need for treatment
- Angioplasty is not always 100% effective and drug treatment may still be required even after this
- Always let your physician know if you develop any other medical conditions or are prescribed any other drugs that might interact with your antihypertensive medication

DRUGS AND OTHER THERAPIES: DETAILS
Drugs
BETA-BLOCKERS

- There are a number of beta-adrenoceptor blocking drugs available (details regarding one example are given here)
- Generally all equally effective
- Very effective in patients with elevated plasma renin
- Atenolol is the most commonly prescribed

Dose
Atenolol: 50–100mg once daily.

Efficacy
- Very effective in patients with elevated plasma renin
- Not always sufficiently effective at lowering blood pressure on its own

Risks/Benefits
Risks: Use caution in diabetes mellitus, thyroid disease, renal disease, chronic obstructive pulmonary disease, peripheral vascular disease

Side-effects and adverse reactions
- Cardiovascular system: bradycardia, congestive heart failure, heart block, peripheral vascular disease
- Central nervous system: lethargy, depression, and vivid dreams
- Eyes, ears, nose, and throat: dry eyes, sore throat
- Gastrointestinal: ischemic colitis, nausea, dry mouth
- Hematologic: agranulocytosis, thrombocytopenia
- Metabolism: hyperglycemia, hyperlipidemia, masked hypoglycemia
- Respiratory: bronchospasm, dyspnea, wheezing
- Skin: alopecia, bruising, rash

Interactions (other drugs)
- Adenosine ■ Antacids ■ Anticholinesterases (neostigmine, physostigmine, tacrine)
- Antihypertensives (clonidine, dipyridamole, prazosin) ■ Calcium channel blockers (verapamil, dihydropyridines) ■ Lidocaine ■ Nonsteroidal anti-inflammatory drugs
- Penicillins (amoxicillin, ampicillin) ■ Theophylline

Contraindications
■ Asthma ■ Cardiogenic shock ■ Congestive heart failure ■ Heart block ■ Sinus bradycardia

Acceptability to patient
Side-effects can be troublesome for some groups of patients, e.g. fatigue and reduced exercise tolerance in young patients who are still working or active in sports; peripheral vasoconstriction can be noticeable in cold weather.

Follow up plan
May need to adjust dose according to blood pressure response and development of side-effects.

Patient and caregiver information
■ Needs to be taken regularly as prescribed
■ Some side-effects may decrease over time so it is worth persevering with the treatment
■ Inform physician if taking any other medication or if any new medications are prescribed for other conditions
■ Women must let their physician know if they become pregnant or intend to do so while on treatment

ANGIOTENSIN CONVERTING ENZYME (ACE) INHIBITORS
■ There are a number of ACE inhibitors available (details regarding one example are given here)
■ Generally all equally effective

Dose
Enalapril: 2.5–5mg daily, rising to 10–40mg in single or divided doses according to response.

Efficacy
■ Highly effective in unilateral renovascular hypertension
■ Contraindicated in bilateral renovascular hypertension
■ May be used in combination with other antihypertensives, e.g. diuretics, for enhanced effect

Risks/Benefits
Risks: Use caution in renal impairment, hypotension, aortic stenosis, hyperkalemia, neutropenia

Side-effects and adverse reactions
■ Cardiovascular system: orthostatic hypotension and syncope, angina, palpitations, sinus tachycardia
■ Central nervous system: headache, dizziness, fatigue
■ Eyes, ears, nose, and throat: cough
■ Gastrointestinal: nausea, vomiting, diarrhea, constipation, abdominal pain
■ Genitourinary: renal damage, impotence
■ Hematologic: neutropenia, agranulocytosis, aplastic and hemolytic anemia, pancytopenia, thrombocytopenia
■ Metabolic: hyperkalemia, hyponatremia
■ Skin: angioedema, macropapular rash

Interactions (other drugs)
■ Allopurinol ■ Antihypertensives (loop and potassium-sparing diuretics, prazosin, terazosin, doxazosin) ■ Azathioprine ■ Heparin ■ Insulin ■ Iron ■ Lithium ■ Nonsteroidal anti-inflammatory drugs ■ Potassium ■ Sodium ■ Trimethoprim

Contraindications
- Pregnancy ▪ Angioedema ▪ Hypotension ▪ Children

Acceptability to patient
Generally very acceptable although the side-effects of cough or dizziness may reduce compliance.

Follow up plan
- May need to adjust dose according to blood pressure response and development of side-effects
- Need to monitor renal function regularly

Patient and caregiver information
- Needs to be taken regularly as prescribed
- If dizziness/postural hypotension is a persistent problem it may be alleviated by taking the medication at night
- Caution with salt substitutes containing potassium
- Some side-effects may decrease over time so it is worth persevering with the treatment
- Inform physician if taking any other medication or if any new medications are prescribed for other conditions
- Women must inform their physician if they become pregnant or intend to do so while on treatment

DIURETICS
- Includes loop and thiazide diuretics (an example from each class is given here)
- Loop diuretics are more effective in patients with renal impairment
- Potassium-sparing diuretics should be avoided in renal impairment

Dose
- Furosemide (loop diuretic): 20–80mg per day up to maximum of 400mg
- Hydrochlorthiazide (thiazide diuretic): 12.5–50mg per day

Efficacy
Highly effective either alone or in combination with other classes of antihypertensive drugs.

Risks/Benefits
Risks:
- Use caution with diabetes mellitus, renal and liver disease, systemic lupus erythematosis, hypertension, gout, porphyria
- Use caution with pregnancy and nursing mothers
- Reduces fluid congestion

Side-effects and adverse reactions
- Cardiovascular system: chest pain, circulatory collapse, orthostatic hypotension
- Central nervous system: dizziness, headache, paresthesia, fever
- Eyes, ears, nose, and throat: visual disturbances, ototoxicity, tinnitus, hearing impairment, thirst
- Gastrointestinal: ischemic hepatitis, vomiting, pancreatitis, nausea, diarrhea, anorexia
- Genitourinary: glycosuria, hyperuricemia, bladder spasm, polyuria
- Hematologic: blood disorders
- Metabolic: hyperglycemia, hyponatremia, hypokalemia, hypomagnesemia, hypovolemia, hypochloremia, hypercholesterolemia, hypertriglyceridemia
- Skin: erythema multiforme, exfoliative dermatitis, urticaria

Interactions (other drugs)
- ACE inhibitors - Alpha-adrenergic antagonists - Amphotericin - Antibiotics (aminoglycosides, polymixins, vancomycin, cephalosporins) - Antidiabetics - Antidysrhythmics (amiodarone, cardiac glycosides, disopyramide, flecainide, mexelitine, quinidine, sotalol) - Beta-2-adrenergic agonists - Carbenoxolone - Cholestyramine, colestipol - Cisplatin - Clofibrate - Corticosteroids - Diuretics (thiazides, metolazone, acetazolamide) - Lignocaine - Lithium - Nonsteroidal anti-inflammatory drugs - Phenobarbital - Phenytoin - Pimozide - Reboxetine - Selective serotonin reuptake inhibitors - Terbutaline - Tubocurarine

Contraindications
- Renal failure with anuria - Hepatic coma

Acceptability to patient
The diuresis produced by these drugs may be unacceptable to patients who have problems with bladder control, such as patients with prostatic hypertrophy

Follow up plan
Regular monitoring of:
- Blood pressure to assess efficacy
- Renal function, uric acid, lipids, and blood glucose

Patient and caregiver information
- May need to alter timing of dose to minimize disruption of work or social activities if urinary frequency is a significant problem
- Need to maintain adequate fluid intake to avoid dehydration
- Need to inform physician if prescribed any other medications or if taking any over-the-counter preparations that might interact
- Women must inform their physician if they become pregnant or intend to do so while on treatment

CALCIUM CHANNEL ANTAGONISTS
- Effective in the treatment of hypertension
- Newer, longer-acting preparations preferable to short-acting preparations
- Three basic types: dihydropyridines (such as amlodipine), diphenylalkylamines (such as verapamil), and benzothiazepines (diltiazem). Details regarding examples from the first two classes are given here

Dose
- Amlodipine (dihydropyridine calcium channel blocker) 5–10mg once daily by mouth
- Verapamil (diphenylalkylamine calcium channel blocker) 80mg twice daily by mouth up to 480mg daily in divided doses (sustained release preparations are also available)

Efficacy
Very effective if tolerated.

Risks/Benefits
Risks:
Amlodipine
- Use caution in congestive heart failure, hypotension, hepatic insufficiency, aortic stenosis
- Use caution in elderly

Verapamil
- The vasodilatory effects of verapamil may cause hemodynamic complications in patients with a substantial outflow gradient or markedly elevated pulmonary pressure

- Use caution with congestive heart failure and hypotension, renal and hepatic disease, Duchenne's muscular dystrophy,
- Use caution in acute phase of myocardial infarction and in concomitant beta-blocker therapy
- Use caution in children

Side-effects and adverse reactions
Amlodipine:

- Cardiovascular system: bradycardia, arrhythmias (including ventricular tachycardia and atrial fibrillation), hypotension, palpitations, chest pain, peripheral edema, syncope, tachycardia, postural dizziness
- Central nervous system: anxiety, asthenia, depression, fatigue, headache, insomnia, malaise, tremor
- Gastrointestinal: constipation, dyspepsia, diarrhea, flatulence, pancreatitis, vomiting, gingival hyperplasic
- Genitourinary: nocturia, polyuria
- Musculoskeletal: arthralgia, arthrosis, muscle cramps, myalgia
- Skin: angiodema, erythema multiforme, pruritus, rash, rash erythematous, rash maculopapular

Verapamil:

- Gastrointestinal: nausea, constipation, vomiting, abdominal pain
- Central nervous system: dizziness, flushing, headache, fatigue
- Ears, eyes, nose, and throat: tinnitus
- Genitourinary: impotence, nocturia, polyuria, gynecomastia
- Cardiovascular system: tachycardia, bradycardia, palpitations, congestive heart failure, atrioventricular block, hypotension, peripheral edema
- Skin: rash

Interactions (other drugs)
Amlodipine:

- Barbiturates ▪ Diltiazem ▪ Erythromycin ▪ Fentanyl ▪ H2-blockers ▪ Grapefruit juice ▪ Proton pump inhibitors ▪ Quinidine ▪ Rifampin ▪ Vincristine

Verapamil:

- Antidysrhythmics (amiodarone, digoxin, disopyramide, dofetilide, encainide, flecainide, procainamide, quinidine) ▪ Antihypertensives (particularly alpha- and beta-blockers) ▪ Antivirals ▪ Aspirin ▪ Azole antifungals ▪ Barbiturates ▪ Benzodiazepines ▪ Buspirone ▪ Calcium ▪ Carbamazepine ▪ Cardiac glycosides ▪ Cimetidine ▪ Cisapride ▪ Clarithromycin, erythromycin ▪ Cyclosporine, tacrolimus ▪ Dantrolene ▪ Diclofenac ▪ Doxorubicin ▪ Ethanol ▪ Fentanyl ▪ General and local anesthetics ▪ Grapefruit juice ▪ Histamine H2-antagonists ▪ Imipramine ▪ Lithium ▪ Neuromuscular blockers ▪ Statins ▪ Phenytoin ▪ Rifampin ▪ SSRIs ▪ Theophylline

Contraindications
Amlodipine:

- Sensitivity to amlodipine ▪ Cardiogenic shock ▪ Unstable angina ▪ Pregnancy and breast-feeding ▪ Significant aortic stenosis

Verapamil:

- Cardiogenic shock ▪ Porphyria ▪ Hypotension ▪ Pregnancy ▪ Sick sinus syndrome ▪ Severe heart failure, history of heart failure ▪ Heart block

Acceptability to patient

- Longer-acting once-daily preparations are better tolerated and increase patient compliance
- Lower-extremity edema may be better tolerated by men than women

Follow up plan
Regular review for monitoring of blood pressure response and adjustment of dose.

Patient and caregiver information
- Some side-effects may lessen with time so it is worth persevering with treatment
- Tell your physician if you are taking any other prescribed or over-the-counter medication
- Avoid grapefruit and excess alcohol
- Women must inform their physician if they become pregnant or intend to do so while on treatment

ALPHA-ADRENERGIC ANTAGONISTS
- Selective alpha-adrenergic antagonists, e.g. doxazosin, have replaced nonselective antagonists, e.g. phenoxybenzamine, in the treatment of hypertension
- There are some recent concerns regarding possible worsening of heart failure in patients using doxazosin

Dose
- Doxazosin: 1–16mg daily by mouth usually as a single dose
- Prazosin: 1–20mg in two or three divided doses daily by mouth
- Terazosin: 1–20mg daily by mouth
- Should all be started at lowest possible dose then titrated up according to response

Efficacy
Highly effective if tolerated.

Risks/Benefits
Risks:
- Orthostatic hypotension – particularly in patients taking other antihypertensive, diuretic, vasodilator medications
- Use caution in hepatic disease
- Use caution in nursing mothers and children

Benefits:
- Improved bladder control
- Can improve lipid profiles
- Has a beneficial effect in coexisting benign prostatic hypertrophy
- Can improve Raynaud's vasospasm

Side-effects and adverse reactions
- Cardiovascular system: edema, chestpain, palpitations, hypotension (particularly orthostatic), dysrhythmia
- Central nervous system: dizziness, headache, fever, paresthesia, vertigo, fatigue, somnolence
- Eyes, ears, nose, and throat: visual disturbances, tinnitus, rhinitis
- Gastrointestinal: abdominal cramps, dry mouth, vomiting, constipation, diarrhea
- Genitourinary: urination difficulties
- Respiratory: dyspnea
- Skin: rash

Interactions (other drugs)
- ACE inhibitors ■ Adrenergic neurone blockers (both alpha and beta) ■ Corticosteroids
- Antipsychotics ■ Aldesleukin ■ Alcohol ■ Alprostadil ■ Amifostine ■ Estrogens
- Diuretics ■ Angiotensin-II receptor antagonists ■ Anxiolytics and nypnotics ■ Levodopa
- Calcium channel blockers ■ General anesthetics ■ Nonsteroidal anti-inflammatory drugs
- Skeletal muscle relaxants (baclofen, tizanidine) ■ Antihypertensives (clonidine, diazoxide, methyldopa, minoxidil, nitrates, nitroprusside)

Contraindications
- Breast-feeding ■ Closed-angle glaucoma

Acceptability to patient
Generally well tolerated unless side-effects occur.

Follow up plan
Regular review for monitoring of blood pressure response and uptitration of dose as required.

Patient and caregiver information
- Alert patient and family members where appropriate regarding the first-dose hypotensive response in case of accident/injury
- If daytime dizziness is a problem can try taking medication at bedtime instead
- Tell physician if taking any other prescribed or over-the-counter medication which may interact
- Women must inform their physician if they become pregnant or intend to do so while on treatment

Surgical therapy
REVASCULARIZATION OF RENAL ARTERIAL SUPPLY
This can involve saphenous-vein bypass grafting of the renal arteries or more complicated microvascular techniques with autotransplantation of the kidney.

Efficacy
In carefully selected patients can be up to 90% effective in restoring normal blood flow to the affected kidney(s).

Risks/Benefits
- Risks: Hazards of general anesthesia and major surgery; especially risky in older patients with coexisting atherosclerotic disease of other major vessels because of increased perioperative risk of myocardial infarction and stroke
- Benefits: Can restore or preserve renal function in severe disease and resolve hypertension, thereby removing or reducing the need for medication

Acceptability to patient
Despite the risks of surgery this procedure may be very acceptable if the alternative could be renal failure and subsequent dialysis or transplantation.

Follow up plan
Routine, immediate, postoperative care followed by regular review to monitor blood pressure and renal function.

- Procedure may not be successful
- May still require some antihypertensive medication postoperatively

Other therapies
PERCUTANEOUS TRANSLUMINAL ANGIOPLASTY (PCTA)
- Treatment of choice in younger patients with fibromuscular dysplasia
- Also effective in atherosclerotic lesions but recurrence rate is high and may be technically more difficult
- Ostial lesions more difficult to treat by this method

Efficacy
- Up to 60% effective in improving blood pressure in patients with fibromuscular dysplasia
- Only 20–30% effective in patients with atherosclerotic disease, and these patients can have up to 50% chance of recurrence within 2 years

Risks/Benefits
- Risks: Hemorrhage, dissection/intimal tear or rupture of the renal artery, thrombosis, cholesterol emboli to kidney
- Benefits: If successful can reduce or remove need for antihypertensive medication and preserve renal function

Evidence
Renal angioplasty is the treatment of choice in the management of renal artery stenosis secondary to fibromuscular renal-artery disease, renal-artery transplant stenosis, and atherosclerosis (unilateral and short, not involving the renal artery ostium) [1] *Level C*

Acceptability to patient
- May be reluctant to undergo invasive procedure unless chances of success are good
- Prospect of reduced need for medication may increase acceptability

Follow up plan
Regular review for monitoring of blood pressure and renal function.

Patient and caregiver information
- Procedure may require hospitalization for up to 24h
- Will still need to have blood pressure monitored regularly

EFFICACY OF THERAPIES

- Whenever possible percutaneous transluminal angioplasty (PCTA) or surgical revascularization should be attempted, particularly in younger patients with fibromuscular dysplasia as the success rate can be as high as 60%
- PCTA and surgery are less successful in older patients with atherosclerotic lesions, particularly at the ostium, and success rates are only between 20% and 30%, with a possible recurrence rate of 50% in 2 years
- Drug therapy to control hypertension associated with renal artery stenosis can be very effective and should be used when PCTA or surgery are not considered feasible

Evidence
PDxMD are unable to cite evidence that meets our criteria for evidence.

Review period
Patients should have their blood pressure and renal function reviewed at no less than 6-monthly intervals.

PROGNOSIS

- If blood pressure is well controlled by whatever therapeutic means are used and renal function is preserved, then the prognosis is the same as for well-controlled essential hypertension
- If the stenosis cannot be corrected or if blood pressure control is poor, then there is an increased risk of chronic renal failure, particularly in bilateral disease or if there is only one functioning kidney
- Recurrence of atherosclerotic stenoses following PCTA can occur in as many as 50% of cases within 2 years

Clinical pearls
In elderly patients (>70 years) with generalized atherosclerosis and renal artery stenosis contributing to hypertension and/or renal insufficiency, surgical therapy is often not possible because of the severity of associated cardiac and metabolic diseases. Therefore, conservative medical treatment is primarily indicated.

Therapeutic failure
If surgical therapy is contraindicated and PCTA (percutaneous transluminal angioplasty) cannot be done or fails to be effective, intensive treatment with antihypertensive agents is necessary. It may take five medications or more to make the patient normotensive. The patient must be closely monitored for decline in renal function when there is bilateral disease.

Recurrence
There is a 30% risk of recurrence in renal artery stenosis treated with PCTA. There is increased incidence of bilateral renal-artery stenosis in patients with the unilateral disease.

Deterioration
A decline in renal function, manifested by elevation of BUN (blood urea nitrogen) and creatinine, should prompt immediate referral to a nephrologist.

COMPLICATIONS

- These are generally the same as for essential hypertension, with myocardial infarction and stroke being the most serious
- There is also a significant risk of chronic renal failure
- Acute renal-artery occlusion may occur as a result of invasive investigation or treatment of chronic renal-artery stenosis

CONSIDER CONSULT

- If blood pressure control deteriorates following PCTA (percutaneous transluminal angioplasty) or surgery
- If renal function begins to deteriorate

- It is doubtful whether renal artery stenosis, particularly the fibromuscular dysplastic type, can be prevented
- Prevention of atherosclerotic disease of the renal arteries involves the same processes as preventing atherosclerosis of any other vessels. Patients should be encouraged to stop smoking, keep their weight under control, keep their serum cholesterol within normal limits, etc.

RISK FACTORS
- Smoking: There is a definite association between smoking and atherosclerosis
- Diet: Encourage a diet which is low in saturated fats and high in fruit and vegetables
- Familial hypercholesterolemia: May predispose to atherosclerosis of any vessel, with development of renal artery stenosis in later life
- Diabetes: Types I and II diabetes should be treated aggressively to keep hemoglobin A1c < 8%

MODIFY RISK FACTORS
Lifestyle and wellness
- The atherosclerotic form of renal artery stenosis has the same etiology as atherosclerosis affecting other parts of the arterial circulation
- The same advice regarding lifestyle should therefore apply to renal artery stenosis patients as to patients with other atherosclerotic disease

TOBACCO
Stop smoking.

DIET
- Low-sodium diet, particularly in the presence of renovascular hypertension and/or renal impairment
- Low saturated fat diet with recommended quantities of fruit and vegetables
- Lipid-lowering drugs if required

DRUG HISTORY
Avoid any over-the-counter or alternative medications that may interact with prescribed medication for hypertension or which may be contraindicated in the presence of renal impairment.

PREVENT RECURRENCE
- The risks of recurrence following PCTA (percutaneous transluminal angioplasty) in fibromuscular dysplasia are quite small but can be minimized by inserting a stent at the time of angioplasty
- This is less effective in the atherosclerotic type of stenosis as these lesions are more often at the ostium and it is technically difficult to insert and maintain a stent at this site
- Strictly speaking recurrence cannot therefore be prevented, but regular follow-up will identify it early and allow time for modification of treatment to prevent worsening of the condition

ASSOCIATIONS

National Kidney Foundation
30 East 33rd St., Suite 1100
New York, NY 10016
Phone: (800) 622-9010
or (212) 889-2210
Fax: (212) 689-9261
http://www.kidney.org

KEY REFERENCES

- Safian RD, Textor SC. Renal-artery stenosis. New Engl J Med 2001;344:431–442
- Dustan HP. Essential hypertension, Part I – Renal arterial disease and hypertension. Med Clin North Am 1997;81(5):1199–212
- Ramsay LE, Waller PC. Blood pressure response to percutaneous transluminal angioplasty for renovascular hypertension; an overview of published series. BMJ 1990;300(6724):569–72
- National High Blood Pressure Education Program Working Group. 1995 update of the working group reports on chronic renal failure and renovascular hypertension. Arch Intern Med 1996;156:1938–47

Evidence references and guidelines

1   Guidelines for percutaneous transluminal angioplasty. J Vasc Interv Radiol 1990;4:5–15. Guidelines developed by the Society of Cardiovascular and Interventional Radiology. Also available at the National Guideline Clearinghouse

FAQS
Question 1

In primary care practice, in which patients should significant renal artery stenosis be suspected as contributing to their clinical problems?

ANSWER 1

Although renal artery stenosis can occur at all ages, practically it is most commonly seen in patients over age 50 (particularly diabetics) who have evidence of generalized atherosclerosis. This may be manifested by severe, difficult to control, diastolic hypertension (with high plasma renin levels) and/or ischemic nephropathy with progressive renal failure.

Question 2

How effective are angiotensin-converting enzyme (ACE) inhibitors in the management of renal artery stenosis?

ANSWER 2

They can be quite effective in helping to control hypertension (in combination with other antihypertensive drugs), and this type of medical therapy is generally indicated prior to attempting invasive, corrective procedures. ACE inhibitors are contraindicated, however, in patients with renal artery stenosis who have renal insufficiency or who have bilateral disease.

Question 3
In patients with severe hypertension and unilateral renal-artery stenosis, what is the status of various types of revascularization procedures?

ANSWER 3
The type of procedure to be attempted depends on the age of the patient, the etiology of the stenosis, and the presence of concomitant cardiovascular and metabolic diseases. Angioplasty and surgery have been the major therapeutic approaches. Angioplasty is more likely to correct hypertension in young patients with fibrous dysplasia than in elderly patients with atherosclerosis. However, recent use of intravascular stents appears to have improved success rates in elderly patients. In general, if feasible, angioplasty with stents should be attempted first. Surgical revascularization may be quite effective in selected patients. Surgery may not be feasible in elderly patients who are at risk of myocardial infarction and stroke.

Question 4
What are the most important clues for the primary care physician that should trigger referral and evaluation for possible, treatable renal vascular stenosis?

ANSWER 4
The 3 most important clues are:
1. Asymmetry of size between the two kidneys in a hypertensive patient.
2. Renal insufficiency in a patient over age 50 who has evidence of generalized atherosclerosis (coronaries and/or peripheral arteries) with a relatively benign urinalysis.
3. Severe, difficult to control, diastolic hypertension at any age that is not associated with a primary renal disease, particularly with a negative family history of hypertension.

CONTRIBUTORS
Gordon H Baustian, MD
Martin Goldberg, MD, FACP
Jennifer E Weil, MD

ACUTE RENAL FAILURE

DESCRIPTION

- Three types are recognized: prerenal, intrinsic, and postrenal
- Prenal failure is more common in hospitalized patients; intrinsic and postrenal failure are seen in both hospitalized patients and those in the community
- Most common subtype of intrinsic acute renal failure is acute tubular necrosis (ATN)
- In favorable circumstances, almost complete recovery is possible
- Prognosis is more guarded in elderly or chronically ill patients

URGENT ACTION

- Commence intravenous fluids (normal saline usually satisfactory in emergency situations) for patients with volume depletion, acute blood loss, major trauma, or burns prior to urgent transfer to hospital. This may reduce incidence and severity of prerenal failure and ATN
- Insert urinary catheter if patient has retention of urine
- If transfer to hospital is delayed, patient may require emergency treatment for hyperkalemia with intravenous insulin and dextrose. Discuss first with admitting physician if possible
- Arrange urgent transfer for all patients with rapid deterioration of renal function, oliguria, life-threatening comorbidity, evidence of urinary tract obstruction, or hyperkalemia (particularly if ECG changes are present)

KEY! DON'T MISS!

Carefully obtain recent history of potentially causative factors, such as vomiting, diarrhea, hemorrhage, exposure to nephrotoxins (especially antibiotics and radiocontrast media).

BACKGROUND

ICD9 CODE
584.9 Acute renal failure, unspecified

SYNONYMS
ARF.

CARDINAL FEATURES
- Impairment of renal function leading to retention in blood of substances normally eliminated by the kidneys
- Prerenal failure follows renal hypoperfusion due to a reduction in effective arterial blood volume
- Intrinsic renal failure is most commonly associated with ATN following severe systemic insult, e.g. surgery, trauma, burns, hypotension
- Postrenal failure is usually caused by urinary tract obstruction
- Clinical features are a combination of the signs and symptoms of renal failure and of the underlying cause
- Prerenal failure is seen more commonly in hospitalized patients
- Intrinsic and postrenal failure are seen in both hospitalized patients and those in the community
- ATN may be associated with oliguria (<400–500mL urine/24h) or nonoliguria
- Prognosis depends on severity and duration of causative factors of acute renal failure, presence of comorbidity, and age of patient; prognosis is worse in oliguric form of ATN and is more guarded in elderly or chronically ill patients
- In favorable circumstances, almost complete recovery is possible

CAUSES
Common causes
Prerenal failure:
- Hypovolemia (e.g. hemorrhage, gastrointestinal losses, burns)
- Volume overload with reduced renal perfusion (e.g. severe congestive heart failure)
- Peripheral vasodilation

Intrinsic renal failure:
- ATN: ischemic-prolonged prerenal state, sepsis syndrome, systemic hypotension; nephrotoxic-aminoglycoside antibiotics, methotrexate, cisplatinum, myoglobin (rhabdomyolysis), hemoglobin, radiocontrast media

Postrenal failure:
- Ureteric obstruction
- Bladder outflow obstruction (prostatism)

Rare causes
Prerenal failure:
- Renal vessel occlusion

Intrinsic renal failure:
- Acute glomerulonephritis, particularly in adults (e.g. due to vasculitis, systemic lupus erythematosus)
- Renal infarction (bilateral renal artery stenosis, renal vein thrombosis)
- Hemolytic uremic syndrome (thrombotic thrombocytopenic purpura)

Postrenal failure:
- Urethral obstruction

Serious causes

All causes of acute renal failure are potentially serious since overall mortality rate is 40–50%.

Contributory or predisposing factors

Prerenal failure:

- Advanced heart disease with very low cardiac output
- Bilateral renal artery stenosis due to reduced renal perfusion
- Systemic sepsis, especially if peripheral vasodilation has occurred
- Extracellular volume depletion: children and the elderly are particularly susceptible
- Acute blood loss following, for example, major trauma or gastrointestinal or postpartum hemorrhage
- 'Third space' fluid loss in patients with intestinal obstruction or ileus
- Severe burns
- Hepatic failure may cause hepatorenal syndrome with intense renal vasoconstriction

Intrinsic renal failure:

- Administration of nephrotoxic drugs, commonly aminoglycoside antibiotics. Rare in outpatient setting
- Administration of radiographic contrast media; patients with diabetes or impaired renal function are particularly susceptible
- Acute glomerulonephritis. Most common type in children is following a streptococcal infection. In adults, other causes predominate with poorer prognosis
- Previous renal transplant with acute or chronic rejection
- Systemic sepsis

Postrenal failure:

- Renal calculi. A large calculus can cause obstruction at the ureteropelvic junction
- Ureteric calculi. May cause obstruction at any level in the ureter. Bilateral obstruction can cause renal failure, but this is uncommon
- Benign prostatic hyperplasia. Prostatic enlargement may lead to bladder outlet obstruction
- Prostatic carcinoma. Prostatic enlargement may lead to bladder outlet obstruction or distal ureteric obstruction, which is often bilateral
- Bladder carcinoma. Tumor adjacent to the ureteric orifices may cause obstruction. Less commonly, urothelial cancer can also involve the ureters at any level. Again this may cause obstruction
- Cervical carcinoma. In advanced disease, distal ureters may be compressed by tumor
- Posterior urethral valves: in young boys
- Urethral stricture. If severe and long-standing, obstructive renal failure may occur
- Retroperitoneal fibrosis. May cause bilateral obstruction at any level of the ureters

EPIDEMIOLOGY

Incidence and prevalence

INCIDENCE

Incidence of acute renal failure severe enough to require dialysis is 0.05 per 1000.

Demographics

AGE

May occur at any age, although the various underlying causes are more common in specific age groups.

DIFFERENTIAL DIAGNOSIS
Chronic renal failure
Chronic renal failure is the most important differential diagnosis.

FEATURES
- Usually develops progressively over several months to years
- Signs and symptoms similar to those of acute renal failure
- Renal ultrasound scan may demonstrate small, shrunken kidneys
- Recognized complication of a number of chronic conditions, especially diabetes, accelerated hypertension, and chronic glomerulonephritis

SIGNS & SYMPTOMS
Signs
- Skin pallor
- Ecchymoses
- Peripheral edema
- Tachypnea
- Tachycardia
- Confusion
- Seizures

Symptoms
- May be asymptomatic
- Lethargy, weakness
- Anorexia
- Nausea
- General malaise
- Muscle cramps

ASSOCIATED DISORDERS
- Patients with acute renal failure are especially susceptible to bacterial infections and sepsis
- Urinary tract infection is often associated with postrenal failure

KEY! DON'T MISS!
Carefully obtain recent history of potentially causative factors, such as vomiting, diarrhea, hemorrhage, exposure to nephrotoxins (especially antibiotics and radiocontrast media).

CONSIDER CONSULT
All patients with evidence of impaired renal function should be referred. Degree of urgency depends on:
- Patient's age: children and the elderly are often more seriously ill
- Rapidity and severity of deterioration in renal function
- Presence of life-threatening comorbidity
- Evidence of urinary tract obstruction
- Presence of hyperkalemia (with or without ECG changes)

INVESTIGATION OF THE PATIENT
Direct questions to patient
Q How long have you felt unwell? May give an indication of length of time patient has suffered from renal failure.
Q What medications are you taking? A number of drugs, particularly antibiotics, may cause renal failure, although this is less common in the outpatient setting.

Q Do you have any pain in your abdomen or back? May indicate presence of urinary tract calculi, retention of urine, or other intra-abdominal pathology, particularly malignancy.

Q Do you think you are passing less urine than normal? May indicate onset of oliguria.

Q Do you think you have any difficulty passing urine? May indicate bladder outflow obstruction.

Q Does your occupation involve exposure to potentially nephrotoxic substances? e.g. ethylene glycol, carbon tetrachloride.

Contributory or predisposing factors

Q Do you have any history of heart disease? Particularly ischemic heart disease, cardiomyopathy, or valvular heart disease.

Q Do you have any history of kidney problems, protein, or blood in the urine? Especially glomerulonephritis, nephritis of any other type, or renal vessel occlusion.

Q Have you had a kidney transplant? Transplanted kidneys are more vulnerable to systemic insult. Deterioration may also indicate rejection of the allograft.

Q Have you ever had a kidney stone? Recurrent stone disease may be present.

Q Have you recently had any X-rays involving an injection of dye? Risk of radiographic contrast nephropathy.

Q Are you diabetic? Risk of renal disease is greater in diabetic patients.

Q Have you had any other serious illnesses in the past? Particularly malignancy, which can cause postrenal failure.

Examination

▪ Check temperature: pyrexia may be observed if patient has systemic sepsis

▪ Check blood pressure: hypertension may indicate pre-existing chronic intrinsic renal disease; hypotension may be present if patient has prerenal failure due to volume depletion

▪ Assess volume status: patients with prerenal failure may be volume depleted. Check for orthostatic hypotension, tachycardia, low jugular venous pressure (JVP), dry mucous membranes, absence of axillary sweat

▪ Auscultate heart and lungs for signs of congestive cardiac failure

▪ Examine the abdomen: a palpable bladder indicates bladder outflow obstruction; palpable kidney may indicate ureteric obstruction; any unexplained abdominal mass may indicate malignancy. A bruit may be heard in renovascular disease

▪ Perform bimanual vaginal examination if pelvic or intra-abdominal malignancy suspected

▪ Perform digital rectal examination if pelvic or intra-abdominal malignancy suspected and to assess size and consistency of prostate gland

Summary of investigative tests

▪ Urinalysis (dipstick) should be performed in all patients; provides rapid confirmation of a variety of abnormalities, including hematuria and proteinuria

▪ Urine microscopy: microscopic examination of urine sediment may be extremely useful in differential diagnosis of acute renal failure: confirms presence or absence of red (RBCs) or white blood cells (WBCs), RBC casts characteristic of glomerulonephritis, and WBC casts seen in acute pyelonephritis; in acute tubular necrosis, muddy brown, coarsely granular casts are typical, associated with large numbers of tubular epithelial cells and occasionally epithelial cell casts

▪ Chemical analysis of spot urine specimen for sodium, osmolality, and creatinine: extremely helpful in differential diagnosis of oliguria; enables calculation of fractional excretion of sodium (FENa) by renal consultant.

For urinary chemical findings in acute renal failure see below*.

▪ Urine culture should be performed because urinary tract infection may be associated, particularly with obstructive (postrenal) failure

- Full blood count should be performed in all patients because anemia and leukocytosis of infection may be present
- Blood urea nitrogen (BUN) and serum creatinine: serial estimation of serum creatinine and BUN is mandatory for diagnosis and monitoring of renal failure
- Serum sodium, potassium, and bicarbonate should be checked in all patients because hyperkalemia and metabolic acidosis are commonly associated with acute renal failure and hyponatremia due to impaired water excretion is common in oliguric states
- 24h urine collection to examine a variety of parameters, including actual volume produced and amount of protein excreted over 24h. This test would usually be supervised by a specialist
- Liver function tests are required in patients with known or suspected malignancy or if patient has any clinical evidence of liver failure
- Blood cultures: for patients with systemic sepsis. These would only be performed in hospital
- Chest X-ray: perform if congestive cardiac failure is suspected
- Abdominal X-ray: perform if renal or ureteric calculi are suspected
- Renal ultrasound scan: imaging investigation of choice in renal failure; measures size of each kidney and determines presence or absence of hydronephrosis and of postmicturition residual volume
- Antegrade or retrograde pyelogram to evaluate ureteric obstruction. This would be performed by a specialist
- ECG: significant disturbances of electrolyte balance may result in ECG changes, particularly hyperkalemia
- Renal biopsy may be performed in cases of intrinsic renal failure where the underlying diagnosis is in doubt. Would be performed by a specialist

*Prenal: Urine [Na] <20mEq/L; FENa <1%; urine osmolality >500mOsm/kg.
ATN: Urine [Na] >40mEq/L; FENa >1%; urine osmolality 200–400mOsm/kg.

DIAGNOSTIC DECISION
- Usually based on an accurate history; careful physical examination; serial analysis of BUN, serum creatinine, and serum electrolytes; and careful monitoring of urine output
- Microscopic examination of urine sediment and chemical analysis of a spot urine specimen for sodium, osmolality, and creatinine are essential in establishing the correct diagnosis

Guidelines
An official publication of the Scientific Advisory Board of the National Kidney Foundation [1]

CLINICAL PEARLS
- It is important to differentiate oliguric from nonoliguric ATN. In the oliguric form, severity of initial renal insult is greater and complications of fluid overload, hyperkalemia, and hyponatremia are more likely and more severe than in the nonoliguric form
- Examination of urine sediment is essential to the diagnosis and differential diagnosis. Most clinical laboratories do not have the time or experience to seek out and recognize the critically important and nearly pathognomonic findings of RBC casts in acute glomerulonephritis or muddy brown granular and tubular epithelial cells and casts in ATN. If primary care physician is inexperienced in this procedure, he/she must make sure that a fresh urine specimen is available for the nephrology consultant
- Interpretation of results of urine sodium, osmolality, and creatinine tests is critical to establishing the correct diagnosis in acute renal failure. The primary care physician bears the responsibility for ordering these tests simultaneously with the request for the nephrology consultation

THE TESTS
Body fluids
URINALYSIS (DIPSTICK)
Description
Midstream urine specimen.

Advantages/Disadvantages
Advantages:
- Quick and simple to perform at office level
- Provides information about a variety of urinary constituents very quickly

Disadvantage: very nonspecific; any abnormalities found are not diagnostic of a particular disorder

Normal
- No RBCs or WBCs
- No or only small amount of protein

Abnormal
- RBCs and/or WBCs, and/or large amount of protein present. If significant proteinuria suspected, patient requires a 24h urine collection so that this may be quantified. Normal result is <150mg/day (<0.15g/day). Specialist referral is usually required for this
- Keep in mind the possibility of a false-positive result

Cause of abnormal result
The glomerular membrane, which in a healthy kidney prevents large molecules from escaping into the urine, can no longer do so.

Drugs, disorders and other factors that may alter results
If patient is a woman of childbearing age, check that she is not menstruating because this may lead to a false-positive result.

URINE MICROSCOPY
Description
Centrifuged urine specimen.

Advantages/Disadvantages
Advantages:
- Presence of dysmorphic RBCs or RBC or WBC casts is highly suggestive of an underlying intrinsic renal disorder, such as glomerulonephritis
- Large numbers of tubular epithelial cells, epithelial cell casts, and muddy brown, coarsely granular casts are compatible with diagnosis of ATN

Disadvantages:
- Procedure is not standardized, and degree of urinary sediment concentration may vary
- Quantitative reports can be difficult to interpret
- None of the findings is absolutely pathognomonic

Normal
- 0–2 RBCs per high-power field (hpf)
- 0–5 WBCs per hpf
- Occasional cast only

Abnormal
- >2 RBCs/hpf
- >5 WBCs/hpf
- Casts: hyaline casts in prerenal failure; muddy brown granular casts in ATN; cellular casts in glomerulonephritis

Cause of abnormal result
- The glomerular membrane, which in the healthy kidney prevents large molecules from escaping into the urine, may no longer do so
- Casts are aggregates of protein, blood cells, or both. They may develop secondary to urinary stasis in renal tubules in the presence of proteinuria

Drugs, disorders and other factors that may alter results
If patient is a woman of childbearing age, check that she is not menstruating because this may lead to a false-positive result

URINE CULTURE
Description
Midstream urine specimen.

Advantages/Disadvantages
Advantages:
- Confirms or refutes diagnosis of urinary tract infection
- Identifies bacteria responsible

Disadvantage: presence of a urinary tract infection may be incidental and unrelated to underlying cause of patient's renal failure

Normal
No bacteria cultured.

Abnormal
Bacteria cultured.

Cause of abnormal result
Presence of infection.

Drugs, disorders and other factors that may alter results
Urine sample may be contaminated, e.g. by skin or bowel commensal organisms.

FULL BLOOD COUNT
Description
Cuffed venous blood sample.

Advantages/Disadvantages
Advantages:
- Confirms or excludes anemia
- Mandatory for evaluating severity of acute blood loss (although this would not be appropriate in the primary care situation)

Disadvantages:
- Does not indicate underlying cause of anemia
- Children particularly may find venepuncture distressing

Normal

Hemoglobin:

- Men: 13–17g/dL (130–170g/L)
- Women: 12–15g/dL (120–150g/L)

Abnormal

Hemoglobin:

- Men: <13g/dL (<130g/L)
- Women: <12g/dL (<120g/L)

Cause of abnormal result

- Acute blood loss
- Reduced RBC production

Drugs, disorders and other factors that may alter results

- Anemia is seen as part of many disorders
- Anemia with no obvious explanation may require investigation itself

SERUM BLOOD UREA NITROGEN (BUN) AND CREATININE

Description

- Cuffed venous blood sample
- May be combined with measurement of serum electrolytes

Advantages/Disadvantages

Advantages:

- Mandatory for assessing whether renal function is impaired
- Serial measurements may be used to monitor patient's progress
- BUN:creatinine ratio may help differentiate type of renal failure

Disadvantage: invasive procedure; children especially may find repeated venepuncture distressing

Normal

- BUN: 10–20mg/dL (3.6–7.1mmol/L)
- Creatinine: <1.5mg/dL (<133mcmol/L)
- Note that reference ranges can vary; check with local laboratory
- Also, since serum creatinine level is a function of body muscle mass, normal levels for males are higher than those for females

Abnormal

- BUN: >20mg/dL (>7.1mmol/L)
- Creatinine: >1.5mg/dL (>133mcmol/L)
- Keep in mind the possibility of a false-positive result
- BUN:creatinine ratio >20:1 in prerenal failure but not extremely sensitive regarding diagnosis

Cause of abnormal result

Impaired clearance of nitrogenous waste products from blood.

Drugs, disorders and other factors that may alter results

Laboratory technique can affect results.

SERUM POTASSIUM

Description

- Cuffed venous blood sample
- May wish to combine with measuring BUN and serum creatinine

Advantages/Disadvantages

- Advantage: allows identification of hyperkalemia, which has important bearing on patient's cardiovascular status
- Disadvantage: invasive procedure; children especially may find repeated venepuncture distressing

Normal

- 3.3–5.0mEq/L (3.3–5.0mmol/L)
- Note that reference ranges vary; check with local laboratory

Abnormal

- <3.3mEq/L (<3.3mmol/L) or >5.0mEq/L (>5.0mmol/L)
- Keep in mind the possibility of a false-positive result

Cause of abnormal result

Impaired clearance of excess potassium from the blood.

Drugs, disorders and other factors that may alter results

- Hemolyzed blood sample
- Significant delay between taking and analyzing sample

SERUM SODIUM

Description

- Cuffed venous blood sample
- May wish to combine with measuring BUN and serum creatinine

Advantages/Disadvantages

- Advantage: allows identification of hyponatremia, which is a manifestation of positive water balance, especially in oliguric states
- Disadvantage: invasive procedure; children especially may find repeated venepuncture distressing

Normal

- 135–145mEq/L (135–145mmol/L)
- Note that reference ranges vary; check with local laboratory

Abnormal

- <135mEq/L (<135mmol/L) or >145mEq/L (>145mmol/L)
- Keep in mind the possibility of a false-positive result

Cause of abnormal result

Impaired water excretion relative to body sodium content due to renal failure.

Drugs, disorders and other factors that may alter results

- Severe hyperlipidemia or hyperproteinemia
- Significant delay between taking and analyzing sample

SODIUM BICARBONATE
Description
- Cuffed venous blood sample
- May wish to combine with measuring BUN and serum creatinine

Advantages/Disadvantages
- Advantage: allows identification of metabolic acidosis, which has important bearing on patient's metabolic status
- Disadvantage: invasive procedure; children especially may find repeated venepuncture distressing

Normal
- 23–28mEq/L (23–28mmol/L)
- Note that reference ranges vary; check with local laboratory

Abnormal
- <23mEq/L (<23mmol/L) or >28mEq/L (>28mmol/L)
- Keep in mind the possibility of a false-positive result

Cause of abnormal result
Impaired renal excretion of fixed acid due to diffuse renal damage.

Drugs, disorders and other factors that may alter results
- Administration of sodium bicarbonate
- Significant delay between taking and analyzing sample

Tests of function
LIVER FUNCTION TESTS
Description
Cuffed venous blood sample.

Advantages/Disadvantages
Advantage: provides information regarding a number of aspects of liver function

Disadvantages:
- Results are mainly nonspecific and not diagnostic of a particular disorder
- Invasive procedure; children particularly may find venepuncture distressing

Normal
Many parameters are measured. Some of the most useful are:
- Alkaline phosphatase: 30–120U/L (0.5–2.0mckat/L)
- Alanine aminotransferase: 0–35U/L (0–0.58mckat/L)
- Albumin: 3.5–5.5g/dL (35–55g/L)
- Bilirubin: direct (conjugated) 0.1–0.3mg/dL (1.7–5.1mcmol/L); indirect (unconjugated) 0.2–0.7mg/dL (3.4–12mcmol/L); total 0.3–1.0mg/dL (5.1–17mcmol/L)

Abnormal
- Alkaline phosphatase: >120U/L (>2.0mckat/L)
- Alanine aminotransferase: >35U/L (> 0.58mckat/L)
- Albumin: <3.5g/dL (35g/L)
- Bilirubin: direct (conjugated) >0.3mg/dL (>5.1mcmol/L); indirect (unconjugated) >0.7mg/dL (>12mcmol/L); total >1.0mg/dL (>17mcmol/L)
- Keep in mind the possibility of a falsely abnormal result

Cause of abnormal result
Abnormal liver function.

Drugs, disorders and other factors that may alter results
- Excessive alcohol consumption
- Many disease processes
- If cause of abnormal liver function not apparent, this may require investigation in itself

Imaging
ABDOMINAL X-RAY
Description
Radiograph of abdomen.

Advantages/Disadvantages
Advantages:
- Quick and simple to perform
- May identify presence of urinary tract calculi

Disadvantages:
- Involves exposure to radiation
- Whether normal or abnormal, will not diagnose acute renal failure or its underlying cause

Abnormal
In the context of acute renal failure, abnormalities that may be seen include:
- Renal calculi
- Ureteric calculi
- Keep in mind the possibility of a false-positive result

Drugs, disorders and other factors that may alter results
Phleboliths in the pelvis may resemble ureteric calculi.

CHEST X-RAY
Description
Radiograph of chest.

Advantages/Disadvantages
Advantages:
- Quick and simple to perform
- Variety of conditions may be diagnosed

Disadvantage: involves exposure to radiation

Abnormal
Abnormalities that may be seen include:
- Cardiomegaly
- Pulmonary edema

Cause of abnormal result
Congestive cardiac failure.

RENAL TRACT ULTRASOUND SCAN

Description

- Ultrasound scan of kidneys, ureters, and bladder
- May be combined with measurement of postmicturition residual urine volume

Advantages/Disadvantages

Advantages:

- Noninvasive
- No exposure to radiation
- May be performed in pregnancy
- May be repeated as often as required, with no risk to patient
- In patients with obstructive renal failure, may indicate level and/or cause of obstruction

Disadvantage: specialist knowledge required for interpretation

Normal

Normal renal tract anatomy.

Abnormal

- Small kidneys (suggests chronic rather than acute process)
- Calculi
- Hydronephrosis
- Hydroureter
- Postmicturition residual volume (of urine)

Cause of abnormal result

- Hydronephrosis, hydroureter, and significant postmicturition residual volume are caused by urinary tract obstruction
- Keep in mind possibility of false-positive result

Drugs, disorders and other factors that may alter results

- Congenital megaureter (hydroureter)
- If patient's bladder is overfull prior to scan, a falsely high postmicturition residual volume may be obtained

Other tests
ELECTROCARDIOGRAPH (ECG)
Description
Noninvasive test of cardiac function.

Advantages/Disadvantages
Advantages:
- Simple to perform
- Provides evidence of a wide variety of cardiac abnormalities
- If patient has hyperkalemia, abnormalities may be identified that require emergency treatment

Disadvantages:
- Special equipment required
- Experience required to interpret results

Abnormal
Many abnormalities may be identified, especially in relation to acute renal failure; peaked T waves may be seen in hyperkalemia.

Cause of abnormal result
Abnormal cardiac function.

Drugs, disorders and other factors that may alter results
- Movement artifact if patient does not lie still
- Presence of cardiac pacemaker will alter appearance of trace

TREATMENT

CONSIDER CONSULT

Patients with evidence of prerenal or intrinsic failure should be referred to a nephrologist. Patients with evidence of postrenal failure should also be referred to a urologist.

IMMEDIATE ACTION

- Commencement of intravenous fluids if evidence of hypovolemia or dehydration
- Insertion of urethral catheter if evidence of bladder outflow obstruction
- Patients with severe hyperkalemia who cannot be transferred to hospital immediately should receive, if possible, an ECG and then be given emergency treatment with intravenous insulin plus glucose

PATIENT AND CAREGIVER ISSUES
Forensic and legal issues

Acute renal failure may cause confusion, especially in the elderly. Emergency treatment, particularly commencement of intravenous fluids, may be lifesaving but may need to be done without patient's consent.

Impact on career, dependants, family, friends

Patients may develop a chronic illness, which can severely impact on their ability to go to school, go to work, or undertake sporting or social activities. Treatment regimens may interfere with these aspects and disrupt family life in general.

Patient or caregiver request

Most patients with acute renal failure have potentially reversible renal disease. Ultimate prognosis depends on severity and persistence of causative factors, which typically are multiple.

Health seeking behavior

Has patient delayed seeing a doctor? Patients may not recognize potential seriousness of their symptoms and delay seeking medical advice; symptoms may be more advanced at time of diagnosis, and irreversible kidney damage may have occurred.

MANAGEMENT ISSUES
Goals

- To recognize need for referral early
- To provide support for patient and caretakers if patient has, or subsequently develops, a chronic illness

Management in special circumstances

Many patients have significant comorbidity that requires concurrent treatment.

COEXISTING DISEASE

In patients with systemic sepsis, potentially nephrotoxic antibiotics (particularly aminoglycosides) should be avoided or the dose reduced.

COEXISTING MEDICATION

Dosages of many drugs need to be modified in the presence of renal failure; some need to be discontinued. Review all of patient's coexisting medication.

SPECIAL PATIENT GROUPS

- Pregnant women: choice of medications (particularly antibiotics) limited to those that are not known to be harmful to the fetus, unless mother's survival requires them

- Patient with trauma or burns: treatment for renal failure will be undertaken concurrently with emergency treatment of injuries. Early treatment likely to lessen severity of acute renal failure
- Patient with a renal allograft: any treatment commenced in the community should first be discussed with patient's nephrologist. Patient should then be referred as soon as possible

PATIENT SATISFACTION/LIFESTYLE PRIORITIES
Patients with significant comorbidity, particularly the elderly, may opt for the simplest, least-invasive treatment options.

SUMMARY OF THERAPEUTIC OPTIONS
Choices
- Treatment may need to be concurrent with that for an underlying condition
- Specific treatment depends on type of renal failure present, although some modes will be common to all types
- Some treatments require patient to be hospitalized before they can be commenced
- Prerenal failure: hypovolemia, if present, is treated with intravenous fluids, which should be commenced prior to transfer to hospital
- Intrinsic renal failure: few effective treatments are available, but aggressive fluid resuscitation to restore intravascular volume may reduce incidence of ATN
- Postrenal failure: immediate treatment consists of relieving obstruction. Patients with lower urinary obstruction should be catheterized, and patients with upper urinary tract obstruction require insertion of a nephrostomy or ureteric stent
- Hyperkalemia may be treated orally with sodium polystyrene sulfonate or in an emergency with intravenous insulin and dextrose
- Dietary modification may be necessary in ATN to provide adequate calories while minimizing accumulation of toxins by moderate short-term protein restriction. Prolonged protein restriction is inadvisable and may delay recovery
- Doses of potentially nephrotoxic drugs may need to be modified or drug discontinued
- All patients with acute renal failure refractory to simple measures may require dialysis

Guidelines
- A summary of established guidelines on management of acute renal failure.[2]

Clinical pearls
- In the early phases of acute renal failure, once ATN is diagnosed, careful fluid and dietary management is essential. Once patient has been appropriately volume-repleted, forcing the administration of additional large quantities of intravenous or oral fluids is not indicated and may produce life-threatening complications of fluid overload and hyponatremic water intoxication. Furthermore, the dietary potassium load closely parallels the protein intake in addition to catabolism of endogenous protein. Hence moderate protein restriction (0.6–0.8g/day) is indicated. If it appears that the patient will enter a long course of renal failure with repeated dialytic treatments, then protein intake needs to be sharply increased
- If patient has acute prerenal failure associated with volume depletion and exhibits a low urine sodium level, i.e. <20mEq/L (<20mmol/L), then diuretics should be avoided and fluid replacement should be initiated until central hemodynamics are restored. This type of therapy mandates admission to a critical care facility
- In the emergency therapy of hyperkalemia, sodium polystyrene resins (Kayexalate) play no role since it takes several hours for sufficient potassium to be exchanged onto the resin in the gut. Resins are useful in the prevention of hyperkalemia and in the maintenance of normal potassium levels in patients with impaired renal potassium excretion

Never
Never commence treatment for hyperkalemia without a recent serum potassium level, a facility to monitor the ECG, and preferably not before discussion with a nephrologist.

FOLLOW UP
Plan for review
- Initially, when the patient is usually in hospital, daily (or even twice daily) estimation of BUN, serum creatinine, and serum electrolytes
- Selected patients require repeated measurements after discharge from hospital.

Information for patient or caregiver
- Patients with acute renal failure require close observation, especially if they are very ill and/or are commencing treatment; daily blood tests may be required
- Different treatments may be required depending on underlying cause of acute renal failure
- It is very important that the patient heeds any advice given regarding changes to his/her medications and diet

DRUGS AND OTHER THERAPIES: DETAILS
Drugs
SODIUM POLYSTYRENE SULFONATE
Dose
Adult:
- 15g given orally up to four times each day
- 30–50g/100mL sorbitol warmed to body temperature every 6h, given rectally

Child:
- 1g/kg every 6h, given orally or rectally

Administer in approximately 25% sorbitol suspension or concurrently treat with 70% oral sorbitol syrup 10–20mL every 2h to produce one or two watery stools per day

Efficacy
- High, but not effective acutely (i.e. <4–6h)
- Effective in all age groups for treating nonlife threatening hyperkalemia

Risks/Benefits
Risks:
- Use caution in patients who need to restrict sodium intake (hypertension, congestive heart failure, edema)
- Use caution in pregnancy

Benefits:
- Reduces serum potassium
- May be used on an outpatient basis

Side-effects and adverse reactions
- Cardiovascular system: congestive heart failure
- Gastrointestinal: nausea, vomiting, anorexia, abdominal pain, gastric irritation, diarrhea, constipation, bowel obstruction, bowel necrosis (after rectal administration)
- Metabolic: hypocalcemia, hypokalemia, sodium retention, hypomagnesemia

Interactions (other drugs)
- Antacids ▪ Calcium salts ▪ Digoxin (may enhance toxic effects of digoxin on the heart)
- Insulin ▪ Loop diuretics ▪ Sodium bicarbonate

Contraindications
- Hypokalemia ▪ Hypocalcemia ▪ Neonates ▪ Bowel obstruction

Acceptability to patient
Some find it unpalatable.

Follow up plan
- Monitor serum potassium, calcium, magnesium, sodium, acid-base balance
- Monitor bowel function

Patient and caregiver information
Do not administer mixed with orange juice.

INSULIN AND DEXTROSE
Normally used in hospitalized patients but may occasionally be used in the community in an emergency situation.

Dose
5–15U of regular insulin and 50mL of 50% dextrose over 5–15min, followed by a continuous infusion of 5% dextrose at 100mL/h to prevent late hypoglycemia.

Efficacy
- Highly effective for rapidly reducing serum potassium
- Most reliable agent for promoting transcellular shift of potassium

Risks/Benefits
- Risk: renal or hepatic impairment may require dose adjustment
- Benefit: produces rapid reduction in serum potassium

Side-effects and adverse reactions
- Metabolic: hypoglycemia, decreased ion concentrations (Ca, PO_4, K, Mg), insulin resistance, hyperglycemic rebound reaction
- Skin: flushing, rash, fat hypertrophy, pruritus, urticaria, anaphylactoid reactions

Interactions (other drugs)
- Anabolic steroids - Angiotensin-converting enzyme (ACE) inhibitors - Beta-blockers
- Cigarette smoking - Clonidine - Corticosteroids - Diazoxide - Ethanol - Fibrates
- Lithium - Monoamine oxidase inhibitors (MAOIs) - Nifedipine - Octreotide
- Salicylates - Sex hormones - Thiazides

Contraindications
Hypoglycemia.

Follow up plan
- Serum potassium should be reassessed 1h after intravenous insulin and dextrose therapy, and the infusion should be repeated if serum potassium is still dangerously elevated.
- Twice daily, or even more frequent serum potassium estimation thereafter

Endoscopic therapy
URETERIC STENT
- Accepted treatment for patients with benign underlying pathology and for selected patients with malignant underlying pathology
- To be inserted by experienced specialist-interventional radiologist or urologist

Efficacy
Highly effective for relieving upper urinary tract obstruction.

Risks/Benefits

Risks:

- General anesthetic usually required
- May be technically impossible in some patients
- May block
- May become encrusted with stone
- May migrate up or down ureter

Benefits:

- Can be used on a long-term basis if necessary
- Patient is not required to wear any form of external appliance
- May be inserted in an antegrade or retrograde fashion

Acceptability to patient

Well tolerated in most patients, although some do have significant side-effects: urinary frequency, flank pain, and hematuria.

Follow up plan

- Most stents need to be changed at 6–12 monthly intervals depending on type
- Some permanent stents are available

Patient and caregiver information

Stent commonly causes flank discomfort while passing urine.

PERCUTANEOUS NEPHROSTOMY

Efficacy

Highly effective for relieving upper urinary tract obstruction.

Risks/Benefits

Risks:

- May migrate outside kidney
- Discomfort at nephrostomy site

Benefits:

- Can be inserted under local anesthetic
- Can be used on a long-term basis if necessary
- Can be inserted prior to antegrade insertion of ureteric stent

Acceptability to patient

Variable; some patients find the need to wear an external appliance unacceptable and/or uncomfortable.

Follow up plan

- Regular estimation of BUN and serum creatinine
- Regular inspection of nephrostomy site

Patient and caregiver information

If tube stops draining urine, consult your doctor because it may mean that the tube is blocked or has become dislodged from the kidney.

Other therapies
URINARY CATHETER (URETHRAL OR SUPRAPUBIC)
Efficacy
High.

Risks/Benefits
Risks:
- Increased risk of urinary sepsis
- Can block
- Can become encrusted
- Patient may develop hematuria
- May promote development of bladder calculi

Benefits:
- Relief of bladder outflow obstruction
- Permits accurate monitoring of urine output

Acceptability to patient
Younger patients particularly may find this unacceptable on anything other than a short-term basis.

Follow up plan
- Regular inspection of catheter
- Regular serum creatinine and BUN estimation
- Depending on cause of obstruction, patient may remain catheterized until definitive treatment takes place
- If catheter is required on a long-term basis, it will need changing every 10 weeks

Patient and caregiver information
If catheter stops draining, it may be blocked. Consult your doctor because it may require changing.

DIETARY MODIFICATION
- Limit protein intake to 0.6g/kg/day on short-term basis
- Total caloric intake of 35–50kcal/kg/day
- Restrict sodium intake depending on urine volume; if 24h volume <400mL, give <80mEq (<80mmol/l) sodium daily
- Restrict potassium intake to 40mEq (40mmol/l)/day
- Restrict phosphorus intake to 800mg/day
- Avoid magnesium-containing foods altogether

Efficacy
Dietary manipulation is used as an adjunct but is not suitable for treating acute renal failure on its own.

Risks/Benefits
Benefits:
- Reduces nitrogenous waste production
- Reduces catabolism

Acceptability to patient
Some patients find the diet very restrictive.

Follow up plan

Regular monitoring to ensure that patient is adhering to diet and to identify any problems relating to diet so that they can be dealt with promptly.

Patient and caregiver information

All dietary advice should be strictly adhered to.

DIALYSIS

- Indicated when severe hyperkalemia, acidosis volume overload, or uremia cannot be controlled by conservative means
- Options are intermittent hemodialysis (IHD), peritoneal dialysis (PD), or continuous renal replacement therapy (CRRT)

Efficacy

High.

Risks/Benefits

Benefit: PD is relatively 'portable' and can be used in remote areas, if required.

Evidence

- Three of four randomized controlled trials (RCTs) comparing nonbiocompatible with biocompatible membrane dialysis in the management of critically ill patients with acute renal failure found that survival was significantly higher in patients treated with biocompatible membranes [3] *Level P*
- An RCT compared different doses of continuous renal replacement therapy. Mortality rate was significantly greater in the lower-dose arm [4] *Level P*

Acceptability to patient

Patients may find dialysis regimen restrictive but must be encouraged to comply.

Follow up plan

Regular monitoring of serum BUN and creatinine.

Patient and caregiver information

- Depending on cause of renal failure, dialysis may be needed for a short or long period of time
- Dialysis needs to be performed regularly to be effective

EFFICACY OF THERAPIES
- Conservative therapy results in complete recovery in many cases
- Relief of urinary tract obstruction is necessary for resolution of postrenal failure
- Dialysis is almost always effective for patients in whom initial conservative therapy fails

Evidence
PDxMD are unable to cite evidence that meets our criteria for evidence.

Review period
- Patients usually need to remain in hospital until renal function is stabilized or returned to normal
- Follow-up after discharge depends on individual patient and any underlying pathology. Those with a chronic underlying disorder need review initially every few days, and then weekly to monthly, depending on their condition

PROGNOSIS
- Depends on underlying cause
- Many cases resolve completely with conservative measures
- Dialysis may be considered for patients in whom initial conservative therapy fails and is almost always effective
- Patient with chronic underlying disease may recover from renal failure but remain unwell due to their underlying condition
- A few progress to chronic renal failure
- Overall, mortality rate is variable because it depends on underlying disease

Clinical pearls
- Overall mortality rate for ATN is 40–50%. Rate varies with etiology and clinical setting in which the renal insult occurs. It approaches 80% in elderly and/or diabetic patients who develop acute renal failure postoperatively, especially following major abdominal or vascular surgical procedures, and is similarly high following renal failure due to traumatic 'crush' injuries. Much lower rates are seen in patients under 60 years of age who develop nephrotoxic ATN (antibiotics, radiocontrast media, pigment nephropathy)
- Not all patients who recover from a prolonged period of ATN recover normal renal function. Mean recovery rate is probably 80%, and in a minority it may be as low as 30–40% of normal
- Patients who recover from oliguric ATN first enter an early diuretic phase in which urine output may rise to polyuric levels and yet overall renal function is poor. In this polyuric phase, patient is still subject to the complications of infection and hemorrhage and a significant morbidity and mortality rate. Prognosis improves considerably after patient enters the late diuretic phase, and BUN and creatinine decrease sharply

Recurrence
All types of acute renal failure may recur; patients with a chronic underlying disorder are particularly at risk.

Terminal illness
In patients with a terminal illness (e.g. advanced malignancy), acute renal failure may develop in final stages of the disease. Treatment choices are as for other patients, but in some cases, especially if patient's quality of life is poor, it may be appropriate not to commence any additional treatment. This should be discussed, as necessary, with the patient, their other physicians, and their caretakers.

COMPLICATIONS

- Chronic renal failure may occasionally occur as a consequence of acute renal failure
- Hemorrhages may occur, particularly if patient has a prolonged bleeding time. This may be due to accumulation of nitrogenous waste products in the blood or a deficiency of von Willebrand factor

CONSIDER CONSULT

Patients may require reconsultation if there is any further deterioration in renal function.

- Prerenal and intrinsic renal failure may be prevented or their severity reduced by early recognition and appropriate management of risk factors
- Obstructive renal failure can be prevented by permanent nephrostomy, ureteric stent, indwelling urinary catheter, or surgical treatment of bladder outflow obstruction

RISK FACTORS

- Cardiovascular disease of any pathology may lead to renal hypoperfusion
- Systemic sepsis
- Dehydration, children, and the elderly are particularly vulnerable
- Pre-existing renal disease
- Renal or ureteric calculi: ureteric calculi particularly may cause obstruction
- Prostatic enlargement is a risk factor for onset of acute urinary retention, which leads, in some cases, to obstructive renal failure
- Intra-abdominal or pelvic malignancy may cause ureteric obstruction
- Urethral obstruction

MODIFY RISK FACTORS

- Early recognition and treatment (medical or surgical) of cardiovascular disease of any pathology reduces risk of acute renal failure
- Prompt and aggressive treatment of systemic sepsis
- Prompt recognition and treatment (with intravenous fluids if necessary) may prevent onset of acute renal failure
- Pre-existing renal disease should be carefully monitored, although onset of acute renal failure may be difficult or impossible to prevent and may be a poor prognostic sign
- Early treatment of renal or ureteric calculi, by shock wave lithotripsy or endoscopic removal, may avoid an obstructive episode
- Pharmacologic or surgical treatment of prostatic enlargement may prevent onset of acute urinary retention, which can lead to obstructive renal failure
- Intra-abdominal or pelvic malignancy cannot be prevented, but regular monitoring of serum BUN and creatinine should ensure early recognition and treatment, which may reduce risk of permanent renal damage
- Surgical correction of urethral obstruction should reduce or prevent onset of complications, including acute renal failure

Lifestyle and wellness
DRUG HISTORY

Care should be taken when prescribing potentially nephrotoxic drugs, particularly to patients who already have impaired renal function or those with other risk factors for acute renal failure.

SCREENING

Screening is not appropriate for acute renal failure, but it is important to be aware of those groups of patients at high risk of developing it.

PREVENT RECURRENCE

- Obstructive renal failure may be prevented if cause of obstruction can be removed (e.g. calculus) or circumvented (e.g. by insertion of a ureteric stent or nephrostomy)
- Prerenal and intrinsic renal failure may be avoided by early recognition and treatment of potential risk factors; e.g. dehydration, cardiac failure, sepsis

Reassess coexisting disease

In patients being treated for a coexisting disease with a potentially nephrotoxic drug, it may be necessary to modify the dose or avoid the drug altogether.

ASSOCIATIONS
National Kidney Foundation
30 East 33rd Street, Suite 1100
New York, NY 10016
Phone: 800-622-9010, 212-889-2210
Fax: 212-689-9261
www.kidney.org

National Kidney and Urologic Diseases Information Clearinghouse
Box NKUDIC
Bethesda, MD 20893
http://www.niddk.nih.gov

KEY REFERENCES
- Brady HR, Brenner BM, Clarkson MR, Lieberthal W. Chapter on acute renal failure. In: Brenner BM, ed. Brenner & Rector's the kidney, 6th edn. Philadelphia: WB Saunders, 2000, p1201–46
- Greenberg A. Hyperkalemia: treatment options. Semin Nephrol 1998;18:46–57
- Paul AB, Love C, Chisholm GD. Management of bilateral ureteric obstruction and renal failure in advanced prostate cancer. Br J Urol 1994;74(5):642–5

The following information is from an official publication of the Scientific Advisory Board of the National Kidney Foundation:
1. Holley JL. Clinical approach to the diagnosis of acute renal failure. In: Greenberg A, ed. Primer on kidney diseases. New York: Academic Press, 2001
2. Hutchison FN. Management of acute renal failure. In: Greenberg A, ed. Primer on kidney diseases. New York: Academic Press, 2001

Evidence references and guidelines
3. Kellum JA, Leblanc M. Acute renal failure: kidney disorders. Clinical Evidence 2001;6:634–48. London: BMJ Publishing Group
4. Ronco C, Bellomo R, Homel P, et al. Effects of different doses in continuous veno-venous haemofiltration on outcomes of acute renal failure: a prospective randomized trial. Lancet 2000;356:26–30. Reviewed in Clinical Evidence 2001;6:634–48

FAQS
Question 1
If one sees a patient who is excreting absolutely no urine (total anuria), is the approach different from that of the oliguric and polyuric patients?

ANSWER 1
The approach is modified by altering the priority list of possible etiologies. The physician must always ensure that hypovolemia and renal hypoperfusion are not playing major contributory roles. If, after restoring central hemodynamics and repairing fluid deficits, anuria persists, then the most likely cause to be ruled out is obstructive uropathy. The site of obstruction can be anywhere in the urinary tract affecting the outflow of both kidneys. Make sure that a palpably enlarged bladder is not present on physical examination.

Question 2

What measures or drugs have been proven to be effective in reversing the progression of prerenal failure to intrinsic ATN?

ANSWER 2

Many drugs and procedures have been proposed and utilized, including volume expansion, intravenous mannitol, loop-acting diuretics, atrial natriuretic peptide, and 'renal-dose' dopamine. To date, with the possible exception of immediate volume re-expansion to restore central hemodynamics, none has been shown to be effective in the amelioration or prevention of ATN in any carefully performed study. Furthermore, volume expansion is only effective early in the course when there remains a significant prerenal component. Repeatedly attempting volume overexpansion, when it is clear that the effects on urine flow are minimal and central hemodynamics are normalized, may produce disastrous consequences related to fluid overload and acute pulmonary edema.

Question 3

For a patient with acute renal failure, what are the most important actions that the primary care physician should take in preparation for the visit by the consulting nephrologist?

ANSWER 3

The following are the most critical and are too often either omitted or incompletely performed:

- Obtain from the patient and/or patient's family a detailed history of possible causative factors, especially drugs, potential toxins, cardiac disease, liver disease, malignancies
- Obtain a fresh urine specimen from the bladder (not the catheter tubing) for microscopic examination by the physician. Do not send all of the scant 'precious fluid' to the hospital laboratory
- Send a portion of the urine (20–30mL if possible) to the chemistry laboratory for sodium, osmolality, and creatinine, while simultaneously sending blood for BUN, creatinine, and electrolytes. The results of these studies may be extremely helpful in differentiating the types of acute renal failure and determining the appropriate therapy
- Make sure an ECG is performed to help evaluate the cardiac impact of hyperkalemia

CONTRIBUTORS

Fred F Ferri, MD, FACP
Martin Goldberg, MD, FACP
Rakesh Gulati, MD

CHRONIC RENAL FAILURE

SUMMARY INFORMATION

DESCRIPTION

- Progressive deterioration in renal function of >3 months' duration
- Must be distinguished from end-stage renal disease; glomerular filtration rate (GFR) <15mL/min with uremic syndrome
- Must be distinguished from acute renal failure

URGENT ACTION

Urgent referral for dialysis is indicated when chronic renal insufficiency progresses to end-stage renal disease, as manifested by a creatinine clearance <15mL/min and the presence of one or more of the following uremic manifestations:

- Symptoms of uremic syndrome (e.g. incessant vomiting, encephalopathy)
- Overload of fluid in the lungs that cannot be removed by diuretics
- Metabolic acidosis
- Electrolyte abnormalities (especially hyperkalemia)

ICD9 CODE
585 Chronic renal failure

SYNONYMS
- Chronic renal insufficiency, CRI
- CRF
- Kidney failure

CARDINAL FEATURES
- Progressive deterioration in renal function of >3 months' duration
- Includes chronic renal insufficiency but not end-stage renal disease
- Accumulation of nitrogenous waste products in the blood (e.g. urea, creatinine)
- Electrolyte disturbances
- Metabolic acidosis
- Volume overload
- Anemia
- Most patients will progress to end-stage renal disease
- Typically, the above features do not become clinically evident until glomerular filtration rate (GFR) drops to <15mL/min

CAUSES
Common causes
- Diabetes mellitus type 1 or type 2
- Hypertension (severe)
- Chronic glomerulonephritis
- Polycystic kidney disease
- Obstructive nephropathy: due to e.g. benign prostatic hypertrophy, nephrolithiasis

Rare causes
- Tubular interstitial nephritis
- Drug toxicity
- Renal artery stenosis (bilateral)
- Viruses: hepatitis B, hepatitis C, HIV
- Autoimmune diseases, particularly systemic lupus erythematosus

EPIDEMIOLOGY
Incidence and prevalence
INCIDENCE
0.2 per 1000 per year.

Demographics
AGE
May occur at any age, although the various underlying causes are themselves more common in specific age groups.

RACE
African-Americans are more commonly affected by chronic renal insufficiency than Caucasians, although it is unclear whether this difference results from genetic or socioeconomic causes.

GENETICS
- Various inherited diseases result in chronic renal insufficiency (e.g. polycystic kidney disease, Alport's disease)
- Renal failure associated with type 1 diabetes mellitus has a strong genetic component

DIAGNOSIS

DIFFERENTIAL DIAGNOSIS
Acute renal failure
The most common differential diagnostic entity is acute renal failure.

FEATURES
- Three types are distinguished: prerenal (due to inadequate renal perfusion), intrinsic (due to disease of the kidney itself), and postrenal (due to obstruction of the renal tract that results in impairment of renal function)
- Many possible underlying conditions
- Clinical features are combined with those of underlying disease
- May resolve completely
- Small number of patients progress to chronic renal failure
- A long history and the lack of any acute insult, injury, or illness point to the likelihood of chronic disease rather than acute renal failure

SIGNS & SYMPTOMS
Signs
Signs of chronic renal insufficiency except hypertension do not appear until the glomerular filtration rate (GFR) is <15ml/min and, when present, suggest end-stage renal disease:
- Skin pallor
- Ecchymoses
- Skin excoriation
- Muscle wasting
- Subcutaneous skin nodules
- Asterixis
- Hypertension
- Edema
- Dyspnea, secondary to volume overload
- Hyperpnea or tachypnea secondary to severe metabolic acidosis

Symptoms
Symptoms do not begin until the GFR is <15mL/min and, when present, suggest end-stage renal disease:
- Fatigue
- Nausea
- Anorexia
- Pruritus
- Insomnia
- Breathlessness
- Taste disturbances
- Altered mental status

CONSIDER CONSULT
- All patients with serum creatinine persistently above normal levels (i.e. higher than the normal range for the laboratory on two or more successive laboratory determinations) should be referred to a nephrologist as early as possible. This facilitates the development of a plan for further diagnostic procedures when indicated (e.g. renal biopsy to determine etiologic diagnosis and pathologic extent of the disease) and recommendations for indicated specific and/or supportive therapy (e.g. angiotensin-converting enzyme inhibitors in diabetic nephropathy or immunosuppressive therapy in vasculitis, lupus)

INVESTIGATION OF THE PATIENT
Direct questions to patient

Q Have you ever been told you have blood or protein in your urine? May indicate a longer history of kidney disease than is perceived by the patient.

Q Have you ever been told your kidney tests are abnormal? May indicate a longer history of kidney disease than is perceived by the patient.

Q What medications or over-the-counter drugs do you take and for how long? This may provide clues to possible analgesic nephropathy from combinations of drugs such as NSAIDs, aspirin, and phenacetin.

Q Do you have difficulty initiating your urinary stream, increased frequency of urination, increased urination at night after retiring? Possible obstructive symptoms of prostatism in males; recurrent or chronic urinary tract infection in females.

Contributory or predisposing factors

Q Do you have any history of kidney problems? Especially inherited conditions.

Q Are you diabetic? Risk of renal disease is greater in diabetic patients.

Q Do you have high blood pressure? Risk of renal disease is greater in patients with hypertension.

Q Do you have hepatitis B, hepatitis C, or HIV? All of these can predispose to chronic renal insufficiency.

Q Do you have lupus? This is another disease that can predispose to chronic renal insufficiency.

Family history

Q Do any diseases run in your family? Inherited renal diseases (e.g. polycystic kidney disease, Alport's syndrome) can lead to renal failure.

Examination

- Check blood pressure. Hypertension is frequently associated with chronic renal failure
- Auscultate heart and lungs. Listen for signs of pulmonary edema, pleuritis, and pericarditis (pleural or pericardial rub), which occur in end-stage renal disease
- Skin. Look for excoriations caused by the patient scratching (may indicate uremic pruritus); indicates end-stage renal disease
- Abdomen. Kidneys may be palpable if enlarged (e.g. in polycystic kidney disease or ureteric obstruction). Presence of a palpable bladder may indicate bladder outflow obstruction
- Vascular. Check for bruits of carotid arteries and renal arteries, and examine for diminished peripheral pulses (femoral, dorsalis pedis, posterior tibial). The presence of generalized atheromatous disease increases the likelihood of renal artery stenosis

Summary of investigative tests

- Urinalysis (dipstick) should be performed in all patients and will provide rapid confirmation of a variety of abnormalities, including hematuria (if microscopic) and proteinuria
- Urine microscopy: microscopic examination of urine sediment will confirm the presence or absence of red or white blood cells and casts
- Creatinine clearance: must be an accurate, 24-h collection of urine, performed by a specialist; from this, the GFR can be estimated
- Complete blood count should be performed in all patients since anemia may be present
- Blood urea nitrogen and serum creatinine: serial estimation of serum creatinine and BUN is mandatory for diagnosis and monitoring of this condition
- Serum potassium should be measured, and serial measurements may be required, since patients are at risk of hyperkalemia when they reach end-stage renal disease
- 24-h urine protein: must be an accurate, 24-h collection of urine; the magnitude of proteinuria can be assessed and the nephrotic syndrome can be diagnosed

- A chest X-ray should be performed if there is dyspnea or if pulmonary edema is suspected
- A renal ultrasound scan is the imaging investigation of choice, since it can measure the size of each kidney and determine the presence or absence of hydronephrosis
- Renal biopsy is occasionally performed, but it is generally not recommended in patients with small kidneys or advanced renal disease since they are unlikely to respond to any form of specific medical therapy. If indicated, it would be performed by an experienced nephrologist or an invasive radiologist. If this is not feasible, an open renal biopsy might, on rare occasions, be performed by a urologist
- Early morning spot urine specimen for protein and creatinine assays. The albumin:creatinine ratio is a good predictor of rate of progression of renal disease
- Microalbuminuria screening in diabetics: elevated in early diabetic nephropathy

DIAGNOSTIC DECISION

- Presence of small, shrunken kidneys on renal ultrasound
- Evidence of impaired renal function for >3 months
- Presence of known underlying kidney disease, e.g. diabetes, glomerulonephritis, polycystic kidney disease

CLINICAL PEARLS

- Renal ultrasonography is most helpful in the differential diagnosis of chronic renal failure. Bilateral small kidneys definitely indicate chronic, long-standing renal disease, but normal-sized or large kidneys are also compatible with some important chronic renal diseases including diabetic nephropathy, myeloma kidney, and amyloidosis
- In the assessment of patients with chronic renal failure, prior to end-stage, it is useful to identify the category of renal disease, i.e. glomerular vs tubulointerstitial. It is important, therefore, to have available a reliable urinalysis with microscopy in these patients. In chronic glomerulopathies, the urine usually contains significant numbers of red blood cells and a variety of casts, and usually moderate to heavy proteinuria (>2.0g/24h). Chronic tubulointerstitial disease (which includes toxic nephropathy and obstructive nephropathy) is characterized by minimal to moderate proteinuria (<2.0g/24h) and minimal hematuria
- The most important predictor of the rate of progression of chronic renal disease to end-stage is the magnitude of proteinuria. In fact, estimation of the protein and creatinine in an early morning spot urine specimen, and calculating the albumin:creatinine ratio, appears to be as useful a predictor as a 24-h urine protein measurement

THE TESTS
Body fluids
URINALYSIS (DIPSTICK)
Description
Midstream urine specimen.

Advantages/Disadvantages
Advantages:
- Simple to perform in the office
- Inexpensive
- Provides information about a variety of urinary constituents very quickly

Disadvantage: very nonspecific – any abnormalities found are not diagnostic of a particular disorder

Normal
No red blood cells, white blood cells, or protein identified.

Abnormal
- Red blood cells, white blood cells, or protein present
- Dipstick tests can be highly sensitive and a false-positive result is possible

Cause of abnormal result
The glomerular membrane, which in a healthy kidney prevents large molecules and red blood cells escaping into the urine, can no longer do so in a failing kidney.

Drugs, disorders and other factors that may alter results
If the patient is a woman of childbearing age, check that she is not menstruating as this may lead to a false-positive result.

URINE MICROSCOPY
Description
Centrifuged urine specimen.

Advantages/Disadvantages
- Advantage: presence of dysmorphic red blood cells, red blood cell casts, or white blood cell casts is highly suggestive of an underlying intrinsic renal disorder, such as glomerulonephritis
- Disadvantage: procedure is not standardized and the degree of urinary sediment concentration may vary. It can, therefore, be difficult to interpret quantitative reports

Normal
- 0–2 red blood cells/high power field
- 0–5 white blood cells/high power field
- Occasional cast only

Abnormal
- >2 red blood cells per high power field
- >5 white blood cells per high power field
- Presence of casts

Cause of abnormal result
- The glomerular membrane, which in the healthy kidney prevents large molecules escaping into the urine, can no longer do so in the failing kidney
- Casts are aggregates of protein, blood cells or epithelial cells, or both. They may develop secondary to urinary stasis in renal tubules and significant proteinuria
- Keep in mind the possibility of a false-positive result

Drugs, disorders and other factors that may alter results
If the patient is a woman of childbearing age, check that she is not menstruating as this may lead to a false-positive result.

COMPLETE BLOOD COUNT
Description
Cuffed venous blood sample.

Advantages/Disadvantages
Advantages:
- Simple, readily available, and inexpensive test
- Confirms or excludes anemia

Disadvantage: nonspecific

Normal
- Hemoglobin: men 13.6–17.7g/dL; women 12.0–15.0g/dL
- Mean corpuscular volume: 76–100mcm^3

Abnormal
Values outside the normal range; in chronic renal failure there is likely to be a normocytic, normochromic anemia.

Cause of abnormal result
Reduced erythropoietin production in chronic renal insufficiency.

Drugs, disorders and other factors that may alter results
- Anemia is seen as part of many disorders
- Anemia with no obvious explanation may require investigation itself

BLOOD UREA NITROGEN AND SERUM CREATININE
Advantages/Disadvantages
Advantages:
- Simple, readily available, and inexpensive test
- Mandatory for assessing whether renal function is impaired
- Serial measurements may be used to monitor progress

Normal
- Blood urea nitrogen (BUN): 8–18mg/dL (3.0–6.5mmol/L)
- Creatinine 0.6–1.2mg/dL (50–110mcmol/L)
- Note that the reference ranges can vary; check with the laboratory

Abnormal
- BUN >18mg/dL (>6.5mmol/L)
- Creatinine >1.2mg/dL (>110mcmol/L)
- Keep in mind the possibility of a falsely abnormal result

Cause of abnormal result
Impaired clearance of waste products from blood.

SERUM POTASSIUM
Description
- Cuffed venous blood sample
- Can be combined with measuring urea and serum creatinine measurement

Advantages/Disadvantages
Advantages:
- Simple, readily available, and inexpensive test
- Will identify hyperkalemia with its attendant risks to the cardiac status

Normal
- 3.3–5.0mEq/L (3.3–5.0mmol/L)
- Note that reference ranges vary; check with the laboratory

Abnormal
- Values outside the normal range
- Keep in mind the possibility of a falsely abnormal result

Drugs, disorders and other factors that may alter results
- Hemolyzed blood sample
- Significant delay in analysis of the blood sample

Tests of function
MICROALBUMINURIA SCREENING
Description
Small volume urine sample.

Advantages/Disadvantages
Advantage: useful as a screen for diabetic nephropathy in patients with type 1 or type 2 diabetes mellitus in whom the standard dipstick test is negative for protein.

Normal
Little or no albumin in the urine.

Abnormal
Positive amounts of microalbuminuria; laboratories vary in how they perform the measurements.

Cause of abnormal result
Albumin is leaking out of the glomeruli and into the urine. The most common reason for microalbuminuria is diabetes mellitus, both type 1 and type 2, but other diseases may cause microalbuminuria such as essential hypertension.

Drugs, disorders and other factors that may alter results
Angiotensin-converting enzyme (ACE) inhibitors may reduce the amount of albumin found in the urine after 1–2 weeks of therapy. The test for microalbuminuria should first be done with the patient off of ACE inhibitors for 2 weeks and then repeated with the patient on ACE inhibitors for a 2-week period to monitor the amount of reduction of albumin in the urine by the drug.

Imaging
CHEST X-RAY
Advantages/Disadvantages
Advantages:
- Quick, readily available test
- A variety of conditions may be diagnosed

Disadvantage:
- Involves exposure to ionizing radiation

Abnormal
Abnormalities which may be seen include:
- Cardiomegaly
- Pulmonary edema
- The above abnormalities suggest volume overload in a patient with chronic renal failure
- Infiltrates compatible with pneumonitis, common in patients with advanced renal failure

Cause of abnormal result
- Congestive heart failure caused by fluid overload
- Other pulmonary lesions or infiltrates that may complicate renal failure, particularly pneumonitis
- Certain uncommon diseases may cause both renal and pulmonary lesions such as Wegener's granulomatosis and Goodpasture's disease. The changes in the chest radiograph in these conditions, however, are neither pathognomonic nor diagnostic

RENAL TRACT ULTRASOUND SCAN
Description
Ultrasound scan of kidneys, ureters, and bladder.

Advantages/Disadvantages
Advantages:
- Noninvasive
- No exposure to radiation
- May be performed during pregnancy
- May be repeated as often as required with no risk to patient
- In patients with obstructive renal failure, may indicate level or cause of obstruction

Disadvantages:
- Specialist knowledge required for interpretation
- Many potential abnormal findings are not diagnostic of chronic renal failure

Normal
Normal renal tract anatomy.

Abnormal
- Small kidneys (highly suggestive of chronic renal disease)
- Renal tract calculi
- Hydronephrosis
- Hydroureter
- Postmicturition residual volume of urine

Cause of abnormal result
- Hydronephrosis, hydroureter, and significant postmicturition residual volume are caused by urinary tract obstruction. Although these findings may be seen in chronic renal failure, they may also be seen in acute renal failure, or in the presence of normal renal function
- Hydroureter is occasionally congenital
- Small kidneys are seen in chronic renal insufficiency, particularly as end-stage renal disease approaches, unless the patient is diabetic, has HIV, myeloma, amyloidosis, or other rare causes of chronic renal insufficiency

Drugs, disorders and other factors that may alter results
- Congenital megaureter (hydroureter)
- If patient's bladder is overfull before the scan, a falsely high postmicturition residual volume may be obtained

TREATMENT

CONSIDER CONSULT

- Diabetic patients may be referred even before a rise in serum creatinine is evident on the basis of microalbuminuria
- Degree of urgency of referral depends on the severity of the renal damage and rapidity of the deterioration of renal function, and whether the patient is approaching end-stage renal disease soon as manifested by: serum creatinine level >6.0mg/dL; 24-h creatinine clearance <15mL/min; uremic symptoms of nausea, vomiting, severe anorexia, bleeding, encephalopathy, intractable congestive heart failure, metabolic acidosis; hyperkalemia

IMMEDIATE ACTION

Patients with end-stage renal disease with overt signs and symptoms of renal failure urgently requiring dialysis require emergency admission to the hospital where therapies can be administered and the patient monitored.

PATIENT AND CAREGIVER ISSUES
Forensic and legal issues

Emergency treatment can be life-saving; occasionally this may need to be carried out without the patient's consent.

Impact on career, dependants, family, friends

Chronic renal failure is a long-term illness. As it progresses to end-stage renal disease, it may have a severe impact on a patient's ability to attend school, to work, or to undertake sporting or social activities. Treatment regimens may also be very disruptive.

Health-seeking behavior
Has there been a delay in seeking medical attention?

- The symptoms of chronic renal failure are often nonspecific (e.g. fatigue, general malaise, anorexia), and renal insufficiency is often long-standing by the time it comes to medical attention
- Many patients are told that they have hypertension, diabetes, or a rise in serum creatinine. Failure to obtain adequate medical care at an early stage often means that they present with severe renal insufficiency or with end-stage renal disease. Adequate medical care early in the illness could often slow or prevent the decline in renal function

MANAGEMENT ISSUES
Goals

- Provide support for patient and caretakers
- Regularly monitor patient's condition so that any deterioration can be quickly recognized and advice sought

Management in special circumstances
COEXISTING DISEASE

- Coexisting disease that has caused or contributed to the poor renal function (e.g. diabetes, hypertension, bladder outflow obstruction, hyperlipidemia) should be treated vigorously with the aim of slowing the decline in renal function
- Some coexisting diseases add to the complexity of managing patients who reach end-stage renal disease and require dialysis (notably congestive heart failure, chronic obstructive pulmonary disease)

COEXISTING MEDICATION

Drugs that are renally excreted may need to have their doses reduced in patients with renal insufficiency or end-stage renal disease:

- Patients with a glomerular filtration rate (GFR) >50mL/min can, in general, have the same dosing as patients with normal renal function
- Patients with a GFR of 10–50mL/min need reduced doses
- Patients with a GFR <10mL/min need substantially reduced doses
- Nephrotoxic drugs may need to be stopped altogether
- The situation may change if a patient with end-stage renal disease starts dialysis, since some drugs will be removed by the dialysis

Drugs to which particular attention must be given include:

- Many antibiotics
- H$_2$ blockers
- Digoxin
- Anticonvulsant agents
- Nonsteroidal anti-inflammatory drugs (NSAIDs) in diabetic patients

SPECIAL PATIENT GROUPS

Patients with renal allograft: any change in a patient's renal function should be discussed with the patient's nephrologist before treatment is changed.

PATIENT SATISFACTION/LIFESTYLE PRIORITIES

- Children and adults of working age are likely to request treatment that will allow them to have as normal life as possible and interfere as little as possible with schooling, ability to work, etc
- Elderly patients may frequently prefer simpler, less invasive treatments

SUMMARY OF THERAPEUTIC OPTIONS
Choices

Treatment of chronic renal insufficiency generally involves measures that slow the progression towards end-stage renal disease:

- Control of underlying factors that may be the cause of the renal disease or may worsen it (e.g. hypertension, diabetes mellitus type 1 or type 2, urinary obstruction, hyperlipidemia, smoking)
- Angiotensin-converting enzyme (ACE) inhibitors (e.g. captopril, enalapril), which can be useful early in the course of chronic renal insufficiency; in addition to controlling blood pressure, ACE inhibition delays the time until dialysis is needed, especially in diabetic nephropathy and other proteinuric diseases
- Dietary modification is often necessary to provide adequate calories while minimizing accumulation of uremic toxins; dietary recommendations vary depending on individual circumstances. Dietary advice would normally be given by a specialist nephrologist or a dietitian with an interest in renal disease
- Doses of nephrotoxic or potentially nephrotoxic drugs need to be reduced or the drug(s) discontinued

When the GFR drops below 15–20mL/min, some of the following special measures may be necessary before dialysis can be started. They should be provided by or in consultation with a nephrologist:

- Management of fluid overload, generally with a loop diuretic (e.g. furosemide) as the drug of first choice
- Management of hyperkalemia, which can be treated orally with sodium polystyrene sulfonate or, in an emergency, with intravenous insulin and dextrose; loop diuretics can also be used to help reduce potassium levels

- Management of hyperphosphatemia with calcium acetate
- Replacement of vitamin D with calcitriol
- Management of anemia, which, if severe, may require treatment with erythropoietin or its analogs; this therapy will work only if serum iron levels are adequate

Treatment of end-stage renal disease revolves around:
- Dialysis, which may take the form of peritoneal dialysis or hemodialysis
- Renal transplantation, which benefits selected patients on long-term dialysis

Clinical pearls
- Control of the level of serum phosphate is very important in the treatment and prevention of renal osteodystrophy. This is accomplished by strict dietary phosphate restriction and the use of phosphate-binding medications in the intestinal tract. Because of the risk of aluminum intoxication, aluminum-containing binders are used with much less frequency, and calcium acetate and similar drugs are currently the treatment of choice
- ACE inhibitors are now established as playing an important role in retarding the rate of progression to end-stage in patients with proteinuric renal disease of diverse etiologies, independent of their antihypertensive action. There are some risks in their use, however. If the patient has renal vascular disease with bilateral renal artery stenosis, he/she is vulnerable to developing acute renal failure following the initiation of ACE inhibitor therapy. Also, while on ACE inhibitors, patients are intolerant to even moderate increases in dietary potassium intake
- Remarkable progress has been made in the management of diabetic nephropathy, the major cause of chronic renal failure in the US. The following measures are most important in retarding progression to end-stage: early referral to a nephrologist once the urinary dipstick is positive for protein or microalbuminuria is detected; initiation of therapy with ACE inhibitors once the diagnosis is made; rigorous control of blood pressure; if feasible, tight control of glycemia

Never
- Never commence treatment for hyperkalemia without knowing a recent serum potassium result and preferably not without discussing it with a renal physician
- Never change the drug regimens of patients who have had renal transplants without discussing with a renal physician first

FOLLOW UP
Plan for review
All patients require regular (often life-long) review with serum potassium, blood urea nitrogen, and creatinine estimation. Factors affecting frequency of review include the severity of the condition and the age of the patient.

Information for patient or caregiver
The chronic nature of the condition and the need for life-long therapy will need to be discussed with the patient.

DRUGS AND OTHER THERAPIES: DETAILS
Drugs
SODIUM POLYSTYRENE SULFONATE
Dose
- Adult: 15–60g orally once daily, depending on the degree of hyperkalemia, the time to next dialysis, and any other potassium-lowering therapies being used
- Administer in approx. 25% sorbitol suspension or concurrently treat with 70% oral sorbitol syrup 10–20mL every 2h to produce one or two watery stools per day

Efficacy
High – removes potassium by exchanging sodium for body potassium; exchange occurs mainly in the large intestine.

Risks/Benefits
Risks:
- Use caution in patients who need to restrict sodium intake (hypertension, congestive heart failure, edema)
- Use caution in pregnancy

Side-effects and adverse reactions
- Cardiovascular system: congestive heart failure
- Gastrointestinal: nausea, vomiting, anorexia, abdominal pain, gastric irritation, diarrhea, constipation, bowel obstruction, bowel necrosis (after rectal administration)
- Metabolic: hypocalcemia, hypokalemia, sodium retention, hypomagnesemia

Interactions (other drugs)
- Antacids ■ Calcium salts ■ Digoxin (may enhance toxic effects of digoxin on the heart) ■ Insulin ■ Loop diuretics ■ Sodium bicarbonate ■ Magnesium hydroxide ■ Aluminium carbonate

Contraindications
- Hypokalemia ■ Hypocalcemia ■ Neonates ■ Bowel obstruction

Acceptability to patient
- Some patients find it unpalatable
- Diarrhea, caused by the sorbitol, and other gastrointestinal side-effects limit its acceptability

Follow up plan
- Monitor serum potassium, calcium, magnesium, sodium, and acid-base balance
- Monitor bowel function

Patient and caregiver information
Do not administer mixed with orange juice.

INSULIN AND DEXTROSE
Although this is normally used in hospitalized patients, it may occasionally be used in the community in an emergency situation.

Dose
One ampule of 50% (50g/100mL water) dextrose in water followed by 10 units of regular insulin intravenously.

Efficacy
Highly effective for rapidly reducing serum potassium level.

Risks/Benefits
Risk (insulin):
- Renal or hepatic impairment may require dose adjustment

Risks (dextrose):

- Use caution in patients receiving corticosteroids
- Prolonged administration of dextrose can result in electrolyte deficiencies, particularly phosphate and potassium
- Do not withdraw abruptly as rebound hypoglycemia may occur

Side-effects and adverse reactions
Insulin:

- Metabolic – hypoglycemia, decreased ion concentrations (calcium, phosphate, potassium, magnesium), insulin resistance, hypoglycemic rebound reaction
- Skin – flushing, rash, fat hypertrophy, pruritus, urticaria, anaphylactoid reactions

Dextrose:

- Venous irritation, thrombophlebitis

Interactions (other drugs)
Insulin:

- Anabolic steroids ▪ Angiotensin-converting enzyme (ACE) inhibitors ▪ Beta-blockers ▪ Cigarette smoking ▪ Clonidine ▪ Corticosteroids ▪ Diazoxide ▪ Ethanol ▪ Fibrates ▪ Lithium ▪ Monoamine oxidase inhibitors ▪ Nifedipine ▪ Octreotide ▪ Salicylates ▪ Sex hormones ▪ Thiazides

Dextrose:

- No known interactions

Contraindications

- Insulin: hypoglycemia ▪ Dextrose: no known contraindications

Follow up plan
Patient must have blood glucose level checked by finger prick every hour until dialysis can be initiated to ensure that hypoglycemia does not develop.

CAPTOPRIL
Dose
Dose depends on the individual clinical circumstances of the patient:

- 25mg three times daily for diabetic nephropathy (in patients with type 1 diabetes)
- 6.25–12.5mg three or four times daily for hypertension

Efficacy
ACE inhibitors have been demonstrated to slow the progression of diabetic kidney disease as well as other proteinuric renal diseases. This effect is independent of a drop in blood pressure.

Risks/Benefits
Risks:

- Use caution in patients receiving diuretics
- First dose may cause hypotension in those on diuretics, a low sodium diet or dialysis, those who are dehydrated or have heart failure
- Use caution in atherosclerosis where renal artery stenosis could be present, renal impairment, and angioedema
- Use caution in breast-feeding

Side-effects and adverse reactions
- Cardiovascular system: hypotension, angioedema, vasculitis
- Central nervous system: headache, dizziness, fatigue, paresthesias, fever, malaise
- Gastrointestinal: nausea, vomiting, diarrhea, constipation, dyspepsia, hepatitis, altered liver function tests, cholestatic jaundice, pancreatitis
- Genitourinary: renal impairment
- Hematologic: blood cell dyscrasias
- Musculoskeletal: myalgia, arthralgia
- Respiratory: dry cough, upper respiratory tract infections
- Skin: rash, photosensitivity

Interactions (other drugs)
- Adrenergic neurone blockers ▪ Alcohol ▪ Alpha-blockers ▪ Alprostadil ▪ Angiotensin II receptor antagonists ▪ Antacids ▪ Antidiabetics (insulin, metformin, sulphonylureas) ▪ Antihypertensives (beta-blockers, clonidine, diazoxide, hydralazine, methyldopa, minoxidil, nitrates, nitroprusside) ▪ Anxiolytics and hypnotics ▪ Baclofen, tizanidine ▪ Calcium channel blockers ▪ Corticosteroids ▪ Cyclosporine ▪ Diuretics ▪ Estrogens ▪ Heparins ▪ Levodopa ▪ Lithium ▪ NSAIDs ▪ Phenothiazines ▪ Potassium salts

Contraindications
- Pregnancy ▪ Aortic stenosis ▪ Renovascular disease

Acceptability to patient
Generally acceptable.

Follow up plan
Potassium levels and blood pressure should be monitored.

Patient and caregiver information
Be aware that ACE inhibitors can cause marked reductions in blood pressure, which may cause dizziness, especially when standing up after sitting or lying down.

FUROSEMIDE
Dose
20–80mg/day in single dose or divided doses.

Efficacy
- Effective diuretic even in advanced renal disease that can help to reduce volume overload, and therefore is especially useful in patients with pulmonary or peripheral edema
- Tends to reduce serum potassium levels
- Has antihypertensive effect (although not generally the first-line treatment for hypertension)

Risks/Benefits
Risks:
- Excessive diuresis may cause dehydration and blood volume reduction with circulatory collapse and possibly vascular thrombosis and embolism, particularly in elderly patients
- Use caution with diabetes mellitus, renal and liver disease, systemic lupus erythematosis, hypertension, gout, porphyria
- Use caution with pregnancy and nursing mothers

Side-effects and adverse reactions
- Cardiovascular system: chest pain, circulatory collapse, orthostatic hypotension
- Central nervous system: dizziness, headache, paresthesia, fever

- Eyes, ears, nose, and throat: visual disturbances, ototoxicity, tinnitus, hearing impairment, thirst
- Gastrointestinal: ischemic hepatitis, vomiting, pancreatitis, nausea, diarrhea, anorexia
- Genitourinary: glycosuria, hyperuricemia, bladder spasm, polyuria
- Hematologic: blood disorders
- Metabolic: hyperglycemia, hyponatremia, hypokalemia, hypomagnesemia, hypovolemia, hypochloremia, hypercholesterolemia, hypertriglyceridemia
- Skin: erythema multiforme, exfoliative dermatitis, urticaria

Interactions (other drugs)
- ACE inhibitors ▪ Alpha-adrenergin antagonists ▪ Amphotericin ▪ Antibiotics (aminoglycosides, polymixins, vancomycin, cephalosporins) ▪ Antidiabetics ▪ Antidysrhythmics (amiodarone, cardiac glycosides, disopyramide, flecainide, mexelitine, quinidine, sotalol) ▪ Beta-2 adrenergic agonists ▪ Carbenoxolone ▪ Cisplatin ▪ Corticosteroids ▪ Cholestyramine, colestipol ▪ Clofibrate ▪ Diuretics (thiazides, metolazone, acetazolamide) ▪ Lignocaine ▪ Lithium ▪ NSAIDs ▪ Phenobarbital ▪ Phenytoin ▪ Pimozide ▪ Reboxetine ▪ Selective serotonin reuptake inhibitors ▪ Terbutaline ▪ Tubocurarine

Contraindications
- Renal failure with anuria ▪ Hepatic coma

Acceptability to patient
Generally good, although an occasional patient may experience intestinal cramps and diarrhea.

Follow up plan
Serum potassium levels should be monitored.

CALCIUM ACETATE
Dose
Two tablets (1334mg) with meals; increase gradually as required up to three to four tablets with each meal.

Efficacy
Effective at reducing the serum phosphate level.

Risks/Benefits
Risks:
- Patients with end-stage renal failure may develop hypercalcemia when given calcium with meals. No other calcium supplements should be given concurrently with calcium acetate
- The serum calcium level should be monitored twice weekly during the early dose adjustment period
- Excessive dosage of calcium acetate induces hypercalcemia

Side-effects and adverse reactions
- Gastrointestinal: nausea
- Metabolic: hypercalcemia

Interactions (other drugs)
Tetracyclines.

Contraindications
- Patients with hypercalcemia ▪ Pregnancy category C ▪ Safety and effectiveness in pediatric patients have not been established

Acceptability to patient
Generally good.

Follow up plan
Follow serum phosphate and adjust dose as necessary.

VITAMIN D (CHOLECALCIFEROL)
Dose
0.25mcg 1,25-dihydroxycholecalciferol/day. Other forms of vitamin D are not acceptable as the diseased kidney cannot perform the second hydroxylation necessary to activate the drug.

Efficacy
Effective in vitamin D deficiency.

Risks/Benefits
Risks:
- The therapeutic range is narrow
- Use caution in cardiac disease or arteriosclerosis, renal disease and kidney stones, sarcoidosis and other granulomatous diseases, hypoparathyroidism
- Use caution in pregnancy and breast-feeding

Side-effects and adverse reactions
- Cardiovascular system: dysrhythmias, hypertension
- Central nervous system: anorexia, overt psychosis, headache, hyperthermia
- Gastrointestinal: nausea, vomiting, pancreatitis, constipation, dry mouth
- Genitourinary: decreased libido, nocturia, and polyuria
- Metabolic: hypercholesterolemia, mild acidosis, hyperphosphatemia, vitaminosis D, hypercalcemia
- Musculoskeletal: muscle and bone pain

Interactions (other drugs)
- Antacids, magnesium, calcium salts - Anticonvulsants (phenobarbitol, phenytoin, primidone, carbamazepine, barbiturates) - Cardiac glycosides - Cholestyramine, colestipol, mineral oil, orlistat - Phosphorus salts - Thiazide diuretics - Vitamin D analogs

Contraindications
- Hypercalcemia - Hypervitaminosis D - Hyperphosphatemia - Metastatic calcification

Acceptability to patient
Good.

Follow up plan
Follow the serum calcium and phosphate, and adjust dose as necessary.

Surgical therapy
RENAL TRANSPLANTATION
Efficacy
High (in selected patients).

Risks/Benefits
Risks:
- Rejection of the transplant
- Need for life-long immunosuppressant agents to try to avoid rejection, which may involve complicated drug regimens and dosages

- Infection as a result of immunosuppression
- Side-effects of immunosuppressants (e.g. diabetes, hypertension, hirsutism, dental problems, toxicity to transplanted kidney by cyclosporine)

Benefit: avoids the need for life-long dialysis

Acceptability to patient
High, although the possibility of rejection and the need for life-long immunosuppression limit acceptability for some patients.

Follow up plan
Regular, life-long follow up, so that complications (particularly rejection) can be recognized early.

Patient and caregiver information
- If patient becomes unwell in any way, medical advice should be sought quickly
- Take any medications (particularly immunosuppressive agents) exactly as prescribed. Do not miss any doses
- The risks and benefits of renal transplantation must be discussed fully with the patient before it is decided to aim for this therapy

Other therapies
DIALYSIS
The timing of initiation of dialysis depends on individual circumstances, but it is usually required when the glomerular filtration rate (GFR) is <15–20mL/min; dialysis may be required urgently if there is a sudden deterioration in the patient's condition.

The main options are:
- Intermittent hemodialysis
- Continuous ambulatory peritoneal dialysis

The type of dialysis chosen depends on individual patient circumstances, and the patient must be involved in the decision-making process when it is decided to embark on long-term dialysis.

Efficacy
High.

Risks/Benefits
Risks
Hemodialysis:
- Blood-borne infections, including hepatitis B (rare)
- Necessity of permanent vascular access
- Blood pressure lability
- Strict adherence to diet and fluid restriction necessary

Peritoneal dialysis:
- Peritonitis
- Weight gain
- Pancreatitis

Benefits
Dialysis:
- Except for transplant, the only available treatment for patients with end-stage renal disease
- Patients who require dialysis generally feel better once regular dialysis is started
- Can be performed on an outpatient basis, either at home or in a dialysis unit outside a hospital

Hemodialysis:
- Most frequently performed at a dialysis center where trained personnel administer the treatment
- Can sometimes be administered at home if the patient is interested

Peritoneal dialysis:
- Easy for most patients to learn the techniques involved
- Special equipment is not necessary
- Less expensive than hemodialysis
- Permanent vascular access is not required
- Produces 'continuous' corrections of biochemical profile
- Blood pressure is often easier to control than in patients having hemodialysis
- Relatively 'portable' so, for example, vacations are relatively easy to arrange

Acceptability to patient
Dialysis is very time-consuming and some patients find that it interferes greatly with work, school, and social activities. Often, however, there is no alternative for patients with end-stage renal disease.

Follow up plan
Long-term, regular, and frequent follow up by a specialist nephrologist is required.

Patient and caregiver information
If dialysis is performed on a long-term basis, it needs to be performed regularly, as prescribed by the nephrologist. Patient should not miss any sessions.

EFFICACY OF THERAPIES

Efficacy of treatment of chronic renal insufficiency varies by underlying etiology, patient compliance, and comorbidities.

Review period

Frequency of review varies between patients. However, all patients with chronic renal insufficiency or end-stage renal disease should be under the care of a nephrologist, who will advise on the need for follow-up and review.

PROGNOSIS

Depends on individual variables, and comorbidities and compliance with therapy.

Therapeutic failure

- Patients with chronic renal insufficiency who do not respond to simple measures (diet, diuretics, antihypertensive agents) are likely to progress to end-stage renal disease
- Selected patients on long-term dialysis may be considered for renal transplantation
- All patients should be referred to a nephrologist

Terminal illness

- Some patients with chronic renal failure fail to respond to treatment, some repeatedly reject donor kidneys, and for some a suitable donor never becomes available. In such cases further treatment choices are usually very limited
- If a patient's quality of life is poor with no likelihood of improvement, it may not be appropriate to continue with treatment or to initiate any new therapies
- This should be discussed, as appropriate, with the patient, other physicians caring for the patient, and the patient's family or caregivers

COMPLICATIONS

Fertility is substantially reduced in female patients with end-stage renal disease, and male erectile dysfunction is common.

CONSIDER CONSULT

- Patients with chronic renal failure should have a plan for long-term specialist follow-up

PREVENTION

RISK FACTORS

■ **Pre-existing renal disease:** should be carefully monitored. It may not be possible to prevent renal failure from occurring but if recognized early, its long-term effects may be lessened. Early referral is strongly advised

■ **Diabetes mellitus:** all aspects of this disease should be treated promptly and patients monitored to reduce the risk of complications such as renal failure

■ **Hypertension:** should be treated aggressively to prevent permanent renal damage

MODIFY RISK FACTORS
Lifestyle and wellness
TOBACCO

Patients with progressive renal disease should be advised to stop smoking.

FAMILY HISTORY

Those with a family history of hereditary renal disease should be monitored regularly, so that any deterioration in renal function can be recognized early and the potential for permanent renal damage may be reduced. (It may not be possible to prevent renal failure from occurring.)

DRUG HISTORY

Care should be taken when prescribing potentially nephrotoxic drugs to at-risk patients. Reduce the dose or use alternative medication if possible.

SCREENING

Screening for microalbuminuria is appropriate for patients with diabetes mellitus.

PREVENT RECURRENCE

■ Once permanent renal damage has occurred, a return to completely normal renal function is unlikely to occur

■ Thus, recurrence as such does not occur; however, all patients should be followed so that any deterioration in their condition can be recognized early

■ Early referral is strongly recommended

ASSOCIATIONS

National Kidney and Neurologic Disease Information Clearing House
Box NKUDIC
Bethesda, MD 20893

National Kidney Foundation
30 East 33rd Street, Suite 1100
New York, NY 10016
Tel: (800) 622-9010 or (212) 889-2210
Fax: (212) 689-9261
E-mail: info@kidney.org
http://www.kidney.org/

KEY REFERENCES

- Pisoni P, Remuzzi G. Pathophysiology and management of progressive renal failure. In: Greenberg A, ed. Primer on kidney diseases. New York: Academic Press, 2001, p385–96
- Peterson JC, Adler S, Burkart LM, et al. For the Modification of Diet In Renal Disease (MDRD) Study Group: blood pressure control, proteinuria, and progression of renal disease. Ann Int Med 1995;123:754–62
- Lakkis FD, Martinez-Maldonado M. Conservative management of chronic renal failure and the uremic syndrome. In: Jacobson HR, Striker GE, Klahr S, eds. The principles and practice of nephrology. St Louis: Mosby, 1995, p614–20
- Tee Wee PM. Initial management of chronic renal failure. In: Cameron S, Davison AM, Grunfeld JP, Kerr D, Ritz E, eds. Oxford textbook of clinical nephrology. New York: Oxford Medical Press: 1992, p1173–91

FAQS

Question 1

How does one advise a patient approaching end-stage renal disease on the best mode of renal replacement therapy, dialysis vs transplantation?

ANSWER 1

First, make it absolutely clear that, regardless of the ultimate mode of therapy, most patients start out on a form of dialysis. This is due to the limitation on the availability of cadaver donor kidneys. On average, even if the patient and physician agree that transplantation is desirable, the average wait for a cadaver kidney in most parts of the US is 12–18 months. If a living related donor is available and is found to be a suitable donor immunologically and medically, then the wait is much shorter. Regarding dialysis, the patient's wishes and the home environment are the major factors in deciding between peritoneal dialysis at home and hemodialysis in a center. Home hemodialysis has not proven to be popular or common in the US for a number of socioeconomic reasons.

Question 2

How does a physician manage congestive heart failure effectively in patients with advanced renal disease?

ANSWER 2

The best two-word answer to this question is 'with difficulty'. If the creatinine clearance is <15mL/min, the best decision is to initiate dialysis and rectify the fluid overload, since the native kidneys no longer have the capacity to handle the sodium and fluid excesses even with potent diuretic therapy. On the other hand, at earlier phases of chronic renal failure (GFR >30mL/min), many compliant patients can be effectively treated with a combination of measures including: rigorous dietary sodium restriction, careful control of hypertension, and the use of loop-acting diuretics such as furosemide. Thiazide diuretics as first-line drugs are essentially ineffective in advanced renal failure, but occasionally they are effective in combination with loop-acting drugs.

Question 3

In view of the potential nephrotoxicity of common analgesic medications, how does one ameliorate headaches, muscular aches, and other types of common discomforts in patients with chronic renal failure?

ANSWER 3

First, it should be emphasized that non-narcotic analgesics (aspirin, acetaminophen, and NSAIDs) are not fundamentally nephrotoxic when taken intermittently in appropriate doses. Analgesic nephropathy, when it occurs, is related to the ingestion of relatively large doses of combinations of analgesic agents over long periods of time (years). It is true that rarely there are acute reactions with renal failure related to hypersensitivity with all three types of drugs, but these are no different in renal patients than in the general population. Thus, one shouldn't hesitate to recommend intermittent ingestion of moderate doses of acetaminophen or aspirin or even ibuprofen when indicated, but avoid combinations and avoid aspirin in the presence of uremia and its hemorrhagic propensities.

CONTRIBUTORS

Fred F Ferri, MD, FACP
Martin Goldberg, MD, FACP
Jennifer E Weil, MD

RHABDOMYOLYSIS

SUMMARY INFORMATION

DESCRIPTION

- Characterized by damage to skeletal muscle with the consequent release of toxic intracellular muscle constituents (myoglobin and muscle enzymes) into the circulation, with or without dark (red or brown) urine (myoglobinuria)
- The disease can be serious, with myoglobin-induced acute renal failure (ARF) developing in 30% of patients with rhabdomyolysis
- Hyperkalemia and metabolic acidosis result from muscle breakdown
- Early intervention with volume expansion is critical for the prevention of acute renal failure (ARF) but the therapeutic window is narrow (approximately 6h)
- Overall prognosis depends on the primary cause and the ability to manage any complications of ARF, and is good with appropriate care

URGENT ACTION

- Any patient with impending or ongoing rhabdomyolysis should be treated immediately with intravenous fluids
- If an individual with trauma is trapped, intravenous fluids should be administered before a limb and the rest of the body are released

KEY! DON'T MISS!

- Rhabdomyolysis should be suspected in any patient with muscle injury or damage, even if obvious symptoms and signs are not evident
- Nontraumatic rhabdomyolysis may occur, in which muscle involvement may be mild
- In one study of patients with rhabdomyolysis, only 50% had muscle pain and only 5% had muscle swelling on admission, emphasizing the need for continued careful evaluation of individuals with a suggestive history

ICD9 CODE
728.89 Idiopathic rhabdomyolysis

SYNONYMS
- Myoglobinuria
- Myoglobin-induced acute tubular necrosis
- Pigment-induced acute tubular necrosis
- Pigment nephropathy

CARDINAL FEATURES
- Clinical features of the underlying muscle damage often predominate the presentation
- Myalgia and reddish-brown urine are important features of the history
- Urinary sediment contains coarsely granular reddish-brown casts (seen in hemoglobinuria) and no red blood cells (differentiating rhabdomyolysis from hematuria)
- Characteristic is marked elevation in the skeletal muscle fraction of creatine kinase (CK-MM) in the serum
- Marked hyperkalemia, hyperphosphatemia, hypocalcemia, hyperuricemia, and metabolic acidosis are serious complications of muscle breakdown
- Serum and urine myoglobin levels can be normal or elevated as myoglobin is rapidly metabolized and filtered
- Acute renal failure (ARF) is a frequent complication of rhabdomyolysis
- The goal of therapy is to prevent or minimize ARF with vigorous hydration, forced diuresis, and urinary alkalinization (only vigorous hydration has been shown to improve outcome in this form of renal failure)
- Overall prognosis depends on the primary cause and the ability to manage any complications of ARF, and is good with appropriate care

CAUSES
Common causes
- Muscle trauma and compression: motor vehicle accidents, occupational accidents, collapsed buildings (earthquakes), individuals struggling against restraints, victims of violence or physical abuse, war injuries, prolonged immobilization as occurs in coma, alcoholism, orthopedic traction, and complex surgical procedures
- Muscle ischemia: extensive thrombosis, multiple embolism, prolonged vessel clamping during orthopedic or vascular surgical procedures, generalized shock, sickle cell crisis, burns
- Muscle exertion: strenuous exercise, marathon runners, exercise in hot humid conditions, exercise in individuals with an inherited myopathy or with poor physical training, status asthmaticus, status epilepticus, delirium tremens, tetanus, psychotic agitation
- Alcohol and drugs: amphetamines, cocaine, ecstasy, PCP, heroin, and alcoholism
- Drugs: antimalarials, carbon monoxide, central nervous system depressants, colchicine, corticosteroids, diuretics, haloperidol, clofibrate, fenofibrate, gemfibrozil, HMG-CoA reductase inhibitors (statins) such as lovastatin, fluvastatin, simvastatin, atrovastatin, cerivastatin (removed from the market); isoniazid, licorice, narcotics, phenothiazines, succinylcholine, zidovudine (AZT), tolcapone (removed from the market), mibefradil (removed from the market), cyclosporin
- Use of statins with concomitant use of a medication which inhibits the CYP450 (cytochrome P450) (e.g. lovastatin with itraconazole)
- Toxins: snake venoms, insect venoms, hemlock, buffalo fish
- Electrical muscle injury: high-voltage electric shock, lightning, repeated cardioversion
- Hyperthermia (heatstroke): neuroleptic malignant syndrome from phenothiazines or haloperidol; malignant hyperthermia from inhalation anesthetics or succinylcholine

Rare causes

- Inherited myopathies: carnitine palmitoyl transferase (CPT) deficiency, myophosphorylase deficiency (McArdle's disease), phosphofructokinase deficiency, alpha-glucosidase deficiency, phosphohexoseisomerase deficiency
- Collagen vascular disorders: polymyositis, dermatomyositis
- Infections: coxsackievirus, herpesviruses, HIV, influenza, Legionnaires' disease, leptospirosis, pyomyositis, salmonellosis, shigellosis, tetanus, toxic shock syndrome, tularemia, gas gangrene, falciparum malaria, *Bacillus cereus*
- Electrolyte disorders: hypokalemia; hypophosphatemia (during treatment of diabetic ketoacidosis or during the use of total parenteral nutrition), hypocalcemia, hyponatremia, hypernatremia, hyperosmolar states
- Endocrine disorders: hypothyroidism, diabetic ketoacidosis, diabetic coma
- Massive blood transfusions
- Mushroom poisoning (*Tricholoma equestre*)

Serious causes

The majority of causes are serious, and appropriate attention should be paid to the underlying etiology.

Contributory or predisposing factors

- Viral infections, fasting or exertion can precipitate rhabdomyolysis in individuals with inherited myopathies
- Exercise in hot humid climate or with poor physical conditioning can precipitate rhabdomyolysis

EPIDEMIOLOGY
Incidence and prevalence

The precise incidence and prevalence are unknown.

FREQUENCY

- The frequency of acute renal failure (ARF) in the setting of rhabdomyolysis is 30%
- Rhabdomyolysis accounts for 10–15% of ARF cases

Demographics
AGE

- Inherited myopathies present with recurrent episodes of rhabdomyolysis during childhood
- Traumatic rhabdomyolysis is most common in young adults; frequently seen in military recruits doing isometric exercises such as squat jumps in hot and humid weather

GENDER

Males are more frequently affected because they have a higher incidence of trauma.

GENETICS

There are several inherited causes of rhabdomyolysis including:
- Carnitine palmitoyl transferase (CPT) deficiency
- Myophosphorylase deficiency (McArdle's disease)
- Phosphofructokinase deficiency (Tarui's disease)
- Alpha-glucosidase deficiency
- Phosphohexoisomerase deficiency

DIFFERENTIAL DIAGNOSIS
Hemoglobinuric ARF
Hemoglobinuric acute renal failure (ARF) closely resembles myoglobinuric ARF.

FEATURES
- ARF with reddish-brown urine, pigmented casts, and no urinary red blood cells
- The history often reveals a cause for intravascular hemolysis
- Major causes include G6PD deficiency, malaria, snake or insect venoms, transfusion reactions, disseminated intravascular coagulation, prosthetic valves, extracorporeal circulation, and heat stroke, massive blood transfusions
- Hemolytic anemia is evident on peripheral smear
- Plasma acquires a reddish-brown discoloration as hemoglobin is a bigger molecule and is not as readily cleared by the kidneys as compared with myoglobin
- Serum creatine kinase and myoglobin levels are normal
- Treatment is similar to that for myoglobinuric ARF

Systemic lupus erythematosus
Systemic lupus erythematosus is a chronic multisystem disease with autoantibody production leading to clinical manifestations.

FEATURES
- Renal manifestations develop in two-thirds of cases, with edema, hypertension, proteinuria, hematuria, urinary red blood cells (RBCs), granular and RBC casts, and varying degrees of renal failure
- More common in young adult females
- Fever, anorexia, malaise
- Malar rash
- Joint and muscle symptoms
- Headaches, psychosis
- Pancytopenia
- Depressed C3 and C4 complement levels
- Elevated erythrocyte sedimentation rate, antinuclear antibodies, anti-double-stranded DNA, anti-Sm (Smith) antibody is specific for lupus
- May respond to steroids and cytotoxic agents

IgA nephropathy
IgA nephropathy is a renal disease caused by IgA autoantibodies.

FEATURES
- Recurrent episodes of gross hematuria following upper respiratory infections or stressful exercise
- Proteinuria, hematuria, urinary red blood cells (RBCs), granular and RBC casts, and varying degrees of renal failure
- More common in males during the second and third decades of life
- Normal serum complements
- Serum IgA level may be elevated in up to 50% of adult and 15% of pediatric patients
- May respond to steroids, fish oil, and cytotoxic agents

Henoch-Schönlein purpura
Henoch-Schönlein purpura is a multisystem disorder that primarily affects the skin, joints, and gastrointestinal and renal systems.

FEATURES

- Most commonly seen in young children
- Purpuric rash over the extensor surface of lower extremities and buttocks
- Arthralgias and periarticular edema
- Abdominal colic
- Renal manifestations develop in two-thirds of cases, and can vary from microscopic urinary abnormalities to varying degrees of renal failure, with edema, hypertension, proteinuria, gross hematuria, urinary red blood cells (RBCs), and granular and RBC casts

Acute post-streptococcal glomerulonephritis

Antecedent streptococcal pharyngitis or impetigo can lead to acute post-streptococcal glomerulonephritis.

FEATURES

- Most commonly seen in children 5–10 years of age
- Typically presents with edema, hypertension, hematuria, urinary red blood cells (RBCs) and RBC casts, and varying degrees of proteinuria and renal failure
- Streptozyme is positive
- Complement levels are low during the acute phase of the illness, but usually return to normal within 2 months
- Therapy is supportive

Hemolytic-uremic syndrome

Hemolytic-uremic syndrome usually follows infection with *Escherichia coli* O157:H7 or *Shigella dysenteriae*.

FEATURES

- Most commonly occurs in children
- Abdominal pain, vomiting, bloody diarrhea
- Hemolytic anemia with microangiopathy (schistocytes) and thrombocytopenia
- Most patients develop irritability, somnolence, behavioral changes
- Approximately 50% of patients develop oligoanuric ARF with urinary red blood cells and hemoglobinuria
- Treatment is supportive

Thrombotic thrombocytopenic purpura (TTP)

Thrombotic thrombocytopenic purpura is a form of thrombotic microangiopathy characterized by thrombocytopenia with thromboses in terminal arterioles and capillaries.

FEATURES

- Often lethal, high morbidity
- Pathophysiology relates to deposition of fibrin and platelet thrombi
- Associated with connective tissue diseases, cancer, pregnancy
- Can occur in younger adults
- Hemolytic anemia, thrombocytopenia, renal failure
- Neurologic status changes (confusion, seizures, coma), and fever
- Treated with plasmapheresis and fresh frozen plasma

Ischemic acute tubular necrosis

Ischemic acute tubular necrosis usually follows prolonged renal hypoperfusion.

FEATURES

- Common causes include hemorrhage, gastrointestinal fluid losses, burns, third-space losses, sepsis, shock, and impaired cardiac output

- ARF with edema, hypertension, urinary red blood cells, and broad brown granular casts
- Can be confused with rhabdomyolysis, but creatine kinase levels are usually normal
- Treatment is supportive, and depends on the cause

Nephrotoxic acute tubular necrosis

Nephrotoxic acute tubular necrosis is similar to rhabdomyolysis, but creatine kinase levels are usually normal.

FEATURES

- Follows administration of a variety of drugs
- Common agents include aminoglycosides, amphotericin, cisplatin, contrast agents, and cyclosporine
- ARF with edema, hypertension, urinary red blood cells and broad brown granular casts
- Treatment is supportive, and depends on the cause

SIGNS & SYMPTOMS

Signs

- Signs relating to the underlying cause usually predominate
- Affected muscles may be swollen and tender, with erythema of the overlying skin
- Muscle weakness is often present in severe cases
- Compartment syndrome may be present or develop after fluid administration, with worsening swelling of the limb and distal neurovascular compromise
- Signs of myoglobinuric ARF include reddish-brown urine, oliguria, hypertension, edema, and congestive heart failure

Symptoms

- Symptoms relating to the underlying cause usually predominate
- Myalgia and muscle swelling may range from mild to severe, and may worsen following fluid therapy
- Symptoms of myoglobinuric ARF may include reddish-brown urine, decreased urine output, edema, and headaches secondary to hypertension

ASSOCIATED DISORDERS

- Rhabdomyolysis is frequently associated with ARF from acute tubular necrosis
- Rhabdomyolysis-induced renal failure may be associated with hypertension, hyperkalemia, hyperphosphatemia, and metabolic acidosis
- As hyperuricemia occurs during rhabdomyolysis, a concurrent acute urate nephropathy can also be present and worsen the ARF

KEY! DON'T MISS!

- Rhabdomyolysis should be suspected in any patient with muscle injury or damage, even if obvious symptoms and signs are not evident
- Nontraumatic rhabdomyolysis may occur, in which muscle involvement may be mild
- In one study of patients with rhabdomyolysis, only 50% had muscle pain and only 5% had muscle swelling on admission, emphasizing the need for continued careful evaluation of individuals with a suggestive history

CONSIDER CONSULT

- The underlying cause frequently necessitates referral to an appropriate specialist
- Patients with recurrent rhabdomyolysis should be referred to a geneticist to evaluate the possibility of an inherited myopathy

INVESTIGATION OF THE PATIENT
Direct questions to patient
Q Have you recently had any muscle pain or swelling? A history of myalgia, ranging from very mild to severe, is frequently available.

Q Have you recently had an injury to your body? Muscle trauma is a common cause of rhabdomyolysis.

Q What has the color of your urine been? Reddish-brown discoloration of the urine is an important symptom in rhabdomyolysis, but may also be present in hemoglobinuria and the glomerulopathies.

Q Are you urinating less than usual? Oliguria in the presence of rhabdomyolysis should be treated rapidly to prevent or reverse the ARF.

Q Are you taking any medications, drugs, or alcohol? Several drugs can result in rhabdomyolysis.

Q Have you taken herbal remedies or over-the-counter medication? Medications can cause rhabdomyolysis and need to be excluded as a cause.

Q Have you had muscle pains and red-brown urine before? Recurrent episodes of rhabdomyolysis, especially triggered by exercise, fasting, or infections, should prompt a search for inherited myopathies.

Q Have you recently had a sore throat, skin rash, joint pains, or abdominal pain? Answers to these questions help to eliminate the other causes of hematuria.

Q Have you recently had any swelling around the eyes or ankles, or headaches? These are symptoms suggestive of edema and hypertension.

Contributory or predisposing factors
Q Do you get muscle pain and red-brown urine following exercise, fasting, or infections? These are known precipitating factors that may point to an inherited myopathy.

Family history
Q Do you have a family history of similar problems? Inherited myopathies are transmitted in an autosomal-recessive pattern

Examination
▪ Examine the patient's general condition. Depending on the cause of rhabdomyolysis, the patient's condition can range from normal to critical

▪ What is the blood pressure? Patients with rhabdomyolysis may present with hypertension secondary to renal failure and/or pain, or hypotension from intravascular volume depletion

▪ Is there any peripheral edema? This may be a sign of renal failure

▪ Is there any muscle swelling or tenderness? The degree of muscle involvement may be variable, and may change with time and fluid therapy

▪ What is the neurovascular status distal to the involved muscles? It is important to assess for compartment syndrome on a continual and ongoing basis

Summary of investigative tests
▪ Urinalysis (dipstick): should be performed in all patients with muscle injury or other clinical features suggestive of rhabdomyolysis. Heme-positive urine suggests myoglobinuria, hemoglobinuria, or hematuria. Significant proteinuria suggests a glomerulopathy. Lack of myoglobinuria does not necessarily rule out rhabdomyolysis

▪ Urine microscopy: should be performed in all patients with an abnormal urine dipstick. Heme-positive urine with absence of red blood cells (RBCs) and presence of pigmented casts by microscopy suggests myoglobinuria or hemoglobinuria. Presence of several RBCs and RBC casts suggests a glomerulonephritis

▪ Complete blood count (CBC): should be performed in all patients to look for anemia of renal failure, and for signs of hemolysis (to rule out hemoglobinuria) or thrombocytopenia (hemolytic-uremic syndrome). The supernatant in plasma is clear in myoglobinuria

- Blood urea nitrogen (BUN) and serum creatinine: should be checked in all patients to look for renal insufficiency
- Serum electrolytes: should be checked in all patients to detect associated hyperkalemia, hyperphosphatemia, hypocalcemia, hyperuricemia, hyponatremia, and metabolic acidosis. The anion gap is increased
- Serum creatine kinase: should be checked in all patients with muscle injury or other clinical features suggestive of rhabdomyolysis. The skeletal muscle fraction (CK-MM) is characteristically elevated in rhabdomyolysis. Serum calcium may be low early in the disease. Serum phosphorus may be high later in disease process. Serum uric acid can be markedly elevated
- Serum and urine myoglobin: should be checked when the diagnosis of rhabdomyolysis is unclear, but is usually performed by a specialist. Elevated levels are diagnostic, but normal values do not rule out rhabdomyolysis
- Serum complement: should be checked when the diagnosis of rhabdomyolysis is unclear, but is usually done by a specialist. Complements are normal in rhabdomyolysis, and low in a variety of glomerular diseases
- Electrocardiography (ECG): may be performed in order to detect cardiac changes in patients with hyperkalemia
- Urine toxicology screen: should be performed in patients with rhabdomyolysis and suspected drug or toxin exposure
- Renal ultrasound: should be performed in patients with renal insufficiency when the diagnosis of rhabdomyolysis is unclear, especially to rule out obstruction. Renal ultrasound is typically performed in the radiology department of the hospital by a radiology technician
- Renal biopsy: a specialist investigation – should be considered in patients with renal insufficiency when the diagnosis is unclear

DIAGNOSTIC DECISION

- In most cases the history of skeletal muscle injury or myalgias, along with reddish-brown urine and elevated CK-MM levels, are sufficient to establish the diagnosis
- In some cases, the skeletal muscle involvement is covert and the differential diagnosis of reddish-brown urine includes myoglobinuria, hemoglobinuria and hematuria
- In such cases, hematuria is confirmed by the presence of RBCs in the urinary sediment, and hemoglobinuria is established by the presence of hemolysis and normal CK-MM levels

CLINICAL PEARLS

Hyperuricemia can occur in rhabdomyolysis due to increased release from the breakdown of muscles and to decreased excretion secondary to renal failure.

THE TESTS
Body fluids
URINALYSIS (DIPSTICK)
Description
Midstream urine collection.

Advantages/Disadvantages
Advantages:
- Quick
- Inexpensive
- Easy to perform
- Semiquantitative

Disadvantages:
- Nonspecific
- Not diagnostic

Normal
Negative for blood and protein.

Abnormal
- Heme-positive (trace to large) urine suggests hematuria, hemoglobinuria or myoglobinuria
- Protein (trace to 3+) in urine is a nonspecific marker of renal disease, but may also be detected in individuals with normal kidneys
- Keep in mind the possibility of a falsely abnormal result

Cause of abnormal result
Heme-positive urine in rhabdomyolysis is due to the presence of myoglobin.

Drugs, disorders and other factors that may alter results
- Reddish-brown urine may also be encountered in porphyria and following ingestion of beets, rifampin or pyridium
- The urine dipstick may be falsely positive for protein in patients with gross hematuria, alkaline urine, and use of pyridium or local antiseptics
- The urine dipstick may be transiently positive for protein in individuals with fever, stress, exercise, and seizures

URINE MICROSCOPY
Description
Centrifuged urinary specimen.

Advantages/Disadvantages
Advantages:
- Direct visualization of RBCs and their morphology
- Distinguishes between hematuria and pigmenturia
- Detection of white blood cells (WBCs) and casts may be diagnostic

Disadvantages:
- Requires microscope and experience
- Requires standardization

Normal
- 0–2 RBCs per high-power field
- 0–5 WBCs per high-power field
- Occasional hyaline cast

Abnormal
- >2 RBCs per high-power field
- >5 WBCs per high-power field
- Casts
- Keep in mind the possibility of falsely abnormal results

Cause of abnormal result
- Urine in rhabdomyolysis is devoid of RBCs because the glomerular membrane is intact and prevents entry of RBCs into the urine
- The glomerular membrane can be damaged in a variety of glomerulopathies, leading to the appearance of RBCs in the urine
- Casts in rhabdomyolysis are aggregates of desquamated tubule cells in a protein matrix that become pigmented due to the presence of myoglobin

Drugs, disorders and other factors that may alter results
Menstruation is an important cause of urinary RBCs.

COMPLETE BLOOD COUNT (CBC)
Description
Venous blood sample.

Advantages/Disadvantages
Advantages:
- Rapid
- Easily available in local laboratories

Disadvantages:
- Nonspecific
- Major utility is to exclude hemolytic disease

Normal
Hematocrit: 0.45+/-0.05 in males; 0.41+/-0.05 in females.

Abnormal
- Low hematocrit may be seen in renal failure
- Keep in mind the possibility of a falsely abnormal result

Cause of abnormal result
Anemia of ARF is due to erythropoietin deficiency and hemodilution.

BLOOD UREA NITROGEN (BUN) AND SERUM CREATININE
Description
Venous blood sample.

Advantages/Disadvantages
Advantages:
- Most sensitive and specific indicators of renal function
- Easily available in local laboratories
- Serial measurements can indicate worsening or recovery

Disadvantages:
- Values may be normal during the early phase of renal failure
- Values may be falsely elevated

Normal
- BUN: 9.2–18.8mg/dL (3.3–6.7mmol/L)
- Creatinine: 0.7–1.4mg/dL (60–120mcmol/L)

Abnormal
- BUN >18.8mg/dL (>6.7mmol/L)
- Creatinine: >1.4mg/dL (>120mcmol/L)

Cause of abnormal result
- Impaired clearance of waste products from the blood
- Release of creatine and creatinine from damaged muscle
- Keep in mind the possibility of a falsely abnormal result

Drugs, disorders and other factors that may alter results
- Elevations in BUN can also result from steroid therapy, parenteral nutrition, gastrointestinal bleeding, and catabolic states
- Spurious elevation in serum creatinine may be seen following the use of cimetidine, trimethoprim and cephalosporins

SERUM ELECTROLYTES
Description
Venous blood sample.

Advantages/Disadvantages
Advantages:
- Easily available in local laboratories
- Important for timely recognition of life-threatening emergencies such as hyperkalemia

Normal
- Serum potassium: 3.3–5.0mEq/L (3.3–5.0mmol/L)
- Serum sodium: 135–145mEq/L (135–145mmol/L)
- Serum phosphorus: 2.8–4.9mg/dL (0.9–1.6mmol/L)
- Serum calcium: 8.8–10.4mg/dL (2.2–2.6mmol/L)

Abnormal
- Serum potassium: >5.0mEq/L (>5.0mmol/L)
- Serum sodium: <135mEq/L (<135mmol/L)
- Serum phosphorus: >4.9mg/dL (>1.6mmol/L)
- Serum calcium: <8.8mg/dL (<2.2mmol/L)
- Keep in mind the possibility of falsely abnormal results

Cause of abnormal result
- Excessive release of potassium and phosphate from damaged muscle
- Impaired clearance of potassium and phosphate from renal insufficiency
- Hyponatremia is usually dilutional
- Hypocalcemia is secondary to the hyperphosphatemia, calcium entry into damaged muscle, and impaired absorption of calcium from the gastrointestinal tract due to inadequate production of active vitamin D by the diseased kidneys

SERUM CREATINE KINASE
Description
Venous blood sample.

Advantages/Disadvantages
- Advantage: diagnostic for rhabdomyolysis if the skeletal muscle fraction (MM isoenzyme) is elevated
- Disadvantage: available only in specialized laboratories

Normal
100–200U/L.

Abnormal
- >200U/L; in rhabdomyolysis, values of 10,000–100,000U/L are frequently encountered
- Keep in mind the possibility of a falsely abnormal result

Cause of abnormal result
Excessive release from damaged muscle.

SERUM AND URINE MYOGLOBIN

Description

- Performed when the diagnosis of rhabdomyolysis is unclear
- Performed by a specialist
- Elevated levels are diagnostic, but normal values do not rule out rhabdomyolysis

Advantages/Disadvantages

Advantages:

- Elevated levels are diagnostic
- Abnormal values are often seen in initial rhabdomyolysis

Disadvantages:

- Test requires specialist knowledge to perform and interpret the results
- Normal values can occur even in rhabdomyolysis because of rapid metabolism and filtration of myoglobin

Normal

Absent.

Abnormal

Present.

Cause of abnormal result

- Rhabdomyolysis
- Keep in mind the possibility of a falsely abnormal result

Imaging

RENAL ULTRASOUND

Description

- This is done by a radiology technician
- It is performed to diagnose certain causes of renal disease
- Abscesses can be seen in bacterial renal disease

Advantages/Disadvantages

Advantages:

- Renal size and abscesses can be ascertained and monitored. Hydronephrosis, if present, would be seen
- Noninvasive
- May diagnose the cause of rhabdomyolysis

Disadvantages:

- Test requiring specialist to perform and interpret the result
- Not diagnostic for rhabdomyolysis

Normal

Normal renal size and appearance.

Abnormal

- Renal abscess
- Enlarged renal size

Cause of abnormal result

Renal disease.

Special tests
URINE TOXICOLOGY SCREEN
Description
- Performed in patients with rhabdomyolysis and suspected drug or toxin exposure
- Specialist investigation

Advantages/Disadvantages
Advantages:
- Drugs or toxins will be diagnosed through this screen
- Noninvasive
- May diagnose the cause of rhabdomyolysis

Disadvantages:
- Specialist test
- Not diagnostic for rhabdomyolysis, but only for a specific cause

Normal
Negative.

Abnormal
Positive.

Cause of abnormal result
Drugs include amphetamines, cocaine and heroin.

Other tests
ELECTROCARDIOGRAPHY (ECG)
Advantages/Disadvantages
Advantages:
- Important for the detection of cardiac changes in patients with hyperkalemia
- Noninvasive
- Inexpensive and easy to perform
- Repeated ECG allow for monitoring

Normal
Normal ECG pattern.

Abnormal
- Mild hyperkalemia: tenting of T waves, PVC
- Severe hyperkalemia: tall peaked T waves, prolonged PR interval, widened QRS, depressed ST
- Terminal events: ventricular tachycardia, ventricular fibrillation
- Keep in mind the possibility of a falsely abnormal result

Cause of abnormal result
Depolarizing effect of hyperkalemia on cardiac conduction pathways.

TREATMENT

CONSIDER CONSULT
- Patients with acute renal failure (ARF) should be referred to a nephrologist

IMMEDIATE ACTION
- Any patient with rhabdomyolysis should be treated immediately with intravenous fluids
- If an individual with trauma is trapped, then intravenous fluids should be administered before a limb and the rest of the body are released
- Need for cardiac monitoring should be considered if there is clinical hyperkalemia, or cardiac arrhythmias

PATIENT AND CAREGIVER ISSUES

Patient or caregiver request
- **Will I recover from this disease?** Most patients recover with appropriate management
- **Will the disease be recurrent?** If the cause is found then management will include preventive measures
- **Will I need to have dialysis for the rest of my life?** Dialysis for ARF caused by rhabdomyolysis is normally transient, and the majority of patients will recover adequate renal function

MANAGEMENT ISSUES
Goals
- To prevent ARF
- Early recognition of the need for referral to a specialist
- To treat the underlying cause
- Careful follow-up of the patient to prevent complications

Management in special circumstances
Early referral to a specialist is advisable in:
- Children
- Patients with recurrent episodes
- Patients whose underlying etiology is not obvious

COEXISTING DISEASE
- Patients with pre-existing renal disease or dehydration are more prone to developing ARF secondary to rhabdomyolysis
- The renal failure may exacerbate a pre-existing hypertension

COEXISTING MEDICATION
Patients with impending or established renal failure should avoid nephrotoxic drugs including:
- Nonsteroidal anti-inflammatory drugs
- Contrast agents
- Aminoglycoside antibiotics
- Angiotensin-converting enzyme (ACE) inhibitors/angiotension receptor blockers (ARBs)

PATIENT SATISFACTION/LIFESTYLE PRIORITIES
- Some patients with rhabdomyolysis may develop chronic renal failure, especially with prolonged hypovolemia, hypotension, or use of nephrotoxic agents
- Chronic renal failure will require long-term dialysis
- Lifestyle issues such as alcohol and recreational drug use must be addressed in order to prevent future episodes

SUMMARY OF THERAPEUTIC OPTIONS
Choices
The aim of therapy in rhabdomyolysis is to prevent myoglobin precipitation leading to ARF.

- The first step is hydration with intravenous fluids (intravenous normal saline)
- The second step is forced diuresis with intravenous mannitol; however, this has not been shown to improve outcome in randomized controlled trials. Forced diuresis with mannitol aims to: increase renal blood flow and glomerular filtration; increase urine flow and prevent obstructive casts; prevent myoglobin precipitation; and reduce muscle swelling and cellular injury by scavenging free radicals
- However, renal failure will be worsened if not properly volume resuscitated before the onset of therapy, and volume overload may occur. Mannitol should be discontinued if adequate urine flow rate cannot be established, or if signs of volume overload supervene. Nephrology guidance is highly recommended
- The third step is urinary alkalinization with intravenous bicarbonate; this also has not been shown to improve the outcome clinically
- Specialized therapy may be required for the control of ARF with dialysis
- Treatment of the underlying cause is important and ongoing
- Fasciotomy is indicated in compartment syndrome for preservation of muscle and nerve function. Fasciotomy can lead to rapid decompression of compartment syndrome. This surgical procedure should be performed as an emergency for preservation of muscle and nerve function. Prevention of rhabdomyolysis is the aim of this procedure

In addition to the above measures, patients should be counseled regarding the importance of avoiding behaviors that may precipitate rhabdomyolysis (lifestyle adjustments).

Clinical pearls
In deconditioned trekkers the condition is more commonly seen during the descent from the mountains than during the ascent because of the greater isometric component of the descent.

Never
- Never delay administration of intravenous fluids
- Never administer potassium-containing fluids or potassium-containing foods to individuals with suspected renal insufficiency

FOLLOW UP
Plan for review
During the acute phase, close monitoring is required for deteriorating muscle manifestations and renal function.

DRUGS AND OTHER THERAPIES: DETAILS
Drugs

INTRAVENOUS NORMAL SALINE
Rapid and vigorous hydration with intravenous normal saline is crucial for the prevention of acute renal failure.

Dose
Recommended dosages vary depending on source; some authorities recommend using a rate determined by the severity of intravascular volume depletion. Guidance from a nephrologist is highly recommended.
- Infuse normal saline. Recommended rates for the initial bolus vary in the literature between 200 and 1000mL/h

- Subsequent fluids at a rate determined by the urine flow rate, blood pressure, hematocrit and in severe cases invasive monitoring. Subsequent fluids may include 5% dextrose in water and bicarbonate solution
- The goal is to achieve a urine output of 2–3mL/kg/h

Efficacy
- There is overwhelming support in the literature for the efficacy of early hydration
- Vigorous hydration with isotonic crystalloid is the mainstay of treatment of rhabdomyolysis
- Prevention of acute renal failure is imperative, with liberal use of intravenous fluids
- Myoglobinuria usually resolves within 3–4 days

Risks/Benefits
Benefit: the ability to prevent renal failure via a modality that is universally available, even in a rural setting.

Follow up plan
- Vigorous hydration should be continued until myoglobinuria disappears (usually in 3–4 days), and the patient is able to take in oral fluids
- Close monitoring is required to prevent volume overload

INTRAVENOUS BICARBONATE
- Bicarbonate enhances urinary excretion of myoglobin
- It also reduces the risk of hyperkalemia

Dose
Recommended dosages vary depending on source. Guidance from a nephrologist is highly recommended.

Efficacy
Bicarbonate prevents myoglobin precipitation by making the urine alkaline.

Risks/Benefits
Risks:
- Myoglobin precipitation leads to renal failure
- Does not have a role to play in the management of diabetic ketoacidosis
- Should not be administered as single dose intravenous injection
- Prolonged use not recommended due to hypernatremia
- Use caution in Cushing's syndrome, Bartter's syndrome and hyperaldosteronism
- Use caution in cardiac disease, and hepatic and renal impairment
- Use caution in the elderly, pregnancy, neonates and children under 2 years of age
- Use caution in respiratory acidosis, hypokalemia, and patients receiving corticosteroids

Benefits:
- Bicarbonate aids in alkaline diuresis
- Alkaline diuresis prevents myoglobin precipitation in the urine

Side-effects and adverse reactions
- Cardiovascular system: peripheral edema
- Central nervous system: tetany, tremor, seizures
- Gastrointestinal: flatulence, bloating, abdominal pain, acid rebound
- Metabolic: metabolic alkalosis, hypernatremia, hyperosmolarity, lactic acidosis, milk-alkali syndrome
- Skin: injection site reaction

Interactions (other drugs)
- Dextroamphetamine ▪ Ephedrine, pseudoephedrine ▪ Flecainide ▪ Iron salts
- Ketoconazole ▪ Lithium ▪ Methenamine ▪ Methotrexate ▪ Quinidine ▪ Salicylates
- Sulfonylureas ▪ Sympathomimetics ▪ Tetracyclines

Contraindications
- Caution should be exercised when using sodium bicarbonate in congestive cardiac failure, hypertension, hypocalcemia, and renal failure ▪ Contraindicated in cirrhosis and toxemia
- Metabolic alkalosis ▪ Respiratory alkalosis

Follow up plan
- Should be determined by a nephrologist. In general, bicarbonate should be discontinued if adequate urine flow rate cannot be established, or if signs of volume overload supervene
- Serum calcium should be closely monitored since bicarbonate therapy can precipitate hypocalcemia

Surgical therapy
FASCIOTOMY
Indicated in compartment syndrome for preservation of muscle and nerve function. The aim of this procedure is prevention of rhabdomyolysis.

Efficacy
Good.

Risks/Benefits
Benefit: fasciotomy can lead to rapid decompression of compartment syndrome.

Follow up plan
- Careful follow-up is required to prevent further episodes of compartment syndrome
- Postsurgical care is necessary to prevent sepsis or hemorrhage
- Low index of suspicion for compartment syndrome
- A very good tool is the intracompartmental pressure monitor used in most modern intensive care units to detect the first sign of increased pressure

Patient and caregiver information
Full patient consent is necessary, although it may be an emergency procedure.

LIFESTYLE
Counsel and treat patients to stop alcohol and drug consumption, as both are causes for rhabdomyolysis.

ACCEPTABILITY TO PATIENT
Addiction to alcohol or recreational drugs may be difficult to treat, especially if the patient is noncompliant.

FOLLOW UP PLAN
Urine toxicology and blood alcohol levels should be undertaken to check on compliance.

PATIENT AND CAREGIVER INFORMATION
The patient and their family should be given information and support regarding substance addiction.

EFFICACY OF THERAPIES
- There is good evidence in the literature on the prevention of acute renal failure in rhabdomyolysis for the efficacy of early hydration (intravenous normal saline)
- Although no proven benefit to outcome exists in the literature, there are anecdotal reports and theoretical advantages to using forced diuresis (intravenous mannitol) and urinary alkalinization (intravenous bicarbonate)

Review period
12 months.

PROGNOSIS
- Early hydration, forced diuresis and urinary alkalinization are efficacious in preventing ARF
- Prognosis in ARF is good with institution of appropriate therapy
- Overall prognosis depends on the underlying etiology

Clinical pearls
- Low index of suspicion for muscle injury due to any cause should prompt a urinalysis and lab evaluation of CK
- Recurrent episodes of rhabdomyolysis may occur in children with inherited myopathies

Therapeutic failure
Hemodialysis is usually required when ARF occurs.

Recurrence
Recurrent episodes of rhabdomyolysis may occur in children with inherited myopathies.

COMPLICATIONS
Complications are related to the muscle breakdown and to the underlying etiology including:
- Hyperkalemia
- Acute renal failure
- Disseminated intravascular coagulation (DIC)
- Metabolic acidosis

CONSIDER CONSULT
- Referral is warranted as soon as creatinine increases to more than 1.2mg/dL, urine output starts to decrease, or CPK starts to rise

PREVENTION

RISK FACTORS
- Pre-existing renal disease: increases the risk for myoglobin-induced ARF
- Alcohol and drug use

MODIFY RISK FACTORS
Pre-existing renal disease: ensure adequate control of renal disease.

Lifestyle and wellness
ALCOHOL AND DRUGS
- Alcoholism: causes rhabdomyolysis from prolonged immobilization, hypokalemia, hypophosphatemia, and agitation
- Drugs that may cause rhabdomyolysis from direct myotoxicity and/or agitation include heroin, amphetamines, ecstasy and cocaine
- Counsel and support patients to stop alcohol and drug consumption

PHYSICAL ACTIVITY
- Excessive exercise can lead to muscle necrosis causing rhabdomyolysis, especially in hot humid climates and with poor physical conditioning
- Patients should be advised against excessive exercise regimens
- If exercise is unavoidable, adequate water and salt must be provided

ENVIRONMENT
Prevention in a bed-bound obese patient: frequent turning and frequent examination of lower extremities/buttocks are required, especially in a postoperative patient.

FAMILY HISTORY
Inherited myopathies increase the risk of recurrent rhabdomyolysis associated with exercise, infections, or fasting.

DRUG HISTORY
Avoidance of the following drugs is imperative in preventing rhabdomyolysis:
- Antimalarials
- Clofibrate
- Central nervous system depressants
- Colchicine
- Corticosteroids
- Diuretics
- Fenofibrate
- Gemfibrozil
- Haloperidol
- HMG-CoA reductase inhibitors (statins): lovastatin, fluvastatin, simvastatin, atrovastatin
- Isoniazid
- Narcotics
- Neuroleptics
- Phenothiazines
- Succinylcholine
- Zidovudine

SCREENING
Screening for rhabdomyolysis in the general population is not necessary.

ASSOCIATIONS
National Kidney Foundation
30 E 33rd Street, Suite 1100
New York, NY 10016
Phone: (800) 622-9010 or (212) 889-2210
Fax: (212) 689-9261
www.kidney.org

KEY REFERENCES

- Better OS, Stein JH. Early management of shock and prophylaxis of acute renal failure in traumatic rhabdomyolysis. N Engl J Med 1990;322:825–829
- Zager RA. Rhabdomyolysis and myohemoglobinuric acute renal failure. Kidney Int 1996;49:314–326
- Vanholder R, Sever MS, Erek E, Lameire N. Rhabdomyolysis. J Am Soc Nephrol 2000;11:1553–1561
- Sinert R, Kohl L, Rainone T, Scalea T. Exercise-induced rhabdomyolysis. Ann Emerg Med 1994;23:(6):1301–6
- Ellsworth AJ. Mosby's medical drug reference, 2001–2002. St Louis: Mosby, 2001
- Eneas JF, Schoenfeld PY, Humphreys MH. The effect of infusion of mannitol sodium bicarbonate on the clinical course of myoglobinuria. Arch Intern Med 1979;139:801–5
- Humphreys MH. Pigment and crystal induced acute renal failure. In: Jacobson HR, Striker GE, Klahr S, eds. The principles and practice of nephrology. St Louis: Mosby, 1991, p650–55
- Wortmann RL. Inflammatory diseases of muscle and other myopathiesl. In: Ruddy, ed. Kelly's textbook of rheumatology. St Louis: Mosby, 2001, p1287–8
- Bolin P Jr. Rhabdomyolysis. In: Wortmann RL, ed. Diseases of skeletal muscle. Philadelphia: Lippincott, Williams and Wilkins, 2000, p245–54
- Staffa JA, Chang J, Green L. Cerivastatin and reports of fatal rhabdomyolysis. N Engl J Med 2002;202;346:539–540
- Bedry R, Baudrimont I, Deffieux G, et al. Wild mushroom intoxication as a cause of rhabdomyolysis. N Engl J Med 2001;345:798–802
- Knochel JP, Moore GE. Rhabdomyolysis in malaria. N Engl J Med 1994;329:1206–12–7
- Lees RS, Lees AM. Rhabdomyolysis and the coadministration of lovastatin and the antifungal agent itraconazole. N Engl J Med 1995;333:664–665
- Mahler H, Pasi A, Kramer JM, et al. Fulminant liver failure in association with the emetic toxin of bacillus cereus. N Engl J Med 1997;336:1142–1148. Note patient developed liver failure with rhabdomyolysis.

FAQS
Question 1
Use of what lipid lowering agents may result in rhabdomyolysis?

ANSWER 1
Clofibrate, bezafibrate, gemfibrozil, lovastatin, pravastatin, simvastatin, niacin.

Question 2
What is the significance of hyperuricemia in these patients?

ANSWER 2
Hyperuricemia resulting from a combination of increased release from skeletal muscle and decreased excretion due to kidney failure may result in a urate nephropathy.

Question 3

What is the CPK in rhabdomyolysis?

ANSWER 3

The CPK is elevated in rhabdomyolysis. Typically levels of greater than 10,000 are found in association with ARF, although both much higher and lower CPK levels may also be found.

CONTRIBUTORS

Thompson H Boyd, III, MD
Maria-Louise Barilla-LaBarca, MD
Ankush Gulati, MD
Rakesh Gulati, MD

TESTICULAR MALIGNANCIES

SUMMARY INFORMATION

DESCRIPTION

- The most common cancer among men between 15 and 34 years of age
- The overall 5-year survival rate has increased from 63% in 1963 to 95% today
- Germ cell tumors account for 95% of testicular cancers
- Delay in diagnosis is associated with a worse prognosis

KEY! DON'T MISS!

- A painful scrotal or testicular mass is often misdiagnosed as epididymitis or epididymo-orchitis and the patient treated for long intervals with antibiotics
- Studies have shown that symptoms last 17–87 weeks before correct diagnosis is made
- Early diagnosis of testicular cancer is crucial because of the rapid doubling time of the tumor, generally estimated at between 10 and 30 days

ICD9 CODE
186 Malignant neoplasm of testis.

CARDINAL FEATURES
- Most common presentation is a painless scrotal mass, although many patients initially report pain, swelling, or 'heaviness' in testis
- On ultrasound, any hypoechoic area within the testis should be considered cancer until proved otherwise
- Although the incidence of testicular cancer is rising, the 5-year survival rate now exceeds 95%
- Depending on the cell type and the stage of the disease, treatment is with chemotherapy, radiation therapy, or both after initial radical orchiectomy
- For treatment planning, testicular tumors are broadly divided between seminoma and nonseminoma because seminomas are more sensitive to radiation therapy
- Testicular cancers grow rapidly with a doubling time of 20–30 days and, as a general rule, have a high risk of metastatic spread

CAUSES
Common causes
- The direct cause of testicular cancer is unknown
- The rise in overall incidence suggests an environmental factor, but one has not been identified

Contributory or predisposing factors
- A male with a history of cryptorchidism, even if corrected, has a 2.5- to 8.8-fold risk of developing testicular cancer than a male without an undescended testicle
- Approximately 10% of testicular cancers are diagnosed in men with a history of cryptorchidism
- In patients with unilateral cryptorchidism, there is also an increased risk of tumor in the contralateral descended testis (5–10% develop the malignancy in the contralateral descended testis)
- Genetic disorders such as testicular feminization, >30 years of age, or gonadal dysgenesis with Y chromosome
- Isochromosomal deletions on the short arm of chromosome 12 have been found in many patients with both seminomatous and nonseminomatous germ cell tumors
- A second important risk factor in the development of testis cancer is the presence of a contralateral tumor. Up to 5% of patients with testis cancer will develop a contralateral testis tumor, most often metachronously
- Trauma, or rather the traumatic event that forces the patient to seek medical consultation, that leads to the discovery of the tumor
- Nonspecific or mumps-associated atrophy is associated with a higher likelihood of developing testis cancer
- Hormonal factors have been associated with the development of testis tumors (diethylstilbestrol [DES] exposure)
- Prenatal factors include maternal severe nausea, unusual bleeding during pregnancy, low birth weight, and early birth order
- HIV infection

EPIDEMIOLOGY
Incidence and prevalence
- Testicular cancer accounts for 1% of all cancers in men
- Testis cancer tends to occur in three distinct age groups: infants and children (0–10 years), young adults (15–40 years), and older adults (>60 years)
- It is the most common cancer in men between 15 and 34 years of age

INCIDENCE

- In the US, the incidence is 0.042 per 1000
- Accounts for 6600 new cases per year, with a lifetime probability of developing testis cancer of 0.2%

FREQUENCY

Primary cell types in germ cell tumors and incidence:

- Seminoma – 42% ranging from 34–55%
- Embryonal cell carcinoma – 26% ranging from 23–34%
- Teratocarcinoma – 26% ranging from 9–32%
- Teratoma – 5% ranging from 1–6%
- Choriocarcinoma – 1%
- Intratubular germ cell neoplasia is a precursor lesion that may precede both seminomatous and nonseminomatous germ cell tumors
- Approximately 25% of testis cancers are composed of multiple cell types, with embryonal cell carcinoma and teratoma being the most common
- Seminoma remains the most common germ cell tumor. It was commonly divided into typical, anaplastic, and spermatocytic cell types
- Spermatocytic seminoma occurs at a later age and is unlikely to metastasize

Demographics

AGE

- The median age for new cases is 32 years
- The incidence in the US peaks between 25 and 34 years of age
- Incidence declines markedly after 40 years of age

GENDER

Males only.

RACE

- Variable incidence rates are noted between different ethnic groups within a given geographic region
- The incidence of testicular tumors in African-Americans is approximately one-third that in Caucasians but 10 times that in Africans
- Lower incidence among Asians and Hispanics

GENETICS

Primary relatives of patients with testicular cancer have a 6- to 10-fold increased risk of contracting it.

GEOGRAPHY

- The incidence in the US between 1940 and 1947 was 2.88 cases per 100,000, whereas the incidence in Great Britain during the same time interval was 2.33 per 100,000
- In 1995, the incidence of testis cancer in the US increased to 4.5 per 100,000
- In England, Scotland, the Nordic countries, Australia, and New Zealand, the incidence has also increased
- The increasing incidence appears to be due to more than just increasing patient awareness and cancer registries, but the exact etiology remains uncertain

SOCIOECONOMIC STATUS

- Men of higher socioeconomic status appear to be more commonly affected
- Men living in rural areas have a higher incidence of testis cancer

DIFFERENTIAL DIAGNOSIS
Epididymitis
Patients with painful scrotal swelling are often misdiagnosed with epididymitis or epididymo-orchitis and may be treated for long intervals with antibiotics (up to 10% of testis tumors present with epididymitis).

FFATURES
- Tender swelling of scrotum with erythema
- Dysuria and/or urethral discharge
- Fever and signs of systemic illness
- Take a 'first catch' urine sample and look for urethral discharge
- Pain and redness on scrotal examination
- Hydrocele or even epididymo-orchitis, especially late

Orchitis
Inflammation of the testicle(s) often due to infections, including *Escherichia coli*, mumps, gonococcal infection, or tuberculosis. The main features of orchitis are as follows:

FEATURES
- Testicular pain and swelling, which may be unilateral or bilateral
- May be associated with epididymitis, prostatitis, fever, scrotal edema, erythema cellulitis
- Inguinal lymphadenopathy
- Nausea and vomiting
- Acute hydrocele
- Possible spermatic cord tenderness

Hydrocele
Collection of fluid in the tunica vaginalis around the testicle. 5–10% of testis tumors present with hydrocele.

FEATURES
- Scrotal enlargement and distention
- Scrotal heaviness or discomfort radiating to the inguinal area
- Back pain
- Primary hydroceles are more common, are larger, and usually develop in younger men
- Secondary hydroceles may be caused by testicular tumors, trauma, or infection
- Ultrasound will help confirm the diagnosis
- Hydroceles may be treated by aspiration or surgery

Testicular torsion
Testicular torsion is a surgical emergency because prompt surgery saves the testicle.

FEATURES
- Sudden onset of pain in one testis only
- Abdominal pain and nausea/vomiting also common (but without fever or urinary symptoms)
- Inflammation of one testis (usually follows pain, but swelling is painless in 10% of cases)
- Most common in 15- to 30-year-olds, although testicular torsion can develop at any age
- Acute hydrocele
- Possible spermatic cord tenderness
- Ultrasound will help confirm the diagnosis
- Surgery includes reducing the torsion and bilateral fixation (orchidopexy)
- Certain cases will require an orchidectomy

Hematoma
Collection of blood within the tunica vaginalis due usually to trauma or surgery.

FEATURES
- Usually follows a history of trauma to the scrotal region
- Occasionally bleeding will occur spontaneously associated with bleeding disorders
- Ultrasound will help confirm the diagnosis
- Aspiration or surgical drainage may be necessary

Spermatocele
Spermatocele is a swelling in the scrotum adjacent to the testicle.

FEATURES
- Generally occurs above or adjacent to the upper pole of the testis and represents a cyst of the rete testis or epididymis
- Tends to transilluminate
- Ultrasound will help confirm the diagnosis

Varicocele
Varicocele are varicosities of the venous plexus attached to the testicle.

FEATURES
- Varicoceles are implicated in male infertility, hypogonadism, and cases of inferior vena cava obstruction on the right and left renal vein obstruction
- Changes in the size of the spermatic cord between the standing and the supine positions or when using the Valsalva maneuver with the patient in the upright position indicate presence of a varicocele
- Ultrasound will help confirm the diagnosis

Hernia
An indirect inguinal hernia can lead to a scrotal lump.

FEATURES
- Hernia passes through both the internal and external inguinal rings to cause a scrotal swelling
- Indirect hernias represent 80% of inguinal hernias
- Indirect inguinal hernias can strangulate
- In the standing position, palpation of the inguinal canal may be carried out
- Increasing intra-abdominal pressure by asking the patient to cough or by using the Valsalva maneuver will help define the presence of an inguinal hernia
- Ultrasound will help confirm the diagnosis
- Patients should be advised to stop smoking and lose weight if applicable prior to surgery

SIGNS & SYMPTOMS
Signs
- The cardinal sign is a painless intratesticular mass
- Other signs include fullness in the scrotum, dull ache, pain, or infertility
- Up to 19% of patients demonstrate signs or symptoms of metastatic disease at first presentation
- Signs of metastases may include neck mass, neurologic findings consistent with spinal cord compression, unilateral or bilateral leg swelling secondary to inguinal node spread, or abdominal mass
- Between 5% and 10% of patients have gynecomastia from tumors that secrete beta-human chorionic gonadotropin (HCG)

Symptoms

- Approximately 50% of patients present with a painless scrotal mass found during self-examination, after testicular trauma, or by a sexual partner
- Between 30% and 40% of patients present with scrotal pain, often initially misdiagnosed as epididymitis
- Symptoms of metastases may include low back or bone pain, cough, dyspnea, hemoptysis, anorexia, nausea, or vomiting
- Remember that trauma is not a cause of tumor but often prompts medical evaluation

KEY! DON'T MISS!

- A painful scrotal or testicular mass is often misdiagnosed as epididymitis or epididymo-orchitis and the patient treated for long intervals with antibiotics
- Studies have shown that symptoms last 17–87 weeks before correct diagnosis is made
- Early diagnosis of testicular cancer is crucial because of the rapid doubling time of the tumor, generally estimated at between 10 and 30 days

CONSIDER CONSULT

- Painless scrotal mass is a cancer until proved otherwise, and men with a painless lump should proceed immediately to ultrasound and blood testing
- Patients with a suspicious scrotal mass should be referred for scrotal ultrasound
- If ultrasound reveals an intratesticular mass, the patient generally will be referred for surgery
- Biopsy should never be done

INVESTIGATION OF THE PATIENT
Direct questions to patient

Q For how long has swelling been present? The prognosis of testicular cancer worsens as the interval between onset and diagnosis lengthens.

Q Is it painful? Although testicular cancer most commonly presents as a painless scrotal mass, between 30% and 40% of cases have pain.

Q Do you have symptoms suggestive of metastases (low back or bone pain, cough, dyspnea, hemoptysis, anorexia, nausea, or vomiting)? Metastatic disease has a worse outcome.

Contributory or predisposing factors

Q Is there a history of undescended testicle? There is an increased risk of testicular cancer in males with a history of cryptorchidism. About 10% of testis tumors arise from an undescended testis. The undescended testis is 35–48 times more likely to undergo malignant degeneration than the normal testis.

Q If so, at what age was it detected and repaired? Early correction of undescended testis does not change the malignant potential but allows for easier examination and follow-up.

Family history

Q Is there a family history of testicular cancer? Primary relatives of cases have a 6- to 10-fold increased risk of testicular cancer.

Examination

- Bimanual examination of the scrotal contents should be done first
- Start with the unaffected testis to get a baseline
- Check the spermatic cord and epididymis for thickening and pain
- Palpate for inguinal, neck, and supraclavicular lymph nodes
- Palpate the abdomen for masses
- Check for gynecomastia

Summary of investigative tests

- A persistent scrotal mass should be evaluated initially with ultrasound. Scrotal ultrasound is virtually 100% accurate in distinguishing between intratesticular and extratesticular masses
- Any intratesticular mass should be considered cancer until proved otherwise, and patients with intratesticular hypoechoic masses should be considered to be candidates for biopsy
- Because of the risk of local recurrence of tumor if a trans-scrotal biopsy is performed, the biopsy method of choice is radical inguinal orchiectomy with high ligation of the spermatic cord
- Patients with proven testicular tumor should be assessed for the presence of the serum tumor markers alpha-fetoprotein, beta subunit of human chorionic gonadotropin, and lactate dehydrogenase; also placental-like alkaline phosphatase
- Computed tomography (CT) is the imaging procedure of choice to assess the clinical stage of the retroperitoneal lymph nodes in patients with testicular cancer
- Retroperitoneal lymph node dissection is an alternative to CT scan in staging patients and is a form of treatment depending on histologic cell type and clinical stage, especially in nonseminomatous cancers

DIAGNOSTIC DECISION

- The diagnosis of testicular cancer is based on radical orchiectomy results
- For treatment planning it is important to distinguish seminomatous from nonseminomatous tumors
- Mixed cell type tumors are considered nonseminomatous cancers
- Pure seminomas that secrete alpha-fetoprotein (AFP), which is detectable in the blood, are considered nonseminomatous cancers

TNM staging system is used for testicular cancer:

- T_0 represents no apparent primary
- T_1 represents testis only (excludes rete testis)
- T_2 represents beyond the tunica albuginea
- T_3 represents rete testis or epididymal involvement
- T_4 represents spermatic cord (1) and (2) scrotum
- N_0 represents no nodal involvement
- N_1 represents ipsilateral regional nodal involvement
- N_2 represents contralateral or bilateral abdominal or groin nodes
- N_3 represents palpable abdominal nodes or fixed groin nodes
- N_4 represents juxtaregional nodes
- M_0 represents no distant metastases
- M_1 represents distant metastases present

Clinical stages are recorded for each patient:

- Stage A – tumor confined to the testis and cord structures
- Stage B – tumor confined to the retroperitoneal lymph nodes
- Stage C – tumor involving the abdominal viscera or disease above the diaphragm

CLINICAL PEARLS

- Different testis cancer histologies tend to occur at different ages. The median age range at diagnosis for a nonseminomatous germ cell tumor (25–29 years) is about 10 years earlier compared with that for seminoma (35–39 years)
- Yolk sac tumors are the most common testis malignancy in children
- A high index of suspicion, proper scrotal examination, and radiologic imaging are necessary to make the diagnosis
- Up to 90% of patients with testis cancer will have an elevated AFP or beta-HCG level

THE TESTS
Body fluids
HUMAN CHORIONIC GONADOTROPIN (HCG)
Description

- A blood test used in the diagnosis and follow-up of nonseminomatous testicular cancer, especially choriocarcinoma (100%), teratocarcinoma (57%), and embryonal (60%). 7% of seminoma also secrete
- Not detectable in healthy men
- To avoid cross-reactivity with luteinizing hormone, follicle-stimulating hormone, and thyroid-stimulating hormone (seen with the alpha subunit of HCG), the beta subunit is measured
- Serum half-life is 24–36h
- After a tumor is eliminated, HCG should return to normal in 5–8 days

Advantages/Disadvantages
Advantages:

- Not detectable in healthy men
- More commonly secreted by nonseminomatous tumors
- A recurrence of measurable levels may occur while a recurrent tumor is too small to be detected on physical examination or by imaging studies

Normal
HCG is normally not detectable in healthy men.

Abnormal

- Any detectable level of HCG is abnormal
- A detectable HCG level after the elimination of an HCG-secreting tumor suggests that not all of the cancer was eradicated
- A return of detectable HCG suggests tumor recurrence

Drugs, disorders and other factors that may alter results

- Stomach, pancreatic, small intestinal, and colon cancer
- Bladder cancer
- Bronchogenic cancer
- Breast cancer
- Hodgkin's disease and non-Hodgkin's lymphoma
- Melanoma
- Insulinomas
- Retroperitoneal sarcoma
- Leukemia and myeloma

ALPHA-FETOPROTEIN (AFP)
Description

- A blood test used in the diagnosis and follow-up of nonseminomatous testicular cancer and choriocarcinoma of the testis
- Produced by the fetal liver. Serum AFP levels fall dramatically at birth and become undetectable by one year of age
- Present only in nanogram amounts in healthy males
- Never produced by choriocarcinomas or pure seminomas
- A histologic seminoma that produces AFP should be considered a nonseminomatous cancer
- Serum half-life is 5–7 days
- Should return to normal levels 25–35 days after elimination of tumor

Advantages/Disadvantages
Advantages:
- Almost always elevated in yolk sac tumors, the most common testicular tumor in patients below 15 years of age
- Not secreted by seminomas or choriocarcinomas
- Recurrence of measurable levels may occur while recurrent tumor is too small to be detected on physical examination or by imaging studies

Normal
<25ng/dL (25mcg/L).

Abnormal
- Levels >25ng/dL are abnormal
- An AFP level above baseline after the elimination of an AFP-secreting tumor suggests that not all of the cancer was eradicated
- A return of detectable AFP above baseline suggests tumor recurrence

Drugs, disorders and other factors that may alter results
- Liver damage
- Metastasis
- Gastrointestinal carcinoma
- Hepatocellular carcinoma
- Ataxia-telangiectasia
- Hereditary tyrosinemia

LACTATE DEHYDROGENASE (LDH)
Description
- An enzyme, which can be measured in the blood, that is elevated in half of all patients with testicular cancer
- LDH is normally found in several tissues, including the heart, liver, and skeletal muscle
- Occurs in several isoenzyme forms that can be measured separately

Advantages/Disadvantages
Advantages:
- When elevated, LDH is a useful tumor marker
- Generally elevated proportional to the volume of tumor present
- LDH-1 is most likely to be elevated

Normal
200–680units/mL.

Abnormal
- False-positives result from artifactual hemolysis (poor venipuncture, failure to spin blood sample properly)
- LDH is less specific but has independent prognostic value in patients with advanced germ cell tumors. Serum LDH levels are also increased in approximately 60% of patients with nonseminomatous germ cell tumors and 80% of those with seminomatous germ cell tumors

Drugs, disorders and other factors that may alter results
LDH is also elevated in myocardial infarction, hepatitis, untreated pernicious anemia, other malignant tumors, pulmonary embolus, and skeletal muscle diseases.

PLACENTAL-LIKE ALKALINE PHOSPHATASE (PLAP)
Description
- Useful for diagnosing and following the course of testicular malignancy
- Specialist blood test for tumor marker

Advantages/Disadvantages
Advantages:
- Elevated in 40–100% of seminomas
- Useful in following the course of the disease

Disadvantage: less useful in patients with nonseminomatous germ cell cancers

Abnormal
Raised level of PLAP.

Cause of abnormal result
Testicular tumor.

Drugs, disorders and other factors that may alter results
- May be spuriously raised by tobacco use
- Smokers have a 30% chance of having an elevated PLAP level

Biopsy
RADICAL INGUINAL ORCHIECTOMY
Description
- Biopsy is never indicated if there is a testis mass unless in unusual cases
- All masses are presumed cancer, and the diagnosis is made at surgery via an inguinal, thus radical orchiectomy, approach
- A hypoechoic, intratesticular mass should be excised by means of a radical inguinal orchiectomy with high ligation of the spermatic cord
- Trans-scrotal biopsy is not considered appropriate because of the risk of local tumor spread into the scrotum or ipsilateral inguinal lymph nodes

Advantages/Disadvantages
- Advantage: provides a definitive diagnosis
- Disadvantage: it has the usual disadvantages of surgery, such as bleeding and infection

Normal
No mass detected.

Abnormal
Mass detected and biopsied.

Drugs, disorders and other factors that may alter results
- Infectious mass
- Testicular torsion
- Hematoma
- Spermatocele
- Varicocele
- Hernia

Imaging
ULTRASOUND
Description
- Scrotal ultrasound is used to determine if a scrotal mass is intratesticular or extratesticular
- All masses within the testis should be considered cancer until proven otherwise

Advantages/Disadvantages
Advantage: scrotal ultrasound can distinguish between extratesticular and intratesticular masses with an accuracy that approaches 100%

Normal
Normal scrotal and testicular anatomy.

Abnormal
Testicular mass diagnosed.

Cause of abnormal result
Any intratesticular mass is a cancer until proven otherwise by biopsy.

COMPUTED TOMOGRAPHY (CT)
Description
- All patients with testicular malignancy need an assessment of their retroperitoneal lymph nodes for staging and treatment planning
- CT has essentially replaced lymphangiography as the imaging procedure of choice for the retroperitoneal nodes
- TNM staging is required for all patients to define treatment and prognosis

Advantages/Disadvantages
- Advantage: noninvasive
- Disadvantage: can produce an underestimate or overestimate of the clinical stage in up to 25% of patients

Special tests
RETROPERITONEAL LYMPH NODE DISSECTION (RPLND)
Description
- RPLND is an adjunct to CT as a staging procedure
- Performed more commonly in nonseminomatous cancers

Advantages/Disadvantages
Advantages:
- Although it provides a more invasive stage, it provides a more accurate stage of the cancer
- About 25% of patients with clinical stage I nonseminomatous cancer will receive a higher stage after RPLND
- About 25% of patients with clinical stage II nonseminomatous cancer will be downgraded to stage I after RPLND
- If a patient has microscopic disease that is limited to the retroperitoneal nodes, RPLND can be curative

Disadvantages:
- As an invasive surgical procedure, RPLND carries the usual surgical risks, including bleeding and infection
- Although nerve-sparing procedures are commonly used, the procedure still carries a risk of postoperative retrograde ejaculation and infertility

TREATMENT

CONSIDER CONSULT

- Testicular cancer typically is managed by a multidisciplinary team of urologic surgeons, radiation therapists, and medical oncologists working in conjunction with the primary care provider
- Primary care physicians usually refer patients for further study when the diagnosis of testicular cancer is suspected
- Primary care physicians also follow treated patients for recurrence and complications and, when necessary, provide end-of-life care

PATIENT AND CAREGIVER ISSUES
Impact on career, dependants, family, friends

- Fertility is an issue for patients
- Many patients have either sperm abnormalities or oligospermia before the initiation of therapy
- Almost all patients become oligospermic during treatment, so sperm banking should be offered
- Many survivors of testicular cancer have fathered children
- Studies to date suggest that the children of testicular cancer survivors are not at increased risk of congenital malformations
- There appears to be an increased risk of secondary leukemia, primarily nonlymphocytic, in survivors of testicular cancer
- Risk factors appear to be prolonged use of alkylating drugs and use of the drug etoposide
- The cumulative incidence of secondary leukemia is probably no greater than 0.5% at 5 years
- Some patients experience mild decreases in creatinine clearance during platinum-based therapy
- There does not appear to be significant risk of further renal deterioration over the long term
- Some patients receiving platinum-based therapy develop bilateral hearing deficits outside the usual range of conversation

MANAGEMENT ISSUES
Goals

The goal of treatment is cure.

Management in special circumstances

SPECIAL PATIENT GROUPS

RPLND is not performed in children with testicular cancer because the information obtained is outweighed by the potential risks of surgery.

PATIENT SATISFACTION/LIFESTYLE PRIORITIES

- If preservation of fertility is important, a nerve-sparing technique should be used for patients undergoing lymph node dissection
- This technique appears to be as effective as standard RPLND in preventing recurrence of disease

SUMMARY OF THERAPEUTIC OPTIONS
Choices

- Treatment depends on cell type (seminomatous or nonseminomatous) and the stage at time of diagnosis
- Seminoma is sensitive to radiotherapy
- After the testis is removed by radical inguinal orchiectomy, the retroperitoneal and inguinal areas are irradiated. For stage I and many stage II seminomatous tumors, radiation is curative
- Some stage II and all stage III seminomas are managed with radiation followed by combination chemotherapy

- Nonseminomatous cancers are generally considered highly curable in early stages
- After removal of testis by radical inguinal orchiectomy, patients with stage I nonseminomatous disease are managed by either RPLND or close follow-up without RPLND
- Management of stage II nonseminomatous germ cell tumor usually includes RPLND and platinum-based chemotherapy, although selected patients can be managed by careful follow-up after lymph node dissection with chemotherapy reserved for recurrence
- Stage III nonseminomatous germ cell tumors is usually curable with multidrug chemotherapy

Clinical pearls

- Patients with metastatic disease are classified on the basis of various prognostic factors
- Three groups have been identified (minimal, moderate, and advanced) based on the extent of the disease
- Patients with minimal or moderate disease have a 99% and 90% response rate, respectively, whereas patients with advanced disease have only a 58% chance of response with standard therapy
- Prior to treatment, patients with testis cancer should be offered sperm banking

FOLLOW UP

Because many deaths from testicular cancer are caused by metastatic disease after inadequate follow-up, a monitoring protocol is essential for at least 5 years after primary treatment is completed.

Plan for review

- Protocols for follow-up vary with cell type, stage, and the treating institution
- A typical protocol for patient follow-up in nonseminomatous cancer includes physical examination every month for one year, then every 3 months for one year, followed by every 4 months for one year, then every 6 months for 1–2 years, and finally annually
- Measure serum tumor markers every month for one year, then every 3 months for one year, followed by every 4 months for one year, then every 6 months for 1–2 years, and finally annually
- Chest X-ray (PA/lateral) every month for one year, then every 3 months for one year, followed by every 4 months for one year, then every 6 months for 1–2 years, and finally annually
- For patients undergoing RPLND and radiation therapy, CT scans of the abdomen, pelvis, and chest are performed at intervals ranging from every 2 months to scans at 3 and 12 months post-treatment

DRUGS AND OTHER THERAPIES: DETAILS
Radiation therapy
RADIATION THERAPY

- Radiation therapy without adjuvant chemotherapy is used to treat patients with stage I seminoma following orchiectomy
- Radiation therapy also is used without chemotherapy in stage II seminoma that is classified as nonbulky (tumors <5cm on a CT scan)
- Patients with bulky (tumors >5cm) stage II seminoma may receive either combination chemotherapy or radiation therapy after orchiectomy
- Current treatment protocols do not include the use of radiation therapy in patients with nonseminomatous testicular cancer

Efficacy

- In stage I seminoma, radiation of the para-aortic nodes alone appears to be as efficacious as para-aortic radiation plus radiation to the ipsilateral inguinal area
- In stage II nonbulky seminoma, radiation of the retroperitoneal and ipsilateral pelvic nodes alone is effective; prophylactic mediastinal or neck radiation is not required
- Bulky stage II seminoma requires radiation to both abdominal and pelvic nodes

Risks/Benefits
- Risk: acute toxicity from radiation therapy is usually gastrointestinal (nausea, vomiting, diarrhea, peptic ulcers) and is usually mild

Benefits:
- Because seminoma is very radiosensitive, radiation therapy offers the advantage of cure without the need for chemotherapy
- Because the recurrence rate for bulky stage II seminomas treated with radiation is higher than the rate for nonbulky tumors, some experts recommend chemotherapy in stage II bulky seminoma disease

Acceptability to patient
Side-effects may limit the acceptability of this form of therapy to the patient.

Patient and caregiver information
The patient must comply with the recommended treatment schedule to achieve the maximum therapeutic effect.

Chemotherapy
Chemotherapy is used for recurrent stage I seminomas and nonseminomas, for bulky stage II seminomas and stage II nonseminomas, and for all stage III disease regardless of cell type.

PLATINUM-BASED COMBINATION CHEMOTHERAPY
- Cisplatin-based therapy has revolutionized the treatment of testicular cancer
- Proved efficacious regimens include BEP (bleomycin, etoposide, and cisplatin) for three courses or EP (etoposide and cisplatin) for four courses
- A regimen of cisplatin, vinblastine, and bleomycin (known as PVB) has also been used in stage II and III disease

Risks:
- Must be administered under specialist supervision
- Should not be used in patients with hearing impairment
- Should not be used in myelosuppressed patients
- Use caution with renal impairment
- Peripheral blood counts should be monitored weekly

Side-effects:
- Central nervous system: fatigue
- Eyes, ears, nose, and throat: ototoxicity
- Gastrointestinal: nausea, vomiting, anorexia
- Genitourinary: sexual dysfunction
- Hematologic: bone marrow suppression
- Metabolic: renal toxicity
- Skin: alopecia
- May interact with pyridoxine and hexmethylmelamine (may affect response duration)
- Contraindicated when there is hypersentivity to cisplatin or platinum-containing preparations, or renal impairment

Efficacy
- All of the above regimens are equally efficacious
- A randomized comparison of BEP and PVB showed equivalent antitumor activity but less toxicity than with BEP

Risks/Benefits

Risks:

- Must be administered under specialist supervision
- Should not be used in patients with hearing impairment
- Should not be used in myelosuppressed patients
- Use caution with renal impairment
- Peripheral blood counts should be monitored weekly
- Side-effects common to all chemotherapeutic regimens include fatigue, nausea and vomiting, hair loss, and sexual dysfunction
- Serious side-effects include bone marrow suppression, stomatitis, and anorexia

Benefits:

- Chemotherapy offers significant benefit
- High-volume and recurrent tumors can be successfully treated

Acceptability to patient

Side-effects may limit the acceptability of this form of therapy to the patient.

Patient and caregiver information

The patient must comply with the recommended treatment schedule in order to achieve the maximum therapeutic effect.

EFFICACY OF THERAPIES
- Testicular cancer is considered to be highly curable
- Even advanced disease responds well to platinum-based combination chemotherapy

Review period
Regular follow-up for 1–2 years and then annually thereafter.

PROGNOSIS
- Testicular cancer is highly curable
- If patients are carefully followed and recurrences are detected, the response rate of recurrent disease to treatment is excellent

Therapeutic failure
Some patients require salvage chemotherapy or combination high-dose chemotherapy and autologous bone marrow transplant.

Recurrence
Some patients require salvage chemotherapy or combination high-dose chemotherapy and autologous bone marrow transplant.

Deterioration
Some patients require salvage chemotherapy or combination high-dose chemotherapy and autologous bone marrow transplant.

Terminal illness
Specialists will need to be involved to deal with potential complications such as pain management or ureteral obstruction.

COMPLICATIONS
Untreated metastatic disease is fatal.

CONSIDER CONSULT
- Medical oncologist and urologist should be involved throughout patient's initial care and long-term follow-up

PREVENTION

There are no known preventive strategies applicable to the general population.

RISK FACTORS
- Cryptorchidism
- Certain chromosomal abnormalities

MODIFY RISK FACTORS
- Infant males should be examined for the presence of cryptorchidism
- If found, cryptorchidism should be corrected at an early age
- Patients with gonadal dysgenesis with Y chromosome should undergo prophylactic gonadectomy, and patients with testicular feminization should have testes removed after secondary sexual characteristics develop

SCREENING
According to the National Cancer Institute, there is insufficient evidence to establish that screening would result in a decrease in mortality rate from testicular cancer.

PREVENT RECURRENCE
- Initial diagnostic and treatment decisions (cell type, stage of disease, treatment modality selected) have a strong effect on the development of recurrence
- Most recurrence and treatment failures occur as a result of inadequate follow-up
- Patients must be followed serially with physical examinations, CT scans, and serum tumor markers for at least 5 years following diagnosis and initial treatment

ASSOCIATIONS
American Cancer Society
Local offices throughout the US; provides patient information and support
Tel: 800-ACS-2345
http://www.cancer.org

Cancer Information Service of the National Cancer Institute
Provides frequently updated information about treatment protocols, including clinical trials
Tel: 800-422-6237
http://cis.nci.nih.gov

KEY REFERENCES

- Solomon MC, Sheinfeld J. Diagnostic approaches to testicular cancer. In: Ernstoff MC, Heaney JA, Paschel RE, eds. Urologic cancer. Malden: Blackwell Science, 1997, p536–43
- Pottern LM, Brown LM, Devesa SS. Epidemiology and pathogenesis of testicular cancer. In: Ernstoff MC, Heaney JA, Paschel RE, eds. Urologic cancer. Malden: Blackwell Science, 1997, p498–507
- Kinkade S. Testicular cancer. Am Fam Physician 1999;59:2539–44
- Physician Data Query. Screening for testicular cancer. National Cancer Institute, June 2001, http://www.cancer.gov/cancer_information/
- Physician Data Query. Testicular cancer treatment. National Cancer Institute, July 2001
- Coogan CL, Rowland RG. Testis tumors: diagnosis and staging. In: Oesterlin JE, Richie JP, eds. Urologic oncology. Philadelphia: WB Saunders, 1997, p457–465

FAQS
Question 1
What is the most common type of tumor affecting the testis?

ANSWER 1
>90% of testis tumors are germ cell tumors derived from the germinal epithelium of the mature testis and are divided into the two major categories: seminomatous and nonseminomatous germ cell tumors (embryonal, choriocarcinoma, teratoma, yolk sac), with the most common histologically pre-form being seminoma. However, mixed tumors occur more frequently than pure ones.

Question 2
What is the most common solid tumor in men between 15 and 35 years of age, and which cell type is the most common?

ANSWER 2
Germ cell tumors of the testis and seminoma.

Question 3
What is the most common presenting complaint in patients with testis tumors?

ANSWER 3
The most common presenting complaint is painless unilateral swelling or nodule, usually as an incidental finding by the patient or his sexual partner. Scrotal or lower abdominal pain occurs in about one-third of patients. In 10% of cases, the presenting symptoms are due to systemic metastases (neck mass due to supraclavicular nodal disease, cough or dyspnea due to lung metastases, gastrointestinal symptoms or back pain due to retroperitoneal disease, bone pain, central nervous system symptoms, gynecomastia).

Question 4
What is the *sine qua non* for diagnosis of germ cell tumor?

ANSWER 4
Inguinal orchiectomy with pathologic examination of the testis.

Question 5
What serum markers are important in germ cell tumors?

ANSWER 5
AFP, HCG, and LDH are the principal tumor markers drawn preoperatively and used in the postoperative period to assess clinical course. Other markers, like placental alkaline phosphatase, are also useful but not to the same extent as the others.

CONTRIBUTORS
Fred F Ferri, MD, FACP
Philip J Aliotta, MD, MHA, FACS
Stewart M Polsky, MD

TESTICULAR TORSION

SUMMARY INFORMATION

DESCRIPTION

- Painful twisting of the testis and spermatic cord, resulting in ischemia and testicular necrosis if not corrected promptly
- Sudden onset of severe testicular pain with poorly localized abdominal pain
- A true surgical emergency

URGENT ACTION

- Testicular torsion is a surgical emergency requiring urgent referral
- If caught early, the testis can be untwisted by rotating the testicle, although surgery is later required to prevent recurrence
- Time is of the essence. Prompt diagnosis and treatment are essential if the testicle is to be saved

BACKGROUND

ICD9 CODE
608.2 Torsion of testis

SYNONYMS
Spermatic cord torsion.

CARDINAL FEATURES
- Unilateral severe testicular pain and swelling
- May be associated with poorly localized abdominal pain and vomiting (due to embryological abdominal nerve supply)
- Absence of the ipsilateral cremasteric reflex
- Testis is tender, slightly swollen, and drawn up into the neck of the scrotum (high riding testis)
- Later the scrotal skin becomes red and edematous
- Rapid surgical treatment is required

CAUSES
Common causes
There is a bilateral underlying anatomic abnormality in affected patients. The tunica vaginalis is overly large and inserts high on the spermatic cord. As a result, the cord is redundant and the testis can 'dangle' and move within the scrotum. This is known as a 'bell-clapper' testicular deformity.

There are two types of torsion:
- Extravaginal: does not occur beyond the newborn period, and involves processsus vaginalis, tunica vaginalis, and testis
- Intravaginal: the classic presentation, occurring within the tunica vaginalis

Contributory or predisposing factors
Torsion is ten times as likely in an undescended testis. The diagnosis should be strongly considered in a patient with a painful inguinal mass and an empty hemi-scrotum.

EPIDEMIOLOGY
Incidence and prevalence
INCIDENCE
About 1 in every 4000 males.

Demographics
AGE
- Can occur at any age
- Most common between 12–18 years, peak at 14 years
- Smaller peak during first year of life

GENDER
Males only.

RACE
No racial predilection has been described in the literature.

GENETICS
No genetic component has been described in the literature.

DIAGNOSIS

DIFFERENTIAL DIAGNOSIS
Epididymitis
An infectious disease, epididymitis is the disorder most commonly confused with testicular torsion.

FEATURES
- Uncommon in childhood since the epididymitis is rarely infected in preadolescents who have no urinary tract disease
- Average age of patients is 25 years
- Pain is more gradual (peaks over days rather than hours)
- Urinary symptoms such as dysuria and frequency preceding onset of pain are often present
- Edema and erythema of scrotum usually not seen in early epididymitis
- 95% of patients have fever (average 38 degrees Centigrade or 100.4 degrees Fahrenheit)
- Elevated white blood cell count and pyuria suggest epididymitis, although only 50% of patients with epididymitis will have either

Torsion of testicular appendage
Vestigial appendages of the testicle can sometimes torse and become painful.

FEATURES
- Pain is usually less than that of testicular torsion
- Edema and reactive hydrocele can make it difficult to palpate the torsed appendage, which presents as a small, painful mass
- If patient seen early, scrotal transillumination may reveal a blue-black dot, which is pathognomonic for torsion of testicular appendage

Testicular cancer
Testicular cancer is the most common cancer in young men.

FEATURES
- Key finding is an intratesticular mass
- Can have acute pain secondary to acute hemorrhage within tumor

Orchitis
FEATURES
- Usually results from infection spreading locally to epididymitis
- Signs and symptoms of infection are present

Scrotal trauma
FEATURES
When scrotal pain and swelling are secondary to trauma, the history usually is obvious

Acute inguinal hernia
FEATURES
- Generally painless unilateral swelling
- Onset usually gradual
- Can be distinguished from torsion by physical examination

Acute hydrocele
FEATURES
- Usually painless
- Transillumination helps to distinguish hydrocele from torsion

SIGNS & SYMPTOMS
Signs

- Affected hemiscrotum is swollen, tender, and firm
- Later, the scrotal skin becomes red and edematous
- Testis is high-riding and in a horizontal lie ('bell-clapper deformity'), although this may not always be detectable
- Testis may be drawn up into the neck of the scrotum where the cord is palpably thickened
- Reactive hydrocele may be present
- Cremasteric reflex absent on affected side
- 20% of patients have mild fever
- Infants and young children may show none of the classic signs
- The size of the scrotal mass is an unreliable way to distinguish torsion from other causes of scrotal pain. Prehn's sign (the relief of pain with testicular elevation as evidence for epididymitis) also is an unreliable way to exclude torsion

Symptoms

- The cardinal manifestation of testicular torsion is pain
- Sudden onset of pain usually starts in scrotum but can be localized to central or lower abdomen or inguinal area
- 41% of patients report at least one prior episode of similar pain with spontaneous resolution
- Nausea and vomiting, probably secondary to sudden testicular vascular occlusion, often occur
- Pain commonly begins while the patient is sleeping or after exertion
- Most patients report no urinary symptoms such as dysuria or frequency

CONSIDER CONSULT

If the diagnosis is considered and cannot be excluded, urgent surgical consultation should be obtained.

INVESTIGATION OF THE PATIENT
Direct questions to patient

Q **Did the pain come on suddenly or gradually?** Most often the pain of torsion is sudden, but a more gradual onset is not uncommon.

Q **What were you doing when the pain began?** Typically the onset of pain is at rest or even during sleep, although some patients report the beginning of pain with exertion or even mild trauma.

Q **Are you having a penile discharge, dysuria, or urinary frequency?** These symptoms are rarely seen in testicular torsion and their presence may suggest another diagnosis.

Q **Is there associated nausea, vomiting, or anorexia?** When present, these symptoms increase the likelihood of torsion.

Examination

- **Does the patient appear to be having significant pain?** Pain is the cardinal manifestation of testicular torsion
- **Check for testicular tenderness.** Diffuse tenderness suggests torsion. Tenderness limited to the posterior testis suggest epididymitis
- **Is the painful testis in a horizontal lie?** If so, torsion is suggested
- **Is the scrotal skin red or edematous?** If so, torsion is suggested
- **Check for the cremasteric reflex.** The presence of the reflex in the setting of acute testicular pain suggests a diagnosis other than torsion
- **Check for a urethral discharge.** The presence of a discharge suggests a diagnosis other than torsion
- **Check a urinalysis and complete blood count.** Both studies should be normal in testicular torsion

Summary of investigative tests

Ultrasound has become the imaging modality of choice in suspected testicular torsion. It is more specific, faster, and more readily available than radionuclide imaging. It is normally performed by a specialist.

DIAGNOSTIC DECISION

Torsion should be strongly considered in a male who:

- Has a history and physical examination consistent with the disorder
- Has no urethral discharge or other urinary symptoms
- Does not have a cremasteric reflex. The presence of a cremasteric reflex on the affected side virtually excludes torsion. The examiner should stroke or pinch the inner thigh. The reflex is present if there is a 0.5 centimeter or greater elevation of the ipsilateral testis
- Has a normal complete blood count and urinalysis

CLINICAL PEARLS

Torsion of the testis can occur in any one of four presentations:

- Normal testicular and epididymal lie
- Bell-clapper deformity horizontal lie of an intact testis and epididymitis
- Loose epididymal attachment to the testis
- Torsed testis with transverse lie

THE TESTS
Imaging
COLOR DOPPLER ULTRASOUND
Advantages/Disadvantages

Ultrasound has become the imaging modality of choice in suspected testicular torsion. It is more specific, faster, and more readily available than radionuclide imaging.

Abnormal

- With conventional ultrasound, the torsed testicle shows a non-homogenous pattern. There are both hypoechoic and hyperechoic areas
- Color ultrasound demonstrates the lack of blood flow to a testicle that is torsed
- The increased blood flow associated with epididymitis also is readily seen on color Doppler ultrasound
- False-negatives can occur because the cessation of blood flow to the involved testis is not immediate
- Keep in mind the possibility of falsely abnormal results

RADIONUCLIDE SCANNING
Advantages/Disadvantages
- Allows differentiation between testicular torsion and other diagnoses when patient presents with acute scrotal pain
- Procedure allows minimal exposure to radiation
- Not usually diagnostic but may indicate ischemia

Normal
Uniform distribution of testicular blood flow.

Abnormal
Uneven flow blood, creating high levels of tracer ('hot spots') indicating duct inflammation or tumor, or areas where tracer accumulation is low ('cold spots'), indicating cyst, abscess, tumor, or blood clot.

Cause of abnormal result
Blood flow reduced by blockage of or damage to testicular blood vessels, indicating twisting of the spermatic cord.

TREATMENT

CONSIDER CONSULT

Timely consultation with an urologist is required for testicular salvage. The urologist should be called and asked where he would like to see the patient. The patient must not take anything by mouth, as he will most likely need surgery.

IMMEDIATE ACTION

- Manual detorsion is a temporizing step when immediate consultation or surgery is not available. Usually the anterior portion of the testis twists medially. Place the patient in the supine position and administer parenteral pain medication. (Do not perform a spermatic cord block.) Grasp the affected testis and twist the anterior portion laterally. Stop if this maneuver appears to shorten the cord or make the patient worse. Successful manual detorsion is not a substitute for surgery

- Therapeutic cooling of the affected testicle may be implemented while awaiting surgery. In experimental animal studies there was an 85–90% testicular preservation rate for up to 6 hours. Cooling is accomplished by placing an ice pack on the testicle, with a towel placed between the pack and the patient to protect the scrotum from cold injury

PATIENT AND CAREGIVER ISSUES
Patient or caregiver request

- Did I cause this problem by straining or over-exertion? Testicular torsion is a complication of a congenital anatomic abnormality

- Is the other testicle likely to suffer torsion? The anatomic abnormality is bilateral, and most experts recommend a procedure to 'tack down' the unaffected testis at the same time that the affected side is detorsed

- Is there a chance it could recur? Torsion can recur even after orchiopexy

Health-seeking behavior

Have you had similar episodes of pain in the past? Almost half of the patients with torsion report prior similar episodes with spontaneous resolution.

MANAGEMENT ISSUES
Goals

The goal of therapy is to salvage a viable testis.

SUMMARY OF THERAPEUTIC OPTIONS
Choices
Acute testicular torsion is a surgical emergency, and no alternative to surgery exists. Because the underlying anatomic abnormality is bilateral, specialists recommend orchiopexy for the unaffected testis as prophylaxis. This is customarily done acutely at the time of surgery on the affected testis.

FOLLOW UP
Plan for review
Postoperatively, the patient should be observed for signs of infection, hematoma, and bleeding.

DRUGS AND OTHER THERAPIES: DETAILS
Surgical therapy
DETORSION AND ORCHIOPEXY
The goal of surgery is to salvage the affected testis, if possible, and to prevent future torsion in the other testis.

Detorsion is accomplished in the operating room under direct vision by means of a midline incision through the median raphe of the scrotum. If the testis already is necrotic, it is removed. Orchiopexy of the contralateral testis involves placing several nonabsorbable sutures to anchor the testis to the scrotal wall.

Efficacy
The salvage rate is 80–100% if the patient is operated on within 6 hours of the onset of pain.

Risks/Benefits
There are no unique risks other than those that apply to surgery in general.

Acceptability to patient
- If the testis is viable at the time of surgery, detorsion produces pain relief. If the testis is already necrotic, orchiectomy also produces pain relief
- Postoperative scrotal pain is usually easily managed with ice packs, scrotal support, and analgesics

Follow up plan
Only routine surgical follow-up is required.

Patient and caregiver information
- Wear a scrotal support and brief-style underwear until pain-free
- Notify the surgeon if you experience worsening pain, bleeding, or scrotal swelling

EFFICACY OF THERAPIES

- The salvage rate is 80–100% if the patient is operated on within 6 hours of the onset of pain, but it is less than 20% beyond 12 hours of onset of pain
- Torsion conforms to no classical picture, nor are there any characteristic features by which it can be excluded. The primary factor responsible for the loss of testicular mass is delay in diagnosis leading to an increase in testicular ischemia
- Investigators have shown a progressive loss of germinal epithelium and Sertoli cells over 4–6 hours, with death of the Leydig cells occurring at 10 hours. The degree of torsion initially affects the veins and it is not until later when increasing congestion and edema alter arterial flow to the testis that infarction occurs

The following factors play a role in determining testis survival:

- Failure of the patient to seek immediate attention
- Misdiagnosis on the part of the physician making the initial contact with the patient. Factors playing a role in this include: (1) the nonspecific nature of the history; (2) physical findings that were unclear and made even more difficult because of the tenderness present precluded an adequate examination; and (3) the age of the patient. The misperception here is that torsion of the testis is an adolescent problem. In fact, numerous studies show that 28–45% of cases of torsion occur in men over 20 years of age

Outcomes of torsion are related to duration of testicular ischemia. Possible complications include:

- Loss of testis volume
- Abnormal semen analyses

PROGNOSIS

Clinical pearls

When there is any doubt, explore the scrotum and perform bilateral orchiopexies.

Recurrence

- The underlying 'bell clapper' abnormality is bilateral. For this reason, orchiopexy of the uninvolved testis is recommended
- Repeat torsion can occur despite orchiopexy

COMPLICATIONS

- Infarction of the testis may be noted at surgery, necessitating its removal
- Defects in spermatogenesis can occur even if the testis was viable after detorsion

RISK FACTORS
The 'bell-clapper' testis is a risk factor for testicular torsion.

PREVENT RECURRENCE
An orchiopexy procedure will prevent torsion of the contralateral testis.

KEY REFERENCES

- Wan J, Bloom DA, Pohl J. Abnormalities of the testis and groin. In: Stein BS, Caldamone AA, Smith JA Jr (eds). Clinical Urologic Practice. New York, WW Norton & Co, 1995:1507–1527
- Grechi G, LiMarzi V. Torsion of the testicle. In Graham SD Jr (ed). Glenn's Urologic Surgery, 5th ed. Philadelphia, Lippincott-Raven, 1998:535–8
- Schwartz GR (ed). Principles and Practice of Emergency Medicine, 4th ed. Baltimore, Williams & Wilkins, 1999:757–9
- Rosen P, Barkin R (eds). Emergency Medicine: Concepts and Clinical Practice, 4th ed. St. Louis, Mosby-Yearbook, 1998:2243–5
- Burgher SW. Acute scrotal pain. Emerg Med Clin N Am 1998; 16:781–809
- Rajfer J. Congenital anomalies of the testis and scrotum. In Walsh PC, Retik AB, Vaughn ED Jr, Weir AJ (eds). Campbell's Urology, 7th ed. Philadelphia, WB Saunders, 1998:2184–6
- Ransler CW III, Allen T: Torsion of the spermatic cord. Urol Clin North Am 1982; 9 (2):245–250
- Ross JH. Evaluation of acute scrotal swelling in children. In: Urology Secrets, Resnick MI, Novick AC. Second edition. Philadelphia: Hanley & Belfus, Inc.; 1999

FAQS
Question 1
What other conditions are included in the differential diagnosis of the acute, painful scrotum?

ANSWER 1
Acute epididymitis, torsion of the testis, torsion of the testicular or epididymal appendages, testis trauma, and testis tumor.

Question 2
What are the causes of acute scrotal swelling in children?

ANSWER 2
Spermatic cord torsion, torsion of the appendix testis and appendix epididymis, epididymo-orchitis, hernia, hydrocele, and testis tumor.

Question 3
What is the difference between intravaginal and extravaginal torsion?

ANSWER 3
Testicular torsion is intravaginal, occurring within the tunica vaginalis. On exposure of the testis, the hydrocele sac is opened and the torsed cord and testis are inside. In newborns, the tunica vaginalis is not adherent to the surrounding dartos fascia, and as a result the testis and processus vaginalis and tunica vaginalis can torse as a unit (extravaginal torsion). Because the tunica vaginalis becomes adherent to the dartos fascia within the first weeks of life, extravaginal torsion does not occur beyond the newborn period. (Ross JH. Evaluation of acute scrotal swelling in children. In: Urology Secrets, Resnick MI, Novick AC. Second edition. Philadelphia: Hanley & Belfus, Inc.; 1999.)

Question 4
What laboratory test(s) are essential in a patient with acute scrotal swelling?

ANSWER 4
CBC and urinalysis. An elevated white blood cell count and pus in the urine is seen with epididymo-orchitis.

Question 5
How does torsion of the appendix testis present?

ANSWER 5
Classically described as the 'blue dot sign'. A torsed appendix testis has a bluish hue when viewed through the scrotal skin. A 'blue dot' at the upper pole of the testis on examination suggests the diagnosis.

CONTRIBUTORS
Fred F Ferri, MD, FACP
Philip J Aliotta, MD, MHA, FACS
John Pinski, MD
Stewart M Polsky, MD

URETHRITIS

SUMMARY INFORMATION

DESCRIPTION

- Inflammation of the urethra, of noninfectious or, more often, infectious etiology
- Infectious urethritis may be caused by *Neisseria gonorrhoeae* or, more commonly, by other organisms (particularly *Chlamydia trachomatis* and *Ureaplasma urealyticum*), in which case it is termed non-gonococcal urethritis (NGU)
- Commonly asymptomatic
- Symptomatic infections are characterized by discharge of mucopurulent or purulent material and burning during urination

URGENT ACTION

Empiric therapy is recommended for symptomatic high-risk patients and those who are unlikely to return for follow up

KEY! DON'T MISS!

- Urethritis often coexists with one or more other sexually transmitted diseases; always bear this in mind and look for signs and symptoms of other STDs
- Micturition immediately preceding urethral examination may remove any signs of infection, particularly in men; if possible, patients should be examined at least 2 hours after last micturition

BACKGROUND

ICD9 CODE
098.20 Gonococcal urethritis
597.80 Urethritis, unspecified
099.40 Nongonococcal urethritis
099.41 Chlamydial urethritis

SYNONYMS
NGU, NGNCU, nongonococcal nonchlamydial ureteritis

CARDINAL FEATURES
- Inflammation of the urethra, usually caused by a sexually transmitted microorganism, but occasionally of noninfectious etiology
- Men can be asymptomatic, but when symptoms occur they usually include dysuria and mucopurulent or purulent discharge, often more marked in early morning
- Most women are asymptomatic, but when symptoms do occur they usually include dysuria, frequency and vaginal discharge
- Coinfection with *N. gonorrhoeae* and *C. trachomatis* is not uncommon
- In most patients, symptoms resolve without treatment, but late complications in women are common

CAUSES
Common causes
- *Neisseria gonorrhoeae* causes gonococcal urethritis
- *Chlamydia trachomatis* is the most common cause of nongonococcal urethritis

Rare causes
- *Ureaplasma urealyticum* and *Mycoplasma genitalium* are implicated in up to one-third of cases of nongonococcal urethritis (NGU); specific diagnostic tests for these organisms are not indicated
- *Trichomonas vaginalis*, Papilloma and herpes simplex virus sometimes cause NGU; diagnosis and treatment of these organisms is indicated only when NGU is unresponsive to therapy
- Noninfectious urethritis may be found in Stevens-Johnson syndrome or Wegener's granulomatosis
- Spermicides and some acidic food can cause urethral irritation in some individuals

Contributory or predisposing factors
- Patients with multiple sex partners, especially those who do not practice safe sex, are at increased risk of contracting infectious urethritis
- Patients with one or more existing sexually transmitted disease are at increased risk for urethritis
- Patients who have undergone urethral instrumentation are at increased risk for urethritis

EPIDEMIOLOGY
Incidence and prevalence
The reported prevalence in 1997 is thought to be an underestimation of the extent of the problem due to severe under-reporting of urethritis – largely a result of substantial numbers of asymptomatic persons

INCIDENCE
- Chlamydial infection: 11–14 cases per 1000
- Gonorrhea: 2.4 cases per 1000

PREVALENCE
- Chlamydial infection: 2.07 per 1000 in 1997
- Gonorrhea: 1.22 per 1000 in 1997

FREQUENCY
C. trachomatis infection is the most common bacterial STD and the most frequently reported infectious disease in the United States

Demographics
AGE
- 15–19 year olds are most commonly infected with *C. trachomatis*
- 20–24 year olds are second most commonly infected age group

GENDER
- *C. trachomatis* infection is more often reported in women than in men, largely due to screening
- *N. gonorrhoeae* infection is more commonly reported in men than women, up to 50% of whom are asymptomatic

SOCIOECONOMIC STATUS
Nongonococcal urethritis is more common than gonococcal urethritis in groups of higher socioeconomic status

DIFFERENTIAL DIAGNOSIS
Acute cystitis
FEATURES
- More common in women than men
- Usually caused by *E. coli*; some cases caused by *Staph. saprophyticus*
- Common symptoms include increased frequency and urgency, dysuria and suprapubic pain
- Hematuria occurs in 40% of cases
- Pyuria is almost always present
- Bacteriuria >/= 105 colony forming units/ml urine

Acute pyelonephritis
FEATURES
- Vaginal discharge and odor are almost always present
- No increased frequency or urgency
- External dysuria and pruritus are common
- Dyspareunia often occurs
- Commonly caused by *Gardnerella vaginalis*

Bacterial vulvovaginitis
FEATURES
- Vaginal discharge and odor are almost always present
- No increased frequency or urgency
- External dysuria and pruritus are common
- Dyspareunia often occurs
- Commonly caused by *Trichomonas vaginalis*

Mucopurulent cervicitis
FEATURES
- Often asymptomatic but some women have an abnormal vaginal discharge and vaginal bleeding (especially after sexual intercourse)
- Purulent/mucopurulent endocervical exudate is common
- Increased numbers of polymorphonuclear leukocytes seen on Gram stain of endocervical smear
- *C. trachomatis* or *N. gonorrhoeae* are not isolated in most cases

Prostatitis
FEATURES
- Discomfort during ejaculation is common
- Deep pelvic pain/pain radiating to back may occur
- Systemic symptoms may include fever and chills
- Dysuria is present in some cases
- Usually caused by *N. gonorrhoeae*, *E. coli*, or *Klebsiella* species

Trichomoniasis
FEATURES
- Profuse malodorous vaginal discharge
- Postcoital bleeding
- Dysuria
- Males: asymptomatic or complain of dysuria, urethral discharge, and can present with epididymitis

SIGNS & SYMPTOMS

Signs

In men:
- Meatal erythema is common in gonococcal and nongonococcal urethritis (NGU)
- Frankly purulent urethral exudate, visible without stripping the urethra is characteristic of gonococcal urethritis; clear or mucopurulent exudate produced by stripping the urethra is common in NGU
- Inguinal adenopathy may be present
- Pyuria is common; hematuria is uncommon

In women:
- Cervicitis is common
- Stripping of the urethra may reveal a purulent (suggestive of gonococcal urethritis) or mucopurulent (suggestive of NGU) discharge
- Pyuria is common; hematuria is rare

Symptoms

In men:
- Estimated 50% of men with urethritis caused by *C. trachomatis* are asymptomatic
- Abrupt onset of symptoms is common in gonococcal urethritis; symptoms of nongonococcal urethritis (NGU) usually develop over several days and may wax and wane
- Urethral discharge, which may be clear or mucopurulent (common in NGU), or frankly purulent (common in gonococcal urethritis); it may be white, yellow, green or brown
- Urethral discharge may be scanty, seen only as a small crust on the meatus on arising, or it may be present throughout the day and be sufficient in quantity to stain undergarments
- Dysuria is common in gonococcal and nongonococcal urethritis and can be exacerbated by alcohol
- Increased urinary frequency and urgency may occur
- Pain and heaviness in the genitals is experienced by some men

In women:
- Majority are asymptomatic
- Dysuria is the most common symptom
- Increased frequency and urgency may occur
- Vaginal discharge or odor may be present
- Some women experience pelvic pain and dyspareunia

ASSOCIATED DISORDERS
- Other sexually transmitted diseases often coexist with urethritis
- Persons with urethritis are at increased risk of acquired HIV infection, if exposed
- Nongonococcal urethritis may occur as part Reiter's syndrome, which also includes arthritis, uveitis, and skin or mucous membrane lesions
- Epididymitis
- Proctitis in homosexual men or women engaging in anal intercourse
- Male and female infertility as a long term sequelae is rare
- Nonbacterial prostatitis
- Urethral stricture

KEY! DON'T MISS!
- Urethritis often coexists with one or more other sexually transmitted diseases; always bear this in mind and look for signs and symptoms of other STDs
- Micturition immediately preceding urethral examination may remove any signs of infection, particularly in men; if possible, patients should be examined at least 2 hours after last micturition

INVESTIGATION OF THE PATIENT
Direct questions to patient

Q **Have you recently had intercourse with a new sex partner?** A history of recent intercourse with a new sex partner is common in infectious urethritis.

Q **Does your sex partner have symptoms of urethritis?** Partner with symptoms of urethritis increases the likelihood of infection in presenting patient.

Q **Do you practice safe sex?** Barrier methods help prevent transmission of infectious urethritis.

Q **Do you have multiple sex partners?** Multiple sex partners increase an individual's risk for infectious urethritis.

Q **Have you recently undergone urethral instrumentation?** Instrumentation (including catheter insertion) increases the risk of urethritis.

Q **Have you been treated for any sexually transmitted disease(s) in the past?** Infectious urethritis is found with increased frequency in persons with a history of other STDs.

Contributory or predisposing factors

Q **Are there signs of any other sexually transmitted disease(s)?** Infectious urethritis often coexists with one or more other STDs.

Examination

- **Examine the entire genital area.** Look for signs of urethritis and signs of other STDs, including lesions and nits in pubic hair; palpate inguinal nodes, testes, epididymis and spermatic cords for tenderness or masses
- **Examine the urethra.** Look for spontaneous discharge, redness (in men), and crusting at the meatus
- **Strip the urethra.** If no spontaneous discharge is found at the meatus, stripping usually expels any discharge located further up the urethra
- **Perform a pelvic examination.** Cervicitis is commonly found in women with infectious urethritis; signs of other STDs should be sought

Summary of investigative tests

- Gram staining of smear from urethral swab is performed on all samples from patients with suspected infectious urethritis; finding of more than a few polymorphonuclear leukocytes (PMNs) strongly suggests infectious urethritis; in addition, Gram negative, intracellular diplococci are characteristic of gonococcal urethritis
- Examination of first-void urine for pyuria is performed in all patients with suspected infectious urethritis: either a positive leukocyte esterase test or identification of PMNs on microscopic examination strongly suggests infectious urethritis
- Examination of divided urine specimen is a simple test that can be performed on urine samples from men; mucoid strands in the first-void specimen but not in the second fraction is characteristic of *C. trachomatis* urethritis; sediments of each aliquot may also be examined microscopically for the presence of PMNs
- Culture of urethral discharge on selective media provides a definitive diagnosis of gonococcal urethritis
- Nucleic acid amplification methods, e.g. ligase chain reaction performed on first void urine samples, can identify *C. trachomatis* or *N. gonorrhoeae* as the cause of infectious urethritis
- Direct Fluorescent Antibody (DFA) rapidly identifies *C. trachomatis*. It uses a chlamydia specific monoclonal antibody to identify *C. trachomatis* elementary bodies.
- Another test available to identify *C. trachomatis* is Enzyme ImmunoAssay (EIA). Through the use of a spectrophotometer, a positive test is indicated by a color change.
- Both DFA and EIA tests can be used when results within 24 hours are required. Experience has suggested that DFA testing may be more specific than EIA, but results seem to be comparable.
- Caution is recommended when using these tests in a low prevalence population (less than 7%). Higher specificity and sensitivity using these two tests is appreciably higher in higher prevalence populations.

- Unexpected positive results should be confirmed by additional testing with more specific methods, such as cell culture.
- Reference: [1]

DIAGNOSTIC DECISION

Urethritis can be documented if any of the following signs is present:

- Purulent or mucopurulent discharge
- of urethral discharge demonstrating >/=5 polymorphonuclear leukocytes (PMNs) per oil immersion field; gonococcal urethritis is indicated by the finding of Gram negative diplococci inside PMNs
- Pyuria in first-void urine, indicated by either a positive or >/= 10PMNs per high-power field on
- If none of these is present, treatment should be deferred and the patient should be tested for *N. gonorrhoeae* and *C. trachomatis*, e.g. using a nucleic acid amplification method such as the

Guidelines for the treatment of sexually transmitted diseases [2]

CLINICAL PEARLS

- To obtain the smear in males, hold the penis with a gloved left hand and lift up parallel to the body. Using the thumb and index finger, open the meatus. Gently, insert the Calgiswab in an angle toward the examiner to enter the ampulla with the right hand. Turn 360 degrees to obtain the specimen, send to the laboratory for Gram stain, DNA probes and appropriate cultures. (NB In younger males, erection is not unusual; and can prove embarrassing for both the examiner and the patient.)
- In females, proceed in the usual fashion

THE TESTS
Body fluids
GRAM STAIN
Description

A swab containing material from the urethra is smeared onto a glass slide, air dried or heat fixed, stained with Gram stain and examined using the oil-immersion objective

Advantages/Disadvantages

- Advantage; quick and easy test
- Disadvantage; *C. trachomatis* can not be visualized on Gram stain

Normal

- Absent or very few polymorphonuclear leukocytes (PMNs)
- A variety of Gram negative and positive organisms of random distribution

Abnormal

- Five or more PMNs per oil-immersion field is always abnormal
- Gram negative diplococci may be seen in large numbers inside PMNs
- Keep in mind the possibility of a false positive result

Cause of abnormal result

- Five or more PMNs per oil-immersion field in the absence of intracellular diplococci strongly suggests nongonococcal urethritis
- Five or more PMNs per oil-immersion field with Gram negative intracellular diplococci is virtually pathognomonic of gonococcal urethritis

Drugs, disorders and other factors that may alter results
- Recent micturition reduces the number of PMNs in a specimen
- Sampling and laboratory technique can affect results

LEUKOCYTE ESTERASE TEST
Description
First-void urine, approximately 10ml, is tested with a dipstick for the presence of leukocyte esterase

Advantages/Disadvantages
- Advantage; convenient, noninvasive and inexpensive test
- Disadvantage; does not allow identification of causative microorganism

Normal
- Leukocyte esterase not detected in urine – result is reported as negative
- False negative results are possible; patients with a negative result and symptoms of urethritis should have microscopic evaluation of urine

Abnormal
- Leukocyte esterase is detected in urine – result is reported as positive
- Keep in mind the possibility of a false positive result

Cause of abnormal result
Pyuria, strongly suggesting infectious urethritis

Drugs, disorders and other factors that may alter results
Sampling and laboratory technique can affect results

MICROSCOPIC EXAMINATION OF FIRST-VOID URINE
Description
First-void urine, smeared onto glass slide and examined under high power objective

Advantages/Disadvantages
- Advantage; convenient, noninvasive and inexpensive test
- Disadvantage; does not allow identification of causative microorganism

Normal
<10 polymorphonuclear leukocytes (PMNs) per high-power field

Abnormal
- >/= 10 PMNs per high-power field, indicating pyuria
- Keep in mind the possibility of a false positive result

Cause of abnormal result
Infectious urethritis, UTI

Drugs, disorders and other factors that may alter results
Sampling and laboratory technique can affect results

EXAMINATION OF DIVIDED URINE SPECIMEN
Description
First-void urine (around 10ml) delivered into one container and midstream urine (around 10ml) delivered into a second container are examined macroscopically and microscopically

Advantages/Disadvantages
- Advantage; noninvasive, inexpensive test
- Disdvantage; does not allow identification of infectious microorganism

Normal
- Macroscopic comparison of the two samples reveals no difference
- Microscopic examination of sediment of the two samples reveals <10 polymorphonuclear leukocytes (PMNs) per high-power field

Abnormal
- Macroscopic examination of the two samples reveals mucus strands in the first-void specimen that are not present in the midstream specimen
- Microscopic examination of sediment of the two samples reveals >/= 15 PMNs per high-power field in the first-void sample and fewer PMNs in the midstream sample
- Keep in mind the possibility of a false positive result

Cause of abnormal result
Infectious urethritis – observing equal numbers of PMNs in both samples suggests cystitis or infection higher in the urinary tract

Drugs, disorders and other factors that may alter results
Sampling and laboratory technique can affect results

CULTURE OF URETHRAL DISCHARGE
Description
Material from urethral swab is cultured on Thayer-Martin medium in humidified, carbon dioxide-enriched atmosphere

Advantages/Disadvantages
- Advantage; allows definitive diagnosis of gonococcal urethritis
- Disdvantage; results are not available for several days

Normal
- No growth of colonies
- Note that false negative results are possible

Abnormal
- Growth of colonies
- Keep in mind the possibility of a false positive result

Cause of abnormal result
N. gonorrhoeae present in clinical specimen

Drugs, disorders and other factors that may alter results
- Sampling and laboratory techniques may affect results
- Suboptimal antibiotic therapy (e.g. if patient self-treats) can reduce the number of organisms in the sample

LIGASE CHAIN REACTION (LCR)
Description
First-void urine sample (around 10ml) is centrifuged and subjected to a ligase chain reaction, which amplifies DNA of *C. trachomatis* or *N. gonorrhoeae*, depending on the ligase used

Advantages/Disadvantages
Advantages:
- Noninvasive test
- Allows identification of causative microorganism

Disdvantages:
- Urine samples must be refrigerated until test is performed
- Expensive compared with other laboratory tests
- Tests take several hours to perform

Normal
- *C. trachomatis* or *N. gonorrhoeae* not identified
- False negative results can occur if ligase inhibitors are present in clinical sample

Abnormal
- *C. trachomatis* or *N. gonorrhoeae* identified, depending on ligase used
- Keep in mind the possibility of a false positive result

Cause of abnormal result
- *N. gonorrhoeae* specific pilin present in clinical sample
- *C. trachomatis* specific plasmid present in clinical sample
- False positive results due to amplicon carryover can occur

Drugs, disorders and other factors that may alter results
- Some rare strains of *C. trachomatis* lack the plasmid amplified in this test
- Sampling and laboratory techniques can affect results

TREATMENT

CONSIDER CONSULT

Patients who fail to respond to antibiotic treatment should be referred for urologic evaluation to rule out anatomic abnormalities.

IMMEDIATE ACTION

Empiric treatment of symptoms is recommended only for persons at high risk of infection who are unlikely to return for follow up (e.g. adolescent patient with multiple partners); treatment for gonococcal and nongonococcal urethritis should be administered.

PATIENT AND CAREGIVER ISSUES
Health-seeking behavior

Has the patient tried any self-medication? Patients may take old antibiotics or use antiseptic creams or iodine before seeking professional help.

MANAGEMENT ISSUES
Goals

- Identification of causative organism
- Resolution of infection and symptoms, where present
- Patient education to prevent recurrence or reinfection
- Identification and treatment, where appropriate, of sex partners

Management in special circumstances
COEXISTING MEDICATION

Antacids can affect absorption of azithromycin, doxycycline, ciprofloxacin, and ofloxacin.

SPECIAL PATIENT GROUPS

- Doxycycline and ofloxacin are contraindicated in pregnancy and the safety of azithromycin has not been established; recommended regimens for pregnant women with urethritis include amoxicillin or erythromycin base
- Sex partners of patients with diagnosed urethritis should be referred for evaluation and treatment with recommended regimen, as appropriate; all partners from 60 days preceding onset of symptoms should be referred

PATIENT SATISFACTION/LIFESTYLE PRIORITIES

Some patients may have difficulty complying with multidose regimens.

SUMMARY OF THERAPEUTIC OPTIONS
Choices

- First choice drug for nongonococcal urethritis (NGU), whether or not C. trachomatis is identified as the causative organism, is either a single oral dose of azithromycin or a 7-day course of oral doxycycline
- Second choice regimens for NGU, whether or not C. trachomatis is identified as the causative organism, are erythromycin base, or erythromycin ethylsuccinate, or ofloxacin, each taken orally for 7 days; erythromycin is not as effective as azithromycin or doxycycline; ofloxacin is as effective as the first choice drugs but offers no dosage or cost benefits
- First choice drug for pregnant women with NGU is either erythromycin base or amoxicillin, each taken orally for 7 days
- First choice regimen for gonococcal urethritis is a single dose of either cefixime, ceftriaxone, ciprofloxacin or ofloxacin; this should be combined with a single dose of azithromycin or a 7-day course of doxycycline for presumptive treatment of C. trachomatis infection in populations with a high rate (20–40%)of coexisting infection

Guidelines for the treatment of sexually transmitted diseases [2]

Clinical pearls
When it is suspected that a patient has urethritis and it is uncertain that he/she may not have one agent or more than one, requiring immediate therapy, treat with 250mg IM ceftriaxone (to cover GC) and give a 10-day supply of an oral agent like doxycycline or ofloxacin.

Never
Never give erythromycin estolate to a pregnant woman with urethritis; hepatotoxicity can occur

FOLLOW UP
Plan for review
- Patients with NGU treated with azithromycin or doxycycline should be instructed to return for evaluation only if symptoms persist or recur after completion of therapy
- Consider testing for cure 3 weeks after treatment with erythromycin or amoxicillin
- Patients with gonococcal urethritis treated with one of the recommended regimens should be instructed to return for evaluation by culture only if symptoms persist or recur
- Consider rescreening women in high-risk populations several months after completion of therapy

Information for patient or caregiver
- Explain the importance of compliance with multidose regimens and follow up
- Explain why all sex partners require evaluation and treatment
- Advise patients to abstain from sexual intercourse until therapy is completed

DRUGS AND OTHER THERAPIES: DETAILS
Drugs
AZITHROMYCIN
Nongonococcal urethritis

Dose
Adult oral dose: 1g in a single dose.

Efficacy
Highly effective therapy for NGU.

Risks/Benefits
Risks:
- Use caution in pregnancy and nursing mothers
- Use caution with hepatic, cardiac and renal disease

Benefit: single dose regimen allows directly observed therapy and improves compliance

Side-effects and adverse reactions
- Central nervous system: dizziness, headache, vertigo
- Cardiovascular system: chest pain, palpitations
- Gastrointestinal: abdominal pain, diarrhea, heartburn, hepatotoxicity
- Genitourinary: moniliasis, nephritis, vaginitis
- Skin: allergic reactions including rash, photosensitivity, pruritus angioneurotic edema and anaphylaxis

Interactions (other drugs)
Penicillins

Contraindications
Hypersensitivity to erythromycin

Evidence
Single-dose azithromycin is an effective treatment for chlamydial urethritis and an effective empiric therapy for NGU [3,4].

Acceptability to patient
Single dose means compliance is high.

Follow up plan
Follow up required only if symptoms recur

Patient and caregiver information
Patient should be informed of effective means of avoiding reinfection (including referral of sex partner(s))

DOXYCYCLINE
Nongonococcal urethritis

Dose
- Adult oral dose: 100–200mg daily
- Child oral dose: 2–5mg/kg daily (maximum dose 200mg daily)

Efficacy
Highly effective therapy for NGU

Risks/Benefits
Risks:
- Compliance can be a problem
- Use caution in patients with hepatic impairment
- Use caution with repeated or prolonged doses

Benefit: inexpensive compared with azithromycin

Side-effects and adverse reactions
- Central nervous system: fever, headache, paresthesia
- Cardiovascular system: pericarditis
- Gastrointestinal: abdominal pain, diarrhea, heartburn, hepatotoxicity, vomiting
- Genitourinary: polyuria, polydipsia
- Hematologic: eosinophilia, hemolytic, neutropenia, thrombocytopenia
- Skin: pruritus, rash, photosensitivity
- Miscellaneous: angioedema

Interactions (other drugs)
- Antacids ▪ Barbiturates ▪ Bismuth subsalicylate ▪ Carbamazepine ▪ Ethanol ▪ Iron ▪ Oral contraceptives ▪ Phenytoin ▪ Warfarin

Contraindications
- Pregnancy ▪ Nursing mothers ▪ Children less than 8 years

Evidence
Doxycycline is an effective treatment for NGU [5].

Acceptability to patient
Compliance with the full 7-day regimen can be a problem for some patients

Follow up plan
Follow up required only if symptoms recur

Patient and caregiver information
- Explain importance of complying with full regimen
- Advise patients on methods of avoiding reinfection

ERYTHROMYCIN
- Nongonococcal
- Macrolide

Dose
- Adult oral dose: 250–500mg (base) four times daily for 14 days
- Child oral dose: 30–50mg/kg (ethyl succinate) daily for14 days

Efficacy
Efficacy is lower than that of azithromycin or doxycycline

Risks/Benefits
Risks:
- Dosing regimens and GI side-effects can cause serious problems with compliance
- If only erythromycin can be used and patients cannot tolerate high dose schedules, low dose regimens, as listed above, can be prescribed
- Use caution with hepatic disease
- Use caution with antibiotic hypersensitivity
- Use caution with prolonged or repeated therapy

Benefit: suitable for pregnant and lactating women

Side-effects and adverse reactions
- Cardiovascualr system: ventricular dysrhythmias
- Eyes, ears, nose, and throat: hearing loss, tinnitus
- Gastrointestinal: abdominal pain, anorexia, cholestatic hepatitis, diarrhea, heartburn, vomiting
- Genitourinary: moniliasis, vaginitis
- Skin: pruritus, rash, thrombophlebitis

Interactions (other drugs)
- Alfentanil ▪ Astemizole ▪ Benzodiazepines ▪ Bromocriptine ▪ Lovastatin, atorvastatin ▪ Carbamazepine ▪ Cisapride ▪ Clozapine ▪ Colchicine ▪ Cyclosporin ▪ Disopyramide ▪ Digoxin ▪ Ergot derivatives ▪ Felodipine ▪ Indinavir, ritonavir, saquinavir ▪ Terfenadine ▪ Warfarin ▪ Methylprednisolone ▪ Penicillin ▪ Phenytoin ▪ Tacrolimus ▪ Theophylline ▪ Triazolam ▪ Valproic acid ▪ Zopiclone

Contraindications
Hepatic disease

Evidence
Erythromycin is an effective treatment for *C. trachomatis* urethritis [6].

Acceptability to patient
- GI side-effects, particularly in high dose regimens can be difficult to tolerate
- Length of regimen can cause problems with compliance

Follow up plan
Consider test of cure 3 weeks after completion of treatment

Patient and caregiver information
Explain importance of complying with full regimen

OFLOXACIN
Gonococcal and nongonococcal urethritis
Quinolones

Dose
Adult oral dose: 300mg twice daily for 7 days (nongonococcal): Adult oral dose: 400mg orally in a single dose(gonococcal)

Efficacy
Highly effective treatment for nongonococcal and gonococcal urethritis

Risks/Benefits
Risks:
- Use caution with the elderly
- Use caution in renal disease and seizure disorders

Benefits:
- In NGU, ofloxacin is more expensive than azithromycin or doxycycline
- Effective against most strains of *N. gonorrhoeae*

Side-effects and adverse reactions
- Central nervous system: anxiety, depression, dizziness, headache, seizures
- Eyes, ears, nose and throat: visual disturbances
- Gastrointestinal: abdominal pain, altered liver function, anorexia, diarrhea, heartburn, pseudomembranous colitis, vomiting
- Genitourinary: moniliasis, vaginitis
- Skin: photosensitivity, pruritus, rash

Interactions (other drugs)
- Antacids ■ Didanosine ■ Sucralfate ■ Warfarin

Contraindications
- Pregnancy ■ Nursing mothers

Evidence
Ofloxacin is an effective therapy for nongonococcal and gonococcal urethritis [7,8].

Acceptability to patient
Compliance with multidose regimen for NGU can be difficult for some patients

Follow up plan
Follow up only if symptoms recur

Patient and caregiver information
- Explain importance of complying with full regimen
- Advise patients on methods of avoiding reinfection

AMOXICILLIN
Gonococcal

Dose
Adult oral dose: 500mg orally three times daily for 7 days

Efficacy
Not highly efficacious

Risks/Benefits
Risks:
- Compliance can be a problem
- Use caution with hypersensitivity to cephalosporins
- Use caution with renal disease
- Use caution with mononucleosis
- Use caution with prolonged or repeated therapy

Benefit: one of the few drugs suitable for use in pregnant women

Side-effects and adverse reactions
- Central nervous system: fever, headache
- Gastrointestinal: abdominal pain, pseudomembranous colitis, diarrhea, vomiting
- Hematologic: anemia, bone marrow depression, eosinophilia, increased bleeding time
- Respiratory: respiratory distress, hypersensitivity reactions
- Skin: erythema multiforme, rash, urticaria

Interactions (other drugs)
- Atenolol ■ Chloramphenicol ■ Macrolides ■ Methotrexate ■ Oral contraceptives
- Tetracyclines

Evidence
Amoxicillin prevents vertical transmission of chlamydial infection to neonates and is an acceptable alternative to erythromycin for chlamydial infections in pregnancy [9].

Acceptability to patient
Compliance with full regimen can be difficult for some patients

Follow up plan
Consider repeat testing for infection 3 weeks after completion of therapy

Patient and caregiver information
- Explain importance of complying with full regimen
- Advise patients on means of avoiding reinfection

CEFIXIME
Gonococcal urethritis
Cephalosporin (3rd generation)

Dose
Adult oral dose: 400mg in a single dose

Efficacy
Highly effective therapy for gonococcal urethritis

Risks/Benefits
- Risk: use caution with hypersensitivity to penicillins
- Benefit: single dose allows directly observed therapy and ensures compliance

Side-effects and adverse reactions
- Central nervous system: dizziness, fever, headache
- Gastrointestinal: bleeding, diarrhea, Pseudomembranous colitis, vomiting
- Genitourinary: candidiasis, dysuria, nephrotoxicity
- Hematologic: anemia, bone marrow depression, eosinophilia
- Respiratory: respiratory distress, hypersensitivity reaction
- Skin: rash, urticaria

Interactions (other drugs)
Oral Anticoagulants

Evidence
Cefixime is an effective treatment for gonococcal urethritis [10].

Acceptability to patient
Single dose oral regimen is compatible with high degree of compliance.

Follow up plan
Follow up only if symptoms recur.

Patient and caregiver information
Advise patients on means of avoiding reinfection.

CEFTRIAXONE
Gonococcal
Cephalosporin(3rd generation)

Dose
Adult dose: 125–250mg IM/IV in a single dose.

Efficacy
Highly effective therapy for gonococcal urethritis.

Risks/Benefits
Risks:
- Use caution with hypersensitivity to penicillins
- Use caution with renal disease and anaphylaxis

Benefits:
- Single dose regimen allows directly observed therapy and ensures compliance
- Provides sustained, high bactericidal levels in blood

Side-effects and adverse reactions
- Central nervous system: dizziness, fever, headache, paresthesia,
- Gastrointestinal: abdominal pain, bleeding, impaired liver function, pseudomembranous colitis
- Genitourinary: candidiasis, nephrotoxicity
- Hematologic: anemia, bone marrow depression, eosinophilia
- Respiratory: respiratory distress, hypersensitivity reaction
- Skin: rash, urticaria

Interactions (other drugs)
Warfarin

Evidence
Ceftriaxone is an effective treatment for gonococcal urethritis [11].

Acceptability to patient
Intramuscular administration may not be as acceptable as oral regimens for some patients

Follow up plan
Follow up only if symptoms recur

Patient and caregiver information
Advise patients on means of avoiding reinfection

CIPROFLOXACIN
Fluoroquinolone
Gonococcal and nongonococcal urethritis

Dose
Adult oral dose: 300mg twice daily for 7 days (nongonococcal)

Efficacy
Highly effective treatment for gonococcal urethritis

Risks/Benefits
Risks:
- Use caution with hypersensitivity to penicillins
- Use caution with pregnancy and nursing mothers
- Use caution with renal disease and anaphylaxis
- Use caution with seizure disorders

Benefits:
- Single dose regimen allows directly observed therapy, ensuring compliance
- Provides sustained bactericidal levels in blood

Side-effects and adverse reactions
- Central nervous system: anxiety, depression, dizziness, fever, headache, seizures
- Eyes, ears, nose and throat: visual disturbances
- Gastrointestinal: abdominal pain, diarrhea, heartburn, impaired liver function, pseudomembranous colitis, vomiting
- Skin: rash, photosensitivity, pruritus

Interactions (other drugs)
- Antacids ■ Didanosine ■ Sucralfate ■ Warfarin

Evidence
Ciprofloxacin is an effective therapy for gonococcal urethritis.

Acceptability to patient
Single dose oral regimen is more acceptable than intramuscular administration for some patients

Follow up plan
Follow up only if symptoms recur

Patient and caregiver information
Advise patients on means of avoiding reinfection

LIFESTYLE
Practice of safe sex, use of barrier methods of contraception and abstaining from sex with multiple partners will reduce the risk of becoming infected (or reinfected) with any of the causative organisms of urethritis.

RISKS/BENEFITS
There are no risks associated with these lifestyle changes.

ACCEPTABILITY TO PATIENT
Some patients may find it difficult to change their sex practices.

FOLLOW UP PLAN
Check if patient is adhering to lifestyle changes at any follow up visits.

PATIENT AND CAREGIVER INFORMATION
Patients should be informed that urethritis is a sexually transmitted disease.

EFFICACY OF THERAPIES

In the majority of patients with uncomplicated urethritis, treatment with one of the recommended regimens leads to resolution of symptoms and cure of infection within two weeks (and often less time), providing the patient completes the full regimen. It is necessary that the patient return at 7–10 days for re-evaluation and to have cultures repeated. Counseling of patients with respect to sexual practices should occur at this visit.

Evidence

- Both 1g azithromycin and a 7-day course of doxycycline (100mg twice daily) produced high clinical cure rates within 2 weeks in nongonococcal urethritis and cervicitis. [5]
- Recommended regimens with ceftriaxone, ciprofloxacin and cefixime can eliminate gonococcal infection within 24 hours. [12]

Review period

- Most patients require review only if symptoms recur
- Pregnant patients should be reviewed 3 weeks after completion of therapy and tested for cure, as neither of the is highly effective
- Patients treated with erythromycin should be tested for cure 3 weeks after completion of therapy as this drug is not as effective as azithromycin or doxycycline

PROGNOSIS

The prognosis for patients with urethritis is excellent, providing they complete the full treatment regimen and take appropriate measures to avoid reinfection, including referral of sex partners.

Therapeutic failure

Relapse is usually due to failure to complete the full course of antibiotics; patients should be retreated with the initial regimen.

Recurrence

- Patients with recurrent or persistent urethritis should be retreated with initial antibiotic regimen if they did not comply with treatment or were re-exposed to an untreated sex partner
- Otherwise, culture a urethral swab for *T. vaginalis*. If infection is confirmed (or strongly suspected), treat with metronidazole (2g orally, single dose) plus erythromycin base (500mg orally four times a day for 7 days) or erythromycin ethylsuccinate (800mg orally four times a day for 7 days); this regimen is also effective against Ureaplasma species

Deterioration

If none of the above regimens is successful, refer the patient for urologic assessment for anatomic abnormality; urethral stricture may be present

COMPLICATIONS

- Complications in men include acute epididymitis, prostatic involvement, urethral stricture and an oculogenital syndrome consisting of NGU and conjunctivitis
- Complications in women include pelvic inflammatory disease, with an increased risk of ectopic pregnancy and infertility
- Infants born to mother with *C. trachomatis* infection are at risk for conjunctivitis and pneumonia; those born to mothers with *N. gonorrhoeae* infection are at risk for infection of the conjunctivae, pharynx, respiratory tract or anal canal

CONSIDER CONSULT

Patients whose relapses are not eliminated by antibiotic treatment should be referred for urologic evaluation to rule out anatomic abnormalities.

PREVENTION

RISK FACTORS
Multiple sex partners: the greater the number of sex partners, the higher the likelihood of exposure to *C. trachomatis* and *N. gonorrhoeae*

Untreated sex partner(s): partners who are not referred for evaluation and treatment are a reservoir of infection

Unprotected sex: barrier methods of contraception can reduce the risk of infection

MODIFY RISK FACTORS
Lifestyle and wellness
SEXUAL BEHAVIOR

- Using barrier methods of contraception and refraining from sex with multiple partners will reduce a person's risk for urethritis
- Persons who have received treatment for urethritis must refer all sex partners (from 60 days preceding onset of symptoms) for evaluation and treatment to avoid reinfection

SCREENING
Screening is recommended in the following groups:

- Sexually active adolescents should be screened annually for *C. trachomatis*
- Women at high risk for chlamydial infection – those <25 years, those with multiple partners and those who have been treated previously for an STD- should be screened routinely for *C. trachomatis*
- Pregnant women at high risk for chlamydial infection should be screened in the third trimester
- Women at high risk for gonorrheal infection should be screened routinely
- Pregnant women at high risk for gonorrheal infection and those living in high prevalence areas should be screened for *N. gonorrhoeae* at the first antenatal visit

There are no recommendations for screening men, who can carry *C. trachomatis* asymptomatically and act as a reservoir of infection.

PREVENT RECURRENCE
The most effective means of preventing recurrence are to ensure that all sex partners are referred for evaluation and treatment where necessary, to use barrier methods of contraception and to refrain from sex with multiple partners.

Reassess coexisting disease
Failure to conform to the therapeutic regimen, use of the wrong antibiotic, the right antibiotic but at a suboptimal dose, the right antibiotic but for an inappropriate time interval, and the presence of two distinct infectious organisms with different sensitivities can cause recurrence of urethritis.

RESOURCES

ASSOCIATIONS
American Social Health Association
PO Box 13827
Research Triangle Park
NC27709–9940
Tel: 800-230-6039

CDC National STD Hotline
Tel: 1-800-227-8922

National Institute of Allergy and Infectious Diseases
31 Center Drive (MSC-2520), Building 31, Room 7A50
Bethesda, MD 20892–2520

KEY REFERENCES
- CDC (http://www.cdc.gov) Factsheet: Some facts about chlamydia; 1999.
  http://www.cdc.govnchstp/dstd/chlamydia facts.htm
- CDC (http://www.cdc.gov) 1998 Guidelines for the Treatment of Sexually Transmitted Diseases. MWMR
  1998;47:49–62
- http://www.cdc.gov/mmwr/preview/mmwrhtml/00050909.htm
- Mandell, Douglas, Bennett . Principles and Practice of Infectious Disease 5th edition. Philadelphia:Churchill
  Livingstone; 2000:1208–1218
- National Institute of Allergy and Infectious Diseases. Sexually Transmitted Disease Statistics. MSN Health
  http://content.health.msn.com/content/article/1680.51920
- Woodward C, Fisher MA. Drug treatment of common STDs: herpes, syphilis, urethritis, chlamydia and gonorrhoea.
  American Family Physician 1999
- http://www.aafp.org/afp/991001ap/1387.html

Evidence references and guidelines
1 Berger RE. Sexually transmitted disease; the classic diseases in Walsh PC, Retik AB, Vaughn Jr ED, Wein AJ (eds)
  Campbell's urology WB Saunders Co. 1998 Philadelphia
2 Guidelines for the treatment of sexually transmitted diseases MWMR 1998;47:49–62
3 Martin DH et al. A controlled trial of single dose of azithromycin for the treatment of chlamydial urethritis and
  cervicitis. N Engl J Med 1992;327:921–5
4 Stamm WE et al. Azithromycin for empirical treatment of the nongonococcal urethritis syndrome in men.
  A randomised double-blind study. JAMA 1995;271:545–0
5 Tan HH. An open label comparitive study of azithromycin and doxycycline in the treatment of nongonococcal
  urethritis in males and *Chlamydia trachomatis* cervitis in female sex workers in an STD clinic in Singapore.
  Singapore Med J 1999;40(8):519–23
6 Scheibel JH et al. Treatment of chlamydial urethritis in men and C. trachomatis positive female partners:
  comparison of erythromycin and tetracycline in treatment courses of one week. Sex Trans Dis 1982;9:128–31
7 Mogabgab WJ et al. Randomised comparison of ofloxacin and doxycycline for chlamydia and ureaplasma
  urethritis and cervicitis. Chemotherapy 1990;36:70–76
8 Moran JS. Drugs of choice for treatment of uncomplicated gonococcal infections. Clin Infect Dis
  1995;20(S1):S47–65
9 Crombleholme WR et al. Amoxicillin therapy for *C. trachomatis* in pregnancy. Obstet. Gynecol 1990;75:752–6
10 Handsfield HH. Comparison of single dose cefixime with ceftriaxone as therapy for uncomplicated gonorrhoea.
  N Engl J Med 1991;325:1937–41
11 Handsfield HH et al. Ceftriaxone for treatment of uncomplicated gonorrhoea. Routine use of a single 125mg dose
  in sexually transmitted disease clinics. Sex Trans Dis 1987;14:227–30
12 Haizlip J. Time required for elimination of N. gonorrhoeae from the congenital tract in men with symptomatic
  urethritis; comparison of oral and intramuscular single-dose therapy. Sex Trans Dis 1995;22(3):145–8

CONTRIBUTORS
Martin L Kabongo, MD, PhD
Philip J Aliotta, MD, MHA, FACS

URINARY INCONTINENCE

SUMMARY INFORMATION

DESCRIPTION

- Involuntary loss of urine from the bladder that may result from failure to store urine because of overactivity, and/or low urethral resistance, or failure to empty bladder due to obstruction or inadequate bladder contractility
- Several classifications of incontinence exist based upon symptoms and underlying causes
- Urge incontinence – sudden urge and desire to void associated with involuntary detrusor contractions
- Stress incontinence – loss of urine with coughing, sneezing, or laughing; causes include urethral sphincter weakness or weakness of pelvic floor and poor support of the vesicourethral sphincter unit
- Overflow incontinence – may have frequent dribbling; associated with distension of the bladder
- Functional incontinence – due to immobility, cognitive deficits, paraplegia
- Acute or transient incontinence – caused by a new, treatable medical problem
- Treatments vary and may include bladder training, pelvic floor exercises, pharmacologic therapies, and surgeries

BACKGROUND

ICD9 CODE
788.3 Incontinence of urine.

CARDINAL FEATURES
History of involuntary urine loss – primary component of diagnosis.

CAUSES
Common causes
Urge incontinence
- Detrusor instability is a term that refers to individuals who suffer from involuntary bladder contractions in the absence of neurologic impairment. These patients are referred to as having an "overactive bladder".
- Neurologically impaired individuals (stroke/CVA, Parkinsonism, multiple sclerosis, transverse myelitis, etc.) who suffer involuntary detrusor contraction and incontinence suffer from detrusor hyperreflexia and are described as having a neurogenic bladder.
- Neurogenic bladder secondary to systemic nonneurological disease – diabetes mellitus type 1, diabetes mellitus type 2
- Bladder irritation – cystitis, tumors, stones, diverticula, hematuria
- Infection
- Drugs – diuretics, caffeine, sedative-hypnotics, alcohol

Stress incontinence
- Pelvic floor muscle weakness – commonly seen in females after repeated pregnancies and vaginal deliveries; contributes to stress incontinence
- Urethral sphincter weakness – common after prostatectomy, trauma, radiation, myelomeningocele, or sacral cord lesions; contributes to stress incontinence
- Drugs – alpha-adrenergic antagonists (e.g. doxazosin)

Overflow incontinence
- Hypotonic bladder
- Anatomic obstruction – prostate, stricture, cystocele
- Fecal impaction – underactive detrusor
- Drugs which cause decreased bladder tone – anticholinergics (antidepressants, antipsychotics, sedative-hypnotics, antihistamines), nervous system depressants (narcotics, alcohol, Ca channel blockers)
- Drugs which cause increased sphincter tone – alpha-adrenergic agonists (e.g. pseudoephedrine) and beta-blockers (e.g. atenolol)

Functional incontinence
- Loss of central nervous system control – severe dementia; contributes to functional incontinence
- Depression; pseudodementia in elderly
- Drugs – many classes which may cause confusion and sedation, particularly in the elderly

Rare causes
- Depression
- Diabetes insipidus
- Dehydration

Contributory or predisposing factors

- Increasing age
- Female gender
- Estrogen deficiency – menopause; decline in mucus production weakens urethra's ability to maintain a tight seal when intra-abdominal pressure increases
- Multiparity – perineal trauma during pregnancy and childbirth
- Urinary tract infections
- Atrophic vaginitis or urethritis
- Obesity
- Chronic obstructive pulmonary disease
- L-hyoscyamine
- Prior pelvic surgery (hysterectomy, urethral surgery)

EPIDEMIOLOGY

Incidence and prevalence

FREQUENCY

- Up to 30% of young and middle-aged females – often associated with childbirth
- After age 60, occurs in 30% of females and 10–15% of males otherwise healthy
- 25–30% of hospitalized older adults (over age 65)
- 50–80% of older adults in long-term care institutions

Demographics

AGE

- Increases with aging
- Up to 50% of elderly

GENDER

- Male to female ratio is 1:8
- As many as 1 in 4 females between ages 30–59 have experienced an episode

GENETICS

Genetic predisposition; prevalence in first degree relatives is 20%.

DIAGNOSIS

DIFFERENTIAL DIAGNOSIS
Urinary tract infection
FEATURES
- Urinary urgency and frequency
- Pelvic pain
- Low back pain
- Hematuria
- Dysuria
- Bacteriuria
- Fever

Diabetes mellitus
FEATURES
- Increased urine output
- Diabetic neuropathic bladder
- Hyperglycemia

SIGNS & SYMPTOMS
Signs
- Post void residual volume of greater than 100ml, 5 minutes after voiding, may indicate overflow incontinence
- Small pinpoint urethra (urethral stenosis) may be associated with overflow incontinence
- Leakage of urine with stress maneuvers confirms diagnosis of stress incontinence
- Bladder filling test in which patient experiences involuntary bladder contractions or severe urgency at a relatively low bladder volume is consistent with urge incontinence
- Voiding difficulty (hesitancy, straining, or intermittent stream) may indicate obstruction or contractility problem
- Urinalysis – negative for urinary tract infection

Symptoms
- Involuntary loss of urine
- Urinary urgency
- Small frequent voiding
- Nocturia
- Burning with urination
- Perineal irritation
- Suprapubic discomfort
- Low back pain with pelvic discomfort
- Pain at the urethra, not painful urination
- A sense of incomplete bladder emptying, pelvic fullness
- A lack of awareness that one has to void until one is wet
- Fecal incontinence with urinary incontinence

ASSOCIATED DISORDERS
- Coughing, sneezing – medical conditions such as allergies contribute to stress incontinence
- Obesity – risk factor for urinary incontinence in females due to increased pressure on bladder or urethra; may impair blood flow or nerves to bladder. May alter sphincter position/tone
- Smoking – increases risk of developing all forms of urinary incontinence, especially stress incontinence; a smoker's chronic cough may damage supports to the urethra and vagina; an association may exist between nicotine and overactive bladder symptoms
- High-impact activities – increase the downward force on pelvic floor muscles

CONSIDER CONSULT

- History of recurrent urinary tract infections
- Underlying neuromuscular disease with incontinence
- History of pelvic trauma
- Patient refractory to initial intervention
- Acute urinary retention
- Very small capacity (<100cc) bladder
- Hematuria (gross and microscopic) in the absence of urinary tract infection
- Severe hesitancy, straining, low flow rate or interrupted urinary stream when voiding
- Enlarged prostate (with residual urine) or suspicion of prostate cancer
- Suspicion of urinary tract structural abnormality

INVESTIGATION OF THE PATIENT
Direct questions to patient

Q Do you ever leak urine when you do not want to?
Q Do you lose urine when you cough, sneeze, lift something heavy, walk or sleep?
Q Do you lose urine on your way to the toilet?
Q Do you wet the bed at night?
Q Do you go to the toilet frequently because you fear wetting yourself?
Q Do you use absorbent products or pads to collect urine?
Q Do you dribble after voiding?
Q Do you void in small quantities?
Q Do you have difficulty initiating urination?
Q How often do you urinate?
Q How many times do you awaken at night to urinate?
Q Do you have chronic problems with constipation?

Contributory or predisposing factors

U Is there a history of predisposing factors? Multiparity, neurologic disorders, bladder obstruction, cognitive deficits, immobility, diabetes, any disorder requiring a medication which can alter urodynamics.

Family history

Q Is there a family history of similar problems? 20% prevalence rate among first degree relatives.

Examination

- **Check temperature** – fever suggests infection
- **Check urine** – urinalysis by dipstick testing is an acceptable method to rule out urinary tract infections
- **Assess abdomen** – determine bladder distension, bowel sounds, and suprapubic discomfort
- **Perform a pelvic examination in females** – to determine the presence of atrophic changes or pelvic prolapse (dropped uterus or bladder). May need to examine patient supine and standing
- **Inspect urethral meatus** – postmenopausal women undergoing atrophic changes exhibit urethral and vaginal changes with mucosa having lost its pink color, dry, and tender to touch
- **Rectal examination** – hard stool in rectum indicates fecal impaction; in males, this should include assessment of size, consistency and contour of the prostate
- **Mental status examination** if cognitive impairment is suspected
- **Neurologic examination** – to check for anal wink and bulbocavernous reflex
- **Perform stress maneuver test** – have patient cough or sneeze with a full bladder

Summary of investigative tests

- Urinalysis; may show glycosuria (diabetes), white blood cells (infection) proteinuria (glomerular disease), bacteria (infection), red blood cells (infection or tumor), renal stones

- Stress maneuver confirms diagnosis of stress incontinence
- Normal voiding determines approximate flow rate by dividing amount of urine voided by time required to pass the urine; detects difficulty voiding
- Postresidual void determination may confirm diagnosis of overflow incontinence or urge incontinence if bladder obstruction or bladder contractility are present (normal is <100cc 5 minutes post voiding)
- Bladder filling may confirm diagnosis of urge incontinence (abnormal – urge to void at less than 250–300cc)
- Urodynamics testing – group of tests that measure bladder function, includes uroflow, cystometrogram, urethral profile pressures and electromyogram; normally performed by a specialist
- Imaging – not usually needed unless renal, pelvic, or prostatic pathology is suspected; normally performed by a specialist

DIAGNOSTIC DECISION
- Diagnosis is made largely based upon history
- Physical examination should include palpation of abdomen, neurologic examination, and fecal impaction examination; males should receive a digital rectal examination for prostatic hypertrophy and females should be given a speculum and bimanual pelvic examination for genitourinary pathology
- It is sometimes helpful to ask patient to demonstrate activities that result in urine loss (laughing, sneezing, coughing)
- Postresidual void, stress maneuver, and cystometry may identify type of incontinence

CLINICAL PEARLS
Referral to a urologist for evaluation of the patient with incontinence who does not respond to simple intervention is recommended.

THE TESTS
Body fluids
URINALYSIS
Description
Urine sample.

Advantages/Disadvantages
- Advantage: assists in ruling out infection, hematuria, or diabetes as contributing to incontinence
- Disadvantage: not diagnostic for urinary incontinence

Normal
- Appearance: yellow, clear
- Specific gravity: 1.010
- pH: 5
- Protein: negative
- Glucose: negative
- Blood: negative

Abnormal
- Appearance: straw-colored
- Specific gravity: >1.015
- pH: >6.0
- Protein: positive
- Glucose: positive
- Blood: positive
- Keep in mind the possibility of a false-positive result

Cause of abnormal result
- Bacterial infection
- Diabetes
- Tumors
- Hematuria – stone, tumor, interstitial cystitis

Drugs, disorders and other factors that may alter results
- Antibiotics – negative urinalysis
- Diuretics – low urine specific gravity
- Tumors – hematuria

Tests of function
STRESS MANEUVER
Description
Identification of leakage of urine coincident with stress maneuvers such as coughing.

Advantages/Disadvantages
Advantage: confirms diagnosis of stress incontinence.

Normal
No leakage of urine onto a small pad that physician holds over urethra while patient performs stress maneuver.

Abnormal
Leakage of urine onto pad placed over urethra with stress maneuver

Cause of abnormal result
Stress incontinence.

NORMAL VOIDING
Description
Urine sample.

Advantages/Disadvantages
Advantages:
- Allows approximate flow rate to be calculated
- Can detect signs of voiding difficulty (hesitancy, straining, intermittent stream)

Normal
Flow rate 15–20ml/sec.

Abnormal
- Flow rate <20ml/sec
- Keep in mind the possibility of a false-positive result

Cause of abnormal result
- Bladder obstruction
- Bladder contractility deficit

Drugs, disorders and other factors that may alter results
- Anticholinergic medications – may slow urinary tract function by decreasing bladder tone. Include antidepressants, antipsychotics, sedative-hypnotics, antihistamines, narcotics, alcohol, Ca channel blockers
- Alpha agonists, beta-blockers – may decrease flow by sphincter contraction

POSTRESIDUAL VOID DETERMINATION
Description
Urine obtained from bladder catheterization.

Advantages/Disadvantages
- Advantage: may diagnose bladder obstruction or contractility problem
- Disdvantage: if not performed using sterile technique, catheterization may cause bladder infection

Normal
Less than 100ml remaining in bladder within 5–10 minutes of voiding.

Abnormal
Greater than 100ml remaining in bladder within 5–10 minutes of voiding.

Cause of abnormal result
- Bladder obstruction
- Bladder contractility deficit

Drugs, disorders and other factors that may alter results
- Anticholinergic medications – may slow urinary tract function by decreasing bladder tone. Include antidepressants, antipsychotics, sedative-hypnotics, antihistamines, narcotics, alcohol, Ca channel blockers
- Alpha agonists, beta-blockers – may decrease flow by sphincter contraction

BLADDER FILLING
Description
Bladder is filled with sterile water via catheterization.

Advantages/Disadvantages
- Advantage: may diagnose urge incontinence
- Disdvantage: if not performed using sterile technique, catheterization may cause bladder infection

Normal
- Lack of involuntary contractions
- Lack of urgency at low bladder volumes (250–300ml)

Abnormal
- Involuntary contractions (detected by continuous upward movement of column of fluid, leaking around catheter, expulsion of catheter)
- Urgency at low bladder volume (less than 250–300ml)
- Keep in mind the possibility of a false-positive result

Cause of abnormal result
- Urge incontinence
- Secondary irritants – infection, hematuria, tumor, stone

CONSIDER CONSULT
- Postresidual void volume greater than 100ml
- Pelvic floor prolapse which does not respond to therapeutic interventions
- Recent pelvic floor surgery or radiation therapy
- Stress incontinence nonresponsive to nonsurgical treatment
- Urodynamic evaluation required
- Diagnosis is uncertain

PATIENT AND CAREGIVER ISSUES
Health-seeking behavior
Self-medications tried? Some herbal remedies have been marketed for incontinence including Huang qi, Cypress and Horsetail, but no controlled clinical trials have been conducted.

MANAGEMENT ISSUES
Goals
- Identify and treat any primary conditions contributing to urinary incontinence (urinary tract infections, fecal impaction, prostatic hypertrophy). When possible, discontinue medications that may alter urodynamics
- Provide patient information including biobehavioral information, assistive devices, exercises, and collecting devices if needed
- Attempt to reduce the number of incontinent episodes by pharmacologic therapy

Management in special circumstances
Restricted mobility – may contribute to incontinence and can be improved by treating the underlying problem (i.e. arthritis, orthostatic hypotension). Assistive devices such as raised toilet seats, bathroom grab bars, toilet seat arms or collective devices including urinals or bedpans may also improve continence for patients who have difficulty ambulating.

COEXISTING DISEASE
- Alcoholism – causes increased urine output and bladder spasm contributing to incontinence
- Glaucoma – drugs with anticholinergic properties often used to treat incontinence are contraindicated in patients with elevated intraocular pressure
- Prostatic hypertrophy – drugs with anticholinergic properties often used to treat incontinence are contraindicated in patients with

COEXISTING MEDICATION
- Diuretics – may precipitate incontinence especially in elderly or in those with already impaired continence
- Antihistamines – anticholinergic properties may cause urinary retention and contribute to overflow urinary incontinence
- Antidepressants – anticholinergic properties may cause urinary retention and contribute to overflow urinary incontinence
- Antipsychotics – anticholinergic properties may cause urinary retention and contribute to overflow urinary incontinence; sedation, rigidity and immobility from these agents may also contribute to incontinence
- Sympathomimetics (decongestants) – may contribute to overflow incontinence particularly in older males with enlarged prostates
- Alpha-adrenergic antagonist agents – may contribute to stress incontinence in females
- Calcium channel blockers – may reduce smooth muscle contractility/tone in bladder causing urinary retention and overflow incontinence
- Beta-blockers may cause overflow incontinence due to increase in sphincter tone

SPECIAL PATIENT GROUPS
- Elderly or disabled with limited mobility may benefit from assistive or collective devices
- Children with nocturnal incontinence may lack normal endogenous elevation in vasopressin at night

PATIENT SATISFACTION/LIFESTYLE PRIORITIES
- Anticholinergic agents may cause dry mouth, blurred vision, constipation, orthostatic hypotension and mental confusion; use lowest dose possible in elderly
- Instructions should be provided to patient regarding rational toilet scheduling, bladder training, and pelvic floor exercises to assist in eliminating embarrassing urinary leakage
- Incontinence in the elderly may contribute significantly to social isolation

SUMMARY OF THERAPEUTIC OPTIONS
Choices
- Bladder training, voiding schedules may be helpful in some patients
- Reduce medications which may adversely affect urodynamics
- Limit oral intake of substances which may contribute to incontinence – caffeine, alcohol
- Maximize cognitive functioning in the cognitively impaired

Urge incontinence
- Oxybutynin is the first-line agent for treatment of urge incontinence caused by detrusor instability
- Tolterodine is better tolerated than traditional oxybutynin, but is more expensive
- Other possibilities are imipramine, propantheline and L-hyoscyamine

Stress incontinence
- Physical therapy interventions – Kegel's exercises, biofeedback, vaginal weight training, pelvic floor electrical stimulation
- Pseudoephedrine and phenylpropanolamine are used as first-line therapy for urethral sphincter insufficiency contributing to stress incontinence in individuals with no contraindications to its use; this is an off-label use
- Midodrine may also be used for the treatment of stress incontinence
- Imipramine may be used as a second-line agent for treatment of stress incontinence due to sphincter incompetence, if first-line agents have failed
- Estrogen may be used as adjunctive therapy in postmenopausal women with stress incontinence
- For stress incontinence nonresponsive to pharmacologic interventions, cystourethropexy (surgical procedures, urethral collagen injections, or artificial sphincter implants) may be useful

Overflow incontinence
- Bethanechol is used to treat overflow incontinence caused by atonic bladder resulting in urinary retention
- Doxazosin, and other peripherally-acting antiadrenergic agents, or finasteride may provide effective treatment for overflow incontinence caused by benign prostatic hypertrophy in males

General
- Desmopressin may be useful as adjunctive treatment for nocturnal incontinence
- Medication is often used in conjunction with lifestyle modifications and exercises such as pelvic floor exercises, pessaries, biobehavioral therapy and assistive/collecting devices

Clinical pearls
- 70–80% of some patient populations can be successfully treated with conservative modalities
- Fewer than 50% of patients who suffer from urinary incontinence mention it to their physician

Never
Anticholinergic agents are contraindicated in patients with narrow angle glaucoma or prostatic hypertrophy.

FOLLOW UP
Plan for review
- Biweekly initially while exercises are being learned and medication is being adjusted
- Quarterly once continence is established and medication doses are stable
- Evaluate side-effects of medication, check for orthostatic hypotension, monitor intraocular pressure in high-risk individuals

Information for patient or caregiver
- With alpha-adrenergic blocking agents, change position slowly because orthostatic hypotension may occur
- Constipation, dry mouth, dry eyes, and blurred vision may occur with anticholinergics

DRUGS AND OTHER THERAPIES: DETAILS
Drugs
OXYBUTYNIN
Genitourinary antispasmodic

Dose
- Adult oral dose: 5.0mg three to four times daily
- Child oral dose: 0.2mg/Kg daily

Efficacy
Effective treatment for urge incontinence caused by detrusor instability.

Risks/Benefits
Risks:
- Use caution with the elderly
- Use caution with autonomic neuropathy
- Use caution with cardiac, renal and hepatic disease
- Use caution with hyperthyroidism and prostatic hypertrophy
- Use caution with ulcerative collitis and reflux oesophagitis

Benefit: improved bladder control

Side-effects and adverse reactions
- CNS: dizziness, hallucinations, insomnia
- CV: palpatations, vasodilatation
- EENT: blurred vision, mydriasis, dry mouth
- Gastrointestinal: constipation, decreased GI motility, vomiting
- Genitourinary: impotence, urinary hesistancy and retention
- Metabolic: suppression of lactation
- Skin: decreased sweating, rash

Interactions (other drugs)
No interactions recorded

Contraindications
- Angle glaucoma - Myasthenia gravis - Intestinal obstruction - Obstructive uropathy
- Severe colitis - Unstable cardiac status

Acceptability to patient
Side-effects may lead to compliance difficulties; may be better tolerated by taking controlled release tablets once daily.

Follow up plan
Follow up with patient should be scheduled for 2–4 weeks.

Patient and caregiver information
- Dry mouth is the most common side effect. May result in deterioration of oral health and poor oral intake/poor nutrition. Other side-effects include blurred vision, which often subsides within a few weeks, constipation, heat intolerance, and mental confusion
- Alcohol or sedatives may enhance drowsiness. Use caution while driving or performing tasks requiring alertness or coordination

OXYBUTYNIN EXTENDED RELEASE
Dose
Adult oral dose: 5.0–30.0mg daily.

Efficacy
Effective treatment for urge incontinence caused by detrusor instability. This drug delivery system is characterized by zero-order drug release. The GI environment such as pH and motility do not affect the drug's release nor does the presence of food.

Risks/Benefits
Risks:
- Use caution with the elderly
- Use caution with autonomic neuropathy
- Use caution with cardiac, renal and hepatic disease
- Use caution with hyperthyroidism and prostatic hypertrophy
- Use caution with ulcerative collitis and reflux oesophagitis

Benefit: improved bladder control.

Side-effects and adverse reactions
- CNS: dizziness, hallucinations, insomnia
- CV: palpatations, vasodilatation
- EENT: blurred vision, mydriasis, dry mouth
- Gastrointestinal: constipation, decreased GI motility, vomiting
- Genitourinary: impotence, urinary hesistancy and retention
- Metabolic: suppression of lactation
- Skin: decreased sweating, rash

Interactions (other drugs)
Antidepressants

Contraindications
- Angle glaucoma
- Myasthenia gravis
- Intestinal obstruction
- Obstructive uropathy
- Severe colitis
- Unstable cardiac status

Acceptability to patient
Better tolerated than oxybutynin tablets or syrup due to the drug being absorbed distal to the small bowel.

Follow up plan
Follow up with patient should be scheduled for 2–4 weeks.

Patient and caregiver information
- Dry mouth is the most common side effect. May result in deterioration of oral health and poor oral intake/poor nutrition. Other side-effects include blurred vision, which often subsides within a few weeks, constipation, heat intolerance, and mental confusion
- Alcohol or sedatives may enhance drowsiness. Use caution while driving or performing tasks requiring alertness or coordination

TOLTERODINE
Dose
Adult oral dose:1–2mg twice daily.

Efficacy
Effective for treating urge incontinence associated with detrusor instability.

Risks/Benefits
Risks:
- Use caution with the elderly
- Use caution with autonomic neuropathy
- Use caution with cardiac, renal and hepatic disease
- Use caution with hyperthyroidism and prostatic hypertrophy
- Use caution with ulcerative collitis and reflux oesophagitis

Benefit. better tolerated than oxybutynin due to fewer side-effects

Side-effects and adverse reactions
- CNS: dizziness, hallucinations, insomnia
- CV: palpatations, vasodilatation
- EENT: blurred vision, dry mouth
- Gastrointestinal: constipation, decreased GI motility, dypepsia
- Genitourinary: impotence, urinary hesistancy and retention
- Metabolic: suppression of lactation
- Skin: decreased sweating, rash

Interactions (other drugs)
Antidepressants

Contraindications
- Angle glaucoma ■ Myasthenia gravis ■ Intestinal obstruction ■ Unstable cardiac status
- Urinary retention

Acceptability to patient
Better tolerated than oxybutynin; however it is more expensive.

Follow up plan
Follow up with patient in 2–4 weeks.

Patient and caregiver information
May produce blurred vision which generally subsides within 2 weeks.

IMIPRAMINE
Tricyclic agent for urinary incontinence

Dose
Adult oral dose: 25–50mg three times daily.

Efficacy
- Effective for urge incontinence associated with detrusor instability
- May be used as a second-line agent for treatment of stress incontinence due to sphincter incompetence if first-line agents have failed

Risks/Benefits
Risks:
- Use caution with electroshock treatment, depression and suicidal patients
- Use caution with increased intra-ocular pressure
- Use caution with urinary retention and hepatic disease
- Use caution with hyperthyroidism and surgery
- Use caution in the elderly

Benefit: may assist in achieving bladder control

Side-effects and adverse reactions
- CNS: anxiety, dizziness, headache, paresthesia, tremors
- CV: cardiac abnormalities, hypertension, hypotension, palpatations
- EENT: blurred vision, tinnitus
- Gastrointestinal: dry mouth, diarrhea, hepatitis, paralytic ileus, weight gain
- Genitourinary: acute renal failure, impotence, retention
- Hematologic: bone marrow depression, eosinophilia
- Metabolic: hyperprolactinemia
- Skin: photosensitivity, pruritus, rash
- Miscellaneous: impairment of mental and physical abilities required for the performance of potentially hazardous tasks

Interactions (other drugs)
- MAOIs - SSRIs

Contraindications
- Hypersensitivity to tricyclic antidepressant - Recovery phase of MI - Convulsive disorders
- Prostatic hypertrophy

Acceptability to patient
Side-effects may limit compliance.

Follow up plan
- Follow up with patient in 2–4 weeks
- Obtain periodic electrocardiograms and compare to baseline

Patient and caregiver information
- Avoid prolonged exposure to sunlight or sunlamps due to photosensitivity
- May cause drowsiness, dizziness, or blurred vision; use caution when driving or performing tasks that require alertness or coordination
- Avoid alcohol and other central nervous system depressants
- Do not discontinue therapy abruptly without consulting the physician

PROPANTHELINE

- This is an off-label indication.
- Inhibits hypertonia of neurogenic bladder

Dose
Adult oral dose: 7.5–60mg up to four times daily

Efficacy
Effective as a second-line anticholinergic drug used for treatment of urge incontinence caused by detrusor instability.

Risks/Benefits
Risks:

- Use caution wih hyperthyroidism and hypertension
- Use caution with cardiac, renal and hepatic disease
- Use caution with ulcerative colitis and hiatal hernia
- Use caution with urinary retention and prostatic hypertrophy
- Use caution in the elderly

Benefit: may assist in achieving bladder control

Side-effects and adverse reactions

- CNS: anxiety, dizziness, headache
- CV: palpatations
- EENT: blurred vision, increased ocular tension
- Gastrointestinal: dry mouth, constipation, heartburn, paralytic ileus
- Genitourinary: hesistancy, impotence, retention
- Skin: allergic reactions, pruritus, rash

Interactions (other drugs)
Antidepressants

Contraindications

- Glaucoma ■ Obstructive uropathy ■ Myasthenia gravis ■ Severe ulcerative colitus
- Gastrointestinal obstructive diorders ■ Unstable cardiovascular disorders

Acceptability to patient
Side-effects may lead to compliance problems.

Follow up plan

- Follow up with patient after 2–4 weeks of therapy
- Postvoid urine residuals should be monitored to avoid urinary retention

Patient and caregiver information

- Usually taken 30–60 minutes prior to eating
- May cause drowsiness, dizziness, or blurred vision; use caution while driving or performing other tasks that require mental alertness
- Notify physician if skin rash or eye pain occurs
- May cause dry mouth, difficulty urinating, constipation, or increased sensitivity to light

L-HYOSCYAMINE

Dose

- 0.125–0.25mg/L 3–4 times daily
- 0.375–0.75mg sustained release every 12 hours

Efficacy
Effective for treatment of urge incontinence caused by detrusor instability.

Risks/Benefits
Benefit: may aid in achieving bladder control

Contraindications
Avoid in patients with glaucoma, gastrointestinal obstructive disease, obstructive uropathy, myasthenia gravis, and certain cardiovascular disorders.

Acceptability to patient
Side-effects may lead to compliance problems.

Follow up plan
- Follow up with patient after 2–4 weeks of therapy
- Postvoid urine residuals should be monitored to avoid urinary retention

Patient and caregiver information
- May cause drowsiness, dizziness, or blurred vision; use caution while driving or performing other tasks that require mental alertness
- Notify physician if skin rash or eye pain occurs
- May cause dry mouth, difficulty urinating, constipation, or increased sensitivity to light

PSEUDOEPHEDRINE
This is an off-label indication.

Dose
Adult oral dose: 15–30mg three times daily.

Efficacy
May be effective for treatment of stress incontinence in postmenopausal women when combined with estrogen treatment. In clinical trials has been shown to be no more effective than pelvic floor exercises. Increases bladder outlet resistance through actions on bladder and urethra to achieve continence in individuals with stress incontinence caused by urethral sphincter insufficiency.

Risks/Benefits
Benefits:
- Improved bladder control
- Over the counter medication

Side-effects and adverse reactions
- Elevated blood pressure
- Stomach cramps
- Nervousness
- Respiratory difficulty
- Dizziness
- Tremor, palpitations

Contraindications
- Concomitant monoamine oxidase inhibitor therapy ▪ Use with caution in patients with hypertension, angina, hyperthyroidism, and diabetes

Acceptability to patient
Usually well tolerated.

Follow up plan
- Follow up in 2–4 weeks
- Monitor blood pressure
- Periodically monitor thyroid levels and serum glucose if used in patients with thyroid disease or diabetes

Patient and caregiver information
- Do not exceed recommended dosages
- May cause insomnia, nervousness, or dizziness

PHENYLPROPANOLAMINE
This is an off-label indication.

Dose
25–100mg sustained release three times daily.

Efficacy
May be effective for treatment of stress incontinence in postmenopausal women when combined with estrogen treatment. In clinical trials has been shown to be no more effective than pelvic floor exercises. Increases bladder outlet resistance through actions on bladder and urethra to achieve continence in individuals with stress incontinence caused by urethral sphincter insufficiency.

Risks/Benefits
Benefits:
- Improved bladder control
- Over the counter medication

Side-effects and adverse reactions
- Elevated blood pressure
- Stomach cramps
- Nervousness
- Respiratory difficulty
- Dizziness

Contraindications
- Concomitant monoamine oxidase inhibitor therapy ■ Use with caution in patients with hypertension, angina, hyperthyroidism, and diabetes

Evidence
Acceptability to patient
Usually well tolerated.

Follow up plan
- Follow up in 2–4 weeks
- Monitor blood pressure
- Periodically monitor thyroid levels and serum glucose if used in patients with thyroid disease or diabetes

Patient and caregiver information
- Do not exceed recommended dosages
- May cause insomnia, nervousness, or dizziness

MIDODRINE (POM)
This is an off-label indication.

Dose
2.5–5.0mg two to three times per day.

Efficacy
Effective for treatment of stress incontinence. The active metabolite is an alpha-1 agonist, which may increase bladder outlet resistance through actions on bladder and urethra to achieve continence in individuals with stress incontinence caused by urethral sphincter insufficiency.

Risks/Benefits
Benefit: improved bladder control

Side-effects and adverse reactions
- Elevated blood pressure
- Paresthesia

Interactions (other drugs)
- **Cardiac glycosides – bradycardia** ■ **Beta-blockers – heart block or arrhythmia**

Contraindications
- **Severe heart or renal disease** ■ **Urinary retention** ■ **Pheochromocytoma** ■ **Thyrotoxicosis**
- **Severe hypertension**

Acceptability to patient
Usually well tolerated.

Follow up plan
- Follow up in 2–4 weeks
- Monitor blood pressure and heart rate
- Periodically evaluate renal and hepatic function
- Periodically monitor thyroid levels if used in patients with thyroid disease

BETHANECHOL
Cholenergic stimulant

Dose
Adult oral dose: 10–30mg three times daily

Efficacy
Useful to treat overflow incontinence caused by atonic bladder resulting in urinary retention.

Risks/Benefits
Risks:
- Individuals with tartrazine sensitivity may have an allergic reaction
- When bethanechol contracts the bladder, if sphincter fails to relax, urine may be forced up the ureters. If bacteriuria is present, a reflux infection may occur
- Use caution with urinary retention due to obstruction

Risk: may improve bladder control

Side-effects and adverse reactions
- CNS: dizziness, headache, fainting
- CV: hypotension
- EENT: lacrimation, miosis
- Gastrointestinal: abdominal cramps, diarrhea, vomiting

- Genitourinary: urinary urgency
- Respiratory: asthma attacks
- Skin: flushing, sweating

Interactions (other drugs)
None recorded

Contraindications
- Obstruction of the genitourinary tract ■ Asthma ■ Coronary artery disease ■ Peptic ulcer
- Hyperthyroidism ■ Cardiac conduction defects ■ Hypertension ■ Parkinsonism ■ Seizures
- Intestinal obstruction ■ Peritonitis ■ Surgery

Acceptability to patient
Side-effects may limit use in some patients.

Follow up plan
- Follow up with patient in 2–4 weeks
- Monitor heart rate and blood pressure

Patient and caregiver information
- To avoid nausea and vomiting, take 1 hour before or 2 hours after meals
- If pronounced abdominal discomfort, salivation, sweating, or flushing occur, notify physician
- Dizziness, lightheadedness, or fainting may occur especially when getting up from a sitting or lying down position

DOXAZOSIN
Dose
1–8mg every day.

Efficacy
Has been shown in controlled trials to be effective in improving urine flow in men with prostatic hypertrophy. No controlled studies have been conducted to show it to be effective in treating overflow incontinence in males due to benign prostatic hypertrophy.

Risks/Benefits
Risks:
- Orthostatic hypotension – particularly in patients taking other antihypertensive, diuretic, vasodilator medications
- Use caution in hepatic disease
- Use caution in nursing mothers

Benefit: improved bladder control

Side-effects and adverse reactions
- CNS: dizziness, headache, fever, paresthesia
- CV: chest pain, palpatations, hypotension
- EENT: visual disturbances, tinnitus
- Gastrointestinal: abdominal cramps,constipation, diarrhea, dry mouth, vomiting
- Genitourinary: Incontinence, polyuria
- Respiratory: dyspnea
- Skin: pruritus, rash

Interactions (other drugs)
- ACE inhibitors ■ Indomethacin ■ Calcium channel blockers

Acceptability to patient
Side-effects are more tolerable if taken at bedtime.

Follow up plan
- Follow up with patient in 2–4 weeks
- Monitor blood pressure routinely

Patient and caregiver information
- Possibility of syncopal and orthostatic symptoms especially when initiating therapy
- Avoid driving or hazardous tasks for 12–24 hours after initiating therapy or following a dosage increase
- Use caution when rising from a sitting or lying position
- If dizziness or palpitations are bothersome, contact physician
- Drowsiness may occur. Use caution when driving or operating heavy machinery

FINASTERIDE (POM)
Dose
5mg every day.

Efficacy
Effective in improving symptoms of benign prostatic hypertrophy but is less effective than alpha-adrenergic blockers. No controlled studies have been conducted to show that finasteride is effective in improving overflow incontinence.

Risks/Benefits
- Risk: hepatic function abnormalities
- Benefit: may be beneficial in achieving bladder control

Side-effects and adverse reactions
- Erectile dysfunction
- Decreased libido
- Breast tenderness and enlargement
- Hypersensitivity including lip swelling and skin rash
- Testicular pain

Acceptability to patient
Well tolerated.

Follow up plan
- Follow up with patient in 2–4 weeks
- Monitor postvoid residual volumes
- Monitor for prostate cancer prior to initiating therapy and periodically thereafter by digital rectal examination
- Evaluate any sustained increases in prostate specific antigen carefully

Patient and caregiver information
- Sexual dysfunction may occur, but is usually mild and transient
- Crushed or broken tablets should not be handled by a female caregiver who is pregnant or likely to become pregnant because of potential risk to male fetus

ESTROGEN
Dose
Adult dose: Conjugated estrogens vaginally (2g or a fraction per day) initially for 1–2 weeks; a maintenance dose of 1g one to three times weekly may be used after restoring vaginal mucosa.

Efficacy

May be effective in reducing stress incontinence in postmenopausal women when used with an alpha-adrenergic agonist. Controlled studies have not shown estrogens to be effective in reducing stress incontinence when used alone.

Risks/Benefits

Risks:

- Use caution with estrogen sensitive neoplasms and genital bleeding
- Use caution with hypertension, cardiac, renal and hepatic disease
- Use caution with asthma, gallbladder disease, blood dyscrasia and diabetes mellitus
- Use caution with depression, convulsive disease and headaches

Benefit: may improve bladder control in women with stress incontinence

Side-effects and adverse reactions

- CNS: depression, dizziness, headache
- CV: edema, hypotension, MI, pulmonary embolus, stroke, thromboembolism, thrombophlebitis
- EENT: visual disturbances
- Gastrointestinal: abdominal cramps,constipation, diarrhea, weight gain, jaundice, pancreatitis, vomiting
- Genitourinary: amenorrhoea, vaginal bleeding, dysmenorrhea, impotence, candidiasis, testicular atrophy
- Metabolic: hypercalcemia, hyperglycemia
- Skin: purpura, rash,
- Elevated blood pressure

Contraindications

- Breast cancer ■ Undiagnosed genital bleeding ■ Thrombophlebitis ■ Thromboembolic
- Endometrial cancer ■ Known or suspected pregnancy

Evidence

In a meta-analysis of results from four randomized controlled trials a subjective improvement of 46% was estimated. Uncontrolled trials showed an average improvement rate of 64% after treatment with estrogen [1]

Acceptability to patient

Generally well tolerated.

Follow up plan

- Follow up with patient in 2–4 weeks
- See patient yearly for Papanicolaou smear
- Periodically evaluate thyroid function, cholesterol, and serum glucose

Patient and caregiver information

- Insert cream deeply into vagina
- After 1–2 weeks, a dosage reduction may be attempted
- Notify physician if any of the following occur: sharp chest pain, shortness of breath, abnormal vaginal bleeding, suspected pregnancy, lumps in breast, severe headache, visual disturbance, yellowing of skin or eyes, depression

DESMOPRESSIN
Antidiuretic

Dose
Adult dose: 20–40mcg intranasally at bedtime.

Efficacy
May be useful as adjunctive treatment for nocturnal incontinence.

Risks/Benefits
Risks:
- Use caution with coronary and hypertensive disease
- Use caution with bleeding disorders

Benefit: may assist in achieving bladder control overnight

Side-effects and adverse reactions
- CNS: headache, flushing, drowsiness
- CV: hypertension
- EENT: rhinitis
- Gastrointestinal: cramps, heartburn, nausea
- Genitourinary: vulvar pain

Interactions (other drugs)
None recorded

Contraindications
None recorded

Acceptability to patient
Generally well tolerated.

Follow up plan
- Follow up with patient in 2–4 weeks
- Monitor blood pressure
- Evaluate nasal mucosa changes
- Monitor fluid/electrolyte balance

Patient and caregiver information
- Administer half of daily dose in each nostril
- If abnormal bleeding, shortness of breath, heartburn, nausea, abdominal cramps or vulval pain occurs, notify physician
- Discard any solution remaining after 25 doses (Stimate) or 50 doses (DDAVP); the amount delivered thereafter may be substantially less than prescribed

Physical therapy
PELVIC FLOOR EXERCISES
Kegal exercises, weighted vaginal cones, biofeedback, electrical stimulation, magnetic treatment.

Efficacy
Strengthening the pelvic floor muscles is beneficial in the treatment of stress incontinence.

Of these modalities, in controlled studies biofeedback has been shown to be most effective, followed by pelvic floor exercises. Adequate studies have not been published to demonstrate that vaginal cones or electrical stimulation are more effective than no treatment. Bladder training has been shown to be effective in the short term, but may not have lasting effect.

Risks/Benefits
May result in fewer leakage episodes.

Evidence
In an analysis of 10 studies (four randomized trials, two quasi-experimental studies, four uncontrolled studies) of pelvic floor muscle exercise therapy with or without myofeedback, the percentage of participants who showed improved continence with combined therapy ranged from 74 to 100. The percentage of participants who were completely continent after combined therapy ranged from 38 to 100 [2]

Acceptability to patient
High.

Follow up plan
Follow up with patient in 2–4 weeks or after 8 weeks of magnetic therapy.

Patient and caregiver information
- Patients should be educated on how to "find" and contract their pelvic floor muscles (Kegal exercise) – biofeedback, digital vaginal examination, or stopping urine midstream can be helpful
- Vaginal weights – lightest weight should be put in vagina initially with the tapered stringed portion resting on the pelvis. Insertion is similar to inserting a tampon. Walk for 15 minutes tightening the muscle to keep the cone in place
- Electrical stimulation – probes, surface electrodes, or implantable devices may apply electrical current to stimulate weak muscles or calm muscles of an overactive bladder (urge incontinence)
- Magnetic therapy – pulsing magnetic fields increase pelvic floor muscle strength in stress incontinence and urge incontinence by causing contractions of pelvic floor muscles; treatments last 30 minutes and occur twice weekly for 8 weeks

Surgical therapy
CYSTOURETHROPEXY
Abdominal suspensions, vaginal suspension, slings or artificial sphincter procedures, and periurethral injection procedures.

Efficacy
- Retropubic suspensions and slings appear to be most efficacious invasive procedures for long-term success in treatment of stress incontinence (based on cure/dry rates) in older women who have had vaginal deliveries or are postmenopausal; success rates appear to be of the order of 70–80%
- For stress incontinence related to intrinsic sphincter deficiency:
- Slings placed under the urethra to support and compress have success rates of 81–98%
- Artificial sphincters have a reported success rate of 90%
- Periurethral collagen injections have a success rate of 64–95%

Risks/Benefits
- Risks: transfusions, surgical complications, postoperative complications, urinary tract infection
- Benefit: improved continence

Evidence
Surgical intervention may be an acceptable alternative for treating incontinence either as initial therapy or after other treatments failed [3]

Acceptability to patient
- Most patients consider surgery successful based on either fully cured stress incontinence or a substantial improvement in continence.
- The following predispose to surgical failure: advanced age, postmenopausal, hysterectomy, prior failed continence surgery, detrusor instability, pelvic radiation, and abnormal perineal electromyography

Follow up plan
- Follow up with patient in 4 weeks to determine whether urinary retention is present
- Periodic evaluations should be conducted no less often than 1, 6, and 12 months after surgery, followed by yearly evaluation thereafter

Patient and caregiver information
- Patients should be prepared for hospitalization varying from 0 to 5 days depending upon the procedure
- Surgeries may need to be repeated

Complementary therapy
NUTRITION/HERBS
It is recommended that caffeine, alcohol, and simple sugars are eliminated from the diet. The addition of calcium (1000mg/day) and magnesium (500mg/day) may improve sphincter tone. Horsetail (*Equisetum arvense*) helps connective tissue integrity (30 drops of tincture/day).

Efficacy
Dietary elimination is known to work fairly well; but there are no well designed controlled trials of herbal remedies.

Acceptability to patient
Dietary/lifestyle change is quite difficult for some patients to implement.

Follow up plan
Standard patient care.

Patient and caregiver information
Herbal remedies may be ingested in tea – 1 teaspoon of dried herb per cup of tea, steeped for 10min.

Other therapies
ASSISTIVE/COLLECTING DEVICES
Raised toilet seats, bathroom grab bars, toilet seat arms, urinals, bedside commodes, bed pans, high-absorbency pads, penile compression devices.

Efficacy
May be especially beneficial in older persons for whom environmental barriers, such as the location of the toilet contribute to their incontinence.

Risks/Benefits
Benefit: may improve continence when environmental barriers are a contributing cause.

Acceptability to patient
High

Follow up plan
None

Patient and caregiver information
Patients should be instructed on availability and proper use of the various devices.

BIOBEHAVIORAL THERAPY
Timed toileting, prompted voiding, fluid schedules, avoidance of dietary irritants, biofeedback.

Efficacy
Improvement occurs in 70–80%; particularly beneficial for treating urge incontinence and may also be helpful for treating stress incontinence.

Risks/Benefits
Risk: may experience fewer urinary leakage episodes

Evidence
Most patients will respond to behavioral techniques [4]

Acceptability to patient
High.

Follow up plan
Follow up with patient in 2–4 weeks.

Patient and caregiver information
- Voiding diaries should be used for 2–5 days prior to initiating biobehavioral therapy to aid in creation of voiding schedules and habits; diary should continue to be maintained to assess outcome of therapy
- For bladder training, patients must inhibit urinating until a set time and this amount of time should be progressively increased. Patient should be treated with a reward when this is accomplished
- For habit training, patients should be prompted to void in the morning, after meals, and before bed
- Fluid loads should be restricted; alcohol, coffee and tea limited

PESSARIES
Donut, cube, inflato ball, incontinence ring and dish, Introl, tampons.

Efficacy
May be beneficial in cases of uterine or vaginal prolapse, rectocele, cystocele, or defects in the vaginal structure contribute to incontinence.

Risks/Benefits
- Risks: urinary retention, constipation, pelvic pain, vaginal discharge
- Benefit: may improve continence

Acceptability to patient
High.

Follow up plan
- Follow up in 24 hours, one week and one month with donut style pessaries
- Evaluate periodically for tissue irritation or ulceration

Patient and caregiver information
- Many pessaries must be removed at bedtime (cube, inflato ball, incontinence ring and dish, Introl) and tampons must be removed after 8 hours
- Some pessaries contain latex and must not be used by women with latex allergies
- It is not uncommon to need to re-size a pessary after the first fitting
- Do not miss scheduled appointments and checkups
- Contact your physician immediately if you have: difficulty urinating, constipation, pelvic pain, vaginal discharge
- Douches or vaginal creams may be used to decrease vaginal odor
- Estrogen creams may be prescribed to moisten vaginal and urethral tissue

LIFESTYLE
- Avoid alcohol
- Lose weight
- Stop smoking

RISKS/BENEFITS
- Avoiding alcohol may improve continence by decreasing urine output and detrusor instability
- Losing weight may improve continence by decreasing pressure on bladder and urethra and by improving blood flow to bladder nerves
- Stopping smoking may improve continence by decreasing overactive bladder symptoms and decreasing cough which frequently damages supports to urethra and vagina

ACCEPTABILITY TO PATIENT
Moderate.

FOLLOW UP PLAN
Follow up with patient periodically.

PATIENT AND CAREGIVER INFORMATION
- Alcohol increases urine output and may also act as a bladder irritant
- If alcohol abuse is present, provide patient with information on organizations that can assist
- Provide daily exercise regimen
- May need assistance of dietician for instruction on healthy eating habits
- Provide information on local weight-loss support groups
- Pharmacologic aids may be available to assist in weight loss to be used in conjunction with healthy diet and exercise
- Provide patient with smoking cessation aids such as nicotine patches, inhalers, gums
- Avoid smoking while utilizing nicotine replacement aids
- Other pharmacologic therapies such as bupropion may also be helpful
- Avoid persons, places, or situations that may prompt smoking
- Alternative therapies such as hypnosis may be helpful

EFFICACY OF THERAPIES
Evidence
has been prepared by The Agency for Health Care Policy and Research.

Review period
Generally, reevaluate every 3–6 months; many pharmacologic interventions have diminished efficacy with prolonged usage.

PROGNOSIS
Prognosis is generally good. Most patients can achieve an increase in bladder control with appropriate pharmacologic and medical management.

Therapeutic failure
For stress incontinence nonresponsive to pharmacologic interventions, cystourethropexy (surgical procedures, urethral collagen injections, or artificial sphincter implants) may be useful.

Recurrence
- Medications may have diminished efficacy with prolonged use
- Surgical procedures may not provide long-term results and frequently need to be repeated
- Collagen injections must be repeated periodically; most patients require 2–3 injections within the first 12 months

Deterioration
Cystourethropexy (including surgeries, intraurethral collagen injections, and artificial sphincter replacement) may be considered if pharmacologic interventions fail.

COMPLICATIONS
- Urinary tract infection
- Hydronephrosis (with atonic bladder or outlet obstruction)
- Renal failure (with obstructive hydronephrosis)
- Skin breakdown
- Social isolation
- Dependency
- Medication noncompliance (particularly diuretics)

MODIFY RISK FACTORS
Lifestyle and wellness
TOBACCO
- Tobacco is a bladder irritant; smoker's cough damages supports of urethra and vagina
- Ceasing smoking may improve continence by decreasing overactive bladder symptoms and decreasing cough which frequently damages supports to urethra and vagina
- Provide patient with smoking cessation aids such as nicotine patches, inhalers, gums
- Avoid smoking while utilizing nicotine replacement aids
- Other pharmacologic therapies such as bupropion may also be helpful
- Avoid persons, places, or situations that may prompt smoking
- Alternative therapies such as hypnosis may be helpful

ALCOHOL AND DRUGS
- Avoiding alcohol may improve continence by decreasing urine output
- Alcohol increases urine output and may also act as a bladder irritant
- If alcohol abuse is present, provide patient with information on organizations that can assist

DIET
- Lose weight
- Losing weight may improve continence by decreasing pressure on bladder and urethra and by improving blood flow to bladder nerves
- Provide daily exercise regimen
- May need assistance of dietician for instruction on healthy eating habits
- Provide information on local weight-loss support groups
- Pharmacologic aids may be available to assist in weight loss to be used in conjunction with healthy diet and exercise

PHYSICAL ACTIVITY
- Lose weight
- Losing weight may improve continence by decreasing pressure on bladder and urethra and by improving blood flow to bladder nerves
- Provide daily exercise regimen
- Avoid high-impact physical activities
- Do pelvic floor exercises regularly, especially after childbirth
- Avoid prolonged second stage of labor

FAMILY HISTORY
20% prevalence rate in first degree relative.

DRUG HISTORY
Estrogen replacement therapy utilized postmenopausally.

SCREENING
Screening is not required, but up to 50% of patients with incontinence do not mention it to their physician.

PREVENT RECURRENCE
- Physical therapy – pelvic floor muscle strengthening
- Biobehavioral therapy – habit voiding

Reassess coexisting disease
Pelvic radiation or pelvic surgery can cause recurrent urinary incontinence.

INTERACTION ALERT
- Diuretics – used for hypertension, edema, and congestive heart failure increase urinary output
- Cholinergic agents – used for glaucoma and stimulating gastrointestinal tract motility may contribute to overflow incontinence
- Anticholinergic agents – antihistamines, antidepressants, antipsychotics may contribute to overflow incontinence

PATIENT SATISFACTION/LIFESTYLE PRIORITIES
- Pelvic surgery or radiation may be required in instance of malignancy
- Pharmacologic alternatives may be available to treat coexisting diseases when medications contribute to recurrent incontinent episodes

ASSOCIATIONS
The American Urological Association
1120 N. Charles Street
Baltimore
MD 21201–5559
Phone: 410-727-1100
Fax: 410.223.4374
Website: http://www.amuro.org

The National Association for Continence
P.O. Box 8310
Spartanburg
South Carolina 29305–8310
Phone: 864-579-7900
Toll Free: 1-800-BLADDER
Fax: 864-579-7902
Website: http://www.nafc.org

KEY REFERENCES
- Lightner DJ and Itano NMB (1999) Treatment options for women with stress incontinence. Mayo Clinic Proceedings 74: 1149–1156.
- Rakel: Conn's Current Therapy 2000, 52nd ed., W.B. Saunders Company
- Leach GE et al. (1997) Female stress urinary incontinence clinical guidelines panel summary report on surgical management of female stress urinary incontinence. J. Urol. 158 (3 pt 1): 875–880.
- Riley MR and Kastrup EK. Drugs Facts and Comparison, A Wolters Kluwer Company, St. Louis, MO, 2000.

Evidence references and guidelines
1 Fantl JA, Cardozo L, McClish DK. Estrogen therapy in the management of urinary incontinence in postmenopausal women: a meta-analysis: first report of the Hormones and Urogenital Therapy Committee. Obstetrics and Gynecology 1994; 83(1): 12–18.
2 de Kruif YP, van Wegen EE. Pelvic floor muscle exercise therapy with myofeedback for women with stress urinary incontinence: a meta-analysis. Physiotherapy 1996;82(2): 107–113.
3 Leach GE et al. (1997) Female stress urinary incontinence clinical guidelines panel summary report on surgical management of female stress urinary incontinence. J. Urol. 158 (3 pt 1): 875–880.
4 Lightner DJ and Itano NMB (1999) Treatment options for women with stress incontinence. Mayo Clinic Proceedings 74: 1149–1156.

FAQS
Question 1
What are the causes of pelvic floor weakness?

ANSWER 1
- Anatomic congenital or traumatic (fracture of pelvis, pelvic surgery)
- Hormonal
- Neurologic: congenital or traumatic

Question 2
What causes urethral incompetence?

ANSWER 2
Damage to the sympathetic neural input to the bladder neck and proximal urethra. This is innervated by the hypogastric nerve.

Question 3
What is the Q-tip test?

ANSWER 3
The test is used to determine the amount of urethral hypermobility that occurs with straining. Normally the angle is 10–25 degrees from the horizontal at rest. In the patient with stress urinary incontinence, the angle increases in excess of 25 degrees and suggests that the urethra descends and foreshortens along with the bladder neck due to weakness of anatomic support.

Question 4
When is urodynamic testing indicated?

ANSWER 4
- Failed previous incontinence surgery
- Previous radical pelvic surgery
- Symptoms of mixed incontinence
- No objective evidence of urinary leakage
- Abnormal neurologic examination
- History of neurologic disorder

Question 5
What is the Marshall Bonney test?

ANSWER 5
A non-diagnostic test in which a portion of the vaginal vault is elevated with a clamp applied after administration of topical local anesthetic, in a fashion that does not occlude the bladder neck.

The patient coughs with a full bladder while the examiner observes for incontinence. The examiner manipulates the urethrovesical angle, pushing the bladder base up and anteriorly without compressing the urethra closed. The patient is asked to bear down and or cough while the practitioner observes for leak with cough but no leak with bladder base elevation, indicating true stress urinary incontinence.

The test is presumed to stimulate the results of the planned surgical procedure by elevating and stabilizing the urethra and vesical neck. It is controversial as evidence would show that inadvertent compression of the urethra occurs. Nonetheless it remains a mainstay of the urodynamic assessment.

CONTRIBUTORS
Russell C Jones, MD, MPH
Jane L Murray, MD
Philip J Aliotta, MD, MHA, FACS

URINARY TRACT INFECTION

DESCRIPTION

- Presence of significant bacteria in urinary tract
- Includes lower tract infections (urethritis, cystitis, and prostatitis) and upper tract infections (pyelonephritis)
- May be classified as uncomplicated (without structural abnormalities or altered urodynamics) or complicated (structural abnormality or altered urodynamics, male infection)
- Lower tract infections often associated with urinary frequency and pain upon urination while upper infections commonly involve flank pain and constitutional symptoms – fever, malaise, etc. 30% of clinical lower tract infections have upper tract involvement
- Empirical initial choice of antibiotic should be based on infection type. microorganisms

URGENT ACTION

Antibiotic therapy should be initiated based upon patient's signs and symptoms after obtaining urine culture results. Acute uncomplicated cystitis in women does not require urine culture prior to treatment.

Patients presenting with urinary tract infection who are immunosuppressed due to HIV, cancer or renal failure should be admitted to hospital.

KEY! DON'T MISS!

Flank pain, chills, abdominal pain, or costovertebral tenderness may indicate pyelonephritis; often accompanied by presence of white blood cell casts determined by microscopic urinalysis.

BACKGROUND

ICD9 CODE
599.0 urinary tract infection.

SYNONYMS
- UTI
- Asymptomatic bacteriuria
- Cystitis
- Urethritis
- Pyelonephritis
- Prostatitis

CARDINAL FEATURES
- Pyuria
- Dysuria
- Urinary urgency
- Urinary frequency
- Suprapubic discomfort
- Fever (more common with upper UTI)
- Flank or abdominal pain (more common with upper UTI)
- Significant bacteriuria
- Malodorous, cloudy urine
- New or increase in urinary incontinence
- Altered mentation, agitation in cognitively impaired
- Symptoms typically resolve after short course of antibiotic treatment (2–3 days); if symptoms persist after short course of antibiotics, suggests upper tract infection, which requires a longer course of antibiotic therapy

CAUSES
Common causes
Bacteria usually originate from bowel as normal flora of host

Gram-positive organisms:
- *Staphylococcus saprophyticus* (causative organism in 5–15% of urinary tract infections)
- *Enterococcus faecalis*

Gram-negative organisms:
- *Escherichia coli* – causative organism in 85% of community-acquired infections
- *Klebsiella pneumoniae*
- *Proteus* spp.
- *Pseudomonas aeruginosa*
- *Enterobacter* spp.

Rare causes
- *Salmonella* spp.
- *Mycobacterium tuberculosis*
- *Chlamydia trichomatis*
- *Candida* spp.
- Multiple microbial organisms causing infection may be found in patients with renal calculi, chronic renal abscesses, indwelling urinary catheters

Serious causes

- *Staphylococcus aureus* – commonly a result of bacteremia producing renal, perinephric abscesses
- *Candida* spp. – found in critically ill, immunosuppressed and chronically catheterized individuals

Contributory or predisposing factors

- Female gender is an independent risk factor for UTI
- Recent sexual intercourse
- Use of spermicides or diaphragm
- Pregnancy
- Antecedent antibiotic use – antimicrobials used 15–28 days prior to UTI may alter urogenital normal flora in favor of pathogen-dominated flora
- Obstruction of urinary tract: benign prostatic hyperplasia, tumors, cholinergic drugs
- Residual urine in bladder due to: prostatic hypertrophy , urethral strictures, cystocele, hypotonic bladder, renal calculi, urolithiasis, tumors, bladder diverticula, or anticholinergic drugs
- Incomplete bladder emptying due to neurologic malfunctions including: stroke, spinal cord injuries, and tabes dorsalis
- Vesicoureteral reflux – retrograde urinary reflux – increased risk of acute and chronic pyelonephritis
- Urinary catheterization
- Mechanical instrumentation

EPIDEMIOLOGY

Incidence and prevalence

INCIDENCE
Males: 0.3/1000 Females: 12/1000.

PREVALENCE
Males: <1/1000 Females: 10–40/1000.
Asymptomatic bacteriuria up to 40% in elderly males and females.

Demographics

AGE
- In infants up to 6 months of age, UTI is more common in males due to abnormalities of the urinary tract
- Between 1 and 65 years, UTI is predominantly a disease of females, presumably due to anatomy of the urethra which allows bacteria to access the urinary tract relatively easily
- Over age 65, bacteriuria affects males and females approximately equally (approximately 40%), with the majority of infections being asymptomatic. Routine screening and treatment has not been found to decrease morbidity or mortality in this population

GENDER
Most prevalent in sexually active adult females; after age 65 the ratio of males and females with asymptomatic bacteriuria is equivalent.

GENETICS
Nonsecretors of ABH blood group antigens are 3–4 times more likely to have recurrent UTI.

DIFFERENTIAL DIAGNOSIS
Pyelonephritis
FEATURES
- Frequent urination
- Fever
- Shaking chills
- Chills
- Malaise
- Nausea and vomiting
- Flank pain or abdominal pain
- Costovertebral angle tenderness
- Altered mentation, agitation in cognitively impaired
- New or increased urinary incontinence
- Urinalysis: bacteriuria, white blood cell casts, hematuria

Urothritic
FEATURES
- Onset is gradual
- Urinary urgency and frequency
- Dysuria – through urination and generally localized to urethra
- Nocturia
- Pyuria
- Urethral discharge
- May be absence of bacteria on Gram stain

Prostatitis
FEATURES
- Urinary urgency, frequency, stranguria, and possibly retention
- Dysuria
- Fever – may be high
- Chills
- Malaise
- Myalgias, arthralgias
- Localized pain (perineal, rectal, sacrococcygeal)
- Altered mentation, agitation in cognitively impaired
- New or increase in incontinence – may indicate overflow incontinence/developing obstruction
- Tender, swollen, firm and warm prostate on palpation

Vaginitis
FEATURES
- Dysuria – symptoms tend to be external and at onset of urination
- Vaginal odor, vaginal itching, vaginal discharge

Pelvic Inflammatory Disease
FEATURES
- Lower abdominal or back pain – may mimic menstrual cramps
- Peritoneal signs
- Fever
- Nausea, vomiting
- Vaginal bleeding/discharge

Gonorrhea
FEATURES
- Dysuria
- Urethral discomfort, discharge
- Pain in lower abdomen or right upper quadrant (late)
- Pharyngitis
- Unilateral pain and swelling posterior scrotum (males)
- Characteristic rash, fever with gonococcemia

Renal Calculi
FEATURES
- Urinary frequency and dysuria
- Colicky flank pain (may be severe) radiating into lower abdomen and groin
- Nausea and vomiting
- Urinary retention
- Hematuria – key finding, may be with pyuria
- Obstructive uropathy
- If coexisting infection is suspected, patient requires aggressive evaluation and treatment

Asymptomatic bacteriuria
FEATURES
- Positive urinalysis, culture
- Clinically asymptomatic

SIGNS & SYMPTOMS
Signs
Significant bacteriuria:
- Dipstick urine nitrite positive – will be negative if infecting organism is not nitrate reducing
- Microscopic urine – greater than 20 bacteria/HPF in spun urine

Culture determinants of significant bacteriuria:
- In symptomatic females: greater than 100 colony-forming units (cfu)/ml
- In symptomatic males: greater than 1000cfu/ml
- In suprapubic catheter specimen: any growth
- In pyelonephritis: greater than 100,000cfu/ml
- In complicated UTI: greater than 10,000cfu/ml
- In pregnancy: greater than 10,000cfu/ml
- In urinary catheter specimen: greater than 100cfu/ml

Pyuria:
- Dipstick urine – leukocyte esterase test positive
- White blood cell (WBC) count greater than 5–10 WBC/hpf on a spun urine specimen

Hematuria

Proteinuria

Symptoms
- Dysuria
- Urinary urgency
- Urinary frequency
- Nocturia
- Suprapubic heaviness or pain

- Hematuria (more common in women)
- New or increased urinary incontinence

Elderly patients:
- Often do not experience specific urinary symptoms
- Altered mental status, particularly in cognitively impaired.
- Change in eating habits with gastrointestinal symptoms

Children:
- Fever
- Nausea, vomiting, decreased appetite
- Irritability
- Urine may have unusual smell

ASSOCIATED DISORDERS
Diabetes mellitus type 1 or type 2 (including diabetic ketoacidosis, necrobiosis lipoidica diabeticorum, hyperosmolar coma, hypoglycemia) – UTI may be result of neurological complications and incomplete bladder emptying.

KEY! DON'T MISS!
Flank pain, chills, abdominal pain, or costovertebral tenderness may indicate pyelonephritis; often accompanied by presence of white blood cell casts determined by microscopic urinalysis.

CONSIDER CONSULT
- Evidence or suspicion of obstruction, sepsis/toxicity, hydronephrosis, perinephric abscess, or other structural abnormality requires referral to urologist
- 'Complicated' UTI caused by unusual or multiple antibiotic-resistant organisms may require infectious disease consult

INVESTIGATION OF THE PATIENT
Direct questions to patient
Q **What symptoms are you experiencing?** Presence of chills, fever and severe flank pain should be treated as acute pyelonephritis. 30% of clinical lower tract infections have upper tract involvement.

Q **Have you had this before?** Recurrent infections may indicate presence of predisposing factors or antibiotic-resistant microorganisms. However, 90% of recurrences of uncomplicated lower tract infections are due to exogenous reinfection.

Q **What other diseases do you have or have you had?** Predisposing factors such as stroke or diabetes may be part of patient's medical history. Prostatism, recent catheterization, instrumentation, history of renal stones, congenital urinary tract anomaly all increase risk of complicated infection.

Q **What medications have you used during the past month?** Anticholinergics will reduce bladder tone and may lead to residual urine in bladder; antibiotics may alter normal flora; sulfonamides may predispose to renal calculi which is a contributory factor for UTI. Cholinergic medications make increase sphincter tome and increase risk of outlet obstruction, retention.

Q **Do you have any drug allergies?** Sensitivities especially to penicillins/cephalosporins or sulfonamides must be determined prior to initiating antibiotic therapy.

Contributory or predisposing factors
Q **Is there a history of predisposing factors?** Prostatic hypertrophy, tumors, bladder diverticula, stroke, diabetes type 1 or type 2, spinal cord injuries, tabes dorsalis, urogenital anomalies, surgery.

Family history

Q Is there a family history of similar problems? May be a genetic predisposition for developing recurrent UTI.

Examination

- Does the patient appear toxic? Toxicity suggests pyelonephritis
- Fever suggests pyelonephritis, prostatitis
- Males – If prostate swollen, tender, warm and indurated, suggests prostatitis
- Urinalysis – Criteria based on category of infection

Summary of investigative tests

- Macroscopic urinalysis
- Dipstick nitrite tests: Detection of nitrite in urine indicates presence of nitrate-reducing bacteria. Sensitivity 0.35; Specificity 0.95
- Leukocyte esterase (LE) dipstick tests: Detects pyuria; sensitive and highly specific test for detecting more than 10 white blood cells/mm3 of urine. Sensitivity 0.75–0.90; Specificity 0.70
- Microscopic urinalysis: Greater than 20 bacteria/hpf of spun urine is abnormal. Greater than 5–10 WBC/hpf of spun urine is abnormal. Epithelial cells on microscopy indicate a contaminated urine specimen
- Quantitative urine culture

Additional tests to consider if structural/functional abnormalities of the urinary tract are suspected or with history of recurrent infections:

- Renal and bladder ultrasound: normally performed by a specialist. May demonstrate structural abnormalities
- Voiding cystourethrogram (VCUG): normally performed by a specialist. May demonstrate abnormalities of the collecting system, particularly vesicoureteral reflux
- Intravenous pyelogram. normally performed by a specialist. May demonstrate abnormal renal function, abnormalities of the collecting system, obstruction
- Postvoiding residual: normally performed by primary care physician. May demonstrate significant urinary retention (greater than 100cc is abnormal)
- Radionuclide scan: normally performed by a specialist. May demonstrate abnormal renal function, structure
- Cystoscopy: normally performed by a specialist. Allows direct visualization of bladder and distal collecting system collection of urine from various areas of the renal system

DIAGNOSTIC DECISION

Clinical decision points:

- Clinical urinary tract infection by clinical and laboratory criteria
- New onset or recurrent infection
- Upper or lower tract infection
- Complicated or uncomplicated infection

Empiric antibiotic therapy should be initiated based upon patient symptoms and signs of urinalysis prior to obtaining urine culture results. Culture may not be required for uncomplicated cystitis in women.

Some species (e.g. *Chlamydia* and *Mycoplasma*) require special cultures in order to be detected. Special tests should be ordered if a patient has signs and symptoms of an UTI but a laboratory culture fails to grow bacteria.

Imaging studies are not needed in vast majority of patients with UTI. However, appropriate imaging studies should be done if structural abnormality or altered urodynamics are suspected. Pelvic ultrasound may be indicated in young women with pelvic tenderness, cervical discharge and unilateral adnexal tenderness or elderly patients with abdominal pain and pyuria whose presentation is not classic for UTI.

When a patient has a persistent infection that does not resolve after appropriate antibiotic therapy or suffers from recurrent infections, referral may be necessary for further tests to identify structural or functional abnormalities.

Guidelines
The following guidelines are available at the :
- The American Academy of Pediatrics [1]
- Evidence based clinical practice guideline for patients 6 years of age or less with a first time acute urinary tract infection (UTI) [2]
- Urinary tract infection [3]

The American Academy of Family Physicians has produced the following information on urinary tract infection in adults [4]

CLINICAL PEARLS
'Significant bacteriuria' is a laboratory test, not a disease! As with other tests, interpretation by the clinician requires taking into account all of the clinical conditions of the patient as well as the nature of the organism recovered. Some organisms grow well in urine (Gram-negative enterococci), while others grow slowly reaching concentrations of between 10,000 to 100,000 colony forming units/ml (coagulase-negative staphylococci). It is important for you to have your laboratories list the actual colony forming units/ml count rather than state 'growth less than 100,000 colony forming units/ml'. You must determine what is 'significant'.

Asymptomatic bacteriuria may be present in 40% of elderly patients. Routine screening and treatment is not indicated for this population.

THE TESTS
Body fluids
MACROSCOPIC URINALYSIS
Description
Urine sample.

Advantages/Disadvantages
- Advantage: noninvasive, assists in confirming diagnosis
- Disadvantage: does not identify causative organism

Normal
- Appearance: yellow, clear
- Specific gravity: 1.010
- pH: 5
- Protein: negative
- Glucose: negative
- Blood: negative

Abnormal

- Appearance: straw-colored, turbid. Amorphous urates may cause turbidity if urine is at or near room temperature
- Specific gravity: >1.015
- pH: >6.0
- Protein: positive
- Glucose: positive
- Blood: positive
- Keep in mind the possibility of a false-positive result

Cause of abnormal result

- Presence of bacteria
- Some medications or concomitant diseases may alter urinary color and pH or cause proteinuria/glucosuria. Hematuria may alter dipstick nitrite and leukocyte esterase results.

Drugs, disorders and other factors that may alter results

- Pharmacologic agents and beverages may either acidify or alkalinize urinary pH and alter the appearance of urine
- Glucose may be found in the urine of patients with diabetes
- Protein may be found in the urine of patients with renal disease

Tests of function
DIPSTICK NITRITE
Description
Urine sample.

Advantages/Disadvantages

- Advantage: noninvasive, available without a prescription. Specificity 0.95
- Disadvantage: does not identify causative organism, false-negative results. Sensitivity 0.35–0.85. Enterococci, *Staph. saprophyticus*, and *Acinetobacter* spp. do not reduce nitrate.

Normal
No nitrite in urine.

Abnormal

- Nitrite in urine
- Although rare, keep in mind the possibility of a false-positive result

Cause of abnormal result
Presence of nitrate-reducing bacteria.

Drugs, disorders and other factors that may alter results

- Gram-positive bacteria and *Pseudomonas aeruginosa* do not reduce nitrate, and may produce a false-negative result depending upon urinary tract colonization
- False negatives may also result from low urinary pH, frequent voiding, or dilute urine

LEUKOCYTE ESTERASE
Description
Urine sample.

Advantages/Disadvantages

- Advantage: noninvasive; detects presence of pyuria; sensitive and highly specific for detecting greater than 10 white blood cells/ml of urine. Sensitivity 0.75–0.90. When combined with nitrite test, specificity and sensitivity increase to 98% and 100%, respectively for detection of bacteriuria

- Disadvantage: does not identify causative organism. Specificity 0.70. Pyuria indicates presence of inflammation but not necessarily infection

Abnormal
- Leukocyte esterase found in urine
- Keep in mind the possibility of a false-positive result

Cause of abnormal result
White blood cells in urine.

Drugs, disorders and other factors that may alter results
Presence of white blood cells is nonspecific; indicates inflammation but not necessarily infection.

MICROSCOPIC URINALYSIS
Description
Urine sample.

Advantages/Disadvantages
Advantages:
- Reveals presence of bacteria in urine. Confirms diagnosis if greater than 20 organisms per high power field are observed
- Gram stain may help to identify causative organisms
- Pyuria detected by presence of 5–10 wbc/hpf of spun urine. Presence of white blood cell casts suggests pyelonephritis
- Epithelial cells indicate contamination of urine specimen

Disadvantage: does not identify specific organism or determine microbial sensitivity to antibiotics. Presence of white blood cells suggestive, not indicative of infection, sterile pyuria observed with some infections (tuberculosis, *Chlamydia* spp., fungus)

Normal
- Bacteria: 0 to few per high power field (hpf)
- White blood cells: 0–5 per hpf

Abnormal
- Bacteria: Greater than 20 per hpf
- White blood cells: >10–15 per hpf
- Keep in mind the possibility of a false-positive result

Cause of abnormal result
- Presence of bacteria
- Inflammation without infection – associated with pyuria
- Some pathogens – sterile pyuria (tuberculosis, chlamydia, fungus, etc)
- False-positive results may result if improper collection technique used to capture specimen or if improper storage/handling of specimen

Drugs, disorders and other factors that may alter results
- Presence of white blood cells is nonspecific; indicates inflammation but not necessarily infection
- Some infections have been associated with sterile pyuria including: urinary tuberculosis and chlamydial and fungal urinary tract infections
- Specimens must be obtained by using proper clean-catch technique, suprapubic aspiration, or catheterization and must be examined immediately or stored refrigerated until examination

QUANTITATIVE URINE CULTURE
Description
Urine sample.

Advantages/Disadvantages
- Advantage: non-invasive. Statistically differentiates between contamination of urine and infection by quantification (>100,000 bacteria/ml urine). Allows identification and susceptibility testing of microorganisms. Greater than 3 organisms on culture may indicate a contaminated specimen
- Disadvantage: a significant portion of patients with UTI have <100,000 bacteria/ml and may fail to meet statistically significant diagnostic criteria. Some laboratories may not report colony counts less than 10,000 or 100,000/ml

Normal
<100,000 colonies of bacteria/ml urine.

Abnormal
- In symptomatic females: greater than 100 colony-forming units (cfu)/ml
- In symptomatic males: greater than 1000cfu/ml
- In suprapubic catheter specimen: any growth
- In pyelonephritis: greater than 100,000cfu/ml
- In complicated UTI: greater than 10,000cfu/ml
- In pregnancy: greater than 10,000cfu/ml
- In urinary catheter specimen: greater than 100cfu/ml
- Keep in mind the possibility of a false-positive result

Cause of abnormal result
- Presence of bacteria/infection
- Urine sample left at room temperature for prolonged period
- Contamination of urine sample by improper clean-catch technique

TREATMENT

CONSIDER CONSULT
- Repeated infections require referral to urologist if structural or functional abnormalities suspected, particularly obstructive uropathy (stones, prostatism, urinary retention)
- Repeated infections require referral to infectious disease specialist if antibiotic-resistant organisms implicated
- 'Complicated' infections involving an obstruction of urine or a disorder of the nervous system require referral to urologist

IMMEDIATE ACTION
Antibiotic therapy should be initiated based upon signs and symptoms of UTI.

PATIENT AND CAREGIVER ISSUES
Health-seeking behavior
- **Self-medication?** Urinary analgesics, available without a prescription, have no curative value and may mask some symptoms of UTI. Most UTI respond rapidly to appropriate antibiotic therapy
- **Hydration?** Paradoxically, increased diuresis may also promote susceptibility to infection by diluting normal antibacterial properties of the urine. Generally, patients with inadequate hydration and infrequent urination may be at increased risk for UTI
- **Drink cranberry juice to acidify urine?** The fructose content of cranberry juice acts to interfere with adherence mechanisms of some pathogens, thereby preventing infection. However, acidification by cranberry juice does not appear to play a role in preventing infection

MANAGEMENT ISSUES
Goals
- Prevent (or treat) systemic consequences of infection
- Eradicate pathogenic organisms in urine, vaginal, and rectal flora
- Prevent recurrence of infection

Management in special circumstances
COEXISTING DISEASE

Urinary tract obstruction or reflux: if underlying problem is not corrected (may need surgical correction), patients at risk for kidney damage. Infections of this type tend to arise from a wider range of microorganisms and may be comprised of a mixed population of bacteria, therefore, choosing appropriate antibiotic therapy may be more complex. Urine culture is necessary in this clinical setting.

SPECIAL PATIENT GROUPS
Pregnancy
- Avoid tetracyclines and quinolones in pregnancy and breast-feeding women; avoid sulfonamides and nitrofurantoin in near-term pregnant women or breast-feeding women
- When UTI occurs, it is more likely to extend to pyelonephritis. Must be treated promptly to avoid premature delivery, low birth weight, high blood pressure, and toxemia. Consider effects of antimicrobial therapy on fetus

Children
- Avoid the following medications in children: Sulfonamides and nitrofurantoin in infants, tetracyclines in children under age 7, and quinolones in children under age 16
- Children are at greatest risk for kidney damage including kidney scars, poor kidney growth, poor kidney function and high blood pressure, especially if underlying urinary tract abnormality exists

Guidelines available at the National Guidelines Clearinghouse:

- The American Academy of Pediatrics [1]
- Evidence based clinical practice guideline for patients 6 years of age or less with a first time acute urinary tract infection (UTI) [2]

PATIENT SATISFACTION/LIFESTYLE PRIORITIES

- Urinary symptoms of urgency, frequency, and dysuria generally resolve quickly following initiation of antibiotic therapy
- Urinary analgesics or a heating pad may help relieve pain prior to eradication of infection; best to avoid irritants such as coffee, alcohol, or spicy foods until infection clears
- Lifestyle changes may help prevent recurrences

SUMMARY OF THERAPEUTIC OPTIONS
Choices

Antibiotics are essential to eliminate infection; the choice of drug and length of treatment depends upon patient's history and urine tests that identify the causative microorganism.

- Antifolates: Trimethoprim/Sulfamethoxazole – effective against common urinary tract pathogens except *Pseudomonas aeruginosa*. Inexpensive. Appropriate first choice in uncomplicated UTI in communities where documented prevalence of TMP/SMX-resistant organisms is low
- Fluoroquinolones: Levofloxacin, ciprofloxacin and others – indicated for *Pseudomonas* spp. and multidrug resistant Gram-negative infections. Expensive. Appropriate first-line therapy in communities with documented high frequency of organism resistance to TMP/SMX, sulfa allergy
- Cephalosporins: cephalexin – first generation cephalosporin. 20–30% resistance to usual pathogens is found nationally. Probably less effective than other alternatives for short (3-day) course treatment due to rapid clearance from urine. Is not effective in elimination of *E. coli* from vaginal flora
- Penicillins: Amoxicillin/clavulanic acid – an amino-penicillin plus beta-lactamase inhibitor effective against beta-lactam-resistant organisms. Probably less effective than other alternatives for short (3-day) course treatment due to rapid clearance from urine. High frequency of resistance to usual pathogens is found nationally (20–30%)
- Nitrofurantoin – attains high concentration in bladder because it is excreted unchanged into urine. Documented lower cure rate in short (3-day) course treatment than other alternatives. Resistance to usual organisms 15–20% nationally
- Urinary analgesics: Used for dysuria to relieve pain, discomfort and spasms of the bladder
- Phenazopyridine – provides symptomatic relief
- Phenazopyridine and Hyoscamine sulfate – provides symptomatic relief and reduces secondary bladder irritability and spasm
- Alternative therapies: Cranberry juice and uva ursi may be useful for prophylaxis against UTI
- Some basic lifestyle measures may be helpful in preventing UTI

Guidelines

The following guidelines are available at the :

- The Infectious Disease Society of America [5]
- The American Academy of Pediatrics [1]
- Evidence based clinical practice guideline for patients 6 years of age or less with a first time acute urinary tract infection (UTI) [2]
- Urinary tract infection [3]

The American Academy of Family Physicians has produced the following information on urinary tract infection in adults [4]

Clinical pearls

Based on culture sensitivities, use quinolone therapy to treat patients with simple and complex UTI. The first dose effect is rapid and patients are often rendered asymptomatic within 12 hours of taking the medication. Compliance with other medications is a concern. Don't use cephalosporins as a first line of therapy due to their effect on bowel and vaginal flora. Only use cephalosporins when organisms are resistant to all other forms of therapy.

Trimethoprim-sulfamethoxazole is inexpensive and is an appropriate first line choice in communities with low documented resistance in usual pathogenic organisms.

Patients should be warned that phenazopyridine will stain underwear and may stain contact lenses.

Never

- Never prescribe penicillins, cephalosporins or sulfonamides to patients with history of allergic responses due to risk of anaphylaxis
- Never prescribe sulfonamides to pregnant women near-term or newborns, due to risk of kernicterus

FOLLOW UP
Plan for review

Follow-up urinalysis two days following completion of antibiotic therapy to confirm the urinary tract is infection free; sooner if infection fails to respond to treatment or worsens

Information for patient or caregiver

- Don't put off the urge to urinate when you feel the need
- Wipe from front to back to prevent bacteria from the anus entering the urethra
- Cleanse the area prior to sexual intercourse
- Empty the bladder before and after sexual intercourse
- Avoid feminine sprays and scented douches
- Seek medical attention immediately if you develop any of the following symptoms while taking antibiotics: rash, hives, shortness of breath, difficulty breathing
- Continue full course of antibiotic therapy until finished, even if symptoms have cleared
- When using sulfonamides, good hydration is essential to prevent crystallization in the urine
- Any broad spectrum antibiotic may precipitate a vaginal yeast infection – eating yogurt may help
- Patients who are taking oral contraceptives should be reminded that birth control pills may be less effective during the cycle they are taking antibiotics

DRUGS AND OTHER THERAPIES: DETAILS
Drugs
TRIMETHOPRIM/SULFAMETHOXAZOLE
Dose

- 160/800mg bid for 3 days – acute uncomplicated UTI
- 160/800mg bid for 10–14 days – complicated UTI
- 40/200 or 80/400mg hs or three times weekly for prophylaxis

Efficacy
Symptoms usually resolve within 1–2 days.

Risks/Benefits

- Use caution in the elderly
- Use caution in renal and hepatic impairment
- Use caution in alcoholism, malnutrition, G6PD deficiency

Side-effects and adverse reactions

- CNS: headache, insomnia, anxiety, depression
- Gastrointestinal: nausea, vomiting, abdominal pain, hepatitis, pseudomembranous colititis
- Renal: nephrosis, renal failure
- Skin: Stevens-Johnson syndrome, rashes
- Hematologic: agranulocytosis

Interactions (other drugs)

- Dapsone ▪ Procainamide ▪ Disulfiram ▪ Methotrexate ▪ Metronidazole ▪ Phenytoin ▪ Warfarin ▪ Oral anticoagulants ▪ Hypoglycemic agents

Contraindications

- Pregnancy ▪ Age less than 2 months ▪ Folate deficiency

Evidence

Trimethoprim-sulfamethoxazole should be considered the current standard therapy for uncomplicated acute bacterial cystitis in non-pregnant women [5] *Level C*

Acceptability to patient

High.

Follow up plan

- Repeat urinalysis 2 days after completion of antibiotic therapy to confirm elimination of bacteria from urinary tract.
- If using for prophylaxis, obtain complete blood counts periodically and discontinue therapy if any reduction in counts is observed.

Patient and caregiver information

- Complete full course of therapy unless directed otherwise by primary care physician
- Drink 6–8 glasses of water daily
- Avoid prolonged exposure to sunlight; photosensitivity may occur
- Notify primary care physician if: blood in urine, rash, ringing in ears, difficulty breathing, fever, sore throat or chills

CIPROFLOXACIN

Dose

- 100–250mg bid for 3 days for uncomplicated UTI
- 250–500mg bid for 10–14 days for complicated UTI
- 250mg qd for prophylaxis

Efficacy

Effective for multidrug resistant Gram-negative bacteria and for most *Pseudomonas* spp.

Risks/Benefits

- Not suitable for children or growing adolescents
- Caution in adolescents, pregnancy, epilepsy, glucose-6-phosphate dehydrogenase deficiency

Side-effects and adverse reactions

- CNS: anxiety, depression, dizziness, headache, seizures
- EENT: visual disturbances
- Gastrointestinal: abdominal pain, altered liver function, anorexia, diarrhoea, heartburn, pseudomembraneous colitis, vomiting
- Genitourinary: monoliasis, vaginitis
- Skin: photosensitivity, pruritis, rash

Interactions (other drugs)
- Theophylline ■ Cyclosporin ■ Oral anticoagulants ■ NSAIDs ■ Opiates ■ Beta-blockers
- Phenytoin ■ Antacids ■ Diazepam ■ Caffeine ■ Iron ■ Didanosine

Contraindications
Use is not recommended in children because arthropathy has developed in weight-bearing joints in young animals.

Acceptability to patient
High, except for expense.

Follow up plan
- Repeat urinalysis 2 days after completion of antibiotic therapy to confirm elimination of bacteria from urinary tract
- If used for prophylaxis, periodic evaluations of renal, hepatic, and hematopoietic functions should be conducted

Patient and caregiver information
- Drink fluids liberally
- Do not take any antacids containing magnesium or aluminum or products containing iron or zinc simultaneously, 4 hours prior, or 2 hours following ciprofloxacin
- May cause dizziness; use caution if performing tasks requiring mental alertness
- Discontinue at first sign of rash or other allergic reaction
- Avoid excessive sunlight/artificial ultraviolet light; discontinue if phototoxicity occurs

CEPHALEXIN
Dose
- 250–500mg q6h for 10–14 days for treatment of UTI. Not indicated for short (3-day) treatment course
- 250mg hs for prophylaxis

Efficacy
Effective against susceptible Gram-positive and Gram-negative organisms. Does not eliminate pathogenic E. *coli* from vaginal flora.

Risks/Benefits
Caution in patients with penicillin hypersensitivity.

Side-effects and adverse reactions
- Gastrointestinal: anorexia, nausea, diarrhea, abdominal pain
- CNS: headache, sleep disturbance, confusion, dizziness
- Hematologic: pancytopenia,
- Skin: rashes, erythema multiforme
- Anaphylaxis

Interactions (other drugs)
Warfarin

Contraindications
Cephalosporin hypersensitivity.

Acceptability to patient
High.

Follow up plan
Repeat urinalysis 2 days after completion of antibiotic therapy to confirm elimination of bacteria from urinary tract.

Patient and caregiver information
- Complete full course of therapy unless directed otherwise by primary care physician
- Take with food or milk if stomach upset occurs
- A false-positive reaction for urinary glucose may occur with non-specific urine tests

AMOXICILLIN/CLAVULANIC ACID
Dose
500mg q12 h or 250mg q8h for 10 days for treatment of UTI.

Efficacy
Eliminates beta-lactam resistant bacteria.

Risks/Benefits
- Use caution if history of hypersensitivity to cephalosporins
- Use caution in renal failure
- Aviod use in mononucleosis

Side-effects and adverse reactions
- CNS: headache, nausea
- Gastrointestinal:diarrhea, abdominal pain, psuedomembranous colitis
- EENT: black tongue, oral thrush
- Hematologic: bone marrow suppression
- Respiratory: anaphylaxis
- Skin: allergic rashes, erythema multiforme

Interactions (other drugs)
- Atenolol ■ Chloramphenicol ■ Macrolide antibiotics ■ Methotrexate ■ Tetracyclines
- Oral contraceptives

Contraindications
Penicillin hypersensitivity

Acceptability to patient
High.

Patient and caregiver information
- Complete full course of therapy unless directed otherwise by primary care physician
- Notify primary care physician if skin rash, hives, severe diarrhea, shortness of breath, wheezing, black tongue, sore throat, nausea, vomiting, fever, swollen joints, or any unusual bleeding or bruising occur

NITROFURANTOIN
Dose
- 50–100mg q6h (100 mg bid sustained release) for 3 days in acute uncomplicated infection
- 50–100mg q day for UTI prophylaxis

Efficacy
- Bacteriostatic at low concentrations and bactericidal at higher concentrations
- May not be as effective in short (3-day) course treatment as other alternatives

Risks/Benefits
Caution needed in:

- Glucose-6-phosphate dehydrogenase deficiency
- Renal impairment
- Electrolyte disturbances
- Anemia
- Diabetes mellitus
- Vitamin B dificiency

Side-effects and adverse reactions

- Gastrointestinal: abdominal pain, anorexia, nausea and vomiting, hepatic necrosis and hepatitis, pancreatitis
- Genitourinary: urinary superinfection
- Pulmonary hypersensitivity reactions
- Hematologic: blood dyscrasias
- Skin: erythema multiforme, exfoliative dermatitis, pruritus, transient alopecia
- Musculoskeletal: arthralgia, myalgia
- CNS: confusion, mood changes, dizziness, drowsiness, headache, nystagmus, peripheral neuropathy, psychotic reaction

Interactions (other drugs)

- Anticholinergics delay gastric emptying and increase nitrofurantoin absorption and bioavailability Magnesium-containing antacids decrease nitrofurantoin efficacy by interfering with absorption Probenecid decreases nitrofurantoin clearance and increases nitrofurantoin toxicity

Contraindications

- Hypersensitivity to nitrofurantoin Renal insufficiency (creatinine clearance less than 60ml/min), anuria, or oliguria

Acceptability to patient
High.

Follow up plan
Repeat urinalysis 2 days after completion of antibiotic therapy to confirm elimination of bacteria from urinary tract.

Patient and caregiver information

- Complete full course of therapy unless notified otherwise by primary care physician
- Take with food or milk to reduce gastrointestinal upset
- May cause brown discoloration of urine
- Notify primary care physician if fever, chills, cough, chest pain, difficult breathing, skin rash, numbness or tingling of fingers or toes, or intolerable gastrointestinal upset occur

FOSFOMYCIN
Dose
3g sachet taken as single dose.

Efficacy
77–94% in uncomplicated UTI.

Risks/Benefits
Useful for patients who are unlikely to comply with a longer course of antibiotics.

Side-effects and adverse reactions
- CNS: dizziness, headache
- EENT: pharyngitis, rhinitis
- Gastrointestinal: abdominal pain, diarrhea, indigestion, nausa
- Genitourinary: dysmenorrhea, vaginitis
- Hematologic: aplastic anemia
- Musculoskeletal: back pain
- Skin: rash

Interactions (other drugs)
Metoclopramide.

Contraindications
No absolute contraindications.

PHENAZOPYRIDINE
Dose
200mg tid for 2 days or prn for relief of symptoms.

Efficacy
Relieves pain, burning, urgency, frequency, and other discomforts from irritation of the bladder before antibiotic therapy begins to eradicate infection.

Risks/Benefits
- Caution needed in long term use
- Not suitable for children aged under 12 years

Side-effects and adverse reactions
- Skin: yellow tinryge of skin or sclera in patients with renal insufficiency
- Gastrointestinal: hepatitis
- Genitourinary: acute renal failure (transient), orange discoloration of urine
- Hematologic: hemolytic anemia, methemoglobinemia
- Anaphylactoid reaction
- Interactions – none recorded

Contraindications
Renal impairment.

Acceptability to patient
High.

Patient and caregiver information
- This medication will treat symptoms of infection, but not eliminate infection
- May cause bright orange discoloration of urine
- A full course of antibiotic therapy needs to be completed even after symptomatic relief is provided
- Drug should be taken for only 2 days; there is no evidence that this agent is more beneficial than antibiotics alone following 2 days of therapy
- Therapy should be discontinued and primary care physician notified if skin or sclera acquire yellowish color
- May stain contact lenses
- May permanently stain underwear

Complementary therapy
HERBAL THERAPIES – UVA URSI
Uva ursi (bearberry) leaves, consisting of the dried leaves of *Arctostaphylos uva ursi* and pharmaceutical preparations thereof.

Efficacy
Active ingredient is arbutin; especially useful in preventing recurrent UTIs.

Risks/Benefits
Risk: excessive dose (15g of dried herb) can result in tinnitus, nausea, vomiting, shortness of breath, convulsions, and delirium in susceptible individuals.

Acceptability to patient
Usually fine.

Follow up plan
Usual care – urinalysis/cultures as indicated.

Patient and caregiver information
- Use dried leaves as a tea: 1.5–4.0g (1–2 tsp) three times daily
- Can use tincture (1:5 dilution) 4–6mL (1–1.5 tsp) three times daily
- Powdered solid extract (250–500mg capsules, standardized to 10% arbutin) three times daily

CRANBERRY JUICE
Efficacy
300mL cranberry juice in women with confirmed bacteriuria reduces the level of bacteria and frequency of UTI recurrence. Works best for *Escherichia coli* infection.

Evidence
- A systematic review found no good quality evidence that cranberry juice is effective for the treatment of urinary tract infection [6] *Level M*
- Another systematic review found no conclusive evidence that cranberry juice is effective in the prevention of urinary tract infections [7] *Level M*

Acceptability to patient
Good.

Follow up plan
Follow-up urinalysis as appropriate.

LIFESTYLE
- Wiping. Because of the proximity of the urethra opening to the anus in females, it is important to wipe in the direction of front to back
- Bubble baths. If the patient has a UTI or is prone to getting UTI, they should be advised to take showers rather than baths
- Hot tubs. Hot tubs use may predispose some women to UTIs

EFFICACY OF THERAPIES

Once appropriate antibiotic therapy has been initiated, uncomplicated infections resolve in 1–2 days.

Evidence

PDxMD are unable to cite evidence which meets our criteria for evidence.

Review period

1–2 weeks

PROGNOSIS

Complications of a simple lower tract infection are rare and typically involve resistant microorganisms or may indicate undiagnosed structural abnormalities or anormal urodynamics.

Clinical pearls

Always collect urine for culture first, then have the patient start antibiotic therapy. The culture results can then be reviewed and therapy modified. If the culture results come back as "no growth", the patient should be referred to a urologist for further evaluation. If the patient has multiple infections, referral to a urologist is indicated.

Therapeutic failure

Relapse of symptoms after a 3-day course of antibiotics suggests upper tract involvement and requires 10–14 days of therapy. 30% of clinical lower tract infections have upper tract involvement.

■ Cephalosporins are useful for UTIs that fail to respond to other antibiotics. Cephalexin, cephradine, cefaclor, and cefadroxil may be used and are safe in pregnancy and lactation. Hypersensitivity is main adverse effect

■ Fluoroquinolones should be used in resistant cases, in patients who cannot tolerate other agents, in nosocomial infections, and in complicated UTIs. They should be avoided in pregnancy, lactation, and children due to risk of arthropathy. Quinolones may interfere with plasma concentrations of theophylline and warfarin

■ Tetracyclines are useful primarily for treating infections caused by *Chlamydia*; resistance develops rapidly thus their usefulness is limited. Always avoid in pregnancy and in children under age 7

Recurrence

Recurrent infections not caused by a structural or functional abnormality may be treated prophylactically with preventative antibiotics

The following antibiotic dosing schedules have been used as prophylaxis against UTI recurrence. There is evidence for antibiotic prophylaxis for recurrent cystitis in non-pregnant women (see BMJ Clinical Evidence Online)

- Trimethoprim/Sulfamethoxazole 40/200 mg or 80/400 mg hs
- Cephalexin 250 mg hs
- Ciprofloxacin 250 mg qd
- Nitrofurantoin 50–100 mg hs

When a patient has a persistent infection that does not resolve after appropriate therapy or suffers from recurrent infections, referral may be necessary for further tests to identify structural or functional abnormalities.

Deterioration

Unfavorable prognoses are associated with the following factors: old age, general debility, renal calculi or obstruction, recent hospitalization, urinary tract instrumentation, diabetes mellitus, chronic nephropathy, sickle cell anemia, cancer, chemotherapy, immunosuppression, incontinence, urinary retention.

- Intravenous antibiotic therapy directed against coliform Gram-negative bacteria
- Trimethoprim/Sulfamethoxazole administered intravenously
- Ceftriaxone – a third generation cephalosporin administered intravenously
- Tobramycin – an aminoglycoside antibiotic administered intravenously
- Ampicillin – add a penicillin if urine gram stain reveals presence of gram-positive cocci; administer intravenously
- Adequate fluid resuscitation to restore urinary volumes
- Antipyretic medications to reduce fever
- Imaging studies by referral to urologist

Terminal illness

All patients presenting with UTI who have impaired host defense mechanisms due to HIV, chemotherapy, cancer, or renal failure should be admitted to hospital

COMPLICATIONS

Complications are rare but may include:
- Acute papillary necrosis with potential ureteral obstruction
- Sepsis
- Perinephric abscess

PREVENTION

Some life-style modifications pertaining to diet, sexual activities, and voiding practices may be helpful to prevent UTI

RISK FACTORS

- **Sexual behavior**: UTI are most common in sexually active women, particularly with use of spermicides and diaphragms.
- **Environmental risks**: use of bubble baths or hot tubs may predispose some women to UTI.

MODIFY RISK FACTORS

Changes in diet, sexual practices, and voiding habits may help to protect against UTI.

Lifestyle and wellness

All people should be made aware of the following:
- Bladder should be completely emptied when voiding
- Do not put off the urge to urinate, particularly after intercourse

Women:
- Wipe from front to back

DIET
- Drinking 6–8 glasses of water daily help to prevent UTI
- Cranberry juice may help to prevent UTI

SEXUAL BEHAVIOR
- Urinating before and after sexual intercourse may help to prevent UTI
- Limiting the number of sexual partners may help to prevent UTI

FAMILY HISTORY
If family history of UTI, a genetic predisposition for bacteria adherence to bladder may be present. Awareness of and adherence to lifestyle and wellness issues, sexual behavioral practices, and dietary considerations may offer protection from UTI

SCREENING

Routine urinalysis should only be performed in pregnant women and treatment should be initiated in all pregnant women with bacteriuria, even if asymptomatic.

Guidelines

United States Preventive Services Task Force. Screening for asymptomatic bacteriuria [8]

PREVENT RECURRENCE

Advise patients:

- Drink 6–8 glasses of water per day so that bladder is emptied often
- Don't hold urine once bladder feels full
- Empty bladder completely each time urine is passed
- Urinate before and after sexual intercourse
- Wipe from front to back so bacteria are not transported from anus to urethra
- Change sanitary napkins frequently
- Drink cranberry juice
- Wear cotton underwear and avoid tight-fitting pants
- Use prophylactic antibiotics (see BMJ Clinical Evidence online)

Reassess coexisting disease

Self-catheterization or mechanical instrumentation – may introduce bacteria into urinary tract.

INTERACTION ALERT

Anticholinerigc medications may leave residual urine in bladder, predisposing to UTI.

PATIENT SATISFACTION/LIFESTYLE PRIORITIES

- Assist or instruct patient on self-catheterization technique
- Discontinue anticholinergic therapy if possible; may not be an option in management of a coexisting disease

RESOURCES

ASSOCIATIONS
The American Urological Association
1120 N. Charles Street, Baltimore, MD 21201–5559
Phone: 410-727-1100
Fax: 410.223.4374
http://www.amuro.org

KEY REFERENCES
http://www.stjames.ie/nmic/lowerurinerytract/lut.html

http://www.emedicine.com/emerg/topic626.htm

http://healthlink.mcw.edu/article/943046204.html

http://www.kidney.ca/uri-e.htm

http://www.merck.com/pubs/mmanual/section17/chapter227/227a.htm

Stapleton A. Host factors in susceptibility to urinary tract infections. Advances in Experimental Medicine and Biology 462: 351–8, 1999

Applied Therapeutics: The Clinical use of Drugs. Koda-Kimble MA and Young LY (Eds.), Applied Therapeutics, Vancouver, WA, 1992

Pharmacotherapy: A Pathophysiologic Approach. Dipiro JT, Talbert RL, Yee GC, Matzke GR, Wells BG and Posey Lm (Eds.), Appleton & Lange, Stamford, CT, 1999.

Drug Facts and Comparisons. Riley MR and Kastrup EK (Eds.), A Wolters Kluwer Company, St. Louis MO, 2000

Evidence references and guidelines
1 The American Academy of Pediatrics. The diagnosis, treatment, and evaluation of the initial urinary tract infection in febrile infants and young children. Pediatrics 1999;103:843–52.
2 Evidence based clinical practice guideline for patients 6 years of age or less with a first time acute urinary tract infection (UTI). Cincinnati (OH): Children's Hospital Medical Center (CHMC); 1999.
3 Urinary tract infection. Ann Arbor (MI): University of Michigan Health System; 1999.
4 Orenstein R, Wong ES. Urinary tract infection in adults. American Family Physician 1999;59:1225–34,1237.
5 The Infectious Disease Society of America. Guidelines for antimicrobial treatment of uncomplicated acute bacterial cystitis and acute pyelonephritis in women. Clin Infect Dis 1999;29:745–58.
6 Jepson RG, Mihaljevic L, Craig J. Cranberries for treating urinary tract infections (Cochrane Review). In: The Cochrane Library, 1, 2002. Oxford: Update Software.
7 Jepson RG, Mihaljevic L, Craig J. Cranberries for preventing urinary tracy infections (Cochrane Review). In: The Cochrane Library, 1, 2002. Oxford: Update Software.
8 United States Preventive Services Task Force. Screening for asymptomatic bacteria. Guide to clinical preventive services 2nd edn Baltimore (MD): Williams and Wilkins. 1996.

FAQS
Question 1
What is the pathogenesis of UTIs in women?

ANSWER 1
Most UTIs in women represent ascending infections. Colonization of the perineum by bacteria from the fecal reservoir accesss the bladder through the urethra. The length of the female urethra is believed to be a factor here as well.

Question 2
How is recurrent uncomplicated cystitis treated?

ANSWER 2
Four options for therapy are generally recognized:
- If infections in an otherwise normal female occur after sexual intercourse, then one can take antibiotic (sulfa or low dose quinolone) either before or immediately after intimate sexual activity
- If infections occur after each menstrual cycle, sulfa or low dose quinolone can be used at the end of each cycle. I also review behavioral techniques to reduce autoinfection
- If a woman has recurrent UTIs (3–4 per year) and has been thoroughly evaluated, I will give her a refillable prescription for either a sulfa or low dose quinolone to start and take for 3 days at the first sign of a UTI. I also give them multiple prescriptions (undated) for Urine c+s so that when they suspect the UTI and can do a clean catch for c+s, they do it and then start the antibiotic. This allows me to document that their symptoms are in fact caused by infection and do not represent increased bladder irritability or other pathology
- Long term prophylaxis is used in women with recurrent UTIs. Low dose sulfa or nitrofurantoin taken at bedtime reduces perineal colonization and urethral seeding by bacteria. I always get a CBC on a 6 month basis with patients on long term sulfa therapy

Question 3
Do you treat UTIs occurring in pregnancy?

ANSWER 3
Yes. Symptomatic infection and asymptomatic infections during pregnancy require antibiotic therapy in order to reduce complications of cystitis like pyelonephritis and its' sequelae as well as reducing the risk of premature delivery.

Question 4
What are the most common organisms in a UTI?

ANSWER 4
Of the bacteria, *E. coli* (80%), *Staphylococcus saprophyticus* (10%), while Enterobacteriaceae account for the remainder.

Question 5
What is the occurrence rate for women?

ANSWER 5
1% of women experience UTI before they become sexually active. With sexual activity the rate rises to approximately 5%. After 65 years roughly 33% of women will experience UTI.

CONTRIBUTORS
Russell C Jones, MD, MPH
Jane L Murray, MD
Philip J Aliotta, MD, MHA, FACS

VARICOCELE

DESCRIPTION

- An abnormal dilation of the spermatic venous or pampiniform plexus of the testicle
- Presents as a scrotal mass that feels like a bag of worms
- It is usually painless
- Usually needs no intervention

URGENT ACTION

None needed.

KEY! DON'T MISS!

Examine for varicoceles as part of the initial male infertility consultation.

BACKGROUND

ICD9 CODE
456.4 Varicocele, (scrotum)

SYNONYMS
Varicocele

CARDINAL FEATURES
- Usually asymptomatic
- Presents as a painless mass in the scrotum that feels like a bag of worms
- When supine there is less distention of the mass than on standing
- When the patient performs the Valsalva maneuver, the distention increases
- Usually unilateral and involving the left testicle but can be right sided only or bilateral
- Commonly found as an incidental finding as part of infertility investigations
- Most clinically insignificant varicoceles require no treatment

CAUSES
Common causes
- Varicoceles are dilated tortuous veins of the pampiniform plexus and the internal spermatic vein around the testicle
- 90% are on the left because of the anatomy of the left spermatic vein and the increased likelihood of valvular incompetence. The cremasteric and deferential veins are rarely involved

Rare causes
Rarely, an obstruction of the venous drainage because of retroperitoneal mass, e.g. renal tumors or renal vein thrombosis can cause varicoceles.

EPIDEMIOLOGY
Incidence and prevalence
- Varicocele is common
- 150 per 1000 adult males
- 400 per 1000 males with decreased fertility

INCIDENCE
Increases with age until adulthood.

PREVALENCE
Varies with age:
- 8 per 1000 boys age 2–6 years
- 10 per 1000 boys age 7–10 years
- 78 per 1000 boys age 11–14 years
- 150 per 1000 boys over 15 years

Demographics
AGE
Varicocele is much more common at adolescence and into adulthood. Bilateral involvement is very unusual below 11 years of age. After the age of 11, 100 in 1000 cases may be bilateral.

GENDER
Varicocele solely affects males.

DIAGNOSIS

DIFFERENTIAL DIAGNOSIS

Hydrocele
FEATURES
- Transilluminates and is more homogenous than a varicocele
- Usually differentiated by ultrasound

Hernia
FEATURES
- Wide neck
- Connects with inguinal or femoral ring
- Usually reducible
- Intestinal contents can sometimes be palpated

Hematocele
FEATURES
- Has a history of trauma
- Tender on palpation
- Transilluminates poorly if at all

Testicular Torsion
FEATURES
- Sudden onset
- Severe pain
- Pain changes according to position
- Tenderness and redness of the scrotum

Cystic lymphangioma
FEATURES
- Rare
- Ultrasound will differentiate

SIGNS & SYMPTOMS

Signs
- Large varicoceles may be found by external inspection
- Moderate varicoceles can be felt as a bag of worms by palpation without asking the patient to bear down
- Small varicoceles can only be felt on palpation when the patient bears down or uses the Valsalva maneuver
- In young children, a testis lying horizontal may indicate an underlying varicocele or suggest a predisposition toward torsion

Symptoms
- The majority of varicoceles are asymptomatic
- There is an association with male infertility and most are diagnosed during fertility investigations
- Pain or a dragging heavy feeling in the scrotum may be noticed by the patient

ASSOCIATED DISORDERS

- The association between varicocele and male infertility is a subject of continuing controversy. In 1000 men with fertility problems, 400 will have a varicocele. The precise mechanism for the harmful effect of varicocele on sperm quality or quantity is not known. Theories implicating increased pressure, temperature, oxygen deprivation, and decreased antioxidants have all been put forward
- There is some evidence that clinically palpable varicocele is associated with testicular atrophy, low sperm count, and poor sperm motility. Some of these parameters improve after surgery to the varicocele
- The scientific evidence to support increased fertility as measured by successful pregnancies after varicocelectomy is poor. However, the largest randomized trial showed 31.3% pregnancies in those with treated varicoceles compared to 14.4% in those not treated at 1 year. These results are statistically significant
- There appears to be no evidence in terms of improving fertility to treat subclinical varicoceles

KEY! DON'T MISS!

Examine for varicoceles as part of the initial male infertility consultation.

CONSIDER CONSULT

- If associated with unexplained male infertility
- In the presence of testicular pain or significant discomfort
- Testicular atrophy i.e., more than 20% loss in size compared to the other testicle
- Diagnosis of testicular mass uncertain

INVESTIGATION OF THE PATIENT

Direct questions to patient

Q Is the mass painful? In most patients the condition is asymptomatic. However, a small percentage of patients may experience chronic discomfort or a dull ache in the affected testicle.

Q Are there particular positions that make the mass more noticeable? In the supine position, the varicocele is often missed. The presence of an atrophic testicle may suggest either a previous testicular torsion or a varicocele. A varicocele is usually easily detected in the standing position.

Q Is there a history of infertility? In 30–50% of men with infertility, a varicocele will be detected.

Examination

- Is there a palpable or visible testicular mass that feels like a bag of worms? This classical physical finding is usually conclusive in the diagnosis of varicocele. Scrotal ultrasound performed with cough and Valsalva maneuver will resolve any uncertainty
- Is the mass painless? Normally, the mass is painless to palpation. However, the patient may complain of a dull ache or pressure sensation, especially if they are on their feet for prolonged periods of time
- Is it bilateral or unilateral? Normally, a varicocele will be present on the left side alone. However, the physician should always carefully examine the contralateral side for the presence of a varicocele
- Does it increase in size on standing and on executing the Valsalva maneuver? Varicocele will normally increase in size in the supine position. When performing a Valsalva maneuver, even in the smallest or subclinical or grade 1 varicoceles, an impulse can be felt in the pampiniform plexus. The physical examination should be performed in both the recumbent and upright position
- Is there significant testicular atrophy? In almost all patients with a significant varicocele, significant testicular atrophy will be present

Summary of investigative tests

- Ultrasound, preferably color flow Doppler, with Valsalva and cough maneuvers can confirm diagnosis if it is in doubt. This will also confirm the extent of the varicocele
- If presenting as part of a fertility problem, semen analysis is needed. Anywhere from two to three semen samples should be examined for adequacy
- Other fertility investigations are normally performed by a specialist and may include hormone assays
- If the varicocele is of sudden onset, right sided and unilateral or unchanged in the supine position, a retroperitoneal cause should be excluded. This will involve investigation by ultrasound or CT scanning, which would be performed by a specialist. If the varicocele does not collapse in the supine position, it is no longer a benign varicocele. To exclude the presence of a renal or retroperitoneal tumor, an abdominal CT scan is advised

DIAGNOSTIC DECISION

Diagnosis of clinical varicocele is usually easy. The cardinal sign is a scrotal mass that feels like a bag of worms. No further diagnostic investigation is usually needed. If the varicocele does not collapse in the recumbent position, it needs to be evaluated further as described above. If testicular atrophy is present, a baseline set of semen analyses is advised.

In the evaluation of the infertile male with a varicocele, an FSH level is requested.

An elevated FSH is an indication of testicular insult and compromise.

Ancillary diagnostic tests for varicocele are:
- Doppler stethoscope
- Scrotal ultrasound
- Spermatic venography
- Scrotal thermography
- Radionuclide scanning of the scrotum

A Scrotal Doppler performed at a noninvasive vascular laboratory is a sensitive test of venous incompetence. It should be performed (as should an ultrasound of the scrotum) with cough and Valsalva maneuvers.

Varicoceles are graded in severity from 0 (not present) to 4+ (marked venous incompetence). Subclinical varicoceles (detected only through various technologies) are repaired only when there are abnormal semen analyses, infertility (unsuccessful attempt at pregnancy over an 18 month interval of unprotected sexual intercourse), testicular atrophy on the affected side, and complaints of orchialgia on the affected side.

Adolescent varicoceles are repaired when there is atrophy of the affected testis and pain.

THE TESTS
Body fluids
SEMEN ANALYSIS
Description
Semen for fertility analysis X 2–3. To include a report on motility, the count, and morphology. This is indicated only if the patient presents with fertility problems associated with a varicocele, or if testicular atrophy is present.

Advantages/Disadvantages
- Advantage: this is a cheap and easy test for the primary care physician to organize
- Disadvantage: the specimen needs to be fresh so requires easy access to a laboratory

Normal
- Sperm counts that are preoperatively greater than 40 million per milliliter do not significantly improve after varicocelectomy
- If patients have normal sperm motility preoperatively, 60% are likely to achieve a pregnancy post varicocelectomy

Abnormal
- Sperm counts between 10–40 million per milliliter significantly improve with varicocelectomy
- Sperm counts of less than 10 million per milliliter do not significantly improve post surgery
- Patients with sperm motility of less than 60% preoperatively have a 30% chance of achieving a pregnancy post surgery
- If sperm morphology is abnormal, there is no good evidence that varicocele surgery will improve this parameter
- Keep in mind the possibility of a falsely abnormal result

Cause of abnormal result
The association between varicocele and subfertility is a subject of continuing controversy.

Drugs, disorders and other factors that may alter results
- Alcohol
- Tobacco

Imaging
COLOR FLOW DOPPLER
Advantages/Disadvantages
- Advantage: painless
- Disadvantage: not universally available

Normal
Normal blood flow to normal testis.

Abnormal
Abnormal blood flow to testis:
- In varicocele a homogenous echo pattern with diminished blood flow to the sac contents is seen
- In epididymitis the increased blood flow is readily seen on color Doppler ultrasound
- The torsed testicle shows a non-homogenous echo pattern with diminished blood flow
- In malignancy increased blood flow with a non-homogenous echo pattern is suspicious
- Keep in mind the possibility of a falsely abnormal result

Cause of abnormal result
- Varicocele
- Epididymitis
- Torsion
- Malignancy

TREATMENT

CONSIDER CONSULT
- If the diagnosis is uncertain
- If there is azoospermia and the couple is interested in assisted reproductive technologies i.e., Intracytoplasmic Sperm Insertion (ICSI)

PATIENT AND CAREGIVER ISSUES
Patient or caregiver request
- **Will my fertility be affected?** Some varicoceles do not affect fertility
- **Do varicoceles cause cancer?** Varicoceles are not associated with testicular cancer
- **Do I have to have surgery?** Not all varicoceles need surgery

MANAGEMENT ISSUES
Goals
- To diagnose and reassure the patient
- To alleviate testicular discomfort if present
- To check for an association with infertility

SUMMARY OF THERAPEUTIC OPTIONS
Choices
- First choice is no specific treatment, unless there is progressive testicular atrophy, pain, an increase in the size of the varicocele, or a lack of decompression in the supine position, and infertility
- Second choice is open repair of the varicocele. Repair is either transinguinal (through the groin), retroperitoneal (through the abdomen), or infrainguinal, performed by a specialist
- Third choice is varicocele repair through a laparoscope, sclerotherapy, or percutaneous embolization. Performed by a specialist

Treatment of a varicocele in a subfertile and infertile male is to be considered when:
- The female partner has a normal fertility by evaluation and/or history
- The varicocele is palpable on physical examination
- The male has abnormal semen parameters
- Males with varicocele and normal semen parameters but abnormal sperm function testing, i.e. abnormal sperm penetration assay, etc.
- An adult male not presently trying to achieve a pregnancy with abnormal semen parameters, a palpable varicocele, and a desire for future children
- Reduced testicular size on the affected side. This is the main criterion for varicocele repair in the adolescent male
- Subclinical varicocele with non-obstructive azoospermia (reversible in 43–55% of men with hypospermatogenesis or maturation arrest on biopsy

Varicocele therapy is not indicated when:

- Semen parameters are normal
- Subclinical varicocele is present
- There are female factors that require the utilization of IVF/intracytoplasmic sperm injection methodology

In young men with varicoceles and normal semen parameters, follow them with annual semen analyses, sexual and fertility history (i.e. is the male and his female partner using contraceptive methods) and physical assessment of the testes and cords. If there is a change in the size of the testis and cord, abnormal seminal parameters, or if there is an absence of pregnancy not using a form of prescribed contraception, further evaluation is required.

Never
There is no evidence to perform surgery on men without palpable varicoceles.

FOLLOW UP
Plan for review
- Plan to see the patient 7–10 days post surgery for wound review
- A semen analysis is needed 4 months post surgery

Information for patient or caregiver
- A varicocelectomy is a minor operation and requires anywhere from 1 to 7 days off work
- There might be some discomfort or bruising post operatively
- No change to the sperm analysis is expected for the first 3–4 months
- There is a 12–15% chance of a recurrence

EFFICACY OF THERAPIES

The beneficial effects of surgery on sperm parameters are better proven than are the effects on male fertility and pregnancy as a positive outcome.

Evidence

- The outcomes from varicocele repair on fertility are at best, inconclusive. The studies that have been performed lack adequacy in patient number, randomization, and controls. There is no consensus of research opinion to show an absolute improvement in fertility after varicocele repair. Most studies do, however, show that there is an improvement in fertility after varicocele therapy.
- Schlegel's review of twelve controlled studies on the fertility effect of varicocelectomy showed a pregnancy rate after varicocele repair of 33% compared to 16% in males without varicocele repair.
- Studies have shown that while no increase in fertility was noted in men who underwent varicocelectomy, there was an improvement in testis volume and seminal parameters.
- However, another study showed that the conception rate in otherwise normal couples, where the male underwent varicocelectomy, was 60% within one year following surgery as compared to only 10% in the untreated control group.

PROGNOSIS
Clinical pearls

- Follow varicocelectomy patients with semen analyses every 3 months for the first year or until pregnancy is achieved
- If recurrence of the varicocele occurs, utilize internal spermatic venography to identify the incompetent recurrent or persistent vessels
- For men with persistently abnormal seminal parameters after varicocelectomy, it is recommend that the couple go to intrauterine insemination and other artificial reproductive technologies

Recurrence

Varicocelectomy can be performed again in cases of recurrence. In these cases the retroperitoneal or subinguinal approach is preferred because of the scar tissue from previous surgery. Percutaneous embolization can also be offered.

PREVENTION

Varicocele is not specifically preventable in the general population.

KEY REFERENCES

- Nagler HM, Luntz RK, Martinis FG. Varicocele in Infertility in the Male. Lipshultz LI, Howards SS, editors. St Louis: Mosby Yearbook; 1997:336–359.
- Akbay E, Cayan S, Doruk E et al. The Prevalence of Varicocele and Varicocele-related testicular atrophy in Turkish children and adolescents. BJU Int 2000 Sep;86(4):490–493.
- Grasso M, Lania C, Castelli M et al. Low-grade left Varicocele in patients over 30 years old: the effect of spermatic vein ligation on fertility. BJU Int 2000 Feb; 85(3):305–7.
- Bouchot O, Prunet D, Gaschignard N et al. Surgery of Varicocele; results concerning sperm motility and morphology. Prog Urol 1999 Sep;9(4);703–6.
- Hargreave T.B. WHO Task force on the prevention; management of infertility. The World Health Organization varicocele trial; 160. British journal of Urology 1996;77(1):39.
- Vandekerckhove P, Lilford R, Evers J. Surgery or Embolisation for varicocele in subfertile men. The Cochrane Database of Systematic reviews-Protocol Only.
- Marsman JWP, Schats R. The Subclinical Varicocele Debate. NHS Center for Reviews and Dissemination. Jan 2000;1.
- Hurwitz RS, Shapiro E, Hulbert WC et al. Scrotal Cystic Lymphangioma: The Misdiagnosed Scrotal Mass. Journal of Urology 1997;158(3):1182–1185.
- Coveney EC, Fitzgerald RJ. Varicocele and the Horizontal Testis: a change in position? J Pediatric Surg 1994;29(3):452–3.
- Yamamoto M, Hibi H, Hirata Y et al. Effect of varicocelectomy on sperm parameters and pregnancy rate in patients with subclinical varicocele: A Randomised Prospective Controlled Study. Journal of Urology 1996;155(5):1636–1638.
- Peterson AC, Lance RS, Ruiz HE. Outcomes of Varicocele Ligation Done for Pain. Journal of Urology 1998;159(5):15565–1567.
- Hendin BN, Kolettis PN, Sharma RK et al. Varicocele is Associated with elevated Spermatazoal Reactive Oxygen species production and diminished Seminal Plasma Antioxidant Capacity. Journal of Urology 1999;161(6):1831–1834.
- Softel AD, Rutchik SD, Chen H et al. Effects Of Subinguinal Varicocele Ligation On Sperm Concentration, Motility and Kruger Morphology. Journal of Urology 1997;158(5):1800–1803.
- Lenzi AMD, Gandini L, Bagolan P et al. Sperm Parameters After Early Left Varicocele Treatment. Fertility and Sterility 1998;69(2):347–349.
- Osuna C JA, Temponi SAF, Lozano HJR et al. Repair Versus Observation in Adolescent Varicocele: A Prospective Study. Journal of Urology 1997;158(3): 1128–1132.
- Cowan N. Varicocele Embolisation Urology News Online. Lead Article Vol 2/6.
- Nagar H, Mabjeesh NJ. Decision -making in Pediatric Varicocele surgery: use of color Doppler ultrasound. Pediatric Surg Int 2000;16(1–2):75–6.

FAQS
Question 1
What is the difference between clinical versus subclinical varicocele?

ANSWER 1
On a severity scale of 0–4+, those varicoceles graded 3+-4+ are clearly visible in the scrotum and are easily palpable/identifiable. Grade 1+- 2+ varicoceles can only be appreciated by physical examination with stress maneuvers like cough and Valsalva, or through the use of ancillary testing, i.e. scrotal dopplers.

Question 2

Is there a rationale for correcting varicoceles in the male who is older or just finished having children?

ANSWER 2

If you believe that a varicocele is gonadotoxic and the patient's varicocele is clinically large, there is atrophic changes in the testis, and pain with prolonged standing or vigorous work, then repair those cases. The rationale being that the varicocele repair will contribute to the preservation of testicular endocrine (sexual) function while maintaining organ integrity.

Question 3

What is a 'stress pattern' on semen analysis that has been associated with varicoceles?

ANSWER 3

The 'stress pattern' is an outcome of a varicocele and is characterized by a low sperm count (<20 million/ml), low sperm motility (<50%), and low sperm morphology (<50% WHO criteria or <15% Strict Kruger Criteria).

Question 4

What are the available surgical/interventional approaches to correct varicoceles?

ANSWER 4

The following approaches can be used for varicocele correction:
- Inguinal approach
- Retroperitoneal 'high ligation' approach
- Subinguinal approach
- Laparoscopic approach
- Interventional internal spermatic vein embolization procedure

Question 5

What is the suspected pathophysiology of a varicocele?

ANSWER 5

Actually no one knows for certain. Various theories have been proposed:
- Increased testicular temperature
- Reflux of adrenal and renal metabolites into the testis through the incompetent spermatic vein
- Hypoxia of the testis because of venous stasis
- Small vessel disease leading to Leydig and Sertoli cell dysfunction
- Depressed androgen secretion
- Increased quantity of Reactive Oxygen Species that may damage sperm

CONTRIBUTORS

Gordon H Baustian, MD
Philip J Aliotta, MD, MHA, FACS
Robert James, MD

Index

Index